Workbook for

Advanced EMT

A Clinical-Reasoning Approach

Melissa Alexander

Melissa Alexander, Ed.D., NREMT-P

Lake Superior State University
Sault Sainte Marie, MI

Richard Belle, BS, NREMT-P

Acadian Ambulance/National EMS Academy
Lafayette, LA

Steven Weiss, MD, MS, FACEP, FACP

Medical Editor

PEARSON

Boston   Columbus   Indianapolis   New York   San Francisco   Upper Saddle River   Amsterdam
Cape Town   Dubai   London   Madrid   Milan   Munich   Paris   Montreal   Toronto   Delhi
Mexico City   São Paulo   Sydney   Hong Kong   Seoul   Singapore   Taipei   Tokyo

Publisher: Julie Levin Alexander
Publisher's Assistant: Regina Bruno
Editor-in-Chief: Marlene McHugh Pratt
Acquisitions Editor: Sladjana Repic
Senior Managing Editor for Development: Lois Berlowitz
Project Manager: Jo Cepeda
Assistant Editor: Jonathan Cheung
Director of Marketing: David Gesell
Marketing Manager: Brian Hoehl
Marketing Specialist: Michael Sirinides
Managing Editor for Production: Patrick Walsh
Production Liaison: Faye Gemmellaro

Production Editor: Shyam Ramasubramony, S4Carlisle Publishing Services
Manufacturing Manager: Ilene Sanford
Editorial Media Manager: Amy Peltier
Media Project Manager: Lorena Cerisano
Art Director: Christopher Weigand
Cover Design: Wanda Espana/Wee Design
Cover Images: Thinkstock, 86479750, 200274650, and 200248739; Superstock, 1647R-100295
Composition: S4Carlisle Publishing Services
Interior Printer/Binder and Cover Printer: Bind-Rite Graphics/Robbinsville

Brady
is an imprint of

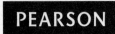

www.bradybooks.com

10 9 8 7 6 5 4 3 2 1
ISBN 13: 978-0-13-503106-3
ISBN 10:   0-13-503106-0

Contents

Introduction vii
About the Author ix
Acknowledgments xi

SECTION 1: Preparing for Advanced Emergency Medical Technician Practice

CHAPTER 1 Introduction to Advanced Emergency Medical Technician Practice 1

CHAPTER 2 Emergency Medical Services, Health Care, and Public Health Systems 5

CHAPTER 3 Workforce Wellness and Personal Safety 12

CHAPTER 4 Ethical and Medical/Legal Considerations in Advanced EMT Practice 21

CHAPTER 5 Ambulance Operations and Responding to EMS Calls 30

CHAPTER 6 Communication and Teamwork 40

SECTION 2: Human Development, Health, and Disease

CHAPTER 7 Medical Terminology 53

CHAPTER 8 Human Body Systems 58

CHAPTER 9 Life Span Development and Cultural Considerations 71

CHAPTER 10 Pathophysiology: Selected Impairments of Homeostasis 79

SECTION 3: Pharmacology

CHAPTER 11 Principles of Pharmacology 90

CHAPTER 12 Medication Administration 96

CHAPTER 13 Medications 112

SECTION 4: Assessment and Initial Management

CHAPTER 14 General Approach to Patient Assessment and Clinical Reasoning 123

CHAPTER 15 Scene Size-Up and Primary Assessment 129

CHAPTER 16 Airway Management, Ventilation, and Oxygenation 139

CHAPTER 17 Resuscitation: Managing Shock and Cardiac Arrest 168

CHAPTER 18 Vital Signs and Monitoring Devices 181

CHAPTER 19 History Taking, Secondary Assessment, and Reassessment 196

SECTION 5: Medical Emergencies

CHAPTER 20 Respiratory Disorders 215

CHAPTER 21 Cardiovascular Disorders 222

CHAPTER 22 Neurologic Disorders 237

CHAPTER 23 Endocrine Disorders 245

CHAPTER 24 Abdominal Pain and Gastrointestinal Disorders 256

CHAPTER 25 Renal, Genitourinary, and Gynecologic Disorders 263

CHAPTER 26 Hematologic Disorders 274

CHAPTER 27 Immunologic Disorders 281

CHAPTER 28 Infectious Illnesses 289

CHAPTER 29 Nontraumatic Musculoskeletal and Soft-Tissue Disorders 299

CHAPTER 30 Disorders of the Eye, Ear, Nose, Throat, and Oral Cavity 305

CHAPTER 31 Mental Illness and Behavioral Emergencies 312

CHAPTER 32 Toxicologic Emergencies 320

SECTION 6: Trauma

CHAPTER 33 Trauma Systems and Incident Command 332

CHAPTER 34 Mechanisms of Injury, Trauma Assessment, and Trauma Triage Criteria 340

CHAPTER 35 Soft-Tissue Injuries and Burns 346

CHAPTER 36 Musculoskeletal Injuries 357

CHAPTER 37 Head, Brain, Face, and Neck Trauma 369

CHAPTER 38 Thoracic Trauma 380

CHAPTER 39 Abdominal Trauma 388

CHAPTER 40 Spine Injuries 394

CHAPTER 41 Environmental Emergencies 404

CHAPTER 42 Multisystem Trauma and Trauma Resuscitation 414

SECTION 7: Special Patient Populations

CHAPTER 43 Obstetrics and Care of the Newborn 420

CHAPTER 44 Pediatric Emergencies 431

CHAPTER 45 Geriatrics 448

CHAPTER 46 Patients with Special Challenges 456

SECTION 8: Rescue and Special Operations

CHAPTER 47 Rescue Operations and Vehicle Extrication 462

CHAPTER 48 Hazardous Materials 468

CHAPTER 49 Response to Terrorism and Disasters 474

Answer Key 480

INTRODUCTION

Overview

The *Advanced EMT: A Clinical Reasoning Approach* Workbook is designed to help you get the most from each textbook chapter. Reading the objective summaries in the workbook before you read the textbook chapter helps prepare you to recognize and mentally organize the chapter content. The objective summaries help you review the textbook material and test your mastery of it after you have read the textbook chapter. Practice using terminology and applying chapter concepts through the exercises provided in the workbook. They are meant to strengthen and enrich your understanding of the chapter material. Finally, the workbook allows you test your understanding and identify areas for additional study.

Features

- *Advanced EMT Education Standards:* The content of each workbook chapter is based on the Advanced EMT level *National EMS Education Standards.* The *Standard* for each chapter is identified at the beginning of the chapter.

- *Summary of Objectives:* The objectives for each chapter are developed from the *Education Standards.* Each objective is summarized to help you check for mastery of the learning objectives for each chapter.

- *Resource Central: Resource Central* provides you with additional review, quizzes, and resources for reinforcement and additional exposure to chapter content to help you better understand the concepts in each chapter.

- *Vocabulary and Concept Review:* Before moving on to more advanced concepts in each chapter, you must have a sound understanding of terminology and basic concepts in the chapter. Each workbook chapter offers you an opportunity to increase your understanding of the terms and concepts through a variety of exercises, including crossword puzzles that give you a fun way to test and review your mastery of terminology.

- *Patient Assessment Review:* The workbook chapters that cover clinical topics provide an application of the patient assessment process for clinical problems covered in the chapter. It is to help you practice adapting your patient assessment skills to various clinical presentations.

- *Check Your Recall and Apply Concepts:* This section of each workbook chapter provides you with opportunities to test your understanding of the major concepts introduced in the chapter and helps you check your ability to apply the concepts in context.

- *Clinical Reasoning:* This section of each chapter presents you with a scenario and questions to help you develop and test your ability to recognize important aspects of patient presentations. You are asked to develop hypotheses about problems and identify what additional information you need in order to test the hypotheses. You are guided through the sense-making process to arrive at clinical impressions and treatment plans. Answers are provided at the end of the workbook to allow you to check your understanding.

- *Project-Based Learning:* This section of the workbook gives you ideas for projects that can enrich your understanding of the chapter content and help you apply the knowledge and share it with others.

- *The EMS Professional in Practice:* In this section, you are presented with real-life problems that often do not have easy answers. These problems help prepare you for the complexities of Advanced EMT practice by giving you an opportunity to think about difficult situations and develop ways of thinking about them before you encounter similar situations in your work.

Melissa Alexander, Ed.D., NREMT-P

ABOUT THE AUTHOR

MELISSA ALEXANDER, Ed.D., NREMT-P

Melissa Alexander began her career in EMS in 1982 and has worked in various prehospital, hospital, and educational settings throughout the United States over the years. She has a BA in Community Health Education from Purdue University, an MS in Health Sciences Education from Indiana University, and an EdD in Human Resources Development from the George Washington University. Dr. Alexander is an assistant professor in the School of Criminal Justice, Fire Science, and EMS at Lake Superior State University in Sault Sainte Marie, Michigan. She has authored and contributed to several EMS texts. Dr. Alexander's research and advocacy interests are in various aspects of EMS education, including improving clinical reasoning skills and EMS workforce issues. She has three daughters, Lindsay, Brittany, and Eleanor, and three grandsons, Asher, Ethan, and Grant. She enjoys spending time with family, organic gardening, and hanging out with her dogs, Sabrina, Benito, and Winston.

ACKNOWLEDGMENTS

We'd like to thank the following contributor for her assistance in preparing the materials for this workbook:

Lyndal M. Curry, MA, NREMT-P
EMS Faculty Instructor
Southern Union State Community College
Opelika, AL

We'd like to thank the following reviewer for her feedback throughout the development process:

Peggy Lahren, NREMT-P
Regional EMS Coordinator
Arizona Bureau of EMS and Trauma System
Phoenix, AZ

Introduction to Advanced Emergency Medical Technician Practice

Content Area

• Preparatory

Advanced EMT Education Standard

• Applies fundamental knowledge of the EMS system, safety/well-being of the Advanced EMT, and medical/legal and ethical issues to the provision of emergency care.

Summary of Objectives

1.1 Define key terms introduced in this chapter.

Knowing and being able to apply the key terms in each chapter is critical to understanding chapter concepts. Write the list of key terms. Then write the definition of each one in your own words. Check your understanding by confirming the definitions in the text glossary. Correct any misunderstandings. Create a study aid by writing each key term on the front of an index card and the definition on the back. Use the cards to quiz yourself, or to have someone quiz you. The exercises under Vocabulary and Concept Review in this chapter will give you additional practice.

1.2 Describe the competencies, roles, responsibilities, and professional characteristics of the Advanced Emergency Medical Technician (Advanced EMT).

Advanced EMTs are health care professionals who provide basic and limited advanced life support interventions to treat ill and injured patients in the prehospital setting, under the direction of a physician medical director. Advanced EMTs have roles and responsibilities in emergency vehicle operations, safety, scene leadership and management, teamwork, patient assessment and management, maintaining current licensure, and working with other health care providers. The professional characteristics of Advanced EMTs include integrity, empathy, self-motivation, appearance and personal hygiene, self-confidence, communication, time management, teamwork, diplomacy, respect, patient advocacy, and careful delivery of service.

1.3 Describe the scope of practice of the Advanced EMT.

In addition to all EMT-level skills, Advanced EMTs (at a minimum) insert airways not intended to be placed in the trachea, perform tracheobronchial suctioning on already intubated patients, start peripheral IVs and administer nonmedicated IV fluids, obtain intraosseous access in pediatric patients, and give nitroglycerin for chest pain, subcutaneous epinephrine for anaphylaxis, glucagon and 50 percent dextrose for hypoglycemia, inhaled bronchodilators for wheezing, naloxone for suspected narcotic overdose, and nitrous oxide for pain relief.

1.4 Place the roles and responsibilities of the Advanced EMT in the larger contexts of emergency medical services, health care, and public health.

Advanced EMTs work with basic-level EMS providers, including emergency medical responders (EMRs) and emergency medical technicians (EMTs), as well as more highly trained personnel, including paramedics, nurses, and physicians. Advanced EMTs may work in the prehospital setting, in the hospital emergency department, and in other health care settings. All EMS personnel have an important role to play in public health in both emergency and nonemergency situations.

1.5 Discuss key issues in the contemporary practice of the Advanced EMT, including professionalism, the focus on patient safety, research, and evidence-based practice.

The Advanced EMT's scope of knowledge must change rapidly to reflect research-based changes in practice. Adequate, current knowledge and a commitment to excellence are required to maintain patient safety. Research continually produces evidence to guide EMS practice and improve patient safety.

Resource Central

Resource Central offers extra practice and review materials in a variety of media. To access it, follow the directions on the Student Access Card provided with the Student Textbook. If there is no card, go to www.bradybooks.com and follow the Resource Central link to Buy Access.

Vocabulary and Concept Review

Write the letter of the correct definition of each term in the blank. Note that there are more definitions than there are terms. (See Resource Central for more vocabulary review.)

1. ___ Advanced EMT

    a. EMS provider who uses minimal equipment to provide immediate lifesaving care to critically ill and injured patients while awaiting the arrival of more highly trained EMS personnel

2. ___ Emergency Medical Responder

    b. Allied health care professional who provides complex assessments and interventions for critical and emergent patients in the prehospital setting

3. ___ Emergency Medical Technician

    c. Obligations associated with a particular position or status

4. ___ Medical Director

    d. Pre-existing written physician's instructions that may be carried out by authorized health care providers without or prior to direct contact with the physician

5. ___ Paramedic

    e. Written procedures that guide the management of specific emergency situations

6. ___ protocols

    f. EMS provider who provides emergency medical care and transportation to the ill and injured, using the basic equipment supplied on an ambulance.

7. _____ responsibilities

    g. Complex patient care assessments and interventions that require in-depth training

8. _____ roles

    h. Licensed physician who assumes an oversight role in an EMS system to provide guidelines for medical treatment and continuous quality improvement activities

9. _____ scope of practice

    i. Systematic investigation that seeks to discover or revise facts, theories, or practical applications

10. _____ standing orders

    j. Functions expected of individuals in particular situations

    k. Occupation or vocation defined by a specialized set of knowledge and code of ethics or conduct

    l. Prehospital emergency care provider who uses basic and limited advanced life support skills to care for acutely ill and injured patients

Check Your Recall and Apply Concepts

Select the best possible choice for each of the following questions.

_____ 1. The knowledge of those engaged in the EMS profession is defined by the:
    a. EMT Oath.
    c. National EMS Education Standards.
    b. EMT Code of Ethics.
    d. EMS Agenda for the Future.

_____ 2. Which one of the following is in the EMT's scope of practice?
    a. Starting an IV
    c. Giving aspirin to patients with chest pain
    b. Pediatric intraosseous infusion
    d. Endotracheal intubation

_____ 3. Whose responsibility is it to meet the EMS provider's requirements to maintain current licensure?
    a. Employer
    c. EMS system medical director
    b. Individual EMS provider
    d. EMS provider's supervisor

_____ 4. When an EMS provider is able to be trusted with confidential information, he demonstrates the professional characteristic of:
    a. integrity.
    c. diplomacy.
    b. careful delivery of service.
    d. empathy

_____ 5. Calling an adult patient "Mrs. Murrow" instead of "hon" demonstrates the professional characteristic of:
    a. patient advocacy.
    c. self-confidence.
    b. respect.
    d. integrity.

Clinical Reasoning

CASE STUDY: HEALTH CAREERS DAY AT WASHINGTON MIDDLE SCHOOL

You and your partner have been asked to talk about EMS to a group of middle school students interested in health careers. You have a week before the date of the presentation, which will last 30 minutes.

1. What are the key things the students should learn about EMS and EMS providers from your presentation?

   _____

   _____

   _____

   _____

   _____

2. How can you explain the differences between the various levels of EMS providers?

   _____

   _____

   _____

   _____

   _____

3. What are the resources you can provide for students who want to learn more about EMS?

   _____

   _____

   _____

   _____

   _____

Project-Based Learning

Put together a one-page information handout for your career day presentation.

The EMS Professional in Practice

What behaviors and observations allow you to identify someone as a professional in his or her field? How can you incorporate those characteristics into your own development as an EMS professional? Jot down your thoughts in a notebook or journal for discussion in class or in your study group.

Emergency Medical Services, Health Care, and Public Health Systems

Content Area

- Preparatory
- Public Health

Advanced EMT Education Standard

- Applies fundamental knowledge of the EMS system, safety/well-being of the Advanced EMT, and medical/legal and ethical issues to the provision of emergency care.
- Uses simple knowledge of the principles of the role of EMS during public health emergencies.

Summary of Objectives

2.1 Define key terms introduced in this chapter.

Knowing and being able to apply the key terms in each chapter is critical to understanding chapter concepts. Write the list of key terms. Then write the definition of each one in your own words. Check your understanding by confirming the definitions in the text glossary. Correct any misunderstandings. Create a study aid by writing each key term on the front of an index card and the definition on the back. Use the cards to quiz yourself or to have someone quiz you. The exercises under Vocabulary and Concept Review in this chapter will give you additional practice.

2.2 Describe key historical events that have shaped the development of EMS systems.

From its birth during the French Revolution, through the development of the early hospital systems to modern-day care and transport of the sick and injured, EMS developed into the sophisticated system we know today. Modern prehospital care began in the mid-twentieth century with the publication of the White Paper, and focused on the care and transportation of trauma patients. Military trauma care has contributed substantially to civilian prehospital care knowledge. EMS has since expanded into a system to provide care to all types of patients. However, the focus has always been on prehospital care, which differentiates it from all other health care providers. The EMS Agenda for the Future and related documents are guiding the continued evolution of EMS.

2.3 Briefly explain each of the components of the Technical Assistance Program Assessment Standards.

In 1988, NHTSA published Statewide Technical Assistance Program Assessment Standards that specify the components of state EMS systems. The 10 components are regulation and policy, resource management, human resources and training, transportation, facilities, communications, public information and education, medical direction, trauma systems, and evaluation.

- *Regulation and Policy:* Each state must have a central EMS agency, legislation, regulations, policies, and procedures in place.
- *Resource Management:* All areas of the state must have access to emergency medical care.
- *Human Resources and Training:* All personnel who staff ambulances must be trained to the EMT level or higher.
- *Transportation:* There must be safe and reliable patient transportation.
- *Facilities:* There must be appropriate emergency facilities within a reasonable distance.
- *Communications:* A communications system must allow public access to EMS and communication among dispatchers, EMS providers, and hospital personnel.
- *Public Information and Education:* Includes activities to educate the public and prevent injuries in their communities.
- *Medical Direction:* A licensed physician medical director is required in every EMS system to oversee patient care.
- *Trauma Systems:* Trauma systems must exist to provide care for trauma patients.
- *Evaluation:* There must be an EMS quality improvement system to assess and improve prehospital care.

2.4 Describe the components of an EMS system that must be in place for a patient to receive emergency medical care.

For patients to receive emergency medical care, the state must set guidelines for EMS services to ensure that there is adequate equipment and enough trained personnel to provide that care. A communication system must be in place to allow the public to access EMS care, and there must be appropriate facilities such as hospitals to care for the patients.

2.5 Discuss the features and benefits of 911 and enhanced 911 emergency access systems.

The number 911, which is widely used to request all emergency services in an area, allows access to a public safety answering point (PSAP) operator. The operator routes the call to the appropriate agency or may dispatch the appropriate resources. The enhanced 911 (E-911) system displays the caller's location on the dispatcher's console, provided the call is placed from a fixed telephone line.

2.6 Explain the importance of Advanced EMTs understanding the health care and public-health resources available in the community.

Advanced EMTs encounter many types of health care facilities including clinics, diagnostic centers, physician offices, rehabilitation centers, and extended-care facilities. The Advanced EMT needs to understand what is provided at each of those facilities. EMS providers are in a unique position because they care for the people in their communities. They enter their patient's homes and see how they live and can see family as well as community problems. This allows Advanced EMTs to better understand the patients' circumstances and educate their patients regarding injury prevention as well as public health resources.

2.7 Discuss the role of EMS as part of the health care system.

Many patients enter the health care setting through EMS and continue to encounter EMS as they move through the health care system. EMS often provides transport between the various facilities—from home to hospital, from hospital to extended-care facility or a specialty hospital, and often returning home via the EMS service.

2.8 Describe the scope of concerns of a public health system.

The public health system exists to promote good health, identify and correct threats to the population as a whole, and to advance public health research.

2.9 Describe the relationship between EMS and public health.

EMS has an important role in public health by helping to identify outbreaks of disease as well as to provide health promotion activities. EMS often goes into neighborhoods and communities that other health care personnel may never see. They may recognize and draw attention to unhealthy circumstances so that they can be improved. Some patients enter the health care system simply because they do not know where to turn for their problems and EMS can be useful in directing them to appropriate resources.

2.10 Discuss the purposes of medical direction and medical oversight in the EMS system.

A physician medical director is an essential and required part of an EMS system. Physicians provide expert input into the clinical operations of an EMS service. Additionally, a physician medical director provides medical oversight that includes specific protocols and standing orders, provider education participation, and continuous quality assurance process supervision.

2.11 Give examples of off-line, on-line, prospective, concurrent, and retrospective medical direction.

Off-line medical direction includes prospective and retrospective medical direction. Prospective medical direction provides direction in advance of patient contact. Examples of prospective medical direction include standing orders and protocols. Concurrent medical direction occurs in the present with personal contact between the provider and the physician. Contact with the physician by radio or phone constitutes concurrent medical direction and is also called on-line medical direction. Retrospective medical direction occurs after patient care has concluded and looks back over records to evaluate and improve overall patient care through continuous quality improvement.

2.12 Describe the purpose of continuous quality improvement (CQI) programs in EMS and the Advanced EMT's role in CQI.

The purpose of CQI is to improve the performance of the EMS system. Evaluation results are used to continually improve the system to ensure high-quality, safe, and efficient patient care. Advanced EMTs have a responsibility to strive to meet system goals, and to work to implement any changes indicated from the evaluation process.

2.13 Identify current issues and trends in EMS.

The EMS Agenda for the Future (NHTSA, 1996) and the IOM report (2006) both call for greater roles for EMS providers in health care and public health, and better integration of EMS into those systems. Some EMS services have experimented with using community paramedics to provide greater roles in public health. This is a possible area of role expansion for EMS.

2.14 Identify resources for learning about issues and trends in EMS.

There are several ways you can learn more about issues and trends in EMS. Become active in EMS professional organizations, attend conferences, and visit the websites of state and national EMS agencies and organizations. Also, subscribe to industry publications and professional journals.

2.15 Given an issue or problem in EMS, suggest changes that could be implemented.

Problem: Many health care professionals have a negative view of the skills and abilities of EMS providers. Most other health care professions have minimum educational standards that begin with an associate's or bachelor's degree. If the EMS profession wants to be respected as much as other health care professions, it can start by raising the educational requirements for licensure. By doing so, other health care professionals will see that EMS also has rigorous standards and is worthy of respect.

Resource Central

Resource Central offers extra practice and review materials in a variety of media. To access it, follow the directions on the Student Access Card provided with the Student Textbook. If there is no card, go to www.bradybooks.com and follow the Resource Central link to Buy Access.

Vocabulary and Concept Review

Complete each sentence with the correct term from the following list. Note that there are more terms than there are sentences. (See Resource Central for more vocabulary review.)

911 system	off-line
certificate	on-line
continuous quality improvement (CQI)	peak load
critical access hospital	private
public safety answering point	enhanced 911
license	reciprocity
National EMS Information System (NEMSIS)	third
National Registry of Emergency Medical Technicians (NREMT)	trauma center

1. The American Red Cross recognizes that certain requirements have been met by issuing a document called a(n) _____.

2. A radio conversation with a physician regarding a patient that you are caring for is an example of _____ medical direction.

3. Your service's medical director examines the patient care reports at the end of the month. That is part of a process known as _____.

4. The nationwide database for collection of uniform data from EMS systems for the purpose of supporting research to improve EMS practices is called the _____.

5. When you transport a critical patient to a smaller community hospital for stabilization and transfer to a higher level of care, you are taking the patient to a(n) _____.

6. The caller's phone number and address appears on the dispatch center call taker's screen when using a(n) _____ system.

7. The permission granted to you by your state to practice as an Advanced EMT is documented by issuance of a(n) _____.

8. A dispatch center that receives emergency calls for assistance, regardless of the nature of the call, is called a _____.

9. When an EMS service is operated by a government, similar to the way police and fire departments are operated by a city or county government, it is called a(n) _____ service.

10. A state issues you an Advanced EMT license because it recognizes your license from another state. By doing so, it can be said that there is _____ between the two states.

Check Your Recall and Apply Concepts

Exercise 1

Being familiar with the history of EMS is an important part of molding the future. Match the event to the dates on the timeline. Write the letter of the correct event on the space provided at the top of the timeline.

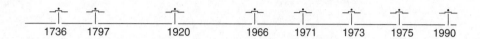

| 1736 | 1797 | 1920 | 1966 | 1971 | 1973 | 1975 | 1990 |

a. The American Medical Association (AMA) recognizes EMT-Paramedic as an allied health occupation.

b. The publication of a White Paper, *Accidental Death and Disability: The Neglected Disease of Modern Society*, by the National Academy of Sciences (NAS) National Research Council (NRC).

c. Napoleon's surgeon-in-chief, Dominique-Jean Larrey, implemented a system of specially designed carriages to quickly retrieve the injured from the battlefields and bring them to surgeons for care.

d. The first National Standard Curriculum (NSC) for training EMTs (called *EMT-Ambulance*) was published.

e. Trauma Care Systems and Development Act focuses on development and implementation of trauma systems.

f. The first U.S. hospital was founded in New York.

g. The first volunteer rescue squads began on the East Coast.

h. Substantial progress in the development of EMS systems began with the Emergency Medical Services Act.

Exercise 2

Match each person listed with his or her contribution to the development of EMS.

a. Nancy Caroline	e. Norman McSwain
b. Jeff Clawson	f. Rocco Morando
c. R. Adams Cowley	g. James O. Page
d. Joseph D. "Deke" Farrington	h. Peter Safar

1. _____ Founder of the *Journal of Emergency Medical Services (JEMS)*, and technical consultant to the television show *Emergency!*

2. _____ Instrumental in the development of the Prehospital Trauma Life Support (PHTLS) course through the National Association of EMTs (NAEMT)

3. _____ Developed the concept of the "Golden Hour" and was instrumental in the development of one of the first air EMS services in the country through the Maryland State Police

4. _____ Introduced the concept of airway, breathing, and circulation (ABCs) in CPR in the 1950s

5. _____ The founding executive director of the NREMT and instrumental in developing the NAEMT

6. _____ Was committed to the idea that people who were not physicians could be taught to deliver lifesaving emergency care outside the hospital

7. _____ Established a first aid training curriculum that served as a prototype for the first EMT-Ambulance curriculum

8. _____ Developed the first set of standardized dispatch protocols in 1978, which have evolved into the widely used Medical Priority Dispatch System

Clinical Reasoning

CASE STUDY: TRAINING NIGHT AT MOUNT PLEASANT EMS

Your EMS service offers training on the third Thursday evening of every month to help you meet your refresher and continuing education requirements. There are a variety of offerings. Some meetings cover current protocols and review your current skills, and while other meetings cover new developments and techniques to improve your patient care. Regardless of the topic, there are always good discussions with the medical director, EMS educators, and your peers, along with sub sandwiches and drinks.

1. Write why refresher and continuing education courses are important professional obligations.

_____

_____

_____

_____

_____

2. What kinds of information could be used to plan refresher and continuing education offerings to make it relevant to your practice as an Advanced EMT?

_____

_____

_____

_____

3. In addition to classes, what are other ways you can ensure ongoing learning?

_____

_____

_____

_____

_____

Project-Based Learning

Check with your state EMS office to determine what is required to renew your Advanced EMT license after your initial license period ends. Most states have some combination of continuing education (CE) hours and refresher training, as well as CPR certification. Make a chart showing each category of education and the number of hours required for your state. Also, check with the National Registry of EMTs for their recertification requirements at http://www.nremt.org. Set goals for obtaining your education requirements throughout your licensure period so that you are not trying in vain to find courses at the last minute. Write down your goals and share them with at least one person; you will be much more likely to keep your goals that way.

The EMS Professional in Practice

You must have your medical director's approval to practice as an Advanced EMT. What does it mean to have a good working relationship with your medical director? What are some ways you can develop a good working relationship with your medical director and earn his or her trust? What are some advantages of having a good working relationship with your medical director? Jot down your thoughts in a notebook or journal for discussion in class or in your study group.

Chapter 3

Workforce Wellness and Personal Safety

Content Area

- Preparatory

Advanced EMT Education Standard

- Applies fundamental knowledge of the EMS system, safety/well-being of the Advanced EMT, and medical/legal and ethical issues to the provision of emergency care.

Summary of Objectives

3.1 Define key terms introduced in this chapter.

Knowing and being able to apply the key terms in each chapter is critical to understanding chapter concepts. Write the list of key terms. Then write the definition of each one in your own words. Check your understanding by confirming the definitions in the textbook glossary. Correct any misunderstandings. Create a study aid by writing each key term on the front of an index card and the definition on the back. Use the cards to quiz yourself or to have someone quiz you. The exercises under Vocabulary and Concept Review in this chapter will give you additional practice.

3.2 Identify aspects of work in EMS that can pose a risk to the health and well-being of EMS providers.

In EMS, there are both physical and emotional stressors that can negatively affect health and well-being. Difficult work schedules and workloads, disrupted sleep patterns, limited access to healthy food choices, exposure to communicable diseases, and long periods of inactivity can jeopardize good physical health. Likewise, poor physical health can increase susceptibility to emotional health problems. Conflicts with coworkers and supervisors, dealing with difficult patients, caring for very sick or dying patients, calls involving children, death of a coworker, or fear of making a wrong decision can be damaging to emotional health.

3.3 Identify specific measures Advanced EMTs can take to protect their health and safety, both on and off the job.

All of the following are important to maintaining good health on and off the job: adequate sleep, proper nutrition, physical exercise, maintaining normal body weight, good body mechanics, limiting alcohol and caffeine intake, immunizations, avoiding tobacco use, frequent handwashing, and using PPE when indicated.

3.4 Discuss the leading health indicators in the United States.

The U.S. Department of Health and Human Services has established leading health indicators as a means to measure the health of the U.S. population. Evaluating those indicators over a period of time can show patterns in the health of the population. The current leading health indicators include physical activity, overweight and obesity, tobacco use, substance abuse, responsible sexual behavior, mental health, injury and violence, environmental quality, immunizations, and access to health care.

3.5 Describe the components of wellness, including considerations for nutrition and physical fitness.

Wellness includes proper nutrition, regular physical exercise, adequate sleep, and the maintenance of a good body weight. Eliminating unhealthy habits, such as smoking or excessive alcohol use, are important to wellness. Because illness prevention contributes to wellness, handwashing and maintaining current immunizations are a part of overall wellness.

3.6 List specific communicable diseases of concern to health care providers.

Tuberculosis, hepatitis B, hepatitis C, bacterial meningitis, pneumonia, staphylococcal infection (including MRSA), HIV-AIDS, rubella, and pertussis are of primary concern to health care providers. Other infections, such as SARS, are not prevalent, but when outbreaks occur, they also can be of concern to health care providers.

3.7 Discuss factors that influence the transmission of communicable diseases.

The route of transmission of the organism, its virulence and dose (number of organisms transmitted), and certain host factors, such as immune status, affect disease transmission.

3.8 Take appropriate standard precautions to protect against communicable diseases in specific situations.

You must wear gloves any time you are performing a procedure with a high likelihood of coming into hand contact with blood, other body fluids, mucous membranes, or nonintact skin. That includes starting an IV and or controlling bleeding. Respiratory and eye protection are used when there is the possibility of airborne droplet contact, such as from a patient with tuberculosis. Fluid-impervious gowns are needed when caring for patients with severe bleeding or during childbirth.

3.9 Recognize situations that may be stressful for EMS providers.

Stressful situations of particular concern to EMS providers include the following: pediatric calls, death or dying patients, injury or death of a coworker, abuse and neglect calls, multiple-casualty incidents, seeing severe or disfiguring injuries, and long work hours with a heavy workload.

3.10 Describe the effects of stress on performance.

Some stress is necessary to good performance, but excess stress interferes with performance. In an acute stress reaction, individuals have difficulty focusing attention, receiving and processing information, performing calculations, and using logic. Chronic stress can interfere with performance through impaired working relationships, irritability, and impaired sleep.

3.11 Explain the effects of stress hormones and the sympathetic nervous system in response to stressors.

A stressor stimulates the sympathetic nervous system, which sets into motion a chain of chemical reactions that prepares the body to mitigate the stress. Stress hormones from the sympathetic nervous system, primarily epinephrine, cause a physiologic response that includes increased heart rate and breathing, a sense of anxiety or nervousness, increased blood pressure, pale skin, sweating, and dilated pupils.

3.12 Explain the general adaptation syndrome model of stress.

The general adaptation syndrome (GAS) divides the stress response into three phases. The initial response is the alarm phase, which prepares the body to respond to the stressor. The next phase, resistance, involves actively coping with the stressor and repairing damage done by the stressor. The final phase, exhaustion, results when the body is exposed to high levels of cortisol over a long period of time, causing physical damage to the body.

3.13 Recognize signs of stress in yourself and others.

Signs of stress include changes in cognition (thinking and processing information), behavior, emotions, and physical signs and symptoms. Difficulty sleeping, irritability, loss of appetite, and general anxiety all may indicate high levels of stress.

3.14 Identify healthy mechanisms for coping with stress.

Emotional wellness, physical wellness (including good nutrition and regular exercise), and a strong social support network (family, friends, coworkers) are important in stress management. Some additional stress management techniques include massage therapy, developing time management and organizational skills, meditation, tai chi, yoga, guided imagery, and counseling.

3.15 Explain the benefits and characteristics of moderate intensity exercise and vigorous exercise.

You should perform moderate to vigorous exercise for at least 30 minutes a day most days per week. Moderate intensity exercise means increasing your heart rate to 60 to 73 percent of your peak heart rate. By stressing your body in a healthy manner (eustress) on a regular basis, your body is better able to handle routine or unexpected job stressors.

3.16 List steps that can reduce the impact of long and irregular shifts on wellness.

The following will help reduce the effects of long or irregular shifts: Maintain the same sleep schedule during both work days and days off, or at least establish an anchor time for sleep. Plan and prepare nutritious meals ahead of time. Get plenty of exercise.

Resource Central

Resource Central offers extra practice and review materials in a variety of media. To access it, follow the directions on the Student Access Card provided with the Student Textbook. If there is no card, go to www.bradybooks.com and follow the Resource Central link to Buy Access.

Vocabulary and Concept Review

Exercise 1

Write the letter of the correct definition in the blank next to the term. (See Resource Central for more vocabulary review.)

1. _____ antioxidant

2. _____ Standard Precautions

3. _____ circadian rhythm

4. _____ communicable illness

5. _____ coping mechanism

6. _____ disinfecting

7. _____ general adaptation syndrome (GAS)

8. _____ homeostasis

9. _____ hypothalamus

10. _____ nosocomial infection

11. _____ phytonutrient

12. _____ sterilizing

13. _____ stressor

a. Three-phase model (alarm, resistance, exhaustion) of the response to stress

b. Part of the brain involved in regulation of endocrine (hormonal) and autonomic nervous system functions

c. Substance that limits cellular damage caused by the breakdown of molecules

d. Psychological response used consciously or unconsciously to reduce the effects of a stressor

e. Maintenance of physiologic equilibrium in the body through a series of complex regulatory mechanisms

f. Naturally occurring plant substances that may play important roles in health through antioxidant and anti-inflammatory properties

g. Infectious disease that can be spread from person to person through direct or indirect contact

h. Something that places a demand on a person psychologically or physiologically

i. Pattern of physiologic and behavioral changes that occur over a 24-hour period

j. Using a steam or chemical process to kill all microorganisms on medical supplies, devices, and equipment

k. Methods to prevent contact with the body fluids of another individual

l. Infection acquired in a health care setting

m. Using a commercial solution or 1:10 bleach and water solution to kill most micro-organisms on a surface

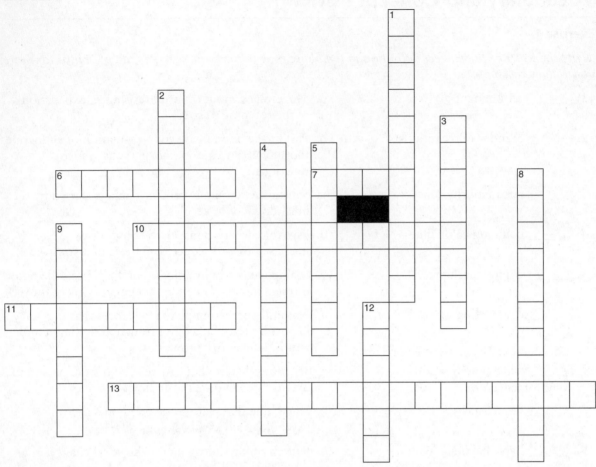

Across

6. Physical and psychological exhaustion from over-exposure to stress.

7. Released from the anterior pituitary and acts on the adrenal glands.

10. Using good posture and proper lifting techniques to prevent injury.

11. A biologic substance that can cause harm or disease.

13. Disease that can be transmitted directly or indirectly from one person to another.

Down

1. Hormone responsible for the fight or flight response.

2. Type of infection acquired in a health care setting.

3. Contact between non-intact skin and potentially infectious body fluids of another person.

4. Physiological equilibrium.

5. Disease-causing microorganism.

8. Occurs immediately in response to a stressor and may last up to four weeks.

9. Type of exercise that increases heart rate to between 74% and 88% of its maximum.

12. A state of complete wellness and not just the absence of disease.

Check Your Recall and Apply Concepts

Select the best possible choice for each of the following questions.

_____ 1. Immediately upon being startled by a loud noise, you experience the _____ phase of the stress response.
- a. adaptation
- b. resistance
- c. post-traumatic
- d. alarm

_____ 2. Prolonged, excessive stress leads to overproduction of _____, leading to long-term health problems, such as diabetes and cardiovascular disease.
- a. norepinephrine
- b. epinephrine
- c. cortisol
- d. glucose

_____ 3. A stress response that is delayed after exposure to a severe stressor and lasts longer than four weeks is categorized as:
- a. post-traumatic stress disorder.
- b. cumulative stress.
- c. burnout.
- d. acute stress.

_____ 4. The most common cause of line-of-duty death and severe injury among EMS personnel is:
- a. communicable disease.
- b. motor vehicle collision.
- c. electrocution.
- d. violence.

_____ 5. Actions taken to protect against infection based on the assumption that all patients' blood and body fluids could be infectious are called:
- a. personal protective actions.
- b. bloodborne substance isolation.
- c. Standard Precautions.
- d. nosocomial precautions.

_____ 6. An animal intermediary in indirect disease transmission is called a(n):
- a. fomite.
- b. pathogen.
- c. vector.
- d. agent.

_____ 7. Which one of the following is a characteristic of a disease-causing organism that can influence its capability for causing disease?
- a. Environment
- b. Acidity
- c. Virulence
- d. Proximity

_____ 8. The lowest, most basic level of human needs according to Maslow's hierarchy of needs are _____ needs.
- a. safety and security
- b. physiologic
- c. social
- d. esteem

_____ 9. Which one of the following statements is true regarding stress?
- a. Up to a certain point, an increase in stress improves performance.
- b. When a stressor results in a negative impact on functioning, it is called *eustress*.
- c. The alarm phase of the stress response stimulates the parasympathetic nervous system.
- d. Prolonged and excessive exposure to cortisol has positive effects on the body.

_____ 10. Conflict with your neighbors is an example of a situation that could have an impact on your _____ wellness.
- a. environmental
- b. occupational
- c. spiritual
- d. social

_____11. Your partner is barbequing chicken behind the station. If the chicken is not cooked to the proper temperature, you should avoid eating it because of the risk of:
  a. salmonella.
  b. hepatitis A.
  c. avian tuberculosis.
  d. SARS.

_____12. The best way to prevent infection when caring for a patient with tuberculosis is to wear:
  a. gloves.
  b. a surgical mask.
  c. protective eyewear.
  d. a particulate respirator.

_____13. Which one of the following is a principle of proper lifting technique?
  a. Lift quickly to minimize the time spent lifting.
  b. Inhale and tighten your leg muscles during the lift.
  c. Use long strides if you must carry a weight over a distance.
  d. Keep your feet approximately shoulder-width apart with one foot slightly in front of the other.

_____14. The primary route of transmission of tuberculosis is:
  a. airborne.
  b. sexual contact.
  c. fomite transmission.
  d. blood and body fluids.

_____15. Any time your skin is contaminated with potentially infectious material, the most effective means of reducing the chances of infection is to immediately:
  a. wash the area with soap and water.
  b. apply antibacterial spray on the area.
  c. wipe the area with an alcohol swab.
  d. receive a tetanus booster shot.

Clinical Reasoning

CASE STUDY: EMPLOYEE WELLNESS AT CITY AMBULANCE

You have just been selected to take part in a committee to design an employee wellness program at work. Your employer has given you a generous budget to work with. List four components that you will propose for the wellness program and give a short justification for each that will convince your employer that your plan is a good idea.

1. _____

   _____

   _____

   _____

2. _____

   _____

   _____

   _____

3. _____

_____

_____

_____

_____

4. _____

_____

_____

_____

_____

Project-Based Learning

Using the Internet, find out all you can about hepatitis B, including answers to the following questions: How is hepatitis B normally transmitted? How long can the virus live on a dry surface? How do you clean a surface contaminated with the hepatitis B virus? What is the effect of alcohol on a patient with hepatitis B?

After you do your research, make an information sheet to share with health care providers such as your classmates. If you were to make an information sheet for patients or for the general public, how would it be different from the one you designed for your classmates?

The EMS Professional in Practice

How do EMS providers act as role models for health in the community? What are some specific observations the public can make about EMS providers that convey values about health? Jot down your thoughts in a notebook or journal for discussion in class or in your study group.

Skills Checklist

The following skill checklist covers the major steps of a selected skill from Chapter 3. Review it prior to your laboratory classes. Practice skills only after they have been demonstrated for you in class and only under the supervision of an authorized instructor or clinical preceptor.

Advanced EMT Skill Checklist: *Handwashing*		
Skill Stimulus: Preparation for providing patient care, after providing patient care, after handling contaminated items, any time hands are contaminated or soiled.		
Step	Performed	Not Performed
Wet your hands with warm water.		
Apply liquid soap.		
Rub your hands together with soap for 20 seconds.		
Include wrists, palms, backs of hands, between fingers, and under fingernails.		
Rinse soap from hands.		
Dry hands with a paper towel.		
Use a paper towel to turn off the faucet.		
Dispose of the paper towel.		
Skill Completion: Hands are dry, water is turned off, paper towel is disposed of.		

Ethical and Medical/Legal Considerations in Advanced EMT Practice

Content Area

- Preparatory

Advanced EMT Education Standard

- The Advanced EMT applies fundamental knowledge of the EMS system, safety/well-being of the Advanced EMT, and medical/legal and ethical issues to the provision of emergency care.

Summary of Objectives

4.1 Define key terms introduced in this chapter.

Knowing and being able to apply the key terms in each chapter is critical to understanding chapter concepts. Write the list of key terms. Then write the definition of each one in your own words. Check your understanding by confirming the definitions in the textbook glossary. Correct any misunderstandings. Create a study aid by writing each key term on the front of an index card and the definition on the back. Use the cards to quiz yourself or to have someone quiz you. The exercises under Vocabulary and Concept Review in this chapter will give you additional practice.

4.2 Describe your responsibilities as an Advanced EMT with respect to scope of practice, standard of care, and medical direction.

An Advanced EMT has a legal responsibility to provide medical care within his or her scope of practice and to an acceptable standard of care. Knowing the medical standards set by the various layers of medical direction at the state, local, and service level is a requirement to practice as an Advanced EMT. All EMS providers are responsible for knowing what is expected and delivering care within those boundaries.

4.3 Given a variety of ethical dilemmas, discuss the issues that must be considered in each situation.

At all times, acting in the patient's best interest will resolve most ethical dilemmas, including the following:

- Consider the instance of providing resuscitative care on an elderly patient in cardiac arrest when his family asks you not to. Do you follow the family's wishes or follow your protocols for resuscitation? Does the patient have a valid do not resuscitate (DNR) order? If you were the patient, what would you want done?

- Consider the instance of providing care for a drunk driver who has caused a wreck that results in the deaths of several people. Do you have an obligation to fully treat this patient? What if your family member was one of the causalities? What if the driver was one of your family members? Does the driver deserve the best care available?

4.4 Discuss the application of the EMT Oath and professional ethics to the practice of EMS.

The EMT Oath was written to assist in the application of ethics to the practice of prehospital care. What is legal is not always ethical, and Advanced EMTs may be called upon to make difficult ethical decisions. Remembering the principles given in the EMT Oath and always having the patient's best interest in mind will guide you in making the best ethical decisions on behalf of the patient.

4.5 Give examples of federal and state laws affecting the practice of EMS.

Federal laws that affect EMS include the Emergency Medical Treatment and Active Labor Act (EMTALA), the Healthcare Information Portability and Accountability Act (HIPAA), the Ryan White CARE Act, and the Social Security Act, which created Medicare. State statutes include areas of EMS regulation, mandatory reporting situations, family law, motor vehicle law, and some areas of employment law.

4.6 Give examples of legal situations involving tort and criminal issues.

Tort law is a form of civil law in which one person is liable for damage to another. Examples of tort law include libel, slander, and negligence. Criminal law covers crimes against society such as murder, embezzlement, and driving while impaired.

4.7 Describe the purpose of and typical protections afforded by Good Samaritan Laws.

The purpose of the Good Samaritan Laws is to encourage health care professionals to provide care in an emergency while they are off duty. Most of those laws apply only when the provider is not being paid for services. They do not protect the provider in the case of gross negligence, but they provide protection when care is rendered in good faith.

4.8 Given a scenario, identify circumstances that may allow a claim of negligence to be established.

A claim of negligence may be upheld if it can be proven that the provider had a duty to act, breached that duty, that the patient suffered harm, and that the actions or omissions were the proximate cause of the patient's harm.

4.9 Discuss several ways to defend yourself against claims of negligence.

Excellent documentation of the facts and observations supporting your patient care will help you defend yourself in the event that the patient makes a claim of negligence. To protect yourself against successful litigation, ensure that you are competent in all of the knowledge and skills required of Advanced EMTs and treat patients compassionately and respectfully.

4.10 Given a scenario, determine the type of patient consent that applies.

A patient who verbally, non-verbally, or in writing accepts treatment has given expressed consent. A patient who is unconscious is unable to give expressed consent, but care is rendered under the doctrine of implied consent, because the patient would most likely consent to care if he could. Patients under the age of 18 are not legally permitted to consent to or refuse medical treatment; therefore, the patient's parent or guardian must give permission for medical treatment.

4.11 Evaluate factors that should be considered when determining a patient's decision-making capacity and in situations in which the use of force or patient restraint are being contemplated.

You must consider many things when evaluating a person's decision-making capacity, including the possibility of mental illness, a behavioral emergency, intoxication by drugs or alcohol, a medical emergency such as a stroke or diabetic emergency, or trauma that alters the patient's mental status. If the patient is a danger to himself or others and it is necessary to restrain him and transport him against his will, you must consult law enforcement and medical direction.

4.12 Apply the concept of the right to self-determination to issues of consent and advance directives.

A competent adult has the right to self-determination, which is the right to decide (consent) whether or not he wants to receive medical care. Many patients will complete legally binding advance directives that guide his medical care in the event of certain medical conditions or circumstances.

4.13 Describe how to avoid claims of assault, battery, abandonment, false imprisonment/ kidnapping, and defamation.

One way to minimize your risk of being involved in a lawsuit is to be empathetic, compassionate, and respectful to all patients, in addition to adhering to the standard of care. When using restraints, only use accepted methods, follow your protocols, and clearly document why restraint was required. When documenting the incident, be sure to describe what the patient was doing or saying that indicated self-harm or harm to another was imminent.

4.14 Identify situations in which Advanced EMTs may be mandatory reporters of suspected crimes or other legally reportable situations.

Mandatory reporting laws vary, but generally include such things as gunshot wounds, child abuse and elder abuse, and animal bites. Some communicable diseases may be reportable, as well.

4.15 Differentiate between instances in which you can and cannot legally share a patient's protected health information.

You may share information without the patient's written consent with other medical care providers who have a need to know, when there is a court order compelling its release, and for billing purposes.

4.16 Discuss the application of EMTALA and HIPAA legislation to the practice of EMS.

EMTALA gives all patients, regardless of the ability to pay, the right to an appropriate screening examination and emergency medical care and treatment (or appropriate emergency transfer). HIPAA specifies the instances in which protected health information (PHI) may be legally provided to others. EMS providers must protect the patient's privacy and not discriminate in providing care.

4.17 Identify presumptive signs of death.

Presumptive signs of death include: decapitation, transsection of the body, decomposition, charring, rigor mortis, and livor mortis.

4.18 Discuss considerations in transport and resuscitation for patients who may be organ donors.

You must be aware of the laws in your area regarding organ donors. Follow your protocols in the treatment of patients who are potential organ donors.

4.19 Identify situations in which law enforcement or the medical examiner's office should be notified.

You may be required to notify the coroner or medical examiner's office in cases where death appears to be natural, but was not expected, as well as in other cases. In cases where there is any suspicion that death was not due to natural causes, you should request law enforcement at the scene.

4.20 Discuss legal considerations in the response to crime scenes and the care of both crime victims and suspects.

Disturb the crime scene as little as possible. Follow the same path into and out of the crime scene with as few providers as possible on the scene. Do not cut through holes in clothing that may be from gunshots or knives and do not touch or remove any weapons from the scene. If the patient is obviously dead, do not enter the crime scene. Fully document your observations and actions.

4.21 Identify items that may be considered evidence at a crime scene.

Weapons, medications, written messages, cell phones, food, clothing, and nearly anything found at a crime scene may be considered evidence.

Resource Central

Resource Central offers extra practice and review materials in a variety of media. To access it, follow the directions on the Student Access Card provided with the Student Textbook. If there is no card, go to www.bradybooks.com and follow the Resource Central link to Buy Access.

Vocabulary and Concept Review

Exercise 1

Write the letter of the correct definition in the blank. (See Resource Central for more vocabulary review.)

1. _____ abandonment

2. _____ competent

3. _____ duty to act

4. _____ expressed consent

5. _____ gross negligence

6. _____ libel

7. _____ proximate cause

8. _____ *res ipsa loquitur*

9. _____ slander

10. _____ standard of care

a. Legal obligation to provide emergency medical services

b. Defamation through a written document

c. Degree of attention and caution that would be exercised by a reasonable person with the same training and in the same circumstances

d. Having the mental capacity to make decisions

e. Termination of patient care without transferring care to a qualified health-care provider, when the patient is still in need of and desires medical care

f. Spoken communication that defames another person

g. Latin term used legally to mean the thing speaks for itself; being self-evident

h. Act or omission of an act that is the cause of injury; an event without which the injury would not have occurred

i. Injury caused by a provider's disregard for the well-being of others

j. Patient's overt acknowledgment that he accepts the medical procedures that are going to be performed

Exercise 2

Complete each sentence with the correct term from the list. Note that there are more terms than there are sentences.

assault	misfeasance
EMTALA	nonfeasance
ethics	plaintiff
Good Samaritan laws	rigor mortis
HIPAA	tort law
livor mortis	

1. Placing a person in fear of imminent bodily harm is _____.

2. The principles of proper conduct within a profession; a branch of philosophy that addresses issues of what is right or good and what is wrong is _____.

3. The type of law that pertains to wrongdoing against an individual and harm done to one party by another is _____.

4. Discoloration of the skin after death caused by pooling of blood from the effects of gravity is called _____.

5. Performing a legitimate act in a manner that causes injuries is known as _____.

6. Laws intended to protect those who volunteer assistance in an emergency against claims of negligence are called _____ laws.

7. Federal legislation that makes it illegal to refuse an appropriate screening examination and, if necessary, treatment or emergency transfer to patients with a medical emergency or in active labor, regardless of their ability to pay, is called _____.

8. Failure to perform an act that one is obligated to perform or wrongdoing by omission is called _____.

9. Performing an improper act that causes injury is known as _____.

10. The party who brings a civil action against someone else is called a(n) _____.

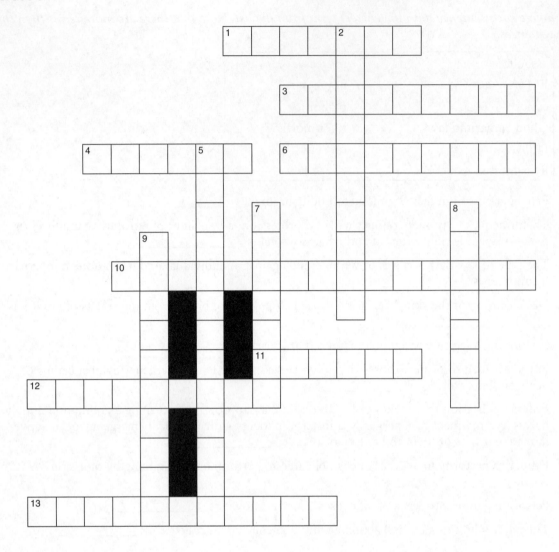

Across

1. Defamation by spoken word.
3. Person against whom a claim of legal wrongdoing is made.
4. Principles of proper professional conduct.
6. Has the capacity to make decisions.
10. Being self-evident.
11. Being legally responsible.
12. Obligation to provide services.
13. Ending patient care without appropriate transfer to a qualified health care provider when the patient is still need of care.

Down

2. Harming the reputation of another person by giving malicious false information.
5. Recognition of accomplishment that can be provided by any party of agency.
7. An act that places a patient in fear of harm.
8. Physical contact without consent of reasonable expectation of physical contact.
9. Having your name listed in a database.

Check Your Recall and Apply Concepts

Exercise 1

1. Write four key considerations in preserving evidence at crime scenes:

   a. _____

   b. _____

   c. _____

   d. _____

2. What four items must be proven for a successful charge of negligence?

   a. _____

   b. _____

   c. _____

   d. _____

3. Describe four situations that would require mandatory reporting to authorities.

   a. _____

   b. _____

   c. _____

   d. _____

4. List four provisions in HIPAA that allow you to reveal a patient's protected health information (PHI).

   a. _____

   b. _____

   c. _____

   d. _____

Exercise 2

Select the best possible choice for each of the following questions.

_____ 1. The standards of conduct expected of persons in a particular profession is called:
   a. morals.
   b. liability.
   c. duty to act.
   d. ethics.

_____ 2. The principle of conduct that means *to do good* is:
   a. advocacy.
   b. justice.
   c. nonmalfeasance.
   d. beneficence.

_____ 3. Not revealing a patient's condition, statements, or other information is an example of:
   a. due diligence.
   b. confidentiality.
   c. self-determination.
   d. objectivity.

_____ 4. If you are accused of negligence and the claim is brought to trial, you are considered the _____ in the case.
   a. defendant
   b. protagonist
   c. plaintiff
   d. advocate

_____ 5. Your lawyer disagrees with the jury's decision in a malpractice trial. He will first request a review and ruling from a(n) _____ court.
   a. supreme
   b. appellate
   c. administrative
   d. circuit

_____ 6. The skills that you are allowed by law to perform are defined by your:
   a. duty to act.
   b. curriculum.
   c. scope of practice.
   d. standing orders.

_____ 7. Legal competence to make decisions is determined by:
   a. on-line medical direction.
   b. a judge.
   c. law enforcement officers at the scene.
   d. the senior EMS provider on the scene.

_____ 8. You have been admitted to the hospital for abdominal pain and vomiting. You are evaluated by a surgeon who says, "I would like to take out your gallbladder. Is that alright with you?" If you agree, you are giving _____ consent.
   a. implied
   b. informed
   c. urgent
   d. expressed

_____ 9. A patient who has had a seizure refuses treatment and transport. If you transport him, you may be charged with:
   a. false imprisonment.
   b. abandonment.
   c. assault.
   d. negligence.

_____ 10. A document that is written by an individual to communicate the types of care he does and does not want at the end of life is called a(n):
   a. do not resuscitate order.
   b. living will.
   c. durable power of attorney for health care.
   d. health care proxy.

_____ 11. You are requested by law enforcement to respond to a residence for a person they believe is deceased. Upon assessing the patient, you find that the muscles are very stiff and you are unable to flex the joints. That condition should be documented as _____ mortis.
   a. rigor
   b. algor
   c. fetor
   d. livor

_____ 12. A civil offense arising from acting with disregard for the well-being of others can be classified as:
   a. defamation.
   b. gross negligence.
   c. due regard.
   d. criminal mischief.

Clinical Reasoning

CASE STUDY: MR. STRUMPH'S DENIAL

You are dispatched to the home of a 68-year-old man, Mr. George Strumph, who is complaining of chest pain. His wife, Henrietta, called 911 when Mr. Strumph became pale and sweaty and complained of difficulty breathing and heaviness in his chest. The patient insists that the problem is his wife's cooking. "She's been giving me heartburn for years," he says, and tells you that he does not need to go to the hospital. His wife is clearly upset and tells you that you have her permission to take her husband against his will. You explain that Mr. Strumph has the right to refuse care because he seems to have decision-making capacity, even though she disagrees with his decision.

1. What observations should you make to determine whether the patient truly does have decision-making capacity?

_____

_____

_____

_____

_____

2. If the patient continues to refuse treatment and transport, what actions should you take and document?

_____

_____

_____

_____

_____

Mr. Strumph ultimately refuses treatment and transport. You inform the night shift that there is a patient with chest pain who refused care to alert them to the possibility of a call to that address. In the morning, the night shift tells you that they responded to the address and, unfortunately, the patient was in cardiac arrest and did not survive.

3. Could you and your partner be sued for negligence? Explain your answer based on the four components of negligence.

_____

_____

_____

_____

_____

Project-Based Learning

Write down three questions about medical/legal and ethical issues to ask your preceptor during your next clinical rotation. Ask about his or her experience with consents, refusals of treatments, do not resuscitate orders, and other issues.

The EMS Professional in Practice

How would you know if you were providing the proper standard of care for your patients? What could you do to be sure you were always providing the very best standard of care? Jot down your thoughts in a notebook or journal for discussion in class or in your study group.

Chapter 5

Ambulance Operations and Responding to EMS Calls

Content Area

- EMS Operations

Advanced EMT Education Standard

- The Advanced EMT applies knowledge of operational roles and responsibilities to ensure patient, public, and personal safety.

Summary of Objectives

5.1 Define key terms introduced in this chapter.

Knowing and being able to apply the key terms in each chapter is critical to understanding chapter concepts. Write the list of key terms. Then write the definition of each one in your own words. Check your understanding by confirming the definitions in the text glossary. Correct any misunderstandings. Create a study aid by writing each key term on the front of an index card and the definition on the back. Use the cards to quiz yourself or to have someone quiz you. The exercises under Vocabulary and Concept Review in this chapter will give you additional practice.

5.2 Give examples of the Advanced EMT's responsibilities during each of the major phases of an ambulance call.

- *Preparations:* Be sure the unit is clean and fully stocked for response and be sure all equipment on the unit is functioning properly.
- *Receiving and responding:* Acknowledge the call promptly, respond with due regard, perform a good scene size-up, and communicate properly with the dispatch center.
- *On-scene care and preparation for transport:* Provide appropriate patient assessment and treatment; properly package the patient for transport; communicate effectively with the patient, his family, and other public safety professional; and dispatch personnel and hospital staff.
- *Transporting the patient:* Select the best destination for your patient and travel the best route as safely as possible. Continue patient care and document pertinent information for inclusion in the patient care report.

- *Transferring patient care:* Appropriately transfer care at the hospital or receiving facility and provide a report about the patient and the care you provided.
- *Terminating the call:* Clean and disinfect equipment, replace supplies used, complete necessary paperwork, and inform the dispatch center that you are back in service.

5.3 Describe the recommendations of the National Association of EMTs with respect to EMS provider security and safety.

- Security briefings should be conducted prior to the start of shifts.
- EMS crews need to be well informed of, and should participate in the development of, operational security measures.
- EMS vehicles should be tracked at all times, including out-of-service vehicles.
- EMS vehicles should not be left running or unattended with the key in the vehicle.
- Out-of-service vehicles should be properly secured to eliminate access to unauthorized persons.
- A key log must be kept to account for all keys to restricted buildings and vehicles.
- Ensure that vehicles off premises for repairs or other reasons are properly secured.
- Vehicles that will be permanently out of service should have all EMS markings and warning devices removed.
- EMS patches, badges, and ID cards must be safeguarded against theft and unauthorized distribution.
- EMS badges and ID cards should be counterfeit resistant and include a photo of the bearer.
- EMS uniforms must be sold only to authorized EMS personnel.

5.4 Describe the legal responsibilities and privileges afforded to Advanced EMTs operating ambulances, and the precautions that must be observed while using those privileges.

Ambulances are allowed to travel with lights and sirens, but it must be done with due regard for the safety of all parties. Ambulances are allowed to break the speed limit, but it should be done safely at no more than 10 mph above the posted speed limit and only when road conditions permit it.

5.5 Give examples of habits and behaviors that improve driving safety.

The emergency vehicle driver must constantly scan the surroundings to include everything outside the front windshield, windows, all mirrors, and blind spots. Do not follow other vehicles too closely. When stopping in traffic, be sure to leave enough room in front for you to leave the lane of traffic if necessary. Simple maneuvers, such as speeding up for a few seconds, slowing down, or changing lanes, can clear the cushion of safety on the sides of your vehicle. Remain alert for tailgaters because they may not see the traffic ahead. Avoid sudden movements of the gas and brake pedals and the steering wheel. Remove your foot from the pedals slowly, and apply your foot to the pedals slowly. Also, turn the steering wheel slowly and smoothly.

5.6 Discuss factors that can affect your ability to maintain control of an ambulance.

Driving too fast for conditions is the primary factor in loss of control of vehicles. To reduce the possibility of crashes, operators should cap their speed at 10 mph over the limit and never exceed 75 mph. Driving too fast for conditions can lead to loss of control of the vehicle.

5.7 Explain precautions that should be taken when operating an ambulance at night or in inclement weather.

Driving at night reduces your visual acuity, so you must adjust your speed and following distance accordingly. You should never activate your high beams when other vehicles are approaching. This includes high beam flashers and emergency lights during emergency responses at night. During inclement weather, increase the normal stopping distance of a 2- to 4-second following distance.

5.8 Describe the appropriate use of emergency warning devices, such as lights and sirens.

The purpose of lights and sirens is to make the ambulance conspicuous and to ask other drivers to pull over and let you pass. Only use emergency warning devices when responding to an emergency or transporting a critical patient. When approaching an intersection or a dangerous stretch, increase your audible warnings by changing the siren tone or activating the horn.

5.9 Describe the safety precautions to be taken when working at scenes on and near roadways.

Position emergency vehicles in order to permit the best access to patients and provide a safe location for all in and around them. The safest place to park an emergency vehicle is on the same side of the road, ahead of the scene, off the road, with an obstacle between the ambulance and traffic. Your vehicle and your uniform should be striped with highly visible, reflective material, regardless of its color. Position your ambulance well before the scene to provide a buffer zone, and turn the wheels to prevent it from being pushed into the scene in the event it is struck from behind.

5.10 Explain precautions to avoid exposing yourself and others to increased levels of carbon monoxide from vehicle exhaust.

You should ensure your ambulance has appropriate preventive maintenance, including tune-ups, and be sure exhaust exits beyond the side of the vehicle, not under it. Always keep ambulance windows shut, and ensure that all doors and windows close tightly. Cover any opening to the outside, such as vents.

Keep the heater or air conditioner on at all times. This creates continuous interior positive pressure. Do not use fuel-powered supplemental equipment inside the ambulance. Carbon monoxide testers and monitors are available, and you should use them to protect patients and providers from this deadly gas.

5.11 Compare the relative risk of ground ambulance operation to other potential risks faced by EMS providers.

A study discovered that the fatality rate of EMS workers is 12.7 per 100,000 workers, which is double the national average of all other occupations. Research on EMS provider injuries found that the ambulance crash injury rate is 10 to 20 times that of civilian vehicles and the primary cause of the line-of-duty deaths is vehicle crashes. The estimated number of injuries and fatalities occurring in and around ambulances, compared to other types of vehicles, make ambulances one of the most dangerous vehicles on the road.

5.12 Relate features of ambulance design to both hazards and safety in ambulance crashes.

Most injuries occur in the patient compartment of ambulances and are caused by improperly restrained occupants and equipment. Type II ambulances have a raised roof that allows providers to stand in the back while providing care, which creates a better working environment in the back, but does nothing to restrain the provider in a vehicle collision. Some ambulances have a pneumatic suspension that allows them to "kneel" or lower to permit loading of stretchers. This feature makes it safer and easier to lift a stretcher and patient into the ambulance.

5.13 Given a high-risk ambulance operation situation, such as negotiating intersections or highway driving, describe actions to reduce the risk as much as possible.

The vehicle driver always must be aware of his surroundings, able to predict potential problems, and prepared to take action to maintain control of the vehicle and prevent crashes. The driver should continually scan outside the front windshield, windows, all mirrors, and blind spots. When traveling emergently through an intersection with a green light, the driver should be at or below the posted speed limit, with his foot covering the brake pedal. When proceeding through a red traffic light, the driver must first come to a complete stop. When the intersection is clear, the driver must proceed slowly and cautiously through. If the intersection has multiple lanes, the driver must treat each lane as a separate intersection. The driver must come to a complete stop at the intersection and evaluate all lanes.

5.14 Explain the impact of speed on both emergency response time and safety.

Speed increases reaction distance and reduces the time available to make evasive maneuvers. Driving too fast for conditions is the primary factor in loss of control of vehicles. Responding to emergency calls or transporting critical patients carries the expectation that your response time or transport time will be expedited.

5.15 Describe the ways of minimizing distractions while driving.

To minimize distractions while driving, your partner should operate the radio, lights, and sirens. The driver should not use his cell phone while driving. Do not eat or drink in the cab of the ambulance for safety as well as cleanliness reasons.

5.16 Explain the impact of fatigue and shift work on the safety of ambulance operations.

Shift work often leads to inconsistent sleep patterns, which can lead to fatigue. Driving an emergency vehicle while fatigued increases the likelihood of crashes. The cause of most crashes is human error by the ambulance operator, commonly due to speed, distractions, and fatigue.

5.17 Discuss situations in which air medical transportation should be considered, disadvantages of air medical transport, and guidelines for setting up a landing zone and interacting with the air medical crew.

Patients who require advanced care with a long transport time to a specialty hospital such as a trauma center or children's hospital are candidates to be transported by air medical providers. Air medical transport units are capable of an advanced level of care above that of ground EMS services. Consider distance to the hospital as well as availability of a landing zone before calling for air medical transportation. However, inclement weather (such as wind, rain, snow, or fog) may prevent air medical units from flying or landing at your destination. Aircraft cabins usually are quite small, so patients who are obese, have extensive deformities, or impaled objects may not be candidates for transport.

When setting up a landing zone, select a large, flat area that is free of obstacles and hazards, at least 150 feet from the scene, and clearly visible from the air. Provide the pilot with large landmarks, cross streets, or GPS coordinates. Mark the landing zone at each corner by highly visible devices, such as large traffic cones, or vehicles.

Some EMS systems will allow direct radio contact, whereas others require a telephone call. Most EMS services have providers request air medical transport through their dispatch center.

5.18 Apply principles of proper body mechanics to lifting and moving patients and equipment.

A variety of techniques and equipment are used to lift and move patients emergently and non-emergently. Proper lifting techniques and skilled use of the proper equipment for each situation are important aspects of patient safety. Before lifting, know your personal limit, and do not be afraid to request additional help. Proper lifting techniques include planting your feet shoulder-distance apart, positioning hands with palms forward, lifting with your legs not your back, and never leaning or twisting as you lift.

5.19 Describe the importance of teamwork and communications in lifting and moving patients.

For your safety and the safety of your partner and patient, good communication is important. When lifting with an assistant, be sure to communicate throughout the lift. Plan the move, including who will lead or initiate the lift and how it will be directed (1-2-3-lift, or 1-2-lift on 3).

5.20 Differentiate among situations that call for emergency, urgent, and non-urgent moves.

Emergency moves are used only when the risks of moving the patient without first assessing or treating him are outweighed by the risks of not moving him. This usually occurs when the environment is unstable, threatening the safety of the patient as well as rescue personnel. Urgent moves are performed when there is a serious mechanism of injury and the patient needs to be moved so you may provide necessary care. Most patients are non-urgent and have no immediate life threats that would require an urgent move.

5.21 Demonstrate the steps required to properly package a patient for transport by ground or by air.

Position the patient appropriately based on his condition. Always secure the patient using the safety straps on the stretcher (placed over the sheet and blanket, so you can access them), and put the side rails up after you have positioned the patient on the stretcher. Next, cover the patient and secure all equipment, blankets, IVs, and clothing. Ensure that there are enough people to move the stretcher safely.

5.22 Describe the proper use, advantages, disadvantages, and techniques for using each of the following: armpit forearm drag, backboard, blanket drag, devices for bariatric patients, direct carry, direct ground lift, draw sheet method, extremity lift, long roll, neonatal isolette, portable stretcher, power grip, power lift, pushing and pulling, rapid extrication, scoop or basket stretcher, shirt drag, squat lift, stair chair, and wheeled stretcher.

- *Armpit forearm drag:* Used for emergency moves but does not allow for spinal protection.
- *Backboard:* Used for patients with possible spine injuries but may also be used to move unconscious patients. Backboards become uncomfortable very quickly.
- *Blanket drag:* Used by a single rescuer for emergency moves but does not allow for spinal protection.
- *Devices for bariatric patients:* Stretchers that have larger wheels for better stability, have wider dimensions, and are made of heavier materials to support the extra weight.
- *Direct carry:* Used to transfer a supine patient from a bed to a stretcher or other device.
- *Direct ground lift:* Used to lift a patient of normal weight from the ground.
- *Draw sheet method:* Used to move a patient from a bed to the stretcher.
- *Extremity lift:* Used to lift a patient from the ground to a carrying device. Do not use on patients with a possible spine injury or extremity injuries.
- *Log roll:* Used to move a patient with a possible spine injury onto a long backboard. Requires at least three rescuers to properly move the patient.
- *Neonatal isolette:* Neonatal isolettes are modified to be secured into the ambulance using the bracket that locks the wheeled stretcher into place. Designed to keep the neonate warm to prevent hypothermia.
- *Portable stretcher:* Used to move a patient in tight quarters where a wheeled stretcher will not fit.
- *Power grip:* Recommended hand position to obtain the best grip on the stretcher.
- *Power lift:* Allows for the optimum technique to lift a stretcher by keeping the weight close to the body and the back straight.
- *Pushing and pulling:* Used to move a patient between two surfaces. Pushing is preferred when possible.
- *Rapid extrication:* Used to quickly move a critical patient to safety so that proper care can be provided.
- *Scoop or basket stretcher:* Used in confined spaces where wheeled or other stretchers will not fit.
- *Shirt drag:* Used as an emergency move. Allows for some support of the patient's head and neck during the move.
- *Squat lift:* Used if the rescuer has a weaker leg or ankle. The weak leg is slightly extended.
- *Stair chair:* Used to move a patient through narrow corridors, through doorways, or up or down stairs. Do not use with patients with altered mental status, spine injuries, or lower extremity injuries.
- *Wheeled stretcher:* Stretcher with wheels, which enables moving without lifting, but is difficult to maneuver on uneven ground.

5.23 Given a scenario involving any of the following types of patients, demonstrate proper patient positioning: chest pain or difficulty breathing; geriatric, pediatric, pregnant, or physical disability; known or suspected spine injury; nausea or vomiting; shock; or unresponsiveness.

- *Chest pain or difficulty breathing:* Patients with respiratory distress or chest pain usually prefer Fowler's position.
- *Geriatric, pediatric, pregnant, or physical disability:* Place these patients in the position of comfort when possible. The elderly are often uncomfortable lying on a long backboard and will require additional padding. Also, you may need to elevate the head of the board for comfort. Do not place pregnant patients in the third trimester supine; instead, use a folded blanket or towels under the right side of the board to slightly tip it to the left. For patients with a physical disability, consider the patient's comfort, chronic conditions, and acute condition when selecting a position for transport.
- *Known or suspected spine injury:* Place patients with possible spine injuries supine on long backboards for spinal immobilization.
- *Nausea or vomiting:* Place patients with abdominal discomfort or nausea and vomiting in the lateral recumbent position.
- *Shock:* Place patients with inadequate perfusion in a supine position to maximize circulation to the vital organs.
- *Unresponsiveness:* Place unresponsive patients with no spine injury who are breathing adequately in the recovery (left lateral recumbent) position.

Resource Central

Resource Central offers extra practice and review materials in a variety of media. To access it, follow the directions on the Student Access Card provided with the Student Textbook. If there is no card, go to www.bradybooks.com and follow the Resource Central link to Buy Access.

Vocabulary and Concept Review

Exercise 1

Write the letter of the correct definition of each term in the blank. (See Resource Central for more vocabulary review.)

1. _____ Fowler's position

2. _____ left lateral recumbent position

3. _____ medium-duty ambulance

4. _____ neonate

5. _____ semi-Fowler's position

6. _____ spotter

7. _____ supine

8. _____ type I ambulance

9. _____ type II ambulance

10. _____ type III ambulance

11. _____ acute illness

12. _____ bariatrics

13. _____ chronic illness

14. _____ due regard

15. _____ defensive driving

a. Newborn infant from birth to 28 days of age

b. Positioned with the head of the bed (ambulance stretcher) elevated at 45 degrees

c. Semi-sitting position with the head of the bed elevated; high-Fowler's position places the torso upright, regular (semi) Fowler's position elevates the torso at a 45-degree angle or higher, and low-Fowler's position elevates the torso at 30 degrees

d. Van with a raised roof and modifications to allow emergency medical care

e. Ambulance box mounted on a pick-up truck chassis

f. Ambulance box mounted on a large truck chassis

g. Position in which the patient is placed lying on his back

h. Position in which the patient is lying on the left side with the arms and legs positioned to prevent rolling forward or backward

i. Modified van chassis with an ambulance box mounted on it

j. Individual who provides instructions and assistance to another individual who cannot see all possible hazards while carrying a patient or backing the ambulance

k. Pertaining to the medical issues related to obesity

l. Techniques of safe driving and crash avoidance that involve anticipating dangerous situations caused by adverse conditions or the mistakes of other drivers

m. Long-standing disease that changes or progresses slowly

n. Appropriate caution and concern

o. Illness with sudden onset, typically of short duration

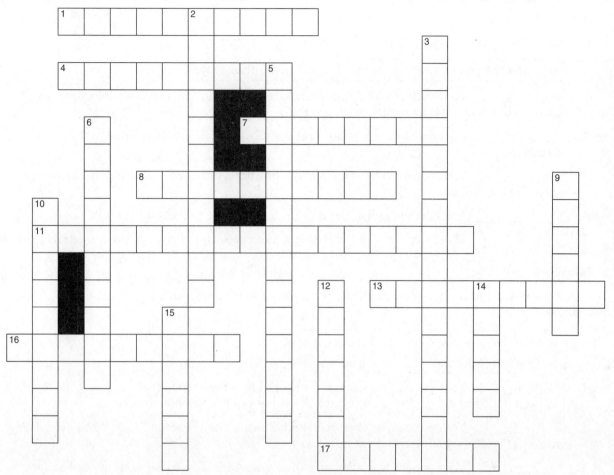

Across

1. Point in the emergency department where arriving patients are usually first evaluated and assigned a priority for care.

4. Medical issues related to obesity.

7. Fixed-wing aircraft.

8. Figure with the Rod of Asciepius at the center that is used to represent emergency medical services.

11. Means by which energy is transmitted to the body, producing the potential for trauma.

13. Process of preparing a patient for transport.

16. Type of driving that improves safety by anticipating adverse conditions and actions of other drivers.

17. Person who provides instructions and guidance to assist another individual and avoid obstacles while moving a patient or driving a vehicle.

Down

2. Process of removing a patient from entrapment, such as from a damaged vehicle.

3. Position in which the patient is lying on his side.

5. Reason a patient states he is requesting medical help.

6. Rotor-wing aircraft.

9. Lying on one's back.

10. Type of move used when a patient is in immediate jeopardy.

12. Position in which a patient is sitting straight up.

14. Having a sudden onset.

15. What is done at the scence to look for potential hazards and determine the nature of the incident.

Check Your Recall and Apply Concepts

Exercise 1

Write the letter of the appropriate patient move beside each scenario.

a. emergency move	b. urgent move	c. non-urgent move

1. _____ Your patient is in a vehicle that has gone off of the road and rests partially submerged in a creek with swiftly moving water.

2. _____ Your patient has a broken ankle and you need to move her downstairs to your stretcher.

3. _____ Your patient is having difficulty breathing after being involved in a low-impact motor vehicle collision.

4. _____ A patient in cardiac arrest needs to be moved to the floor for CPR.

5. _____ The driver of a car involved in a motor vehicle collision complains of back pain.

Exercise 2

Check your recall of moving devices. Write the letter of the appropriate moving device beside each scenario.

a. stair chair	c. basket stretcher
b. portable stretcher	d. scoop stretcher

1. _____ Your patient has sustained a broken leg after she fell from a creek bank. She has been pulled to safety, but she is located at the bottom of a steep ravine.

2. _____ Your patient has chest pain and is located on the second floor of an older home with a very narrow and steep staircase.

3. _____ Your patient has fallen off of her bed and is wedged between the bed and the wall. You suspect she has a broken hip.

4. _____ Your patient is in a back bedroom at the end of a narrow hallway that has stacks of books blocking the passage.

5. _____ Your patient is in the attic and is having difficulty breathing after climbing up the steep stairs.

Clinical Reasoning

Case Study: Dispatch for an Injured Patient on a Hiking Trail

You are dispatched to a residence for a woman who is lying in the grass at the bottom of a moderately sloping hill. She is complaining of pain in her knee but denies any other pain or injuries, and she tells you she has no pertinent medical history. You do not suspect a spine injury.

1. What would be an appropriate device for moving the patient back up to the top of the hill so you can place her in the ambulance?

_____

_____

_____

_____

_____

2. What technique should you use to move the patient onto the device?

_____

_____

_____

_____

_____

3. What are the considerations in determining by what means you should transport the patient and how you should carry out the transport?

_____

_____

_____

_____

_____

Project-Based Learning

Go to your state's department of motor vehicles website to learn more about the requirements and guidelines for emergency driving in your state. Jot down five to seven key points in your notebook or journal.

The EMS Professional in Practice

What behaviors would you consider inappropriate when driving an emergency vehicle? What rules should you set for yourself when driving an emergency vehicle? Jot down your thoughts in a notebook or journal for discussion in class or in your study group.

6 Communication and Teamwork

Content Area

- Preparatory

Advanced EMT Education Standard

- The Advanced EMT applies fundamental knowledge of the EMS system, safety/well-being of the Advanced EMT, and medical/legal and ethical issues to the provision of emergency care.

Summary of Objectives

6.1 Define key terms introduced in this chapter.

In order to understand chapter concepts, it is critical to know, and able to apply, the key terms in each chapter. Write the list of key terms. Then write the definition of each one in your own words. Check your understanding by confirming the definitions in the textbook glossary. Correct any misunderstandings. Create a study aid by writing each key term on the front of an index card and the definition on the back. Use the cards to quiz yourself or to have someone quiz you. The exercises under Vocabulary and Concept Review in this chapter will give you additional practice.

6.2 Describe the components of the communication process, including factors that can interfere with effective communication.

Communication takes place when a message is exchanged between a sender and a receiver. Many characteristics of the environment, sender, receiver, message, and channel or medium through which the message is sent can impact the effectiveness of communication.

6.3 Identify the potential impact of the perceptions of nonverbal behaviors on communication.

Your credibility is communicated through your credentials. Your uniform, patches, and name badge should clearly identify you as an Advanced EMT. Your trustworthiness may be judged on your appearance, and your facial expression, body language, and tone of voice convey empathy and respect.

6.4 Demonstrate effective communications that promote continuity and safety in patient care when communicating with EMS crewmembers, other public safety personnel, and receiving hospital personnel.

All health care team members have the common goal of providing safe, efficient, high-quality patient care, and good communication is the key. Pertinent patient information is handed off from one provider to another to ensure the most thorough information reaches the physicians. Each link in the chain has particular information that is important to the patient's care.

6.5 Given a scenario, demonstrate effective communication that improves team dynamics.

Many EMS responses involve several different agencies and personnel. On the scene of a motor vehicle crash, the Advanced EMT may discuss with the law enforcement officer the best place to park the ambulance to not hinder traffic flow. This shows the officer that the Advanced EMT validates the officer's job responsibilities and appreciates that the officer is protecting the safety of the EMS crew. The Advanced EMT may take a report about the scene and patient condition from a firefighter on scene. By listening carefully and asking questions, the Advanced EMT demonstrates respect and appreciation for the job done by the firefighter. Effective communications validates each person involved in the chain of patient care.

6.6 Describe the responsibilities of the Federal Communications Commission with respect to EMS communication.

The Federal Communications Commission (FCC) is responsible for oversight of EMS radio communication. Some of the responsibilities of the FCC include approving radio equipment, assigning broadcast frequencies, licensing base stations, and assigning radio call signs. The FCC also issues regulations concerning interference with emergency medical broadcasts and bars the use of profane language.

6.7 Discuss the purpose and characteristics of each of the following EMS system communication components: base station, cell phones, digitized radio equipment, interoperability, mobile data terminals, mobile radios, portable radios, and repeaters.

- Base stations are high-powered (up to 150 watts), two-way radios at a fixed site, such as a dispatch center or hospital. Each has a fixed antenna to facilitate transmission and reception.
- Cell phones can provide communication links when traditional radios are limited by range. They use digital transmission systems and are often more reliable than radio waves.
- Digitized radio equipment encodes and decodes sound waves into digital format. It allows more data to be sent over the limited number of available radio frequencies.
- Interoperability is the ability to exchange information between systems. It is important for communication between different agencies working on the same incident.
- Mobile data terminals are electronic communication devices that send and receive a limited amount of data, using a small screen that displays text information. They allow information to be transmitted directly to the unit responding to the call.
- Mobile radios are mounted inside a vehicle and have lower power (20 to 50 watts) than a base station. The range of such a radio is affected by its power, radio frequency used, and geography of the area. The typical range of mobile radios is 10 to 15 miles.
- Portable radios are low-power (1 to 5 watts), two-way radios with a limited range and are carried by EMS personnel to enable communication from outside the vehicle.
- Repeaters enhance transmissions from mobile and portable radios by picking up the lower-power transmissions of portable and mobile radios and retransmitting them at a higher power on a different frequency.

6.8 List the key points in an EMS call at which you should communicate and with whom you should communicate.

Key points in an EMS call at which you should communicate and with whom you should communicate, include dispatch center to EMS crew with call information; EMS crew to dispatch center, confirming receipt of call information and reporting going en route; EMS crew to dispatch, advising arrival on scene; EMS crew communication with patient and family members; EMS crew to dispatch, advising en route to destination; EMS crew to receiving facility with patient information and arrival time; EMS crew to dispatch center with arrival at destination information; EMS crew to hospital staff turning over patient care; and EMS crew to dispatch with return to service information.

6.9 Demonstrate standard rules of radio communications.

Make sure the radio is powered on and you have selected the correct frequency. Listen before transmitting to avoid interrupting other transmissions. Press the "PTT" button and wait 1 second to avoid cutting off the first part of your transmission. Hold the microphone 2 to 3 inches away from your mouth. Speak clearly and in a normal volume. Control voice inflection, aiming for a neutral, professional tone. First state the name of the entity or unit you are calling, followed by your unit identification. Wait for the unit being called to respond: "Go ahead," means proceed with your transmission; "Stand-by," means wait for the unit to let you know they are ready for your transmission. Transmit for no more than 30 seconds without a pause. Deliver information in a concise, organized format.

6.10 Deliver a concise, organized radio report that clearly communicates essential information to medical direction or the receiving facility.

Essential information includes the patient's age, gender, chief complaint or initial presentation, and pertinent history and physical exam findings, including vital signs; any treatment performed and the patient's response to it; any requests for orders; and your estimated time of arrival.

6.11 Demonstrate the ability to receive and confirm an order for medical treatment over the radio.

EXAMPLE:

Dr. Mason: "Copy, Ambulance 21. Give 0.3 mg of epinephrine 1:1,000, IM, and advise us of further problems."

You: "Copy, Dr. Mason. That's 0.3 mg of epinephrine 1:1,000, IM, and advise of further problems. Ambulance 21 clear."

6.12 Discuss the advantages and disadvantages of using radio codes.

The use of codes and signals can communicate some types of information concisely or securely. But, it also can create an opportunity for miscommunication if you or the receiver have not memorized the codes or signals. In general, it usually is best to use plain language in radio communications.

6.13 Convert back and forth between standard clock and military time.

To convert to military time, add 12 to each hour after noon. 1:00 PM is 1300 hours, and 11:00 PM is 2300 hours. To designate minutes after the hour, 3:21 AM is 0321 hours, and 4:06 PM is 1606 hours.

6.14 Explain the importance of establishing rapport with patients and their families in the therapeutic communication process.

You must establish rapport with the patient and efficiently obtain specific pieces of information. Conducting an interview to successfully complete those tasks requires special techniques in addition to knowledge of the general principles of communication. Cultural differences can provide a possibility of misunderstanding and you must consider them, too.

6.15 Given a scenario, engage in effective, empathetic, culturally sensitive communication.

EXAMPLE:

Advanced EMT: "Hello, sir. My name is Monica Benito. I'm an Advanced EMT with the fire department. This is my partner, Connie. What's your name?"

Patient: "I'm Davis Mitchell Nelson, III."

Advanced EMT: "How can we help you today, Mr. Nelson?"

Patient: "I am having a hard time swallowing. I was eating a steak and a piece of it did not go down right. It feels like it stuck right here (indicating a spot in the center of his chest)."

Advanced EMT: "We're here to help. I'd like to ask you some questions while Connie takes your pulse and blood pressure, is that okay?"

6.16 Give examples of the appropriate use of the following communication behaviors: clarification, closed-ended questions, confrontation, empathy, explanation, open-ended questions, reflection, silence, and summary.

- *Clarification:* "I'm not sure I understand. Are you having chest pain now, or is the chest pain something you experienced in the past?"
- *Closed-ended questions:* "How long have you had this cough?"
- *Confrontation:* "You said that you don't have a headache, but you keep rubbing your forehead."
- *Empathy:* "I'm sorry your wife died. It must be hard for you to take care of everything yourself."
- *Explanation:* "Why didn't you call 911 sooner?"
- *Open-ended questions:* "Tell me about your chest pain."
- *Reflection:* "You took five aspirin this morning?"
- *Silence:* "Take your time and think about the last time you felt this way," then remain silent for a spell.
- *Summary:* "Let me make sure I have all the information. You were running on the treadmill when the chest pain started."

6.17 Analyze your communication to avoid the pitfalls of leading or biased questions, interrupting the patient, talking too much, providing false reassurance or inappropriate advice, and implying blame.

- *Leading or biased questions:* Do not suggest answers to the patient.
- *Interrupting the patient:* Let the patient finish his thought before continuing with questions.
- *Talking too much:* You need to gather information from the patient, and that cannot happen if you do all of the talking.
- *Providing false reassurance or inappropriate advice:* You need your patient to trust you and he will not if he feels you are not truthful.
- *Implying blame:* Blame has no value in assessment or treatment of a patient.

6.18 Given a scenario, demonstrate modifications in communication for the following situations: communicating with a patient's family, getting a non-communicative patient to talk, interviewing a hostile patient/using verbal defusing strategies, cross-cultural communication and language barriers, and communicating with children, elderly patients with sensory deficits, and patients with cognitive impairment.

- *Communicating with a patient's family:* "I know you have information for me, but I need to hear the answers to these questions from him."
- *Getting a non-communicative patient to talk:* Encourage him and let him know you are interested by saying something like "You have a history of high blood pressure. That's important for me to know. I'm glad you told me that."
- *Interviewing a hostile patient/using verbal defusing strategies:* Let the patient know you are there to help, and acknowledge his feelings. Stay calm and professional, but take care not to seem condescending, which can provoke an angry patient.
- *Cross-cultural communication and language barriers:* When responding to patients whose culture is different from yours, examine any biases or stereotypes you may hold that can affect communication. Evaluate how your actions may be perceived and how you can best understand the patient's behavior before proceeding.
- *Communicating with children, elderly patients with sensory deficits, and patients with cognitive impairment:* Involve family members in communication as much as the patient is comfortable. "Can you help him find his hearing aids?" or "Do you mind if your mom tells me about your fever?"

6.19 Explain the purposes and importance of documenting patient care.

Documentation is an essential part of continuity of patient care. The assessments, history, treatments, and other information in the PCR communicate critical information to hospital personnel. It also provides a baseline against which to measure changes in the patient's condition. It provides information for billing, insurance claims, and statistical information about the operation of the EMS service. The PCR is a legal document, which may be subpoenaed in criminal or civil cases involving you or the patient. PCRs provide data for research and education and are a key component of continuous quality improvement.

6.20 Describe the elements of the U.S. Department of Transportation (DOT)/National EMS Information System (NEMSIS) minimum data set for patient care reports (PCRs).

Patient information includes the chief complaint; level of responsiveness/mental status; blood pressure; skin perfusion; skin color, temperature, and condition; pulse rate; respiratory rate and effort; and patient demographics. Administrative information includes the incident reported; unit notified; arrived at patient; unit left scene; unit at destination; and patient care transferred.

6.21 Accurately complete the contents of each section of a PCR to include administrative data, patient demographic data and other patient data, vital signs, narrative, and treatment.

- *Administrative data:* EMS unit, crew names, key times, dispatched times, and dispatched address.
- *Patient demographic data and other patient data:* Name, age, gender, ethnicity, date of birth, home address, location where patient was found, insurance and billing information, and care provided before EMS arrival.
- *Vital signs:* Pulse, respirations, blood pressure, and other information, including blood glucose level and pupil assessment.
- *Narrative:* Written account of the call.
- *Treatment:* Documents treatments and responses to treatments.

6.22 Give examples of each of the following types of PCR narrative data: chief complaint, pertinent history, subjective information, and objective information.

- *Chief complaint:* "My chest hurts when I breathe."
- *Pertinent history:* "I had bypass surgery two weeks ago."
- *Subjective information:* "My head hurts."
- *Objective information:* "Patient's skin is pale and moist."

6.23 Explain the importance of using proper abbreviations and terminology in the PCR.

PCRs may be read by people not familiar with the patient or treatment, and they may be confused by nonstandard abbreviations. It is important that anyone who reads the PCR be able to understand what exactly is meant by an abbreviation.

6.24 Describe the SOAP, CHART, and CHEATED methods of PCR narrative documentation.

SOAP Method:

- *Subjective:* Information about the problem as it is given by the patient, including the chief complaint, history of the present illness, and symptoms.
- *Objective:* Information observed in some way by the Advanced EMT, such as vital signs, pupil reaction, response to pain, and other physical findings. Also includes a description of the circumstances in which you found the patient.
- *Assessment:* Your field impression of the patient's problem, based on subjective and objective information.
- *Plan:* Treatment provided and transport information.

CHART Method:

- Usually starts with an introductory statement.
- *Chief complaint (CC):* Describes the patient's chief complaint; also includes associated complaints and pertinent negatives.
- *History:* Includes history of the present illness (HPI) and pertinent past medical history (PMH).
- *Assessment:* Information from primary and secondary assessments and ongoing assessment.
- *Rx (treatment):* Lists treatments provided and the patient's response to them.
- *Transport:* How and where patient was transported, changes in transport, transfer of care.

CHEATED Method:

- Chief complaint
- *History*
- *Exam:* Information from primary and secondary assessments.
- *Assessment:* Field impression, based on chief complaint, history, and exam.
- *Treatment*
- *Evaluation:* Information from ongoing assessment.
- *Disposition:* Transport and transfer of care information.

6.25 Explain each of the following legal concerns with respect to the PCR: confidentiality, documentation of consent and refusal to consent, correction of errors, and falsification of PCR information.

- Confidentiality means that PCR information is provided only to other medical personnel involved in the patient's care, such as receiving hospital staff, and for approved administrative purposes.
- *Documentation of consent and refusal to consent:* When a patient refuses care, there is typically a special additional section of the PCR to be completed. Here, the provider details his actions to ensure a legal refusal.

- *Correction of errors:* For electronic formats, use the features of the program according to your protocols. For written forms, do not scratch out corrections; instead, use correction fluid or otherwise obliterate errors. Draw a single line through the error, initial it, and then write in the correct information.
- *Falsification of PCR information:* Falsification of information on a PCR is a serious violation that can lead to patient harm and disciplinary action against you, including revocation of your license.

6.26 **Discuss how to handle each of the following situations with respect to documentation: transfer of patient care when returning to service before the PCR is complete, multiple-casualty incidents, supplemental reports for special situations, such as exposure to infectious disease and injury to a patient in the course of treatment and transport.**

- *Transfer of patient care when returning to service before the PCR is complete:* You will leave an abbreviated form or a copy of partial PCR information with hospital staff to provide as much information as possible. Ensure that you have given a complete verbal report of patient care information to hospital staff.
- *Multiple-casualty incidents:* The number of patients may not allow completion of a traditional PCR. Typically, you provide a limited amount of information gained in triage, major injuries, and treatments in abbreviated form.
- *Supplemental reports for special situations, such as exposure to infectious disease and injury to a patient in the course of treatment and transport:* You would use a separate incident form provided by your employer. You will mention patient injuries and patient care mistakes in the PCR, but complete documentation of the circumstances usually requires additional documentation.

Resource Central

Resource Central offers extra practice and review materials in a variety of media. To access it, follow the directions on the Student Access Card provided with the Student Textbook. If there is no card, go to www.bradybooks.com and follow the Resource Central link to Buy Access.

Vocabulary and Concept Review

Exercise 1

Write the letter of the correct definition in the blank next to the term. (See Resource Central for more vocabulary review.)

1. _____ active listening

2. _____ clarification

3. _____ close-ended questions

4. _____ confrontation

5. _____ empathy

6. _____ facilitation

7. _____ feedback

8. _____ interference

9. _____ leading questions

10. _____ narrative report

11. _____ nonverbal cues

12. _____ open-ended questions

13. _____ pertinent negatives

14. _____ reflection

15. _____ verbal cues

a. Questions with a narrow range of possible answers, such as "yes" or "no"

b. Written outline of the events of an EMS call, usually following one of several standard formats

c. Factor that is expected to be present in a given type of situation, but not present in the specific situation, the absence of which is notable

d. Listening beyond the sender's words for the meanings behind them

e. Meanings conveyed through written or spoken words

f. Seeking feedback on your understanding of what a patient tells you

g. Questions phrased (usually inadvertently) to exert influence on the patient's answer

h. Mirroring a patient's words back to him to obtain further information

i. Pointing out inconsistencies in information to seek explanation

j. Encouraging a patient to keep speaking

k. Insight into the feelings and situation of another

l. Questions that can lead to a broad range of possible responses

m. Message sent back to the original source of communication about how the message was received

n. Anything that disrupts the transmission or receipt of a message

o. Messages conveyed by means other than spoken or written words

Exercise 2

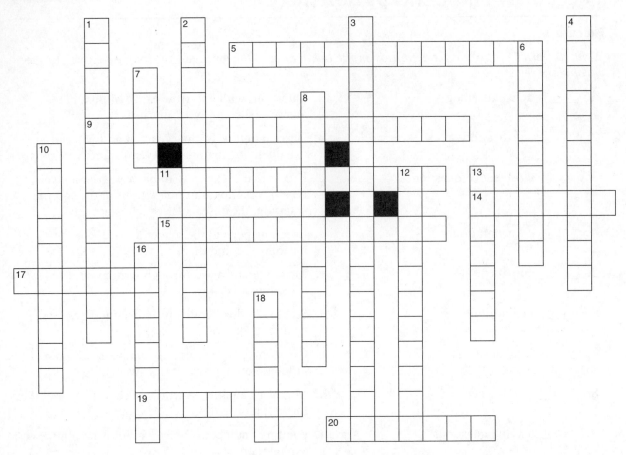

Across

5. Record of an event.
9. Ability to exchange information between different communication systems.
11. Disruption in the transmission of a message.
14. Type of radio mounted in a vehicle.
15. "You said you had some health problems a few months ago. Tell me more about what happened."
17. Type of listening in which you listen beyond the speaker's words for the meaning's behind them.
19. Medium through which a message can be sent.
20. Type of question that influences the patient's answer.

Down

1. Seeking feedback to make sure you understand what the patient tells you.
2. Point out inconsistencies in the information a patient gives you.
3. "The patient complains of nausea but denies vomiting.
4. Believability.
6. Communication through facial expressions, for example.
7. Unit of power used to measure the strength of a radio transmitter.
8. High-power two-way radio in a fixed location.
10. Echoing the patient's words back to him.
12. Possible answers to this type of question are predetermined.
13. Understanding the situation of another person.
16. Message about a message.
18. Person who initiates a message.

Check Your Recall and Apply Concepts

Exercise 1

Select the best possible choice for each of the following questions.

_____ 1. Which one of the following would most likely lead to misunderstanding?
   a. Repeating a medication order back to the physician.
   b. Assuming that all cultures appreciate eye contact.
   c. Asking a patient to spell his name.
   d. Writing down the names of the patient's medications.

_____ 2. Which one of the following should you include in the patient demographic portion of the patient care report?
   a. Dispatched address.
   b. Patient's vital signs.
   c. Written account of the call.
   d. Patient's ethnicity.

_____ 3. When contacting the receiving facility, you should:
   a. report the treatment you have performed.
   b. advise of your arrival time.
   c. give the patient's name and birth date.
   d. pass on insurance information.

_____ 4. Which one of the following is most likely to interfere with good communication?
   a. Making eye contact with the police officer giving you a report.
   b. Placing yourself at eye level with the patient.
   c. Following a predetermined list of questions to ask the patient.
   d. Repeating back to the patient what you heard him say.

_____ 5. When using the "push to talk" radio, you should:
   a. keep your communications about 1 minute in length.
   b. say "thank you" at the conclusion of each transmission.
   c. use 10-codes to shorten your transmission.
   d. wait 1 second before speaking into the microphone.

_____ 6. When you have to repeatedly ask the patient to repeat what he has told you, you are sending a nonverbal message that conveys:
   a. you are trying to get the information straight.
   b. what he is saying is very important to you.
   c. you are not paying attention to what he is saying.
   d. you may possibly have a hearing problem.

_____ 7. Which one of the following would be considered a pertinent negative for a patient with abdominal cramps?
   a. The patient's abdomen is not tender.
   b. The patient has been vomiting for 3 hours.
   c. The patient denies chest pain.
   d. The patient has had his appendix removed.

_____ 8. When requesting orders from a physician over the radio, you should:
   a. let the nurse relay the message.
   b. advise the physician of the patient's vital signs.
   c. question the physician about side effects of the medication.
   d. give the patient's name and list of medications.

Exercise 2

1. List four ways that a patient can tell you are "actively listening" to what he is telling you.

   a. _____

   b. _____

   c. _____

   d. _____

2. List four items of information you will provide to the receiving staff member when you turn over patient care.

   a. _____

   b. _____

   c. _____

   d. _____

Clinical Reasoning

CASE STUDY: A WELL-MEANING MOM

You have been called to the scene of a 15-year-old girl with abdominal pain who also has nausea and vomiting. As you are interviewing and assessing the patient, her mother tells you that her daughter has not been eating well for a couple of days and she thinks she has food poisoning. The mother answers for her daughter each time you ask the patient a question. The teenager is not saying much during the interview.

1. What can you do or say to prevent the mother from answering all of the questions you are asking the patient?

   _____

   _____

   _____

   _____

2. How can you get the patient to open up to you?

   _____

   _____

   _____

   _____

3. What can you do to gain the patient's trust?

_____

_____

_____

_____

Project-Based Learning

With a classmate, simulate a call to a hospital emergency department to give a patient report to the nurse (your classmate). Use a patient scenario that you had in one of your labs or make up a patient in your mind. Be sure to keep the report short, but give all pertinent information. Have your classmate give you feedback on your report.

The EMS Professional in Practice

Being a professional includes making your patients comfortable with you and confident that you know what you are doing. What behaviors or actions can you take to convey professionalism in your communications with your patients? Jot down your thoughts in a notebook or journal for discussion in class or in your study group.

Skills Checklist

Use the following checklist to evaluate your own patient care reports.

Advanced EMT Skill Checklist: *Patient Care Report*		
Skill Stimulus: You have completed an EMS call in which you provided patient assessment and care.		
Documentation	Included	Not Included
Administrative information		
EMS unit		
Crew names		
Times		
Dispatched address		
Patient data and demographics		
Name		
Age		
Gender		
Ethnicity		
Date of birth		
Home address		
Location where patient was found		
Insurance and billing information		
Care provided before EMS arrival		
Vital signs		
Pulse		
Respirations		
Blood pressure		
Pulse oximetry		
Blood glucose level		
Patient care narrative		
Introductory statement		
Chief complaint and associated complaints		
History (history of present illness and past medical history)		
Assessment (primary assessment, secondary assessment, reassessment)		
Treatment		
Transport		
Skill Completion: All pertinent sections of the PCR have been completed.		

Content Area

• Medical Terminology

Advanced EMT Education Standard

• The Advanced EMT uses foundational anatomical and medical terms and abbreviations in written and oral communications with colleagues and other health care professionals.

Summary of Objectives

7.1 Define key terms introduced in this chapter.

Knowing and being able to apply the key terms in each chapter is critical to understanding chapter concepts. Write the list of key terms. Then write the definition of each one in your own words. Check your understanding by confirming the definitions in the textbook glossary. Correct any misunderstandings. Create a study aid by writing each key term on the front of an index card and the definition on the back. Use the cards to quiz yourself or to have someone quiz you. The exercises under Vocabulary and Concept Review below will give you additional practice.

7.2 Use terms of anatomical position, planes, and direction and movement to describe the anatomy of the body.

Anatomical position refers to an erect body with palms facing forward. Distal is away from the midline, while proximal is nearer the midline or point of reference. Adduction is movement toward the body, while abduction is movement away from the body. Anatomical planes include the sagittal (or medial) plane that runs lengthwise, vertically dividing the body into left and right segments. The frontal or coronal plane divides the body into front and back halves. The transverse or horizontal plane is parallel to the ground and divides the body into upper and lower halves. The midline is an imaginary line running through the center of the body beginning at the top, through the nose, past the naval, and down between the legs. The midaxillary line runs from the middle of the armpit down the side to the ankle.

7.3 Apply knowledge of common medical prefixes, suffixes, and roots (combining forms) to determine the meaning of medical terms.

Common prefixes include hyper- (hypertension), brady- (bradycardia), cardio- (cardiology), sub- (subcutaneous), and tachy- (tachycardia). Common suffixes include -genic (cardiogenic),

-rrhea (diarrhea), -trophy (hypertrophy), -ical (neurological), -ostomy (colostomy), and -gram (electrocardiogram). Common combining forms or root words include laryng (laryngeal), hemat (hematology), pulmon (pulmonary), cardi (cardiac), and neuro (neurology).

7.4 Use common medical terminology in communication with other health care providers, including inpatient care documentation.

Members of the health care profession often use a common language to communicate patient information. Terminology such as "denies" merely indicates that the patient answered negatively when asked a question such as "Do you have chest pain?" Other examples include statements such as "the patient was alert and oriented × 3," which means the patient was alert and oriented to person, place, and time. Proper use of medical terminology can more precisely describe a patient's presentation; however, if used incorrectly, it may lead to patient care errors. When communicating with other health care personnel, it is essential that all parties use and understand the same language. It could be confusing to document that the patient had urticaria, when he reported being bitten by an army of ants.

7.5 Differentiate between accepted standard and nonstandard medical symbols and abbreviations.

In patient care documentation, use commonly accepted terminology to avoid confusion. For example, in EMS say the patient complains of "CP," which means chest pain; however, in another setting "CP" might mean cerebral palsy. Any medical symbols or abbreviations used in patient care reports, which are legal documents, need to be readily found in most medical dictionaries to be considered standard. Colloquialisms of a medical nature are not acceptable for legal documents; do not use them in any official capacity.

Resource Central

Resource Central offers extra practice and review materials in a variety of media. To access it, follow the directions on the Student Access Card provided with the Student Textbook. If there is no card, go to www.bradybooks.com and follow the Resource Central link to Buy Access.

Vocabulary and Concept Review

Exercise 1

Write the letter of the correct definition in the blank next to the term. (See Resource Central for more vocabulary review.)

1. _____ anatomical position

2. _____ body planes

3. _____ combining form

4. _____ lesion

5. _____ prefix

6. _____ root word

7. _____ suffix

a. Defined area of injury or diseased tissue

b. Syllables or letters added to the end of a word to modify its meaning

c. Imaginary lines used to divide the body for reference

d. Standing, facing forward, with the palms turned forward

e. Part of a term that provides its basic meaning

f. Syllables or letters added to the beginning of a word to modify its meaning

g. Root word with a vowel added to connect it with another root word or a suffix

Exercise 2

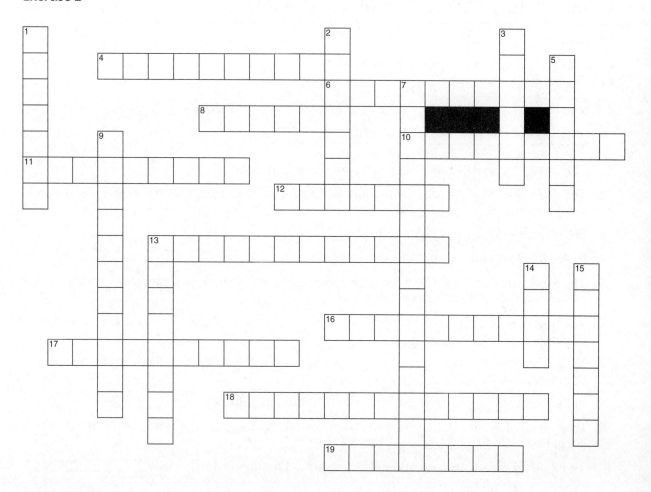

Across

4. Disease process of a gland.
6. Lack of sensation.
8. Pertaining to the back of the body or body structure.
10. Finger bones.
11. Bone cell.
12. Term that refers to the body cavity that houses the brain.
13. Enlargement of the heart.
16. Position in which the patient is partially sitting up.
17. Heart muscle.
18. Physician who specializes in treatment of skin disorders.
19. Loss of appetite.

Down

1. Action of bending a joint.
2. Muscle pain.
3. Location of the fingers with reference to the wrist.
5. Acronyms and idiomatic expressions that are not understood outside a particular group.
7. Above the clavicle.
9. Surgical removal of a kidney.
13. Toward the head.
14. The tip of a structure.
15. Difficult or painful urination.

Check Your Recall and Apply Concepts

Exercise 1

Using the following word list, insert the term that best completes each sentence. Note that some terms may be used more than once.

combining vowel	root word	the study of
prefix	suffix	

1. The word part attached to the end of a combining form is called the _____.

2. The word part that is used at the beginning of a root word and modifies the meaning of the word is called the _____.

3. In the word *neurology*, *-ology* means _____.

4. In the word *cardiology, cardio-* is the _____.

5. The word part that is used between a root word and a suffix to make pronunciation easier and to combine several word parts is called the _____.

6. The word part that indicates the body system or part of the body being discussed or may mean an action is called the _____.

7. In the phrase *bilateral femur fractures*, the word part that tells you the patient has fractures on both legs is the _____.

8. In the word *gastralgia*, the word part, *-algia*, that means pain, is a _____.

9. From the root word *cardi/o*, you could form a word that indicates one who studies the heart by adding a(n) _____.

10. To modify meaning, prefixes and suffixes are added to the word part called _____.

Exercise 2

Using the tables provided at the end of Chapter 7 in the textbook, interpret this patient care report (PCR) and then select the best answer to complete the following questions.

> Called for a 68-year-old man with substernal CP and dyspnea. He recently underwent CABG and is taking a CCB and ASA along with NTG PRN. On assessment, his BS are clear and = to auscultation. Vital signs are WNL and pupils are PEARL. IV placed in left AC with normal saline run KVO. Patient transported to Baldwin Hospital to R/O AMI. Patient transported s̄ Δ.

1. Which of the words or symbols in the PCR indicates the patient has shortness of breath? _____

2. Which of the terms or symbols tells you that the patient's blood pressure is satisfactory? _____

3. Which prefix tells you that the patient has pain below his sternum? _____

4. The symbols, s̄ Δ, tell you that the patient was transported _____

5. The term KVO indicates that the saline is running enough to _____

6. Why type of surgery did this patient have? _____

7. Which root word refers to the patient's respiratory system? _____

8. What do you know about the patient's pupils based on this run report? _____

9. How often is the patient taking his nitroglycerin? _____

10. What do the abbreviations R/O AMI mean? _____

Clinical Reasoning

CASE STUDY: PATIENT TRANSPORTED TO REHABILITATION HOSPITAL

You and your partner were called to transport a patient from an acute care hospital to a rehabilitation hospital. Even though it is just a routine transport, you still have to complete a thorough run report. See what you can discern about this patient's previous medical history based on the medical file that the hospital sent with you to give to the rehabilitation hospital. Use a medical dictionary if necessary.

The report says that the patient was diagnosed with cardiomegaly as a child and has suffered with valvulitis and endocarditis ever since. He was given an antiemetic before he left the hospital.

1. What do you think is his primary problem?

_____

_____

_____

_____

_____

2. Why was he given an antiemetic before your transport?

_____

_____

_____

_____

_____

Project-Based Learning

Put together a one-page "cheat sheet" showing different symbols and abbreviations that you may use when writing the narrative portion of a run report.

The EMS Professional in Practice

An Advanced EMT, tired of transporting patients from the nursing home, to the hospital, and back again, wrote the following in the narrative portion of one of his patient care reports:

"Carried a SOB 83 y/o ♂, hope to get him to the nursing home before he croaks."

How does reading this abbreviated narrative make you feel? What do you think about the quality of medical care this AEMT provides for his patient? How would you feel if he was called to care for your grandmother? Jot down your thoughts in a notebook or journal for discussion in class or in your study group.

8 Human Body Systems

Content Area

- Anatomy and Physiology

Advanced EMT Education Standard

- Integrates complex knowledge of the anatomy and physiology of the airway, respiratory, and circulatory systems to the practice of EMS.

Summary of Objectives

8.1 Define key terms introduced in this chapter.

Knowing and being able to apply the key terms in each chapter is critical to understanding chapter concepts. Write the list of key terms. Then write the definition of each one in your own words. Check your understanding by confirming the definitions in the textbook glossary. Correct any misunderstandings. Create a study aid by writing each key term on the front of an index card and the definition on the back. Use the cards to quiz yourself or to have someone quiz you. The exercises under Vocabulary and Concept Review below will give you additional practice.

8.2 Explain the concepts of metabolism and homeostasis.

The collection of chemical processes that allow the body to grow, reproduce, maintain and repair itself, and respond to its environment is called *metabolism*. Groups of cells form tissues, which in turn form organs and body systems, which function together to support metabolism and maintain homeostasis. Homeostasis is the overall inner balance maintained within the body despite environmental changes.

8.3 Describe each of the levels of organization of the human body.

The basic building block of life is the cell. Individual cells are grouped together both structurally and functionally to create tissues. Tissues come together to form organs, which work together in systems to serve specific functions. Systems are collections of organs and tissues that interact to carry out a complex set of functions.

8.4 Describe the anatomy and physiology of a typical body cell.

The major parts of a cell are the nucleus, cytoplasm, and cell membrane. Other parts of the cell include chromosomes, which hold the cell's DNA in the nucleus; the cytoplasmic organelles, which are compartmentalized structures that perform a specialized function within a cell; and the Golgi apparatus, which moves material around the cell. Other structures include the lysosomes that destroy waste and clean up the cell, the mitochondria that produce energy to power the cell, and the ribosomes that make proteins for the cell. The cell membrane is a selectively permeable structure that envelops the cell and protects the cell's internal environment.

8.5 Explain the physiology and distribution of fluids and electrolytes in the body.

The body is about 60 percent water and is contained within two major compartments in the body—intracellular and extracellular. However, some water is stored as interstitial fluid. Solutes such as electrolytes, carbohydrates, proteins, lipids, and drugs influence the movement of water into and out of the three fluid compartments. Water moves across the cell membrane from lower to higher solute concentration. The difference in concentration of solutes creates osmotic pressure, which has the ability to "pull" water across the cell membrane from the less-concentrated solution to the more-concentrated solution to equalize them. If one side of a cell membrane has a higher quantity of a given electrolyte, there will be a shift of the electrolyte from that side and a shift of water from the other side to maintain fluid balance.

8.6 Describe the regulation of acid–base balance and blood gases.

Acid–base balance is the regulation of hydrogen ions. The more hydrogen ions, the more acidic the environment and the lower the pH. The lower the hydrogen concentration, the more alkaline the environment and the higher the pH. The pH is the potential of hydrogen, which is a measure of acid–base balance in the body. Neutral pH is 7.0; however, the body operates optimally within a pH range of 7.35 to 7.45. When energy production occurs normally (aerobic metabolism), the acid by-products created by the metabolism are easily buffered and removed through the respiratory and renal systems. When energy is produced by anaerobic metabolism, the acid waste products build up in the body and lower the pH. The buildup of acid waste products in the body interferes with normal metabolism and destroys body tissues. Arterial blood gas tests measure the pH and the levels of oxygen and carbon dioxide in the blood from an artery. This test indicates how efficient the respiratory system is in removing excess acid waste products.

8.7 Identify the anatomy and explain the basic physiology of the following body systems: gastrointestinal, genitourinary, integumentary, male and female reproductive, and musculoskeletal.

- The gastrointestinal (GI) system receives and digests food, absorbing nutrients into the body, and excretes waste. The GI system consists of the stomach, small intestine, large intestine, and the rectum.
- The genitourinary system includes all organs involved in reproduction and in the formation and excretion of urine. The major structures of the urinary system are the kidneys, ureters, bladder, and urethra. The major structures of the reproductive system in males are the testes, sperm ducts, urethra, and penis; in females, they are the ovaries, fallopian tubes, uterus, and vagina.
- The integumentary system consists of the skin, or integument, and is the largest organ in the human body. It has the crucial tasks of maintaining body warmth and protecting from external pathogens. The skin is composed of three layers, the epidermis, dermis, and hypodermis or subcutaneous layer.
- The male reproductive system includes the testes, which produce the hormones responsible for sexual maturation and sperm cells. Other parts of the male reproductive system include the epididymis, vas deferens, prostate gland, and the penis, the organ of copulation.
- The female reproductive system is much more complex than the male's. External female reproductive organs include the perineum, mons pubis, labia, and clitoris. Internal genitalia include the vagina, uterus, fallopian tubes, and the ovaries. The male reproductive system is responsible for producing and delivering sperm. The female reproductive is responsible for producing eggs to be fertilized by the sperm and then nurturing and delivering the term fetus.

- The musculoskeletal system consists of two distinct subsystems, which are the skeleton and the muscles. The skeleton provides the structure for the body, protects vital organs, stores salts and other materials needed for metabolism, and produces red blood cells. The muscular system is composed of soft tissues and muscles that protect the body and allow for movement and heat generation.

8.8 Identify the anatomy and explain the functions, including mechanisms for maintaining homeostasis, of the following systems: cardiovascular, with particular attention to cardiac electrophysiology, cardiac output, hemodynamics, and perfusion; endocrine, with particular emphasis on the regulation of glucose; nervous, with particular focus on the autonomic nervous system and its sympathetic and parasympathetic receptors and neurotransmitters; and respiratory, with particular attention to the mechanics of ventilation, and external and internal respiration.

- The cardiovascular system is composed of the heart, blood, and blood vessels that provide blood with access to the tissues and organs of the body for the exchange of gases, nutrients, and other substances. The cardiac conduction system initiates an impulse that spreads through the atria, causing contraction, and then moves through the ventricles, causing contraction. Those contractions force blood through the heart into the systemic circulation. As signals are received in the brain indicating an increased need for oxygen, the heart is stimulated to increase the amount of blood ejected with each contraction as well as an increase in the rate of contractions. As the volume of blood decreases, or the vascular space increases, the heart must speed up contractions to try to meet the demands of metabolism and delivery of oxygen and nutrients to the cells and removal of waste products (perfusion).
- The endocrine system is a collection of ductless glands that secrete hormones into the bloodstream. The pancreas is located behind the stomach and serves several important functions. One important function is the regulation of blood sugar. Alpha cells in the islets of Langerhans secrete the hormone glucagon in response to low blood sugar levels. Glucagon stimulates breakdown of glycogen, a complex carbohydrate in the liver, to glucose. Beta cells secrete insulin, which opposes the actions of glucagon. It is secreted in response to high glucose levels and promotes the uptake of glucose by cells to use in metabolism. Insulin also promotes conversion of excess glucose into glycogen for storage in the liver.
- The nervous system encompasses all the nerve cells, or neurons, in the body. The central nervous system and peripheral nervous system work together to allow both voluntary (somatic) functions and involuntary (autonomic) functions. Autonomic functions are further classified into actions of the sympathetic nervous system and parasympathetic nervous system. The actions of those two divisions of the autonomic nervous system oppose each other to provide both balance and the ability to respond to stimuli to maintain homeostasis. A variety of substances in the body serve as chemical messengers between the synaptic terminals of neurons and adjacent receptors. The neurotransmitters act only on cells that have specific receptors for them. Acetylcholine is the neurotransmitter for parasympathetic nervous system, and norepinephrine is the neurotransmitter for the sympathetic system.
- The respiratory system obtains oxygen needed for cell metabolism and eliminates carbon dioxide produced by cell metabolism. It is divided into external respiration, which occurs in the alveoli, and internal respiration, which occurs at the cellular level. Ventilation relies on basic principles of physics to create the conditions for air to flow into and out of the lungs. The process further relies on the way the lungs are structured and situated in the thoracic cavity. Respiration relies on the microscopic anatomy of the alveoli and capillaries, as well as the principle of gradients—differences in the concentrations of gases from one area to another.

Resource Central

Resource Central offers extra practice and review materials in a variety of media. To access it, follow the directions on the Student Access Card provided with the Student Textbook. If there is no card, go to www.bradybooks.com and follow the Resource Central link to Buy Access.

Vocabulary and Concept Review

Match each term on the left with its definition on the right. Write the letter of the correct definition in the blank next to the term. (See Resource Central for more vocabulary review.)

Exercise 1

1. _____ acid

2. _____ aerobic metabolism

3. _____ alkali

4. _____ anaerobic metabolism

5. _____ bicarbonate

6. _____ buffer system

7. _____ depolarization

8. _____ diffuse

9. _____ electrolyte

10. _____ excitability

11. _____ extracellular fluid

12. _____ glycolysis

13. _____ gradient

14. _____ hydrostatic pressure

15. _____ Krebs cycle

16. _____ metabolism

17. _____ osmolarity

18. _____ osmosis

19. _____ pH

20. _____ repolarization

a. Mechanisms in the body that prevent significant changes in pH

b. Property of being able to respond to a stimulus

c. Graduated change in the degree of a property present

d. Sum of all chemical and physical changes in the body

e. Potential of hydrogen as measured by hydrogen ion concentration; a measure of the acidity or alkalinity of a substance on a scale from 0 to 14

f. Any substance that gives up hydrogen ions in a solution

g. Cellular production of energy that takes place without oxygen, resulting in a small amount of energy with pyruvic acid as a waste product that requires oxygen to be converted to carbon dioxide and water

h. Equalizing a difference in electrical charge across a cell membrane through the movement of ions

i. All fluid in the body that is not within cells

j. Return to a polarized state following depolarization

k. Substance that can accept hydrogen ions in a solution

l. Cellular production of energy that includes the use of oxygen, resulting in production of energy and wastes that are easily eliminated by the body

m. Movement of water across a semipermeable membrane from an area of lower solute concentration to an area of higher solute concentration to achieve equilibrium of solute concentration across the membrane

n. Pressure exerted by nonmoving water

o. Concentration of ions in a solution

p. Anion (HCO_3^-) that can combine with other substances

q. Compound that dissociates into ions in a solution

r. Movement of solutes from an area of higher concentration to an area of lower concentration

s. Breakdown of the sugar molecule glucose ($C_6H_{12}O_6$)

t. Complex series of reactions in the mitochondria of cells in which pyruvic acid (from anaerobic metabolism) is converted to energy

Exercise 2

1. _____ antibody

2. _____ antigen

3. _____ basilar skull

4. _____ Boyle's law

5. _____ cerebrospinal fluid

6. _____ chemoreceptor

7. _____ connective tissue

8. _____ cutaneous

9. _____ endothelium

10. _____ epithelial tissue

11. _____ extracellular fluid

12. _____ foramen magnum

13. _____ hemoglobin

14. _____ millimeters of mercury (mmHg)

15. _____ partial pressure

16. _____ respiration

17. _____ respiratory membrane

18. _____ surfactant

19. _____ suture

20. _____ ventilation

a. Exchange of gases between the body and the environment

b. Movement of air into and out of the lungs

c. Floor of the cranial cavity, which includes portions of the temporal and occipital bones, as well as the sphenoid and ethmoid bones

d. Sensory cells that respond to chemical changes in the body fluids, such as the level of carbon dioxide or oxygen, and send this information to the central nervous system to initiate changes that maintain or restore homeostasis

e. Epithelial tissue that lines the inner surface of a structure

f. All fluid in the body that is not within cells

g. Measure of pressure as determined by the amount of pressure needed to raise a column of mercury 1 mm

h. Tissue layer created by the close proximity of the alveolar sacs and the walls of the capillaries surrounding them, which allows gases to diffuse between the lungs and blood

i. Substance synthesized by the immune system that can recognize specific foreign materials in the body and initiate a specific immune response against it

j. Layers of cells that cover or line a structure, allowing for protection, absorption, secretion, and other specialized functions

k. Iron-containing protein molecule in red blood cells to which oxygen can bind reversibly

l. Large opening at the base of the skull that allows the brainstem to be continuous with the spinal cord

m. Pertaining to the skin

n. States that at a constant temperature, the volume of a gas varies inversely with its pressure

o. One of the four basic tissue types in the body (in addition to muscle, epithelium, and nervous tissue)

p. Partial pressure of a gas in the proportion of the total pressure of a mixture of gases that can be accounted for by an individual gas

q. Immovable joint that joins the bones of the skull

r. Wetting agent that allows fluid to spread across a surface

s. Any substance recognized by the body as foreign, or "not self"

t. Fluid secreted from special cells in the ventricles of the brain that serves to cushion the brain and spinal cord, as well as provide a carefully regulated chemical environment around them

Exercise 3

1. _____ action potential
2. _____ ion
3. _____ excitability
4. _____ perfusion
5. _____ homeostasis
6. _____ insulin
7. _____ serous fluid
8. _____ automaticity
9. _____ villi
10. _____ tidal volume
11. _____ conductivity
12. _____ pulse pressure
13. _____ hemostasis
14. _____ neurotransmitter
15. _____ hormone

a. Process by which the body stops bleeding

b. Finger-like projections of certain cells that increase their surface area for absorption

c. Watery fluid, such as that secreted by the membranes of the peritoneum lining the abdominal cavity

d. Difference between systolic blood pressure and diastolic blood pressure

e. Provision of nutrients, oxygen, and other substances to the cellular level through adequate tissue capillary circulation

f. Particle that carries an electrical charge

g. Temporary change in the electrical charge of the interior of a cell membrane from negative to positive, which allows an impulse to spread to adjacent cells

h. Substances that act as chemical messengers when secreted into the blood by endocrine tissue

i. Property of a structure that allows an electrical impulse to travel along it

j. Substance secreted by the beta cells of the pancreas that decreases blood glucose levels by allowing glucose to enter cells for energy

k. Molecule that acts as a chemical messenger between the axon of one nerve cell and the dendrites of another neuron

l. State of dynamic equilibrium maintained by the body through processes of feedback and adjustment

m. Unique property of cardiac cells that allows them to initiate their own electrical impulse

n. Property of being able to respond to a stimulus

o. Amount of air that is moved into the lungs (and then out) with each normal ventilation

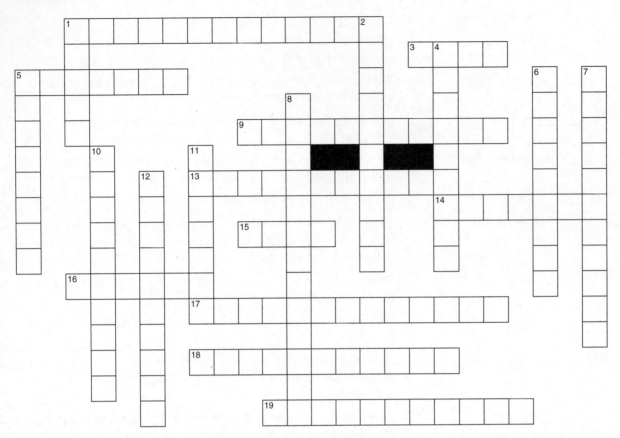

Across

1. Large opening at the base of the skull.
3. Substance that gives up hydrogen ions in a solution.
5. Any substance recognized by the body as foreign.
9. Increased amount in the blood indicates alkalosis.
13. Substances that dissosiates into ions when placed in a solution.
14. Movement of water across a semipermeable membrane to achieve equilibration of solute concentration.
15. Bitter fluid that breaks down fats in the digestive tract.
16. Substance that accepts hydrogen ions in a solution.
17. Sensory cells that respond to chemical changes in the body.
18. Movement of air in and out of the lungs.
19. Exchange of oxygen and carbon dioxide between the body and the environment.

Down

1. Human organism from the eighth week of gestation to birth.
2. Sum of all chemical and physical changes in the body.
4. Pertaining to the skin.
5. Substance synthesized by immune system that recognizes a foreign material and initiates a specific immune response against it.
6. Movement of solutes from an area of higher concentration to an area of lower concentration.
7. Type of pressure exerted by water.
8. Preganglionic sympathetic nervous system neurotransmitter.
10. Iron-containing protein molecule that carries oxygen within red blood cells.
11. Phase of metabolism that occurs when oxygen is present at the cellular level.
12. Substance that acts to prevent collapse of the alveoli.

Check Your Recall and Apply Concepts

Exercise 1

Select the best possible choice for each of the following questions.

_____ 1. The osmolarity of body fluids is between _____ mOsm/L.
  a. 120 and 180
  b. 200 and 240
  c. 280 and 310
  d. 325 and 350

_____ 2. The process of disintegration or dissolution of the cells is called:
  a. crenation.
  b. tonicity.
  c. lysis.
  d. anabolism.

_____ 3. During glycolysis, glucose is broken down into:
  a. lactic acid.
  b. pyruvic acid.
  c. bicarbonate.
  d. glucagon.

_____ 4. The process of aerobic metabolism through which additional energy is produced and by-products are converted into carbon dioxide and water is called:
  a. the Krebs cycle.
  b. crenation.
  c. anabolism.
  d. action potential.

_____ 5. Of the following, the most acidic solution is the one with a pH of:
  a. 4.
  b. 5.
  c. 7.
  d. 10.

_____ 6. The type of muscle found in the walls of blood vessels and in the digestive tract is _____ muscle.
  a. cardiac
  b. skeletal
  c. striated
  d. smooth

_____ 7. The part of the cell in which ATP is produced in aerobic metabolism is the:
  a. nucleolus.
  b. Golgi apparatus.
  c. vacuole.
  d. mitochondria.

_____ 8. What will happen if you give your patient a hypertonic IV fluid such as 2 percent NaCl?
  a. Water will move from within red blood cells to the intravascular compartment.
  b. Water will leave the bloodstream and enter the interstitial fluid and cells.
  c. It will have no immediate net effect on the movement of water between the extravascular and intravascular compartments.
  d. Water will enter the cell in sufficient quantity to cause the cell to burst and die.

_____ 9. Which blood type could theoretically be given to any patient, regardless of his blood type?
  a. O+
  b. O−
  c. AB+
  d. AB−

_____ 10. Electrically, ventricular systole is associated with the _____ on an ECG.
  a. QRS complex
  b. P wave
  c. QT interval
  d. PR interval

Label the anatomical structures.

A.

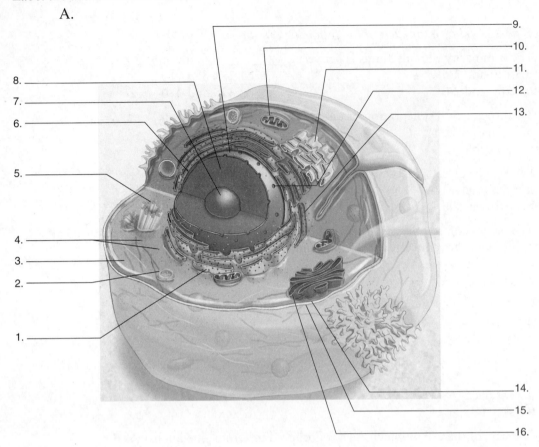

B.

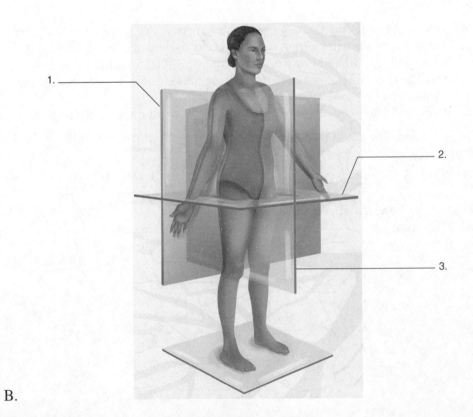

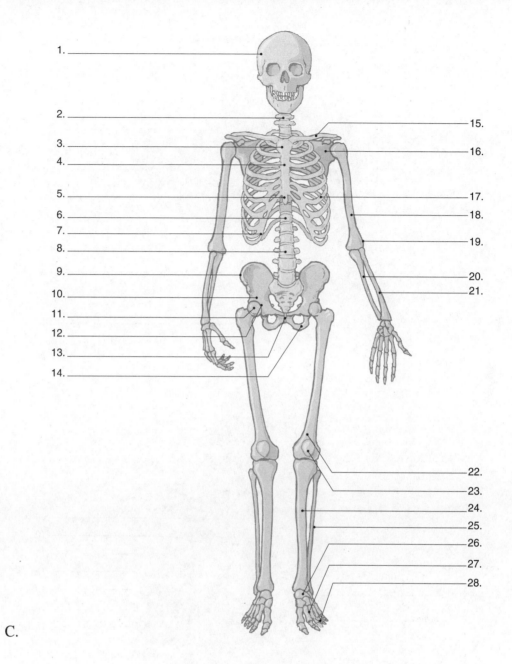

1. _____

2. _____
3. _____
4. _____

5. _____
6. _____
7. _____
8. _____
9. _____

10. _____
11. _____
12. _____
13. _____
14. _____

15. _____
16. _____

17. _____
18. _____

19. _____

20. _____
21. _____

22. _____
23. _____
24. _____
25. _____
26. _____
27. _____
28. _____

C.

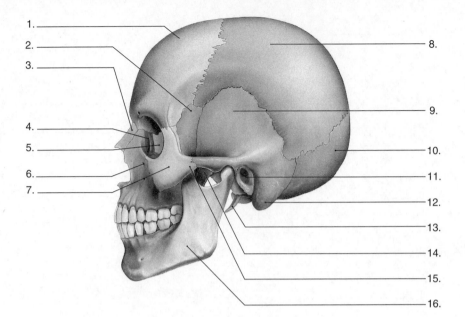

1.
2.
3.
4.
5.
6.
7.

8.
9.
10.
11.
12.
13.
14.
15.
16.

D.

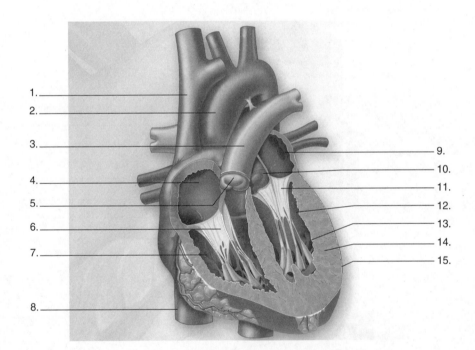

1.
2.
3.
4.
5.
6.
7.

8.

9.
10.
11.
12.
13.
14.
15.

E.

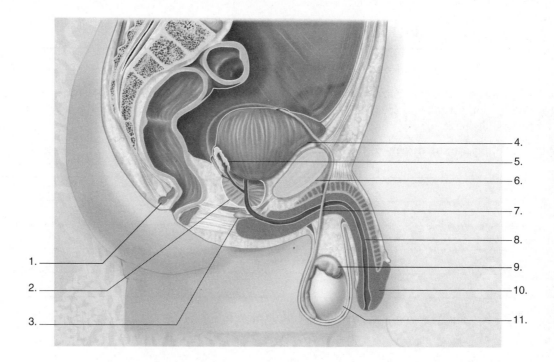

1. _____
2. _____
3. _____
4. _____
5. _____
6. _____
7. _____
8. _____
9. _____
10. _____
11. _____

F.

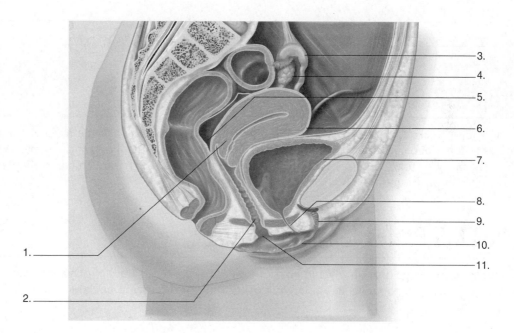

1. _____
2. _____
3. _____
4. _____
5. _____
6. _____
7. _____
8. _____
9. _____
10. _____
11. _____

G.

Clinical Reasoning

CASE STUDY: DROWNING AT MOSQUITO LAKE

You and your partner are dispatched to a campground on Mosquito Lake for a possible drowning. When you arrive, you see that bystanders have pulled a teenage male from the water and are performing CPR.

1. What are the threats to the patient's homeostasis?

_____

_____

_____

_____

_____

_____

2. What is happening at the patient's cellular level?

_____

_____

_____

_____

_____

_____

Project-Based Learning

As a group project, go to the meat counter at your grocery store and ask the butcher for a 7-foot section of butcher paper. Outline the silhouette of one of the group members on the paper. Make a list of all of the body systems and organs studied in this chapter and see if you can correctly place each part in the correct position on the body.

The EMS Professional in Practice

How does knowledge of anatomy and physiology contribute to the quality of patient care you can provide? Jot down your thoughts in a notebook or journal for discussion in class or in your study group.

Life Span Development and Cultural Considerations

Content Area

- Preparatory
- Life Span Development

Advanced EMT Education Standard

- The Advanced EMT applies fundamental knowledge of the EMS system, safety/well-being of the Advanced EMT, and medical-legal and ethical issues to the provision of emergency care.
- The Advanced EMT applies fundamental knowledge of life span development to patient assessment and management.

Summary of Objectives

9.1 Define key terms introduced in this chapter.

Knowing and being able to apply the key terms in each chapter is critical to understanding chapter concepts. Write the list of key terms. Then write the definition of each one in your own words. Check your understanding by confirming the definitions in the textbook glossary. Correct any misunderstandings. Create a study aid by writing each key term on the front of an index card and the definition on the back. Use the cards to quiz yourself or to have someone quiz you. The exercises under Vocabulary and Concept Review below will give you additional practice.

9.2 Identify the age ranges associated with each of the following age classifications: neonate, infant, toddler, preschooler, school age, adolescent, early adulthood, middle adulthood, late adulthood.

- Infancy, birth to 1½ years
- Toddler, 1 to 3 years
- Preschool age, 3 to 6 years
- School age, 5 to 12 years
- Adolescence, onset of puberty to 18 years
- Young adult, 18 to 40 years
- Middle adult, 40 to 65 years
- Older age, greater than 65 years

9.3 Describe the physiological adaptations that occur immediately after birth.

At birth, the lungs must begin to take in air, and blood that was once diverted from the pulmonary circulation must now flow through the lungs for oxygenation and carbon dioxide elimination. Blood that once largely bypassed the gastrointestinal tract must now circulate through it to pick up nutrients and deliver them to the liver for processing.

9.4 Discuss the key physical and psychosocial characteristics and concerns of individuals in each age classification.

- *Infancy:* Infants undergo the greatest physical changes relative to other age groups—they learn to sit up, communicate through cries, and double their birth weight by one year of age. Infants must have their physical and emotional needs met in order to develop trusting relationships. If needs are not met, the individual is less able to feel hope. Overprotectiveness can lead to misplaced trust.
- *Toddler:* Toddlers learn to walk and talk by the age of three years. They must learn the right balance between self-reliance and limits, based on parental reactions. The sense of confidence and independent thought develops if the conflict is resolved successfully and the child develops self-control, resourcefulness, and courage. Without successful resolution, the individual may lack confidence and a sense of self.
- *Preschool age:* Preschoolers gain confidence and skill physically as they learn to run and play games. They continue to grow in height and weight. The approval or disapproval of parents and others either give individuals the ability to take initiative to create and accomplish tasks, or make them feel guilty or incompetent about their ideas and efforts. There must be a balance between allowing the child to experiment and learn through trial and error and keeping the child safe and giving him a realistic view of the consequences of mistakes. Successful resolution at this stage of development leads to a sense of purpose.
- *School age:* School-age children continue growing taller, but their weight gain slows. Their vital signs near those of adults, and brain function increases in both hemispheres. Children who are allowed to find and develop talents and learn skills (including skills needed for academic success) develop a sense of competence, unique strengths, and potential. Children who are denied opportunities feel inferior and develop low self-esteem. Parents remain important at this stage, but children also must be accepted by peers to develop confidence and self-esteem.
- *Adolescence:* A period of rapid growth, commonly called a growth spurt, is characteristic of adolescence. Girls usually finish growing by age 16 years and boys by 18 years, but the teenage brain has not fully developed and adolescents' judgment is not yet the same as in adults. Adolescents strive to develop a sense of who they are and their place in the world. Acceptance by peers and others is important, yet adolescents must develop a sense of independence. Developing morality and a lack of life experience can lead to periods of idealism.
- *Young adult:* Peak physical condition occurs during this period. At the end of it, the body begins showing some of the changes related to the aging process. This is the stage in life in which individuals seek a significant other and start families. Failure to secure stable relationships results in feelings of loneliness and isolation.
- *Middle adult:* The body still functions at a high level with varying degrees of degradation based on the individual. The focus is on successful parenting as children mature and finding satisfying work and ways to express creativity. The challenge is to contribute to family and society and to avoid becoming self-absorbed and self-indulgent. Without an outlet through which to give back, growth stagnates.
- *Older age:* Individual health status determines physiological health at this stage. All systems are deteriorating regardless of a person's efforts. However, a person may feel a sense of satisfaction at life's accomplishments, but also may feel regret about missed opportunities.

9.5 Describe reactions to loss, death, and dying, including stages of grief.

A person's cognitive and emotional development affects how they understand loss and death. Among older children and adults, there is a common sequence of reactions to loss, while younger children are less able to comprehend death. Stages of grief are as follows:

- *Denial:* The initial reaction to the news of death of a loved one, or of one's own impending death, is disbelief.
- *Anger:* Once the reality of death or dying is clear, the person becomes angry.
- *Bargaining:* The dying patient or his family extend promises in an attempt to find out that the diagnosis was a mistake or to buy more time.
- *Depression:* Sadness and cognitive and physical symptoms of depression appear as it becomes clear that death is approaching or that the death of a loved one has occurred.
- *Acceptance:* If the dying person has enough time, or with time after the death of a loved one, the situation is finally accepted.

9.6 Demonstrate awareness of health beliefs of different cultures.

Even among those who do not practice organized religion, the rituals and beliefs surrounding death are influenced by the religious traditions of the culture.

- *Hinduism:* Hindus may believe illness is a result of karma. Taking care of unfinished business in relationships and other matters is an important concern for Hindus at the end of life. Chanting, meditation, prayer, and incense are important parts of the dying and mourning processes. It is preferred that only family touch the body of the deceased, and health care providers should touch the body as little as possible.
- *Judaism:* The eyes of the deceased should be closed, preferably by a relative, and it is preferred that a family member remain with the body until burial. Cremation, embalming, the use of cosmetics or restorative procedures, public viewing, and lavish caskets are forbidden.
- *Buddhism:* It is believed that separations and suffering—such as birth, illness, and death—are inevitable and that suffering results from desire or attachments. Following the Eightfold Path (eight steps for belief and conduct) ends desire and suffering, and leads to Nirvana. Prescriptions for how to handle the body after death, and whether autopsy or organ donation is allowed, are not specific in Buddhism.
- *Islam:* The Qur'an does not provide strict guidance on matters of illness, death, and burial. Important facets of Islam are ritual cleanliness before prayers, prayer while facing Mecca (to the east), dietary guidance, fasting (especially during the holy period, Ramadan), and modesty. It is strongly preferred that health care providers are the same gender as the patient. At death, the patient should be facing Mecca and after death the body should not be touched by non-Muslims.
- *Christianity:* Depending upon particular beliefs, there are many end-of-life sacraments or rites that are desired to be performed by a priest or minister. They may include baptism, confession, holy communion, and last rites (anointing of the sick). Dying patients may wish to read or have read to them passages from the Bible and may wish to pray.

9.7 Adapt communication strategies to patients of different cultural backgrounds.

In Hispanic/Latino culture, maintaining eye contact is important and friendly physical contact, such as a hand on the shoulder, is widely accepted. It is often expected that health care providers will position themselves closer than they might otherwise. Treating others with respect is highly valued, as is the recognition paid to those with official titles.

African Americans tend to have a distrust of the health care system. Those living in urban areas are more subject to certain health problems, such as violence. Female heads of household are common. Economic and educational disparities accompany the health care disparities. Many African Americans are very involved in religious institutions.

In American Indian/Native Alaskan culture, a softer handshake may be seen as more respectful or humble. A comfortable communication distance is several feet and unnecessary contact may not be welcome, especially among elders. Make eye contact, but extended eye contact can be seen as disrespectful. Many medical terms do not have a translation in American Indian/Native Alaskan languages. Silence and slower speech patterns are valued. Listen carefully and do not interrupt.

In Asian culture, self-control, respect for elders, and family loyalty are important. Negative emotions, such as anger, are sometimes not expressed openly, and politeness is highly valued. Patients may prefer a same-sex health care provider. Smiling and nodding may be used out of politeness, despite lack of understanding.

In Middle Eastern culture, same-sex health care providers are preferred (sometimes mandated). In many countries, both men and women cover the head. Women may further be expected to cover the face and not expose the arms or legs. The use of alcohol may be discouraged or forbidden. Muslims may pray several times a day at given times.

9.8 Display cultural sensitivity in interactions with patients of different ethnicities.

Health and medical beliefs of every culture are rich and complex and difficult to summarize. In contrast to the dominant U.S. culture, minority groups tend to place more emphasis on the value of family, including extended family, the community (social group, tribe, village, neighborhood), and respect and deference to elders. Multi-generational families living under the same roof are more common than among White Americans. There is a more holistic view of health and medicine, and many cultures prefer, or even mandate, same-sex health care providers. People of many cultures expect that health care providers will offer some kind of treatment in the form of medications or procedures, rather than just consultation. A number of cultures believe in the importance of prayer by and for the ill, and value the use of plant-based traditional medicines and other alternative and complementary approaches. Many recent immigrants have fled political unrest, corrupt governments, war, and other conditions that may make them distrustful of those in authority.

Resource Central

Resource Central offers extra practice and review materials in a variety of media. To access it, follow the directions on the Student Access Card provided with the Student Textbook. If there is no card, go to www.bradybooks.com and follow the Resource Central link to Buy Access.

Vocabulary and Concept Review

Exercise 1

Write each term from the following list beside its correct definition. (See Resource Central for more vocabulary review.)

adolescent	grief	life expectancy	palliative care	life span
bereavement	hospice	school-age child	preschooler	toddler
fontanel	infant	mourning	proprioception	

1. Opening between the skull bones of an infant where the bones are connected by membranous tissue to allow for compression of the bones during childbirth and rapid growth of the skull and brain after birth._____

2. Child from 3 to 6 years of age._____

3. Child from 6 to 12 years of age._____

4. Maximum biologically determined amount of time human beings could live under ideal conditions._____

5. Philosophy of end-of-life care with a focus on comfort care and social, spiritual, and emotional support for the terminally ill patient and his family._____

6. Child from 12 to 18 years old._____

7. Emotional response to a loss._____

8. Statistical calculation of the length of time a person can expect to live based on his year of birth, where he lives, ethnicity, and other factors._____

9. Child from 1 to 3 years of age._____

10. Experience of a loss._____

11. Care aimed at making patients as comfortable as possible._____

12. Ability to sense the position and spatial orientation of the body or body parts._____

13. Rituals and outward displays associated with grief._____

14. Child from 1 month to 12 months of age._____

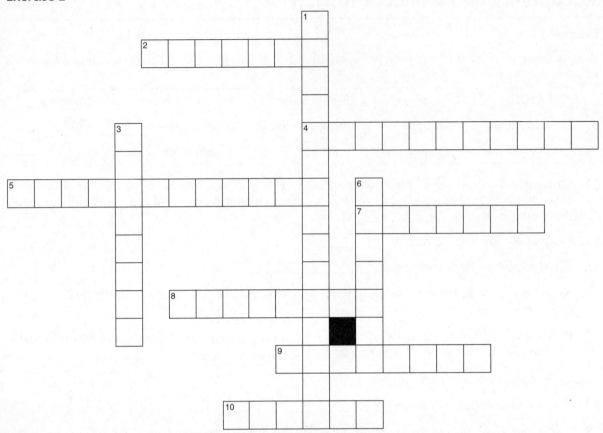

Across

2. Eating disorder characterized by binging and purging.

4. Narrowest part of the infant airway.

5. Type of development based on psychological maturation through interactions in a social context.

7. His eight-stage theory of development is based on the resolution of conflicts at various stages of life from birth through old age.

8. It allows maternal antibodies to be passed to a fetus before birth.

9. About 120 years for human beings.

10. His theory of development explains how people develop cognitively up to adulthood.

Down

1. Toddlers use this to explain things they cannot yet understand.

3. His theory of development explains the moral reasoning behind actions.

6. Individual from birth to one month of age.

Check Your Recall and Apply Concepts

Exercise 1

Write a T (true) or F (false) on the line next to the statement to indicate whether it is true or false.

1. _____ The decline of body structures and functions affect the body's ability to maintain homeostasis.

2. _____ Piaget's theory focuses on the cognitive development of adults.

3. _____ The conflict of trust versus mistrust is part of Kohlberg's Theory of Moral Development.

4. _____ The maximum life span of human beings is about 120 years.

5. _____ Our average life expectancy in the United States is currently 73.9 years.

6. _____ Life expectancy can be influenced by cultural differences.

7. _____ From 1 month of age to 1 year of age, the child is called an infant.

8. _____ In infants, the head comprises about 30 percent of the body weight.

9. _____ Infants have a well-developed thermoregulatory system.

10. _____ Neonates are primarily mouth breathers.

11. _____ Fever in neonates and infants is always concerning.

12. _____ A majority of the elderly live in nursing homes.

13. _____ Bias, stereotypes, and lack of understanding by health care providers contribute to health disparities.

14. _____ Islam is the most common religion for people from Western Asia and the Middle East.

15. _____ Hospice programs help patients and families with assisted suicide.

Exercise 2

Match the characteristics or behaviors with the appropriate age group.

infant	preschooler	adolescent	middle-age adult
toddler	school-age child	young adult	older adult

1. They strive to develop a sense of who they are and their place in the world._____

2. They must be accepted by peers to develop confidence and self-esteem._____

3. Their challenge is to contribute back to family and society and to avoid becoming self-absorbed and self-indulgent._____

4. Their focus is on successful parenting as children mature, and finding satisfying work and ways to express creativity._____

5. They are in the stage in life in which individuals seek a significant other and start families._____

6. They must learn the right balance between self-reliance and limits, based on parental reactions._____

7. They must have their physical and emotional needs met in order to develop trusting relationships._____

8. The approval or disapproval of parents and others give these individuals the ability to take initiative to create and accomplish tasks._____

9. Failure to secure stable relationships results in them feeling lonely and isolated._____

10. They are developing morality, and a lack of life experience can lead to periods of idealism._____

Clinical Reasoning

CASE STUDY: CALL FOR A MOTOR VEHICLE COLLISION

Your crew has been called for a motor vehicle collision (MVC) near the exit from the parking lot of Central High School. Apparently, a teenager pulled out of the parking lot at a high rate of speed and struck a large, older model sedan. The driver of the sedan is an elderly woman, Mrs. Romero. She has a deformed ankle, but was not aware of the injury until you asked her if her ankle hurt. The teenage boy, Caleb, has a small cut on his cheek and he is most concerned about it not leaving a scar.

1. To what do you attribute the fact that Mrs. Romero was unaware of her injury?

_____

_____

_____

_____

_____

2. To what do you attribute Caleb's reckless driving?

_____

_____

_____

_____

_____

_____

Project-Based Learning

Exercise 1

Create flashcards by writing age ranges on one side of index cards and normal vital signs on the other side. Use the cards to study on your own or with a partner.

Exercise 2

During your clinical rotations, reflect on how the various stages of psychosocial and physical development were evident in patients of different ages. What did you observe about an elderly patient that you read about in the text? What differences did you notice in middle-aged and young adults, adolescents, and younger children? Jot down your thoughts in a notebook or journal for discussion in class or in your study group.

The EMS Professional in Practice

When you have a small child as your patient, you really have two (or more) patients because you must consider the needs of the parents, as well. What can you do to meet the needs of both a pediatric patient and his parents? Jot down your thoughts in a notebook or journal for discussion in class or in your study group.

Pathophysiology: Selected Impairments of Homeostasis

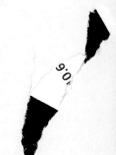

Content Area

- Pathophysiology

Advanced EMT Education Standard

- The Advanced EMT applies comprehensive knowledge of the pathophysiology of respiration and perfusion to patient assessment and management.

Summary of Objectives

10.1   Define key terms introduced in this chapter.

Knowing and being able to apply the key terms in each chapter is critical to understanding chapter concepts. Write the list of key terms. Then write the definition of each one in your own words. Check your understanding by confirming the definitions in the textbook glossary. Correct any misunderstandings. Create a study aid by writing each key term on the front of an index card and the definition on the back. Use the cards to quiz yourself or to have someone quiz you. The exercises under Vocabulary and Concept Review below will give you additional practice.

10.2   Explain the importance of understanding basic pathophysiology.

Understanding pathophysiology for medical emergencies is like recognizing the mechanism of injury for trauma emergencies. Simply knowing how to treat signs and symptoms is not enough. Often, discovering and reversing the cause of the medical problem can be lifesaving.

10.3   Give examples of mechanisms that cause disease and injury in the human body.

Trauma, exposure to extreme environments, lack of oxygen, genetic abnormalities, exposure to excess amounts of various types of energy (heat, radiation, kinetic energy), and lifestyle choices (such as diet, smoking, and other health behaviors) can all lead to illness or injury. Following are some specific examples. (1) After exposure to an allergen, the body may have an anaphylactic reaction causing respiratory distress and widespread vasodilation and shock. (2) A diabetic needs insulin to allow sufficient glucose to enter cells. However, if the patient fails to eat soon after taking insulin, the blood glucose level falls too low and there is not enough circulating glucose to continue to provide fuel for cellular energy production.

10.4 **Describe the composition of ambient air as it relates to ventilation and respiration.**

The concentration of oxygen in the ambient air (21 percent oxygen) determines the partial pressure of oxygen in the alveoli, which must be high enough to result in a gradient (the difference between alveolar oxygen and oxygen in blood returning to the lungs from the body) that allows gas exchange and onloading of oxygen onto hemoglobin.

10.5 **Explain how changes in the compliance of the lungs and chest wall and in airway resistance can affect ventilation.**

Lung compliance, the amount of resistance to air movement, can be affected by decreased surfactant, atelectasis, overinflation, and a number of lung diseases. Too much or too little compliance will result in ventilatory compromise. Chronic exposure to chemical irritants can damage the alveolar walls and cause scarring, ultimately stiffening the lung. This stiffening causes a decrease in compliance that prevents effective inhalation. Excessive compliance is detrimental to ventilation and is the result of the chronic obstructive lung diseases.

Explain how common disease processes can interfere with ventilation and with external and internal respiration.

Decreases in ventilation secondary to disease processes can affect the ability of air to get to the alveoli for gas exchange. Pulmonary edema increases the diffusion distance from alveoli to blood, asthma and COPD narrow the bronchioles, pneumonia prevents ventilation of affected areas, and foreign bodies can obstruct all or some air movement into the lower airway. Any disease that interferes with ventilation will have an impact on external and internal respiration and lead to hypoxia.

10.7 **Describe the homeostatic mechanisms that attempt to correct for changes in ventilation and perfusion.**

Hypoxia and acidosis are detected by chemoreceptors in the body. A drop in blood pressure is detected by sensory receptors called **baroreceptors,** which relay messages to the nervous system and the body's compensatory mechanisms. Compensatory mechanisms include vasoconstriction to shunt blood away from peripheral tissues and increase the perfusion of vital organs, increased heart rate to increase cardiac output, and increased rate and depth of ventilation to improve oxygenation and increase carbon dioxide elimination.

10.8 **Explain the consequences of impaired tidal volume, respiratory rate, and minute volume, as well as increases in anatomical dead space.**

Impaired tidal volume, respiratory rate, or minute volume or an increase in dead space all reduce the amount of air available for gas exchange at the alveolar level, which ultimately leads to cellular hypoxia.

10.9 **Explain the concept of ventilation–perfusion mismatch.**

Ventilation–perfusion mismatch is the term used when either alveolar ventilation or alveolar capillary circulation is impaired. This can occur because part of the lung is not being ventilated, because of pneumonia, for example, so that the blood circulating to the affected area remains deoxygenated; or because part of the lung is not receiving circulation, such as occurs with pulmonary embolism. In pulmonary embolism, air enters the alveoli, but no blood can reach the affected area to participate in gas exchange. Whether the underlying problem is due to a problem with ventilation or with perfusion, hypoxia results.

10.10 **Explain the pathophysiology of shock (hypoperfusion), including the consequences of cellular hypoxia and death.**

Shock reflects the failure of the body's ability to compensate for a problem with blood volume, vascular tone, heart function, circulation, or respiration. When a problem, such as hemorrhage, presents a potential threat to survival, the sympathetic nervous system is stimulated.

Stimulation of the sympathetic nervous system accounts for many of the signs and symptoms of shock. Tachycardia occurs as the heart rate attempts to maintain adequate cardiac output. The body shunts blood away from the skin and gastrointestinal system through vasoconstriction to the core organs most required for life—the heart, brain, and lungs. The skin becomes pale and cool when the color and warmth provided by the circulation of blood has disappeared. Gastrointestinal tract upset—nausea, vomiting, and sometimes bowel incontinence—occurs because the stomach and intestines are deprived of blood. The increase in sympathetic activity causes diaphoresis, as well. If not reversed, the lack of oxygen delivered to the tissues will result in cellular hypoxia and ultimately irreversible end-organ damage and death of the patient.

10.11 Compare and contrast aerobic and anaerobic cellular metabolism, including consideration of the amount of ATP produced and the removal of by-products of energy metabolism.

Aerobic metabolism is the most efficient process to produce energy for the body. Glucose is broken down in the presence of oxygen, which produces 36 ATP molecules through oxidative phosphorylation. Waste products from aerobic metabolism are easily eliminated by the body. In anaerobic metabolism, glucose is broken down without the presence of oxygen, which prevents pyruvic acid from being used for energy. Pyruvic acid is converted to lactic acid, and only a small amount of energy (two molecules of ATP) is produced. Lactic acid cannot be further broken down by the cells into water and carbon dioxide and accumulates in tissues.

10.12 Describe the consequences of failure of the cellular sodium/potassium pump.

ATP is required to pump sodium molecules out of the cell against the concentration gradient. Potassium then moves with the gradient to flow into the cell. Sodium and potassium are exchanged in a continuous cycle that is necessary for proper cell function and water balance. The cycle continues as long as the cells produce energy through aerobic metabolism. When insufficient energy is produced through anaerobic metabolism, the sodium/potassium pump fails and cells die as their water balance is altered, resulting in lysis.

10.13 Describe how inadequate vascular volume, inadequate heart function, and decreased peripheral vascular resistance can each lead to shock.

All forms of shock share a final common pathway of inadequate cellular perfusion to meet metabolic needs. With inadequate vascular volume, the insufficient blood volume within the vascular space prevents tissues and organs from being adequately perfused. When the heart is unable to function properly, either by inefficient stroke volume or inappropriate rate, adequate blood flow is not provided to the lungs or the vascular system to deliver enough oxygen to sustain life. With decreased peripheral vascular resistance, uncontrolled vasodilation creates a vascular container that is too large for the amount of blood in the body. Even when the blood volume is normal, it cannot exert the force needed to maintain blood pressure. Inadequate blood pressure results in inadequate perfusion.

10.14 Give examples of conditions that can lead to the following conditions: loss of vascular volume, inadequate heart function, and decreased peripheral vascular resistance.

- *Loss of vascular volume*: Gastrointestinal bleeding, hemorrhage from trauma, or dehydration from inadequate fluid intake or increased fluid loss (increased urination, vomiting, diarrhea) all lead to loss of circulating blood volume.
- *Inadequate heart function*: Myocardial infarction with electrical abnormalities, such as blockage of electrical conduction, can occur if the infarct affects the electrical pathways. The result may be a nonperfusing dysrhythmia, such as ventricular fibrillation or severe bradycardia. Cardiomyopathy, death of myocardial tissue from infarction, and cardiac valve malfunction can affect the heart's ability to pump.
- *Decreased peripheral vascular resistance*: Causes of distributive shock, which presents with decreased peripheral vascular resistance, include spinal cord injury, anaphylaxis, and septic shock.

10.15 **Explain the mechanisms and pathophysiology of each of the following types of shock: hypovolemic (hemorrhagic and nonhemorrhagic), distributive (anaphylactic, septic, neurogenic), cardiogenic, and obstructive.**

- *Hypovolemic (hemorrhagic and nonhemorrhagic)*: This type of shock presents with low circulating blood volume, which prevents the delivery of adequate oxygen to the tissues. Inadequate oxygen supply leads to anaerobic metabolism.
- *Distributive (anaphylactic, septic, neurogenic)*: Distributive shock presents with widespread vasodilation, which does not allow adequate blood pressure to perfuse the tissues.
- *Cardiogenic*: This type of shock presents with the inability of the heart to contract sufficiently to produce adequate blood pressure to perfuse the tissues.
- *Obstructive*: Obstructive shock occurs when there is a physical obstruction, such as a pulmonary embolism or increased intrathoracic pressure from a tension pneumothorax, blocking the forward flow of blood through the circulatory system, which impairs perfusion of the tissues.

10.16 **Explain how mechanisms such as exposure to carbon monoxide and cyanide can lead to shock.**

Carbon monoxide binds to hemoglobin, preventing oxygen from binding to it. Oxygen is not delivered to the cellular level, impairing cellular metabolism. Cyanide binds to molecules that are part of the electron transport chain in the mitochondria of cells, disabling oxidative phosphorylation. Despite the presence of oxygen, the cell is unable to use it. Without delivery of oxygen to the tissues, tissue death occurs.

10.17 **Explain the body's compensatory reactions to hypoperfusion and how they manifest in the early signs and symptoms of shock.**

The central nervous system reaction to conditions of shock is to increase the respiratory rate to bring in more oxygen to the tissues. Constriction of the peripheral vascular system diverts the circulation of oxygenated blood from the peripheral tissues to provide oxygen for the more vital organs. Vasoconstriction results in cool, pale, and diaphoretic skin and a thready pulse. The heart rate increases (resulting in a rapid pulse) and the contractile force increases to ensure delivery of more oxygenated blood to the tissues.

10.18 **Describe the progression of shock through the compensated, decompensated, and irreversible stages.**

The body's compensatory mechanisms allow maintenance of blood pressure during the early stage of shock, called **compensated shock**. This means that the blood pressure does not drop until the compensatory mechanisms fail and the patient enters decompensated shock. If shock is not reversed before extensive cell death and tissue damage occurs, the patient enters irreversible shock. At that point, regardless of treatment, the patient will die, either within minutes or later, due to organ failure.

10.19 **Discuss the rationales behind the priorities and goals of prehospital management of patients with hypoperfusion.**

Management of shock is limited in the field. The priority of pre-hospital care for shock is to anticipate and recognize it quickly; provide field interventions to support the airway, ventilation, and oxygenation; stop ongoing external hemorrhage; prevent heat loss; and provide transportation to the closest facility capable of providing the care the patient needs.

10.20 **Perform the following for a series of scenarios: recognize patients who are at risk for shock and explain the influence of age on the assessment and management of patients with hypoperfusion.**

To recognize patients who are at risk for shock, analyze the mechanism of injury for the potential for hemorrhage or other causes of shock and recognize medical conditions, such as signs of myocardial infarction, respiratory failure, fluid loss (diabetes, vomiting, diarrhea) and gastrointestinal bleeding that can lead to shock. Maintain a higher index of suspicion for shock in pediatric patients, pregnant patients, the elderly, and those with pre-existing medical conditions.

To explain the influence of age on the assessment and management of patients with hypoperfusion, keep in mind that children's bodies are very healthy and can compensate much better than those of adults, but when the compensation fails, it fails very rapidly. It is critical to anticipate and look for shock in pediatric patients with a history or mechanism of injury that could lead to shock. Elderly and chronically ill patients often take medications that may mask the signs and symptoms of shock. In addition, their bodies can react with decreased effectiveness to conditions of shock. History, nature of the illness, and mechanism of injury are important indicators of shock potential.

10.21 Describe the pathophysiology of cardiac arrest.

In cardiac arrest, there is no cardiac output and no cell perfusion. Cells become hypoxic and stop functioning. Cells with high ischemic sensitivity, such as brain, heart, and lung cells, begin to suffer irreversible damage in just 4 to 6 minutes. Unless circulation is restored, death is almost certain in 10 minutes.

10.22 Differentiate between the electrical, circulatory, and metabolic phases of cardiac arrest.

The first 4 minutes of a cardiac arrest is the electrical phase. During this time, the myocardium is still relatively well perfused and likely to respond to defibrillation. Once this time period has passed, the patient enters the circulatory phase of cardiac arrest, which lasts for approximately 6 minutes. At this point, the cells of the myocardium have become hypoxic through the mechanisms discussed earlier and are unlikely to respond to defibrillation unless circulation is assisted (through chest compressions) in providing oxygen to the cells. Once a patient has been in cardiac arrest for 10 to 15 or more minutes, he transitions to the metabolic phase of cardiac arrest. At this point, cells have been hypoxic for considerable time throughout the body and begin to break down.

10.23 Explain the dependence of cells upon glucose as a source of energy.

All cells require glucose to produce energy (ATP). It is through glycolysis, the breakdown of glucose, that ATP is produced through anaerobic and aerobic metabolism. The body is adept at storing glucose, and can survive for some time without new intake. Some cells can adapt for brief periods of time using alternative mechanisms of energy production. Alternative energy production methods are not as efficient in producing ATP and are all associated with byproduct waste buildups that eventually have toxic effects.

10.24 Explain the consequences of untreated hypoglycemia.

The brain is unable to quickly adapt to fuels other than glucose. A sudden and significant drop in blood glucose level (hypoglycemia) can quickly lead to brain cell damage and death.

10.25 Explain how disruptions of electrolyte balance and pH impact body functions.

The critical function of electrolytes in the cell and in fluid balance means that the levels of electrolytes must be maintained within narrow ranges for normal cellular function and fluid balance. Cardiac rhythm, electrical conduction, and contraction can be affected by disturbances in sodium, potassium, magnesium, and calcium.

10.26 Explain the consequences of inadequate temperature regulation in the body.

The body's physiological activities can only occur within a narrow range of core temperature. When the body cannot compensate for environmental extremes, or its temperature regulation mechanisms are impaired, death can occur. Hypothermia causes blood-clotting mechanisms to become impaired, and the heart and central nervous system malfunction. Hyperthermia has significant consequences for the central nervous system.

Resource Central

Resource Central offers extra practice and review materials in a variety of media. To access it, follow the directions on the Student Access Card provided with the Student Textbook. If there is no card, go to www.bradybooks.com and follow the Resource Central link to Buy Access.

Vocabulary and Concept Review

Exercise 1

Write each term from the following list beside its correct definition. (See Resource Central for more vocabulary review.)

anaphylaxis	atelectasis	hyperpyrexia	pathology	shock
apoptosis	cardiomyopathy	hypoxia	pneumothorax	sign
asphyxiation	defibrillation	ischemia	pyruvate	symptom

1. Airless state (collapse) of alveoli._____

2. Electrical current passed through the heart between two pads or paddles placed on the chest to terminate ventricular fibrillation and pulseless ventricular tachycardia._____

3. Study of disease states._____

4. Initial substance formed in the anaerobic phase of cellular metabolism, which, in the presence of oxygen, is then converted to acetyl coenzyme A for use in the Krebs cycle for further ATP production._____

5. Decreased level of oxygen at the cellular level._____

6. Indication of illness or injury that can be objectively observed._____

7. Severe, life-threatening allergic reaction._____

8. Subjective sensation of an abnormality in body function._____

9. Disorder of the heart in which the muscle is enlarged and unable to function effectively.

10. State in which the level of perfusion to the tissues is not adequate to meet metabolic demands._____

11. Severely diminished or absent blood flow to tissues._____

12. Cell death caused by the genetic programming of cellular function of the cell itself to eliminate damaged cells; essentially, suicide of damaged cells._____

13. Accumulation of air between the pleural layers that occupies space normally filled by the lungs._____

14. Extremely high fever, above 41.1°C or 106°F._____

15. Cellular deprivation of oxygen; suffocation._____

Exercise 2

Write the letter of the correct definition in the blank next to the term. Note that there are more definitions than there are terms. (See Resource Central for more vocabulary review.)

1. _____ dysrhythmia

2. _____ hemorrhagic shock

3. _____ hyperthermia

4. _____ hypothermia

5. _____ ischemic phase

6. _____ pathophysiology

7. _____ pulmonary edema

8. _____ respiratory arrest

9. _____ respiratory failure

10. _____ sodium/potassium pump

11. _____ stagnant phase

12. _____ sudden cardiac arrest (SCA)

13. _____ ventricular fibrillation

14. _____ ventricular tachycardia

15. _____ washout phase

a. Absence of breathing; apnea

b. Cardiac dysrhythmia that produces a rapidly firing ectopic pacemaker in the ventricles

c. Phase of shock in which both the precapillary and postcapillary sphincters constrict to divert blood flow away from the peripheral tissues and gastrointestinal system

d. Mechanism of the cell membrane that uses energy to exchange sodium and potassium ions across the cell membrane

e. Phase of shock in which both the precapillary and postcapillary sphincters have failed and the blood that had stagnated in the capillary beds, along with lactic acid and microscopic blood clots, re-enters the circulation

f. Heart rhythm that may be irregular, too slow, too fast, or arise from a site other than the sinoatrial node; may or may not be life threatening

g. Abrupt, unexpected cessation of heart function that often occurs outside the hospital setting

h. Body temperature that is higher than normal, generally because of factors other than increased metabolism, such as prolonged exposure to an extremely hot environment

i. Shock caused by blood loss

j. Study of the impact of disease on the body and the body's responses to the disease state

k. Phase of shock in which the precapillary sphincter fails, allowing blood to enter the microvasculature; the postcapillary sphincter remains closed, causing blood to pool in the capillary beds, where it collects lactic acid and microscopic blood clots are formed

l. Lethal cardiac dysrhythmia in which multiple ectopic pacemakers in the ventricles create chaotic electrical activity that does not produce mechanical contraction of the heart

m. Increase in interstitial fluid in the lungs, resulting in a greater diffusion distance for oxygen and carbon dioxide across the respiratory membrane

n. Lower than normal body temperature

o. Inability to maintain adequate ventilation and oxygen

Exercise 3

Write the definitions for each of the listed terms.

1. Anatomical dead space

   _____

   _____

2. Clinical impression

   _____

   _____

3. Compensated shock

   _____

   _____

4. Decompensated shock

   _____

   _____

5. Diabetic ketoacidosis

   _____

   _____

6. Irreversible shock

   _____

   _____

7. Lactic acid

   _____

   _____

8. Metabolic acidosis

   _____

   _____

9. Pulmonary embolism

   _____

   _____

10. Ventilation–perfusion mismatch

   _____

   _____

Exercise 4

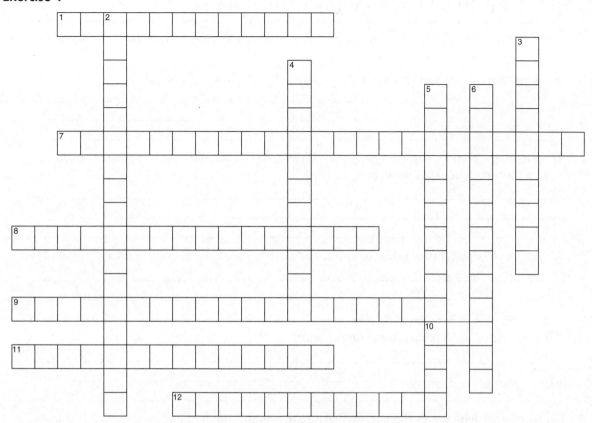

Across

1. Suffocation.
7. Lethal cardiac dysrhythmia in which there is chaotic, ineffective electrical activity.
8. Perfusion is inadequate but the blood pressure is normal.
9. Portion of the airway where air is present but gas exchange cannot occur.
10. State of hyperglycemia, dehydration, and acidosis in a patient with diabetes.
11. Type of enlargement of the heart that results in inadequate heart function.
12. High body temperature resulting from exposure to a hot environment.

Down

2. Blood clot that obstructions circulation through the lungs.
3. By-product of anaerobic metabolism.
4. Abnormal heartbeat.
5. Increase in interstitial fluid in the lungs that interferes with gas exchange.
6. Stage of shock in which both the precapillary and postcapillary sphincters are closed.

Check Your Recall and Apply Concepts

Read each question and think about the information presented in your text. Answer each question with one or two sentences.

1. What happens when a patient takes his insulin in the morning but forgets to eat?

2. What happens to your patient's perfusion status if he has a faulty gas furnace that releases carbon monoxide into his residence?

3. Why does your patient complain of weakness when he becomes hypoglycemic?

4. What can cause a spontaneous pneumothorax?

5. Describe what happens in the lungs when a patient has pulmonary edema.

6. Describe management of a patient with severe respiratory compromise.

7. How does defibrillation convert ventricular fibrillation?

8. How can a patient with carbon monoxide poisoning have an oxygen saturation of 99 percent?

9. When would you give a patient glucagon?

10. What is the purpose of shivering when the body gets cold?

Clinical Reasoning

CASE STUDY: CALL TO A PHYSICIAN'S OFFICE

You respond to a physician's office for a 68-year-old man who is feeling weak and dizzy. The patient says he has had loose stools that are black and grainy. The nurse reports that the patient's vital signs are blood pressure 88/52, pulse 126, and respirations 24.

1. To what do his signs and symptoms point?

_____

_____

_____

_____

_____

2. Based on your assessment, what treatment do you recommend?

_____

_____

_____

_____

_____

3. Explain why this patient has a low blood pressure. What do you think is wrong with him?

_____

_____

_____

_____

_____

Project-Based Learning

Watch a medical drama on television. Pay attention to the signs and symptoms of critically ill and injured patients. Do they make sense based on what you are learning about pathophysiology? If not, what advice would you provide if you were asked to be a technical advisor for the show? Rewrite one of the scenes of the show to portray it more accurately. Have your study group act out the scene for your classmates. Your classmates can act as television critics to determine if they agree with your portrayal of the illness or injury.

The EMS Professional in Practice

A patient who is hypoxic may have an altered mental status as a result of lack of oxygen to the brain. Often, this presents as hostility or combativeness. How will you respond to a patient who is hostile because of a medical condition? Jot down your thoughts in a notebook or journal for discussion in class or in your study group.

Principles of Pharmacology

Content Area

- Pharmacology

Advanced EMT Education Standard

- The Advanced EMT applies fundamental knowledge of medications in the Advanced EMT scope of practice to patient assessment and management.

Summary of Objectives

11.1 Define key terms introduced in this chapter.

Knowing and being able to apply the key terms in each chapter is critical to understanding chapter concepts. Write the list of key terms. Then write the definition of each one in your own words. Check your understanding by confirming the definitions in the textbook glossary. Correct any misunderstandings. Create a study aid by writing each key term on the front of an index card and the definition on the back. Use the cards to quiz yourself or to have someone quiz you. The exercises under Vocabulary and Concept Review below will give you additional practice.

11.2 Give examples of each of the four sources of drugs.

- Plant: atropine (belladonna), morphine (opium poppy)
- Animal: insulin, thyroid hormone oxytocin, vaccines
- Mineral: calcium chloride, magnesium sulfate
- Synthetic: acetaminophen, lidocaine

11.3 Explain the role of the Food and Drug Administration in the development and continued oversight of drugs.

The FDA oversees the development and approval processes for drugs and collects information about drug safety after drugs are marketed.

11.4 Discuss relevant legislation regarding the administration of prescription medications, including controlled substances.

The Pure Food and Drug Act required proper labeling of medications. The Harrison Narcotic Act placed regulations on addicting drugs. The Food, Drug, and Cosmetic Act and its amendments authorized the formation of the FDA and mandated that addicting or potentially harmful medications are dispensed only by prescription. The Controlled Substance Act established five schedules of controlled substances.

11.5 Identify the official, generic, and trade names of drugs in the Advanced EMT scope of practice.

The official name of a drug is the name under which it is listed in the United States Pharmacopeia and is followed by the letters USP. The generic name is usually the official name without those letters. The trade name is the name under which a drug is marketed by a specific company. An example is aspirin USP (official name), aspirin (generic name), and Bayer (trade name).

11.6 Describe the various forms in which drugs are supplied.

Drugs come in solid forms, such as tablets, powders, and capsules; liquids, such as solutions and suspensions; semisolids, such as ointments and gels; and gases, such as oxygen and nitrous oxide.

11.7 Describe the various types of medication packaging.

Medications for pre-hospital use come in vials, ampules, prefilled syringes, metered-dose inhalers, nebules, compressed gas cylinders, and bottles or unit-dose packages (such as blister packs) of tablets or capsules.

11.8 Explain each of the components of a drug profile.

A drug profile consists of the medication name (generic, trade, and chemical), classification (such as body system acted upon or way that the medication works), mechanism of action (the way the medication has its intended effect), indications (reasons the medication is used), pharmacokinetics (how the drug and body interact), side effects (unintended effects), route of administration (the way the medication is given), contraindications (factors that preclude drug administration), dose (amount that can be given), how the medication is supplied (packaging, forms, concentration), and special considerations (such as storage and use in special populations).

11.9 Explain each of the following with respect to pharmacology: drug absorption, drug distribution, mechanism of action, and drug elimination.

Drug absorption is the process by which the drug enters the vascular system. Drug distribution is the process by which the drug is delivered to the target tissues. Mechanism of action refers to the way in which the drug exerts its effects. Most drugs work by binding to a cellular receptor to modify cellular function. Drug elimination is the way in which the drug is broken down and removed from the body.

11.10 Explain the roles of the kidneys and liver in drug metabolism and excretion.

Many drugs are processed by enzymes in the liver, which may either convert a drug from an inactive to an active form or break an active form of a drug down into other components. Many drugs are eliminated (either changed or unchanged) in the urine.

11.11 Explain factors that can affect the concentration of a drug in a patient's body.

Dose, route of administration, perfusion status, presence of other drugs, body weight, hydration status, liver function, and kidney function all can affect drug concentration.

11.12 Describe the concepts of drug receptor sites and protein binding of medications.

Receptors are proteins in cell membranes that can bind with drug molecules. The drug receptor concept is like a key and lock. Drugs that are not specific for a receptor will not affect the cell. Many drugs circulate through the body bound to the plasma protein albumin. As the amount of free drug (drug not bound to proteins) decreases, more bound drug is released. Drugs can compete for both receptors and protein binding.

11.13 Identify special populations in whom the administration of drugs may need to be modified.

Drug dosage and administration may need to be modified in pregnant, pediatric, and geriatric patients; patients with kidney or liver failure; and patients who are taking other drugs.

Resource Central

Resource Central offers extra practice and review materials in a variety of media. To access it, follow the directions on the Student Access Card provided with the Student Textbook. If there is no card, go to www.bradybooks.com and follow the Resource Central link to Buy Access.

Vocabulary and Concept Review

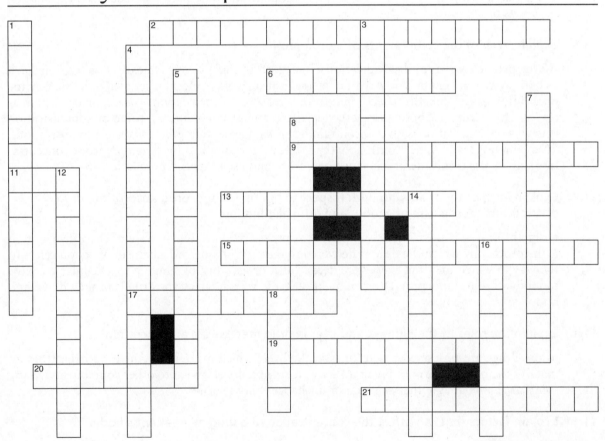

Across

2. Opposes the effects of acetylcholine.
6. Property that affects the strength of cardiac contraction.
9. Drug reaction that is unique to a given individual.
11. Acetaminophen is an example.
13. Adverse reaction caused by medical treatment.
15. A reason a drug must not be given.
17. The need for a larger dose of a drug to get the same effect as before.
19. How a drug moves from the site of administration to the circulation.
20. Drug that stimulates a specific action in the body.
21. Property that affects the speed of cardiac conduction.

Down

1. Drug that acts to break down a blood clot.
3. Causes harm to a fetus.
4. Results in an allergic reaction.
5. Drug that prevents blood from clotting.
7. Enhances the effect of another drug.
8. Drug that increases urination.
12. Increases the function of the parasympathetic nervous system.
14. A reason a drug is given.
16. Degree of attraction between a drug and receptor.
18. Ibuprofen is an example.

Check Your Recall and Apply Concepts

Select the best possible choice for each of the following questions.

_____ 1. The medication diphenhydramine is an example of a(n) _____ name of a drug.
  a. trade
  b. generic
  c. official
  d. chemical

_____ 2. The way a drug has its effects on the body is called the:
  a. indication.
  b. classification.
  c. mechanism of action.
  d. therapeutic index.

_____ 3. The federal agency that provides oversight for drug safety is the:
  a. FDA.
  b. OSHA.
  c. USP.
  d. PDR.

_____ 4. Which one of the following is an example of a solid medication?
  a. Solution
  b. Elixir
  c. Ointment
  d. Tablet

_____ 5. Another term for a sympathomimetic drug is:
  a. cholinergic.
  b. anticholinergic.
  c. adrenergic.
  d. antiadrenergic.

_____ 6. Selective serotonin uptake inhibitors (SSRIs) can be classified as what kind of drugs?
  a. Respiratory
  b. Sedative
  c. Depressant
  d. Psychotherapeutic

_____ 7. Which one of the following is an example of an antidysrhythmic medication?
  a. Diazepam
  b. Calcium channel blocker
  c. Albuterol
  d. Morphine

_____ 8. A glass or plastic container with a sealed rubber stopper through which a needle is inserted to draw up medication is called a(n):
   a. prefilled syringe.   c. vial.
   b. ampule.   d. nebule.

_____ 9. A medication requires repeated dosages to reach the desired concentration in the body and have the intended results. This effect is known specifically as:
   a. cumulative.   c. iatrogenic.
   b. therapeutic.   d. untoward.

_____ 10. When a drug binds to a receptor and blocks the effect of another substance on the receptor, it is known as a(n):
   a. depressant.   c. agonist.
   b. lytic.   d. antagonist.

_____ 11. Your patient requires a higher dose of a drug because he is already regularly taking a drug that has similar effects. This is known as:
   a. synergism.   c. cross-tolerance.
   b. potentiation.   d. hypersensitivity.

_____ 12. The point at which the amount of drug in the body is sufficient to have the desired effect is called the:
   a. LD_{50}.   c. therapeutic threshold.
   b. half-life.   d. therapeutic index.

Clinical Reasoning

CASE STUDY: MRS. MILLER'S MEDICATION

Your neighbor, Mrs. Miller, knocks on your door as you are studying for your pharmacology quiz. "I know you are studying to be an Advanced EMT," she says. "I don't understand the papers that came with my medication at all. Can you help me out?" She has the following questions for you:

1. "What is a mechanism of action?"

_____

_____

_____

_____

2. "How will I know if I am having an idiosyncratic reaction?"

_____

_____

_____

_____

_____

3. "What does it mean when it says that alcohol can potentiate the effects of this drug?"

_____

_____

_____

_____

_____

4. "Where can I find out more about my medications?"

_____

_____

_____

_____

_____

Project-Based Learning

Research possible sources of drug information by looking on-line, visiting your library, searching for smart phone applications, and asking other EMS providers what information sources they find useful. Find out which sources are easiest for you to use. Check with your instructor about the reliability of specific sources. Bookmark reliable information sources that you find especially useful and share them with your classmates at your next class session.

The EMS Professional in Practice

Why is general knowledge of principles of pharmacology important for Advanced EMTs? Jot down your thoughts in a notebook or journal for discussion in class, in your study group, or in the virtual classroom.

12 Medication Administration

Content Area

- Pharmacology

Advanced EMT Education Standard

- Applies fundamental knowledge of medications in the Advanced EMT scope of practice to patient assessment and management.

Summary of Objectives

12.1 Define key terms introduced in this chapter.

Knowing and being able to apply the key terms in each chapter is critical to understanding chapter concepts. Write the list of key terms. Then write the definition of each one in your own words. Check your understanding by confirming the definitions in the textbook glossary. Correct any misunderstandings. Create a study aid by writing each key term on the front of an index card and the definition on the back. Use the cards to quiz yourself or to have someone quiz you. The exercises under Vocabulary and Concept Review below will give you additional practice.

12.2 Explain the medical direction mechanisms by which an Advanced EMT may be authorized to administer a medication.

Advanced EMTs can only give medications by order of a medical direction physician. The orders may be in the form of standing orders or may be received verbally by phone, radio, or in person. Advanced EMTs who work in hospital emergency departments or similar settings may receive written orders for specific patients.

12.3 Explain Advanced EMT practices that are necessary with regard to medication administration safety.

Advanced EMTs must protect their own safety, that of the patient, and others when giving medications. Personal safety includes selecting appropriate Standard Precautions and handling sharps properly. Patient safety includes following the Six Rights of Medication Administration.

12.4 Differentiate between enteral and parenteral routes of drug administration.

Enteral routes are those that allow absorption through the vasculature of the gastrointestinal system. Parenteral routes are those that bypass the gastrointestinal tract circulation.

12.5 Describe each of the following routes of medication administration: inhaled (gases and nebulized medications), intramuscular (IM), intraosseous infusion (pediatric), intravenous bolus, intravenous infusion, oral (PO), subcutaneous (subQ), and sublingual (SL).

- *Inhaled (gases and nebulized medications):* Inhaled medications pass through the upper respiratory system and into the lungs, where they have local effects (such as bronchodilators) or are absorbed across the respiratory membrane to have systemic effects, or both.
- *Intramuscular (IM):* Medication is injected into a large muscle mass, where it is absorbed into the vasculature.
- *Intraosseous infusion (IO) (pediatric):* IO medications are injected through tubing attached to a needle inserted into the bone marrow cavity of a long bone.
- *Intravenous bolus:* A bolus is a single, usually large dose of medication or IV fluid given over a short period of time—in this case, through an intravenous line.
- *Intravenous infusion:* Administration of a specific volume of intravenous fluids or medications over a specific amount of time by calculating an IV drip rate.
- *Oral (PO):* Administration of medications by mouth to be swallowed.
- *Subcutaneous (subQ):* Injection of medications beneath the dermis into the subcutaneous tissues, where they can be absorbed.
- *Sublingual (SL):* Placing medication beneath the tongue to be absorbed through the mucous membranes into the vasculature.

12.6 Properly interpret verbal and written drug orders.

To properly interpret drug orders, you must understand common terminology, abbreviations, units of measure, and the conventions for writing drug dosages.

12.7 Use proper abbreviations and terminology with respect to drug administration.

See Table 12-2 in the Student Textbook.

12.8 Calculate drug dosages from drug orders, including proper use of the metric system.

Standard formulas and approaches are used for translating drug orders.

12.9 Explain the concept of medical asepsis.

All percutaneous medication administration requires proper cleaning of the skin to minimize the chances of infection. All equipment used for percutaneous medication administration must be sterile.

12.10 Demonstrate the following skills under instructor supervision: administering drugs by small-volume nebulizer, administering nitrous oxide, assisting patient with the use of a metered-dose inhaler, intramuscular injection, intravenous access, intravenous and intraosseous fluid administration, intravenous medication bolus, oral medication administration, pediatric intraosseous access, subcutaneous injection, sublingual medication administration, use of an auto-injector device.

Refer to the skill sheets at the end of this workbook chapter.

Resource Central

Resource Central offers extra practice and review materials in a variety of media. To access it, follow the directions on the Student Access Card provided with the Student Textbook. If there is no card, go to www.bradybooks.com and follow the Resource Central link to Buy Access.

Vocabulary and Concept Review

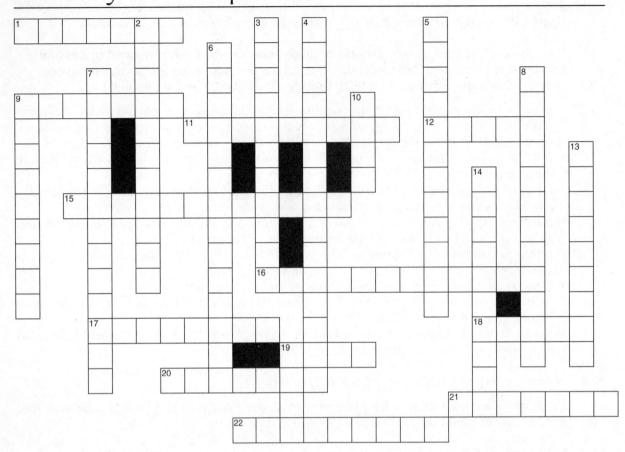

Across

1. Pertaining to the gastrointestinal tract.
9. Substance that causes fever.
11. IV tubing that provides 1 mL per 60 gtts.
12. Metric base unit for volume.
15. Inserting a needle into a vein.
16. Gaseous analgesic.
17. Administration of medication by an intravenous drip.
18. Diameter of a needle.
19. Metric base unit for volume.
20. Without infection.
21. Muscle in which volumes of medication exceeding 2 mL can be injected.
22. The type of container in which used sharps are properly disposed of.

Down

2. Refers to the front of the arm.
3. Point at which two branches merge into a single vein.
4. Drug that regulates the heartbeat.
5. Escape of interavenous fluid into the surrounding tissue.
6. Can be used in place of alcohol to prepare the skin for an IV.
7. One of the six rights of medication administration.
8. Medication routes that go through the skin.
9. Inflammation of a vein.
10. Denominator in the standard drip rate calculation formula.
13. Device that converts liquid medication to a fine mist.
14. Medication route in which medicine is placed beneath the tongue.
19. Metric prefix meaning one thousand.

Check Your Recall and Apply Concepts

Select the best possible choice for each of the following questions.

_____ 1. The most common types of medication errors involve the wrong:
    a. patient.
    b. drug.
    c. dosage.
    d. route.

_____ 2. Which one of the following is an enteral route of medication administration?
    a. Intraosseous
    b. Intravenous
    c. Subcutaneous
    d. Per os

_____ 3. Which one of the following routes of administration results in the fastest absorptions of medication?
    a. Intravenous
    b. Subcutaneous
    c. Sublingual
    d. Intramuscular

_____ 4. Under what circumstances must you report a medication error?
    a. Only if the wrong medication is given
    b. Only if harm comes to the patient
    c. In all cases of medication error
    d. Only if the error involves controlled substances

_____ 5. You have received an order to give a medication "SL." That means you should give the medication by:
    a. injecting it beneath the skin.
    b. instructing the patient to swallow it.
    c. placing it beneath the patient's tongue.
    d. applying it topically to the skin.

_____ 6. One milligram is the same as:
    a. 0.1 gram.
    b. 1,000 micrograms.
    c. 100 kilograms.
    d. 0.01 grams.

_____ 7. You are going to give a patient. 0.4 mg of 1:1,000 epinephrine. How many milliliters of the drug must you administer to complete the order correctly?
    a. 40
    b. 4
    c. 0.4
    d. 0.04

_____ 8. You are going to give 1.2 mg of naloxone to a patient. The medication is supplied in 10-mL vials with a concentration of 0.4 mg/mL. How many milliliters of the medication are needed to achieve the ordered dose?
    a. 1
    b. 2
    c. 3
    d. 4

_____ 9. A patient weighs 185 pounds. How much does he weigh in kilograms?
    a. 72
    b. 84
    c. 97
    d. 0

_____ 10. A patient is to receive IV fluids at a rate of 125 mL/hour. You will be using IV tubing that delivers 15 gtts/mL. What is the drip rate per minute at which you must infuse the fluids?
    a. 15
    b. 30
    c. 45
    d. 60

_____ 11. A patient is to receive a bolus of 20 mL/kg of IV fluid over 1 hour. He weighs 79 pounds. You will be using tubing that delivers 10 gtts/mL. What is the drip rate per minute needed to deliver the correct dosage?

a. 30
b. 60
c. 90
d. 120

_____ 12. You have started an IV on a patient using 60-gtts/mL tubing. What drip rate per minute is needed to deliver fluids at a rate of 50 mL/hour?

a. 15
b. 25
c. 35
d. 50

Clinical Reasoning

CASE STUDY: NIGHT SHIFT IN THE PRESBYTERIAN HOSPITAL EMERGENCY DEPARTMENT

You have just started your new job as an emergency department technician at Presbyterian Hospital. One of your duties is starting IVs. After checking the IV cart assigned to you, you are paged to check a patient whose IV does not seem to be working properly.

1. What are some common complications of IV therapy that could be causing the problem? List at least five complications.

_____

_____

_____

_____

_____

2. What are some things you can do to troubleshoot the IV? Provide at least three of them in the following space.

_____

_____

_____

_____

3. Under what circumstances should you discontinue the IV and start a new IV in a different site?

_____

_____

_____

_____

_____

4. What factors should you consider in selecting a new site and the equipment you will use if you must start a new IV? Write at least three ideas in the following space.

_____

_____

_____

_____

_____

Project-Based Learning

Create an IV drip rate calculation table to help you check your answers when practicing IV drip rates. Include the volume of fluid to be infused on one axis of the table and the tubing drip factor on the other. Clearly label your table. Perform the calculations needed to fill out the table and keep it handy as a reference. What patterns do you see in the following example? How can those patterns help you select the right IV tubing and check the accuracy of your calculations?

Example IV Drip Rate Chart

	30 mL/hr	50 mL/hr	75 mL/hr	100 mL/hr	125 mL/hr	150 mL/hr
10-gtts/mL tubing	5 gtts/min	8 gtts/min	13 gtts/min	17 gtts/min	21 gtts/min	25 gtts/min
15-gtts/mL tubing	8 gtts/min	13 gtts/min	19 gtts/mL	25 gtts/min	31 gtts/min	38 gtts/min
20-gtts/mL tubing	10 gtts/min	17 gtts/min	25 gtts/min	33 gtts/min	42 gtts/min	50 gtts/min
60-gtts/mL tubing	30 gtts/min	50 gtts/min	75 gtts/min	100 gtts/min	125 gtts/min	150 gtts/min

The EMS Professional in Practice

Giving medications is a weighty professional responsibility. How can you make the Six Rights of Medication Administration of practical use in decreasing medication errors? What other practices can help you keep your patients safe when you administer medications? Jot down your thoughts in a notebook or journal for discussion in class or in your study group.

Skills Checklists

The following skill checklists cover the major steps of selected skills from Chapter 12. Review them prior to your laboratory classes. Practice skills only after they have been demonstrated for you in class and only under the supervision of an authorized instructor or clinical preceptor.

Advanced EMT Skill Checklist: *Drawing Up Medication from a Vial*		
Skill Stimulus: Drug order is received (standing order or on-line medical direction); Six Rights of Medication Administration have been confirmed.		
Step	**Performed**	**Not Performed**
Check the medication. (Confirm the name and concentration of the medication. Check the expiration date and inspect the fluid for clarity and absence of particulates. Check the integrity of the container.)		
Assemble all needed equipment and supplies.		
Attach a fill needle to a syringe of the appropriate size.		
Disinfect the rubber stopper of vial with an alcohol swab.		
Remove the cap from the needle on the syringe and pull out the plunger to fill the syringe with just slightly more air than the volume of medication to be injected.		
Pierce the rubber stopper of the vial with the needle and invert the vial. Depress the syringe plunger to inject the air into the vial.		
Making sure the bevel of the needle is below the fluid level in the vial, pull out the syringe plunger to fill the syringe with just slightly more than the volume of medication to be delivered.		
Remove the syringe from the vial and set the vial aside.		
Holding the syringe upright, tap or flick the barrel of the syringe so that all air bubbles migrate to the top of the syringe. Slightly depress the syringe plunger to remove the air.		
If necessary, replace the needle with the appropriate size needle for injection.		
Skill Completion: Medication dosage is confirmed and appropriate needle for administration has been attached to the syringe.		

Advanced EMT Skill Checklist: *Drawing Up Medication from an Ampule*		
Skill Stimulus: Drug order is received (standing order or on-line medical direction); Six Rights of Medication Administration have been confirmed.		
Step	**Performed**	**Not Performed**
Check the medication. (Confirm the name and concentration of the medication. Check the expiration date and inspect the fluid for clarity and absence of particulates. Check the integrity of the container.)		
Assemble all needed equipment and supplies.		
Attach a fill needle or filter straw to a syringe of appropriate size.		
Tap or swirl the ampule to ensure all fluid is in the bottom portion.		
Wrap an alcohol swab or small gauze square around the neck of the ampule.		
Snap open the ampule at the neck. Discard the top of the ampule in a puncture-proof biohazard container.		
Place the tip of the needle or filter straw into the open ampule, ensuring that the tip is below the fluid level.		
Making sure the bevel of the needle is below the fluid level in the ampule, pull out the syringe plunger to fill the syringe with just slightly more than the volume of medication to be delivered.		
Remove the syringe from the ampule and discard the vial in a puncture-proof biohazard container.		
Holding the syringe upright, tap or flick the barrel of the syringe so that all air bubbles migrate to the top of the syringe. Slightly depress the syringe plunger to remove the air.		
If necessary, replace the needle with the appropriate size needle for injection.		
Skill Completion: Medication dosage is confirmed and appropriate needle for administration has been attached to the syringe.		

Advanced EMT Skill Checklist: *Intramuscular Injection*

Skill Stimulus: Drug order is received (standing order or on-line medical direction); Six Rights of Medication Administration have been confirmed.

Step	Performed	Not Performed
Collect all equipment needed for the procedure.		
Draw up the medication in the syringe, ensure proper dose, and expel air.		
Attach a needle of appropriate length and gauge.		
Select the administration site (usually the deltoid for prehospital care).		
Prepare the administration site with an alcohol swab and let it dry.		
Remove the cap from the needle.		
Stabilize the skin around the injection site with the non-dominant hand.		
Hold the barrel of the syringe with a pencil grip, and dart the needle into the skin at a 90-degree angle to the hub of the needle.		
Stabilize the syringe with the non-dominant hand and use the dominant hand to pull back slightly on the plunger of the syringe. Observe for blood in the barrel of the syringe. If blood appears, discontinue the procedure.		
If no blood appears in the barrel of the syringe, depress the syringe plunger smoothly and completely to inject the medication.		
Withdraw the needle and syringe as a unit, engaging any needle safety devices (depending on needle design).		
Dispose of the syringe and needle as a unit in a puncture-proof biohazard container.		
Check the site to see if there is any bleeding. Cover with an adhesive bandage.		
Monitor the patient during administration for desired effect, side effects, and any other changes.		
Skill Completion: Medication has been delivered and patient has been reassessed.		

Advanced EMT Skill Checklist: *Subcutaneous Injection*		
Skill Stimulus: Drug order is received (standing order or on-line medical direction); Six Rights of Medication Administration have been confirmed.		
Step	**Performed**	**Not Performed**
Collect all equipment needed for the procedure.		
Draw up the medication in the syringe, ensure proper dose, and expel air.		
Attach a needle of appropriate length and gauge.		
Select the administration site (usually the skin over the deltoid area for pre-hospital care).		
Prepare the administration site with an alcohol swab and let it dry.		
Remove the cap from the needle.		
Pinch up a fold of skin and subcutaneous tissue, lifting it away from the underlying muscle.		
Hold the barrel of the syringe with a pencil grip, and dart the needle into the skin at a 45-degree angle to the hub of the needle.		
Depress the syringe plunger smoothly and completely to inject the medication.		
Withdraw the needle and syringe as a unit, engaging any needle safety devices (depending on needle design).		
Dispose of the syringe and needle as a unit in a puncture-proof biohazard container.		
Observe the site for bleeding. Cover with an adhesive bandage.		
Monitor the patient during administration for desired effect, side effects, and any other changes.		
Skill Completion: Medication has been delivered and patient has been reassessed.		

Advanced EMT Skill Checklist: *Intravenous Access*

Skill Stimulus: IV order is received (standing order or on-line medical direction); Six Rights of Medication Administration have been confirmed.

Step	Performed	Not Performed
Collect all equipment and supplies needed for the procedure.		
Set up the IV infusion set or saline lock.		
Apply a venous constricting band to the arm proximal to the intended site.		
Select a suitable vein.		
Use an alcohol or povidone-iodine swab to disinfect the skin over the site and allow it to dry.		
Put on gloves if not done previously.		
Remove the plastic cover from the needle/catheter unit and inspect the device.		
Stabilize the vein without contaminating the site.		
Hold the needle/catheter unit bevel-up at a 45-degree angle or lower to the skin, in alignment with the vein.		
Insert the needle, advancing it until there is a flash of blood in the chamber behind the needle. Then advance the needle/catheter unit about 2 mm more to ensure the edge of the catheter is in the lumen of the vein.		
Lower the angle of the needle/catheter unit and advance the catheter over the needle until the hub of the catheter rests against the entry site.		
Release the constricting band.		
Use one finger to occlude the vein proximal to the tip of the catheter.		
Remove the needle, leaving the catheter in place.		
Dispose of the needle in a puncture-proof biohazard container.		
Remove the cap from the end of the IV tubing or saline lock and connect the tubing to the hub of the IV catheter.		
Briefly open the roller clamp on the tubing to check for patency of the IV or inject saline through the saline lock.		
Ensure the area around the insertion site is clean and dry.		
Apply a dressing and secure the catheter and tubing in place.		
Adjust the drip rate of the IV.		

Skill Completion: The IV line is patent and secure, the drip is adjusted correctly, and the patient is being monitored.

Advanced EMT Skill Checklist: *Intravenous Medication Bolus*		
Skill Stimulus: Drug order is received (standing order or on-line medical direction); Six Rights of Medication Administration have been confirmed.		
Step	Performed	Not Performed
Draw up the medication in a syringe or prepare a prefilled syringe by placing the plunger into the barrel or the syringe.		
Disinfect the injection port with an alcohol swab.		
Insert the needle into a rubber injection port or attach a needleless device to the port provided.		
If injecting into an IV infusion set, pinch the IV tubing closed.		
Depress the syringe plunger to deliver the medication at the rate appropriate for the medication being given.		
Monitor the IV site for signs of leakage or infiltration during the injection. Discontinue the injection and the IV if infiltration occurs.		
For an IV infusion set: Release the tubing and open the roller clamp briefly to flush medication through the tubing. Reset the drip rate.		
For a saline lock: Follow the medication injection with a saline flush of at least 3 mL.		
Monitor the patient during administration for desired effect, side effects, and any other changes.		
Skill Completion: Medication has been delivered and patient has been reassessed.		

Advanced EMT Skill Checklist: *Small-Volume Nebulizer Medication Administration*

Skill Stimulus: Drug order is received (standing order or on-line medical direction); Six Rights of Medication Administration have been confirmed.

Step	Performed	Not Performed
Collect all equipment and supplies needed for the procedure. Remove the nebulizer from the plastic packaging.		
Assemble the nebulizer, using the "T" piece to connect the mouthpiece (or, alternatively, attaching the face mask provided with the nebulizer).		
Open the medication container (and additional saline, if it is to be added) and empty the measured amount into the medication cup of the nebulizer.		
Place the cap on the medication cup.		
Attach oxygen tubing to the inlet at the bottom of the medication cup.		
Adjust the flow of oxygen to 8 liters per minute (lpm) to nebulize the medication in the cup. Ensure that mist is being generated.		
Inform the patient about the procedure.		
Instruct patient how to use the mouthpiece to inhale the medication, or place the mask on the patient's face and secure it with the elastic strap.		
Monitor the patient during administration for desired effect, side effects, and any other changes.		

Skill Completion: Medication cup is empty and the patient has been reassessed.

Advanced EMT Skill Checklist: *Metered-Dose Inhaler*

Skill Stimulus: Drug order is received (standing order or on-line medical direction); Six Rights of Medication Administration have been confirmed.

Step	Performed	Not Performed
If not already done, insert the metal medication canister into the plastic dispenser.		
Agitate the container to mix the contents.		
Remove the cap from the mouthpiece on the dispenser.		
Instruct the patient to place the mouthpiece in his mouth and make a seal.		
Instruct the patient to begin to inhale deeply.		
Instruct the patient to depress the canister into the dispenser as he begins to exhale, assisting him in the process if needed, and then to hold his breath for a few seconds before exhaling.		
Repeat the process if a second dose is ordered.		
Monitor the patient during administration for desired effect, side effects, and any other changes.		
Skill Completion: Medication has been delivered and patient has been reassessed.		

Advanced EMT Skill Checklist: *Intranasal Medication Administration*		
Skill Stimulus: Drug order is received (standing order or on-line medical direction); Six Rights of Medication Administration have been confirmed. Check for contraindications to use of a mucosal atomizer device (epistaxis, nasal trauma, nasal congestion, abnormalities of the nasal septum).		
Step	Performed	Not Performed
Draw up the medication in the syringe, ensure proper dose, and expel air.		
Remove the needle or filter straw from the syringe and attach a mucosal atomizer device (MAD).		
With the patient supine, place the MAD into one nare and depress the syringe plunger to deliver half the dose, which must be 1 mL or less.		
Place the MAD into the second nare and depress the syringe plunger to deliver the second half of the dose.		
Monitor the patient during administration for desired effect, side effects, and any other changes.		
Skill Completion: Medication has been delivered and patient has been reassessed.		

Advanced EMT Skill Checklist: *Pediatric Intraosseous Access (EZ IO)*		
Skill Stimulus: IV order is received (standing order or on-line medical direction); Six Rights of Medication Administration have been confirmed.		
Step	**Performed**	**Not Performed**
Collect all equipment and supplies needed for the procedure.		
Set up an IV fluid infusion.		
Prefill the extension tubing with saline and leave the syringe attached.		
Locate the insertion site on the anteriomedial tibia, two fingerbreadths below the tibial tuberosity.		
Select the proper needle length for the patient.		
Prepare the site using a povidone-iodine swab.		
Place the needle on the driver.		
Hold the driver at a 90-degree angle to the leg and depress the trigger mechanism to drill the needle into the bone.		
Remove the stylet (guide) from the needle.		
Attach the prefilled extension tubing and flush with saline. Observe for free flow of fluid and absence of infiltration.		
Attach the IV tubing to the extension tubing and adjust the flow rate.		
Secure the needle and tubing to the leg. Complete and attach the information band.		
Skill Completion: The IO line is patent and secure, the drip is adjusted correctly, and the patient is being monitored.		

13

Medications

Content Area

- Pharmacology

Advanced EMT Education Standard

- The Advanced EMT applies fundamental knowledge of medications in the Advanced EMT scope of practice to patient assessment and management.

Summary of Objectives

13.1 Define key terms introduced in this chapter.

Knowing and being able to apply the key terms in each chapter is critical to understanding chapter concepts. Write the list of key terms. Then write the definition of each one in your own words. Check your understanding by confirming the definitions in the textbook glossary. Correct any misunderstandings. Create a study aid by writing each key term on the front of an index card and the definition on the back. Use the cards to quiz yourself or to have someone quiz you. The exercises under Vocabulary and Concept Review below will give you additional practice.

13.2 Describe the drug profiles for each of the following medications: acetaminophen; activated charcoal; aspirin; dextrose 50 percent, 25 percent, and 10 percent for treating hypoglycemia, and 5 percent in water for intravenous infusion; epinephrine, 1:1,000; glucagon; ibuprofen; inhaled beta$_2$ agonists; lactated Ringer's solution for intravenous infusion; naloxone; nitroglycerin tablets and spray; nitrous oxide; oral glucose; other isotonic intravenous solutions as allowed by medical direction; oxygen; sodium chloride solution 0.9 percent for intravenous infusion.

- Acetaminophen is an analgesic and antipyretic. It is used in both adults and children to relieve minor pain and reduce fever.
- Activated charcoal is an adsorbent, which is sometimes given in cases of overdose and poisoning by ingestion to prevent the toxin from being absorbed from the gastrointestinal tract.

- Aspirin is a nonsteroidal anti-inflammatory drug that is used to reduce minor pain, reduce fever, and prevent further platelet aggregation in patients with acute coronary syndrome or ischemic stroke.
- Following are the uses of the various dextrose solutions: 50 percent dextrose is used in adult hypoglycemic patients to increase the blood glucose level; 25 percent dextrose is used in children; 10 percent dextrose is used in neonates to treat hypoglycemia; 5 percent dextrose is used as an intravenous infusion fluid for patients who can benefit from the administration of a small amount of carbohydrates. The dextrose from 5 percent dextrose solution is quickly metabolized, leaving water in the vascular system, making 5 percent a hypotonic IV solution.
- 1:1,000 epinephrine is a catecholamine that stimulates the sympathetic nervous system to cause increased heart rate, force of contraction, and rate of electrical conduction. It causes vasoconstriction and relaxes bronchial smooth muscle. 1:1,000 epinephrine is indicated for anaphylaxis to increase blood pressure and reduce airway obstruction.
- Glucagon is a catabolic hormone that acts in the liver to cause the breakdown of stored glycogen into glucose. Glucagon is given intramuscularly in hypoglycemia when IV access cannot be obtained to administer dextrose. However, the patient must have adequate liver glycogen stores for glucagon to be effective.
- Ibuprofen is a nonsteroidal anti-inflammatory drug used to treat mild to moderate pain and reduce fever in both children and adults.
- Inhaled beta$_2$ agonists work on the bronchiolar smooth muscle to bring about smooth muscle relaxation and bronchodilation in patients with asthma, COPD, or anaphylaxis.
- Lactated Ringer's solution is an isotonic solution of electrolytes with lactate, which acts as a buffer to reduce acidosis. It is used in patients who need volume replacement, particularly those who may be acidotic, such as patients in shock.
- Naloxone (Narcan) is a narcotic antagonist that competes for opiate receptor sites to reduce the effects of drugs such as morphine, heroin, fentanyl, meperidine, and others. Naloxone is indicated to reduce respiratory depression associated with narcotic overdose.
- Nitroglycerin is a nonselective vascular smooth muscle relaxant. It is used in the prehospital setting to cause coronary vasodilation to improve myocardial blood flow in acute coronary syndrome. Nitroglycerin also reduces afterload through systemic vasodilation. As such, hypotension and headache are common side effects.
- Nitrous oxide is an analgesic gas that is self-administered under the guidance of a health care professional for conditions such as chest pain and musculoskeletal trauma.
- Oral glucose is a source of carbohydrates that can be given to hypoglycemic patients whose level of responsiveness is not impaired.
- Various combinations and concentrations of electrolytes, such as those in lactated Ringer's solution, sodium chloride, and dextrose are available, but are typically not used in the short-term setting of prehospital care.
- Compressed medical grade oxygen is administered by face masks, nasal cannulas, or ventilation devices to increase the SpO$_2$ in patients with hypoxia.
- Normal saline, or 0.9 percent sodium chloride, is an isotonic intravenous fluid used for keep-open IVs for medication administration, as a basis for mixing drugs for intravenous infusion, and for fluid replacement in hypovolemia.

Resource Central

Resource Central offers extra practice and review materials in a variety of media. To access it, follow the directions on the Student Access Card provided with the Student Textbook. If there is no card, go to www.bradybooks.com and follow the Resource Central link to Buy Access.

Vocabulary and Concept Review

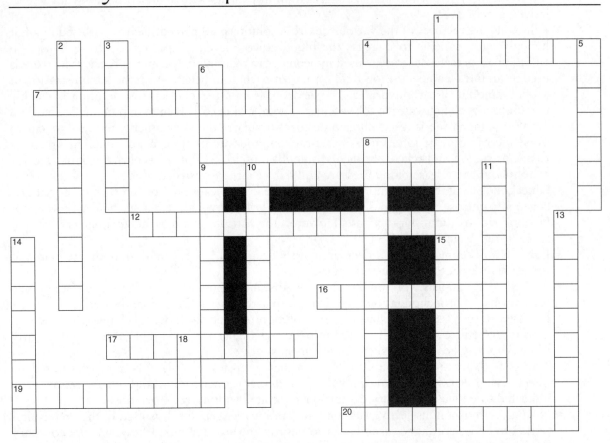

Across

4. Solution with an osmolarity that is higher than that of plasma.

7. Substance that imitates the effects of epinephrine and norepinephrine in the body.

9. Indication for 1:1,000 epinephrine.

12. Condition in which lactated Ringers solution is contraindicated.

16. It is indicated to reverse respiratory depression from narcotic overdose.

17. Aspirin is given to prevent aggregation of these.

19. Beta₂ selective bronchodilator administered by nebulizer or metered-dose inhaler.

20. Reason a medication would be given for treatment.

Down

1. This is given in a concentration of 50 percent to treat hypoglycemia in adults.

2. Solution that contains small particles, such as electrolytes or dextrose.

3. Acetylsalicylic acid.

5. Solution that contains large protein molecules.

6. 0.9 percent sodium chloride solution.

8. Therapeutic effect of nitroglycerin.

10. You must complete a thorough one of these before giving any drug.

11. Medication that provides pain relief.

13. NSAID that is used as an antipyretic in adults and children.

14. What can happen when too much IV fluid is given.

15. Solution with an osmolarity that is in the same range as that of plasma.

18. IV rate of 30 mL/hour.

Check Your Recall and Apply Concepts

Exercise 1

Complete each of the drug profiles in the following charts.

Activated Charcoal

Class	
Mechanism of Action	
Indications	
Contraindications	
Dosage and Administration	
Precautions	
Side Effects	

Albuterol

Class	
Mechanism of Action	
Indications	
Contraindications	
Dosage and Administration	
Precautions	
Side Effects	

Aspirin

Class	
Mechanism of Action	
Indications	
Contraindications	
Dosage and Administration	
Precautions	
Side Effects	

50 Percent Dextrose

Class	
Mechanism of Action	
Indications	
Contraindications	
Dosage and Administration	
Precautions	
Side Effects	

Epinephrine 1:1,000

Class	
Mechanism of Action	
Indications	
Contraindications	
Dosage and Administration	
Precautions	
Side Effects	

Glucagon

Class	
Mechanism of Action	
Indications	
Contraindications	
Dosage and Administration	
Precautions	
Side Effects	

Lactated Ringer's Solution for Intravenous Infusion

Class	
Mechanism of Action	
Indications	
Contraindications	
Dosage and Administration	
Precautions	
Side Effects	

Naloxone

Class	
Mechanism of Action	
Indications	
Contraindications	
Dosage and Administration	
Precautions	
Side Effects	

Nitroglycerin (for Sublingual Administration)

Class	
Mechanism of Action	
Indications	
Contraindications	
Dosage and Administration	
Precautions	
Side Effects	

Nitrous Oxide

Class	
Mechanism of Action	
Indications	
Contraindications	
Dosage and Administration	
Precautions	
Side Effects	

Normal Saline (0.9 Percent NaCl for Intravenous Infusion)

Class	
Mechanism of Action	
Indications	
Contraindications	
Dosage and Administration	
Precautions	
Side Effects	

Exercise 2

Select the best possible choice for each of the following questions.

_____ 1. In which one of the following conditions must you use extreme caution when administering normal saline by intravenous infusion?
   a. Heart failure
   b. Burns
   c. Hemorrhagic shock
   d. Diabetic ketoacidosis

_____ 2. Lactated Ringer's solution is considered to be what kind of an intravenous fluid?
   a. Crystalloid
   b. Hypertonic
   c. Colloid
   d. Hypotonic

_____ 3. Normal saline contains_____ percent sodium chloride.
   a. 0.45
   b. 0.9
   c. 4.5
   d. 9

_____ 4. Lactated Ringer's solution is contraindicated in patients with known or suspected:
   a. diabetic ketoacidosis.
   b. hypovolemia.
   c. hyperkalemia.
   d. dehydration.

_____ 5. Which one of the following is the reason aspirin is given to patients with chest pain suspected of cardiac origin?
   a. It reduces coronary artery inflammation.
   b. It is an analgesic.
   c. It prevents platelets from clumping together.
   d. It treats the fever that can accompany acute coronary syndrome.

_____ 6. Albuterol acts primarily on which one of the following types of cellular receptors?
   a. Alpha$_1$ sympathetic
   b. Parasympathetic postganglionic
   c. Beta$_1$ sympathetic
   d. Beta$_2$ sympathetic

_____ 7. For which one of the following signs is albuterol indicated?
   a. Wheezing
   b. Chest pain
   c. Palpitations
   d. Respiratory depression

_____ 8. The amount of a single dosage of sublingual nitroglycerin is:
   a. 0.04 mg.   c. 0.4 mg.
   b. 40 mcg.   d. 0.4 mcg.

_____ 9. An amount of 25 mL of 50 percent dextrose contains_____ of dextrose.
   a. 12.5 g   c. 25 g
   b. 12.5 mg   d. 25 mg

_____10. An acceptable adult dose of epinephrine 1:1,000, IM is:
   a. 0.04 mg.   c. 0.4 mg.
   b. 40 mcg.   d. 0.4 mcg.

_____11. Which one of the following is an expected side effect of epinephrine?
   a. Wheezing   c. Loss of bowel control
   b. Paralysis   d. Tachycardia

_____12. In which one of the following conditions would you anticipate that glucagon might not
          be effective in increasing the blood glucose level?
   a. Cirrhosis of the liver   c. Aspirin overdose
   b. Type 2 diabetes   d. Obesity

_____13. The typical dose for naloxone to treat respiratory depression caused by narcotic
          overdose is:
   a. 1 to 2 mg.   c. 1 to 2 mcg.
   b. 2 to 4 mg.   d. 2 to 4 mcg.

_____14. A patient has never taken nitroglycerin before. You should let him know
          that_____ is a common side effect.
   a. cardiac arrest   c. anxiety
   b. diarrhea   d. headache

_____15. A contraindication to administration of nitroglycerin is the use of drugs
          for_____ in the past 24 to 48 hours.
   a. acne   c. psoriasis
   b. erectile dysfunction   d. irritable bowel syndrome

Clinical Reasoning

CASE STUDY: MEDICATION MYSTERY

You and your partner, Greg, are on the scene for an elderly man who is complaining of weakness and near syncope. He has a long list of medications. The medications include Cardura, Proscar, Tambocor, Zocor, and Zithromax.

1. How can you find out some basic information about the patient's medications?

   _____

   _____

   _____

   _____

2. What is each of the medications used for and how can it contribute to understanding the patient's medical history?

   _____

   _____

   _____

   _____

3. How could the patient's medications explain his complaints?

   _____

   _____

   _____

   _____

Project-Based Learning

Keep a list of medications that you hear about in your clinical rotations. Select the 10 most common drugs and create index cards to help you learn about them. Write the drug name on one side of the card and basic information about its profile on the other side. Compare your list with a classmate's list to see if your experience with patient prescription medications is similar or different.

The EMS Professional in Practice

While writing down a patient's list of medications, you notice that he has prescriptions from three different physicians that have been filled at two different pharmacies. Why is the situation of concern? Should you say anything to the patient about it? If so, what would you say? Jot down your thoughts in a notebook or journal for discussion in class or in your study group.

14

General Approach to Patient Assessment and Clinical Reasoning

Content Area

• Assessment

Advanced EMT Education Standard

• Applies scene information and patient assessment findings (scene size-up, primary and secondary assessment, patient history, and reassessment) to guide emergency management.

Summary of Objectives

14.1 Define key terms introduced in this chapter.

Knowing and being able to apply the key terms in each chapter is critical to understanding chapter concepts. Write the list of key terms. Then write the definition of each one in your own words. Check your understanding by confirming the definitions in the textbook glossary. Correct any misunderstandings. Create a study aid by writing each key term on the front of an index card and the definition on the back. Use the cards to quiz yourself or to have someone quiz you. The exercises under Vocabulary and Concept Review below will give you additional practice.

14.2 Describe the purpose and goals of patient assessment.

Patient assessment begins with dispatch and continues through arrival at the scene, first contact with the patient, patient care, and patient transport, until patient care is transferred, either on the scene or at the hospital. Other EMS providers and hospital personnel rely on the information, because the Advanced EMT has a unique opportunity to observe the patient's environment and collect clues that can be utilized to decide on mechanism of injury or clinical impressions. The goals in the patient assessment process include answering the following questions:

• Is it safe to approach the patient and begin care in the patient's current location? If not, what must you to do solve this problem?
• What is the nature of the patient's problem?
• How sick is the patient?

- Which interventions, resources, and actions are required immediately?
- Which health care facility can best meet the patient's immediate needs?
- How should you transport the patient to receive that care?
- What do you need to do to support the patient's vital functions from the time you arrive at the scene to the time you transfer the patient care to other health care personnel?
- Is the patient's condition stable, improving, or worsening?

14.3   Describe the components of the patient assessment process.

There are four components to the assessment:

- Scene size-up, in which you look for health and safety hazards, determine the nature of the problem, recognize the need for additional resources, determine the total number of patients, form a general impression, and obtain a chief complaint.
- Primary assessment, in which you assess and, if needed, begin management of the patient's airway, breathing, and circulation.
- Secondary assessment, in which you obtain a medical history and vital signs and perform a physical examination.
- Reassessment, in which you compare the patient's baseline condition with subsequent findings and determine the effects of treatment.

14.4   Discuss the decisions that must be made during the patient assessment process.

You must decide whether additional resources are needed, whether the nature of the problem is medical or trauma, if the patient's condition is critical or noncritical, what interventions and additional information are needed, and how, when, and where you should transport the patient.

14.5   Explain the importance of both a systematic approach and adaptability in patient assessment.

A systematic approach gives the advantage of providing structure so that steps are not omitted. However, you must obtain flexibility to adapt the components of a systematic approach to each unique situation in order to efficiently obtain information that is relevant to the situation. This approach allows you to form hypotheses and test them to develop a short list of differential diagnoses. With experience, you will recognize presenting problems and diagnostic findings as they relate to previously encountered cases or patients, which can make you more efficient in determining the nature of the problem.

14.6   Explain the importance of various decision-making and problem-solving approaches in the patient assessment and patient care process.

Patient assessment is more than just a process of collecting information. You must analyze the information for meaning. Pattern recognition, rule-out-the-worst-case-scenario, hypothetico–deductive reasoning, and other problem-solving methods have advantages and disadvantages. You must be aware of the strengths and weaknesses of each approach and analyze your thinking to avoid pitfalls in clinical reasoning. Obtaining feedback is critical to the development of clinical reasoning and decision making. Clinical problem solving requires an adequate knowledge base of the facts and principles of anatomy, physiology, pathophysiology, and pharmacology.

Resource Central

Resource Central offers extra practice and review materials in a variety of media. To access it, follow the directions on the Student Access Card provided with the Student Textbook. If there is no card, go to www.bradybooks.com and follow the Resource Central link to Buy Access.

Vocabulary and Concept Review

Write the letter of the correct definition of each term in the blank next to the term. (See Resource Central for more vocabulary review.)

1. _____ assessment-based management

2. _____ baseline vital signs

3. _____ chief complaint

4. _____ clinical problem solving

5. _____ critical patient

6. _____ detailed physical examination

7. _____ field impression

8. _____ focused physical examination

9. _____ level of responsiveness

10. _____ mechanism of injury

11. _____ mental status

12. _____ noncritical patient

13. _____ obtunded

14. _____ patient assessment

15. _____ primary assessment

a. Engaging in a systematic reasoning process to identify and plan the treatment of a patient's medical problem

b. Patient's ability to detect and respond to environmental stimuli, such as sound and pain

c. Providing treatments on the basis of the patient's signs and symptoms, without a specific diagnosis of the problem

d. Careful, systematic examination of the body from head to toe

e. Determining the status of a patient's airway, breathing, and circulation

f. Degree to which a patient is aware of and able to respond to the environment, perform higher cognitive functions, and display appropriate emotions and behaviors

g. Initial set of vital signs obtained, which serves as a reference point to evaluate subsequent sets of vital signs

h. Process in which you obtain vital signs, a medical history, and perform a physical examination

i. Having a decreased level of awareness and ability to respond to stimuli

j. EMS provider's provisional diagnosis of a patient's medical problem upon which the medical treatment plan is based

k. Patient's statement of the reason he is seeking medical attention

l. Means by which energy, often mechanical forces, are transmitted to the body, producing the potential for trauma

m. Re-evaluating previous components of the patient assessment process to identify trends in the patient's condition and response to treatments provided

n. Patient who requires or is on the verge of requiring immediate, lifesaving medical attention

o. Systematic process of collecting relevant patient information in order to determine a patient's medical condition and establish priorities for treatment and transport

(continued on the next page)

16. _____ rapid physical examination

p. Quick physical examination performed on critical medical or trauma patients to identify potentially life-threatening conditions not found in the primary assessment

17. _____ reassessment

q. Physical examination that is limited to the anatomical area or body system that is the source of the patient's chief complaint

18. _____ scene size-up

r. Evaluating the setting in which a patient is found for the purposes of obtaining information about operational and clinical aspects of the emergency call

19. _____ secondary assessment

s. Patient who requires medical attention, but who does not have an immediate threat to life or limb

Patient Assessment Review

Scene Size-Up
- Operational aspects: Identify hazards, number of patients, and need for additional resources.
- Clinical aspects: Determine nature of illness/mechanism of injury; and general appearance, including age, sex, and whether the patient is responsive or apparently unresponsive.

Primary Assessment
- Apparently unresponsive: Quickly confirm level of responsiveness and determine presence or absence of breathing.
- Unresponsive and not breathing: Check pulse.
- No pulse: Start chest compressions.
- Pulse: Check for problems with airway, breathing, and circulation.
- Responsive: Confirm level of responsiveness; check for problems with airway, breathing, and circulation; and determine chief complaint.
- Perform interventions for airway, breathing, and circulation and determine whether patient is critical or noncritical.

Secondary Assessment
- Critical medical patient: Obtain history as available, perform rapid medical examination, obtain baseline vitals and use monitoring devices, and perform head-to-toe examination as needed.
- Critical trauma patient: Perform rapid trauma examination, obtain baseline vitals and use monitoring devices, perform head-to-toe examination, and obtain history as available.
- Noncritical medical patient: Obtain history, perform focused physical examination, and obtain baseline vitals and use monitoring devices.
- Noncritical trauma patient: Perform focused physical examination, obtain baseline vitals and use monitoring devices, and obtain history.

Reassessment
- Primary assessment (level of responsiveness, airway, breathing, and circulation)
- Vital signs and monitoring devices
- Aspects of physical examination
- Changes in complaints
- Specific effects of treatment

Check Your Recall and Apply Concepts

Select the best possible choice to answer the following questions.

_____ 1. Looking for clues about the scene to ensure that it is safe for responders to approach is performed in the:
   a. scene size-up.
   b. primary assessment.
   c. secondary assessment.
   d. reassessment.

_____ 2. You verify that the patient has an adequate airway, is breathing efficiently, and has adequate circulation. What else should you have already determined in the primary assessment?
   a. Vital signs
   b. Noncritical treatments
   c. Level of responsiveness
   d. Medical history

_____ 3. Which one of the following criteria should lead a patient to be classified as critical?
   a. Open airway
   b. Alert
   c. Appears to be in pain
   d. Severe difficulty breathing

_____ 4. Which one of the following patient conditions meets the National Trauma Triage Protocol criteria for requiring transport to a trauma center?
   a. Head laceration
   b. Adult who fell 12 feet
   c. Ejection from a motor vehicle
   d. Stab wound to the hand

_____ 5. Which one of the following is part of the primary assessment?
   a. Obtaining a medical history
   b. Baseline vital signs
   c. Determining transport priority
   d. Focused physical examination

_____ 6. What problem-solving approach are you using when you use repetitive process of identifying potential problems, collecting data about them, and creating a list of differential diagnoses?
   a. Pattern recognition
   b. Search satisficing
   c. Heuristics
   d. Hypothetico-deductive reasoning

_____ 7. You should assess a critical patient every _____ minutes or more frequently.
   a. 5
   b. 10
   c. 15
   d. 20

Clinical Reasoning

CASE STUDY: BREAKFAST AT GARCIA'S DINER

You and your partner have finished getting your gear together and checking your vehicle. Now, it is time for a critical decision: where to have breakfast. You agree on one of your favorites, Garcia's Diner. Shortly after ordering, you hear a commotion from the kitchen. The waitress, Christina, rushes out and tells you one of the cooks is choking. In the kitchen you find a middle-aged man on the floor, grabbing his throat and gasping for air. He is unable to talk or cough and is his lips are beginning to turn blue.

1. What do you need to find out from the scene size-up?

_____

_____

_____

_____

_____

2. What have you learned so far about the primary assessment of the patient?

_____

_____

_____

_____

3. At what point should you begin the secondary assessment?

_____

_____

_____

_____

Project-Based Learning

Create a poster that depicts the steps of patient assessment. For each step, outline the goals that you must accomplish.

The EMS Professional In Practice

What kind of preparation will make you more confident in your patient assessment abilities? What actions can you take to increase patients' confidence and trust in you and the decisions you make? Jot down your thoughts in a notebook or journal for discussion in class or in your study group.

15

Scene Size-Up and Primary Assessment

Content Area

- Assessment

Advanced EMT Education Standard

- Applies scene information and patient assessment findings (scene size-up, primary and secondary assessments, patient history, and reassessment) to guide emergency management.

Summary of Objectives

15.1   Define key terms introduced in this chapter.

Knowing and being able to apply the key terms in each chapter is critical to understanding chapter concepts. Write the list of key terms. Then write the definition of each one in your own words. Check your understanding by confirming the definitions in the textbook glossary. Correct any misunderstandings. Create a study aid by writing each key term on the front of an index card and the definition on the back. Use the cards to quiz yourself or to have someone quiz you. The exercises under Vocabulary and Concept Review below will give you additional practice.

15.2   Use information from the scene size-up and initial approach to the patient to formulate a general impression of the nature and seriousness of the patient's condition.

You can assimilate much information before making contact with the patient. Clues found on and around the patient can give you information about the events that preceded the need to call. Develop a general impression from the patient's general appearance and chief complaint or presenting problem.

15.3   Use the primary assessment findings to identify immediate threats to life.

The steps of primary assessment are ABCD, which stand for airway, breathing, circulation, and disability (level of responsiveness). Any problem with airway, breathing, circulation, or level of responsiveness represents a potential threat to life and you must correct it immediately.

15.4   Accurately assess a patient's level of responsiveness using the AVPU approach.

A patient whose eyes are purposefully open and who is aware of the environment around him, including your approach, is alert (A). If the patient's eyes are closed or he seems unaware of your presence, speak to him. If he reacts to your voice by opening his eyes, he is responsive to verbal stimuli (V). If he remains unaware, there are a variety of techniques to apply a light, painful pressure to the patient. Should one of those arouse the patient, he is responsive to painful stimuli (P). If he remains nonarousable despite those efforts, he is unresponsive (U).

15.5   Determine whether a patient's airway is patent.

Absence of air movement or presence of abnormal sounds, such as snoring or gurgling, mean the airway is not patent. If the airway is not patent, begin with manual positioning, suctioning, and simple adjuncts to provide an airway.

15.6   Differentiate between adequate and inadequate breathing.

Patients with normal respiratory effort, normal respiratory rate and quality, no abnormal respiratory noises, and no evidence of hypoxia or respiratory distress have adequate breathing. Inadequate breathing is identified by increased work of breathing, signs of hypoxia (such as altered mental status and cyanosis), abnormal respiratory rate and quality, abnormal respiratory noises, and indications of respiratory distress.

15.7   Determine whether a patient has adequate circulation.

Signs of adequate circulation are normal mental status, warm, dry skin with good color, and a strong, regular pulse with a normal heart rate. Signs of inadequate circulation include altered mental status, significant hemorrhage, pale, cool, sweaty skin, and an absent, slow, irregular, weak, or abnormally fast pulse.

15.8   Integrate the use of manual airway maneuvers, simple airway adjuncts, bag-valve-mask ventilations, supplemental oxygen, CPR, defibrillation, and bleeding control into the primary assessment.

See the skill checklists at the end of this workbook chapter.

15.9   Use the primary assessment findings to re-evaluate the general impression and determine the priority for patient transport.

The initial primary assessment findings serve as a baseline from which to track improvement or deterioration in the patient's condition. The priority for transport can change based on reassessment findings. Reassess patients in critical condition every 5 minutes or more frequently, and reassess patients in non-critical condition every 15 minutes or more frequently.

15.10   Use primary assessment findings to make a decision about the next step in the assessment and management of the patient.

Assessment is a process that evolves from one step to the next, based on your findings. At the completion of the primary assessment, you will have made an initial determination of whether the problem is medical or trauma, and whether the patient's condition is critical or noncritical. Those determinations set the priority for transport and the approach to the secondary assessment.

15.11   Describe the processes of gaining and maintaining control of the scene, teamwork, and reducing the patient's anxiety in preparation for obtaining the history and assessing the patient.

Be calm and confident, taking the time to make observations about the scene and patient. Professionalism and good communication help calm the patient and bystanders and evoke the confidence and cooperation of the team.

Resource Central

Resource Central offers extra practice and review materials in a variety of media. To access it, follow the directions on the Student Access Card provided with the Student Textbook. If there is no card, go to www.bradybooks.com and follow the Resource Central link to Buy Access.

Vocabulary and Concept Review

Exercise 1

Write the letter of the correct definition in the blank. (See Resource Central for more vocabulary review.)

1. _____ agonal respirations

2. _____ apnea

3. _____ bag-valve-mask device

4. _____ blunt force injury

5. _____ cyanosis

6. _____ dyspnea

7. _____ jaundice

8. _____ pallor

9. _____ penetrating trauma

10. _____ rales

11. _____ respiratory distress

12. _____ respiratory failure

13. _____ stridor

14. _____ tidal volume

15. _____ wheezing

a. Trauma caused by mechanisms of injury that do not enter the body cavity

b. Amount of air in a normal exhalation following a normal inspiration

c. Crackling noise heard in the lower airways when fluid is present

d. Ineffective, irregular, gasping attempts at breathing

e. Yellow discoloration of the tissues that may occur in liver disease

f. Manual piece of equipment that delivers artificial ventilations

g. High-pitched inspiratory sound that indicates partial upper airway obstruction

h. Injuries caused by an object that pierces the body tissues

i. Absence of breathing

j. High-pitched musical or whistling sound caused by constriction of the bronchioles

k. Inability to maintain adequate ventilation and oxygenation

l. Difficulty breathing, with increased effort to maintain adequate ventilation and oxygenation

m. Pale skin

n. Dusky blue-purple discoloration of the tissues that occurs as a result of hypoxia

o. Difficulty breathing

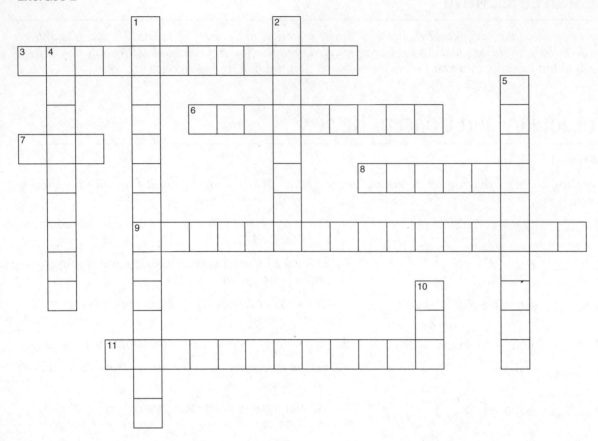

Across

3. Manual device used to deliver positive pressure ventilations.

6. Refers to the higher mental abilities, such as reasoning and problem solving.

7. Device that analyzes the cardiac rhythm in unresponsive, pulseless patients and delivers an electrical shock, if indicated.

8. Paleness of the skin.

9. A patient should be situated like this if he is breathing spontaneously but is at risk for aspirating secretions in the airway.

11. Patient's level of responsiveness and level of cognitive function.

Down

1. Type of simple airway adjunct inserted through the nares and into the throat to provide a channel for air movement through the upper airway.

2. Yellowish discoloration of the skin, often due to liver disease.

4. Muscles in the neck and abdomen that are not used in normal breathing, but are used to assist breathing in respiratory distress.

5. Wide band placed circumferentially around an extremity to compress the blood vessels and control severe hemorrhage.

10. Scale used to assess the level of responsiveness.

Patient Assessment Review

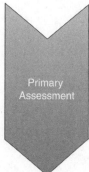

Primary Assessment

- Apparently unresponsive: Quickly confirm level of responsiveness and determine presence or absence of breathing.
- Unresponsive and not breathing: Check pulse.
- No pulse: Start chest compressions.
- Pulse: Check for problems with airway, breathing, and circulation.
- Responsive: Confirm level of responsiveness; check for problems with airway, breathing, and circulation; and determine chief complaint.
- Perform interventions for airway, breathing, and circulation, and determine whether patient is critical or noncritical.

Check Your Recall and Apply Concepts

Select the best possible choice for each of the following questions.

_____ 1. The scene size-up should include looking for indications of scene safety, the number of patients involved, and:
- a. sources of bleeding.
- b. the general nature of the incident.
- c. whether the patient needs transport to the hospital.
- d. signs of inadequate breathing.

_____ 2. The type and amount of energy that a patient was subjected to is known as the _____ of injury.
- a. mechanism
- b. kinetics
- c. force
- d. vector

_____ 3. If your patient is suspected of having a cervical-spine injury, what manual airway maneuver is preferred?
- a. Head-tilt/chin-lift
- b. Recovery position
- c. Modified jaw thrust
- d. Triple airway maneuver

_____ 4. The "D" in the mnemonic ABCD prompts you to check the patient's:
- a. respirations.
- b. level of responsiveness.
- c. pulse.
- d. chief complaint.

_____ 5. Which one of the following are you likely to see when a patient is having difficulty breathing?
- a. Use of neck and abdominal muscles to assist breathing
- b. Patient lying in a supine position
- c. Respiratory rate greater than 12 but less than 20 per minute
- d. Pink, warm, dry skin

_____ 6. A patient with a gunshot wound to his posterior thigh has lost a large amount of blood, and blood loss is continuing. The patient is pale with cool, sweaty skin and a decreased level of responsiveness. You cannot control the bleeding with direct pressure. Which one of the following should you attempt next to control bleeding?
- a. Elevate the extremity.
- b. Irrigate the wound with water or sterile saline.
- c. Apply a tourniquet.
- d. Apply a pressure bandage.

_____ 7. The primary assessment involves looking for information about:
   a. all possible signs and symptoms of illness or injury.
   b. the patient's baseline vital signs.
   c. the patient's past medical history.
   d. immediate threats to life.

_____ 8. Kinetic energy refers to the energy associated with:
   a. movement.   c. chemical bonds.
   b. electricity.   d. heat.

_____ 9. It is best to think of scene size-up as an assessment step that:
   a. is completed before the primary assessment begins.
   b. continues throughout the call.
   c. is performed only when there is a risk of danger to you and your partner.
   d. is useful on trauma calls, but not on medical calls.

_____ 10. You approach a patient who is cyanotic and seems to be unresponsive. He has irregular, gasping respirations. Which one of the following steps should you perform next?
   a. Apply an AED.
   b. Begin ventilations with a bag-valve-mask device.
   c. Open the airway.
   d. Check the carotid pulse.

_____ 11. You are approaching a patient who has normal skin color and who appears to be unresponsive. You can hear regular, snoring respirations that are about 7 to 8 seconds apart. Which of the following steps should you perform next?
   a. Obtain a pulse oximetry reading.   c. Check the carotid pulse.
   b. Open the airway.   d. Apply oxygen by nonrebreather mask.

_____ 12. A patient has her eyes closed and does not respond when you speak to her. When you pinch her trapezius muscle, she flinches and moans. Using the AVPU scale, her level of responsiveness is best described as:
   a. alert.   c. responds to painful stimulus.
   b. responds to verbal stimulus. d. unresponsive.

_____ 13. A patient who does not respond to verbal or painful stimuli would receive a score of _____ on the Glasgow Coma Scale.
   a. 0   c. 5
   b. 3   d. 7

_____ 14. You approach an unresponsive patient who has suffered a gunshot wound to the head. You hear gurgling as he attempts to breathe. The gurgling noise should indicate to you that you must immediately:
   a. place an advanced airway.   c. suction the airway.
   b. elevate the patient's head.   d. place a basic airway adjunct.

Clinical Reasoning

CASE STUDY: THE EVENING NEWS

You, your partner, Kent, and an Advanced EMT student named McKenzie are discussing whether to go to the sandwich shop to get grinders for dinner or get take-out from a salad buffet when you are dispatched to a television studio for an unresponsive person. When you arrive at the back entrance of the studio, an employee lets you in and directs you to one of the news sets, where you see a well-known news anchor collapsed on the floor behind the news desk. He is the only patient and there are no indications of hazards. A co-anchor has placed the patient on his side.

1. What should you look for as you observe the patient?

   _____

   _____

   _____

   _____

2. What directions should you give the team?

   _____

   _____

   _____

   _____

3. What questions should you ask of bystanders?

   _____

   _____

   _____

   _____

The patient appears to be in his late 40s. He is pale and has labored, shallow, rapid breathing. The co-anchor tells you they were preparing for the 6:00 PM newscast when the patient, Dick Winston, grasped his chest and became short of breath. Mr. Winston was weak and unable to sit in his chair, so bystanders helped him to the floor. When McKenzie places her hand on Mr. Winston's shoulder and asks if he can hear her, he opens his eyes, but does not speak. Kent reports a weak, rapid radial pulse and cool, diaphoretic skin.

4. How does the primary assessment inform your initial decision making about the situation?

   _____

   _____

   _____

   _____

5. What are your next actions?

   _____

   _____

   _____

   _____

   _____

Project-Based Learning

Construct a table to compare and contrast the primary assessment approach for adult patients and pediatric patients. Include things such as determining level of responsiveness; assessing the airway, breathing, and circulation; and 9 determining interventions that might be needed. Identify what features are the same (compare) and what features are different (contrast) for each step of the assessment.

The EMS Professional In Practice

The assessment approach that is appropriate to the first patient of the day may not be the one that is best for last patient of the day. The principles remain the same, but you must adapt the way you achieve the principles to each situation. How might your approach to primary assessment change depending on circumstances? What details inform your decisions about how to approach primary assessment? Jot down your thoughts in a notebook or journal for discussion in class or in your study group.

Skills Checklists

The following skill checklists cover the major steps of selected skills from Chapter 15. Review them prior to your laboratory classes. Practice skills only after they have been demonstrated for you in class and only under the supervision of an authorized instructor or clinical preceptor.

Advanced EMT Skill Checklist: *Primary Assessment—Responsive Patient*		
Skill Stimulus: Scene size-up reveals a patient who is responsive.		
Step	Performed	Not Performed
Confirm level of responsiveness using AVPU.		
Observe for problems with the airway, such as indications of partial or complete obstruction.		
Intervene to establish and protect the airway as needed.		
Observe for problems with breathing, such as increased effort, tripod position, abnormal noises, accessory muscle use, or cyanosis.		
Intervene to ensure adequate ventilation as needed.		
Observe for problems with circulation, such as external bleeding, pale or mottled skin, weak, absent, irregular pulse, or abnormal pulse rate.		
Intervene to correct problems with circulation, such as controlling external hemorrhage.		
Determine whether patient is critical (decreased level of responsiveness or problems with airway, breathing, or circulation) or noncritical.		
If not already established in the scene size-up, obtain the chief complaint.		
Skill Completion: AVPU determined and all immediately life-threatening problems with the airway, breathing, and circulation have been identified and corrected and a determination of the transport priority (critical or noncritical) has been made.		

Advanced EMT Skill Checklist: *Primary Assessment, Apparently Unresponsive Patient*

Skill Stimulus: Scene size-up reveals a patient who appears to be unresponsive (patient is critical).

Step	Performed	Not Performed
Quickly confirm level of responsiveness.		
Quickly determine presence or absence of normal breathing.		
If patient is unresponsive and does not have normal breathing, check the carotid pulse for no more than 10 seconds.		
If the patient is pulseless, begin chest compressions.		
If the patient has a pulse, check the airway for signs of obstruction (abnormal noises, lack of air movement)		
Intervene as needed (positioning, manual maneuvers, basic airway adjuncts, suction) to establish and maintain the airway.		
Observe for problems with breathing (shallow, abnormal rate, increased effort, cyanosis).		
Intervene as needed to ensure adequate ventilation (bag-valve-mask ventilations).		
Observe for problems with circulation such as external bleeding; pale or mottled skin; weak, absent, irregular pulse; or abnormal pulse rate.		
Intervene to correct problems with circulation, such as controlling external hemorrhage.		
Skill Completion: Level of responsiveness confirmed and all immediately life-threatening problems with the airway, breathing, and circulation have been identified and corrected.		

16

Airway Management, Ventilation, and Oxygenation

Content Area

- Airway Management, Respiration, and Artificial Ventilation

Advanced EMT Education Standard

- Applies knowledge of upper airway anatomy and physiology to patient assessment and management in order to ensure a patent airway, adequate mechanical ventilation, and respiration for patients of all ages.

Summary of Objectives

16.1   Define the key terms introduced in this chapter.

Knowing and being able to apply the key terms in each chapter is critical to understanding chapter concepts. Write the list of key terms. Then write the definition of each one in your own words. Check your understanding by confirming the definitions in the textbook glossary. Correct any misunderstandings. Create a study aid by writing each key term on the front of an index card and the definition on the back. Use the cards to quiz yourself or to have someone quiz you. The exercises under Vocabulary and Concept Review below will give you additional practice.

16.2   Relate the anatomy and physiology of the respiratory system to oxygenation, perfusion, and removal of carbon dioxide.

Perfusion is the circulation of blood to the cellular level to provide the oxygen and nutrients that support cellular energy metabolism and to remove the waste products of metabolism. The respiratory system provides the required oxygen and removes carbon dioxide through the process ventilation. Ventilation is the mechanical process of moving air in and out of the lungs by way of the upper airway, which begins with the mouth and nose. Ventilation is controlled by the response of the nervous system to levels of oxygen and carbon dioxide. Increased levels of oxygen (and secondarily, decreased levels of oxygen) stimulate the process of inspiration. Inspiration begins when the intercostal muscles and diaphragm contract, increasing the intrathoracic volume, which leads to a decrease in intrathoracic and intrapulmonary pressures. Air moves from the higher pressure of the atmosphere to the lower pressure in the lungs. Once the lungs have expanded to a certain degree, a reflex mediated by the nervous system causes the diaphragm and intercostal muscles to relax, which decreases the intrathoracic volume and increases the intrathoracic pressure. Air moves from the higher pressure in the lungs to the lower pressure of the atmosphere. While the air is in the alveoli of the lungs, oxygen crosses the respiratory membrane to be carried to the cells by binding to hemoglobin within red blood cells and carbon dioxide diffuses across the respiratory membrane in the opposite direction so that it can be exhaled. The process of gas exchange in the lungs is called external respiration. When oxygenated blood reaches the cellular level, oxygen dissociates from hemoglobin and diffuses into the cell and the carbon dioxide produced by metabolism diffuses into the blood for transport. The process of gas exchange at the cellular level is called internal respiration.

16.3 Give examples of complaints and conditions that are associated with the risk of hypoxia and hypoventilation.

Any patient complaining of difficulty breathing is at risk for hypoventilation and hypoxia. Patients with airway obstruction (foreign bodies, swelling, trauma, bleeding in the airway), neurologic problems (altered mental status, paralysis, traumatic brain injury, stroke, drug overdose), respiratory complaints (coughing, wheezing, congestion, shortness of breath, chest pain), or injuries to the airway or chest (pneumothorax, rib fractures) are at risk for hypoventilation and hypoxia.

16.4 Relate findings from the assessment of the airway and ventilation to the patient's need for interventions in airway, oxygenation, and ventilation.

Every patient receives an evaluation of airway, ventilation, and oxygenation in the scene size-up and primary assessment. The goal of this assessment is to rapidly identify life-threatening problems and correct them immediately. Indications of a problem with airway, breathing, or oxygenation include altered mental status (anxiety, confusion, combativeness, decreased responsiveness, unresponsiveness, cyanosis), increased effort to breathe, use of the accessory muscles of breathing, abnormal breath sounds (stridor, coughing, wheezing, crackles [rales], rhonchi), tripod position, decreased chest wall movement or air movement, and cyanosis.

Provide oxygen by face mask or nasal cannula to patients at risk for hypoxia who are breathing adequately. Assist ventilations with a bag-valve-mask device attached to supplemental oxygen for patients who are not breathing adequately. CPAP is an alternative for patients who require ventilatory assistance but who cannot tolerate assistance with a bag-valve-mask device.

16.5 Recognize signs and symptoms of mild, moderate, and severe hypoxia.

Hypoxia has clinical signs and symptoms and also can be indicated by pulse oximetry. SpO_2 from 91 to 94 percent indicates mild hypoxia, SpO_2 from 86 to 90 percent indicates moderate hypoxia, and SpO_2 at 85 percent or less indicates severe hypoxia. Mental status is a sensitive indicator of hypoxia. In mild hypoxia, patients may exhibit anxiety. As hypoxia progresses, the patient may become confused, agitated, hostile, lethargic, or unresponsive. In adults, tachypnea and tachycardia are indications of hypoxia. Children may exhibit bradycardia, rather than tachycardia.

16.6 Distinguish between adequate and inadequate breathing.

The primary assessment provides a gross indication of the presence and adequacy of breathing. Inadequate breathing is characterized by increased work of breathing, use of accessory muscles, noisy breathing, decreased or absent air movement or breath sounds, apnea, a ventilatory rate of less than 8 or greater than 30 per minute in an adult, irregular breathing, or cyanosis. Adequate breathing is characterized by ease of effort, regular rhythm, adequate depth, and normal rate.

16.7 Measure oxygenation by pulse oximetry.

Pulse oximetry uses infrared technology to assess the oxygen saturation of hemoglobin in the peripheral tissues. A noninvasive probe is placed on the finger, toe, or ear lobe, where a light is passed through peripheral capillaries. The device calculates saturation by measuring the amount of light that was absorbed. This reading is a percentage of hemoglobin saturated by oxygen.

16.8 Measure exhaled carbon dioxide by colorimetric capnometry and wave-form capnography.

Colorimetric devices are simple devices used to confirm placement of endotracheal tubes in patients with spontaneous circulation. Essentially, they measure if there is CO_2 in exhaled air. Waveform capnography is measured by way of a sampling port on the end of an LMA or endotracheal tube or by way of a simple mask or nasal cannula. The sample is processed and produces a numerical value as well as a waveform correlating to that numerical value as displayed on a graph.

16.9 Incorporate the values of pulse oximetry and capnometry into decisions regarding management of airway, breathing, and oxygenation.

As with any technology, you must rely upon a thorough patient assessment and good clinical judgment to assess the value of the information provided by capnometry and pulse oximetry. Treat hypoxia by administering supplemental oxygen and, if needed, assisting with ventilation. Treat hypercapnia by ensuring adequate ventilation.

16.10 Demonstrate the proper technique of auscultating breath sounds.

Listen first to one side and then move your stethoscope to the opposite side to compare sounds. Breath sounds should be equally present at each level on both sides. Begin auscultating high in the chest or back and work toward the bases. Listen for abnormal sounds such as wheezing, crackles (rales), and rhonchi.

16.11 Describe the causes of abnormal breathing sounds including decreased and absent breath sounds, gurgling, crackles (rales), rhonchi, snoring, stridor, and wheezing.

Decreased and absent breath sounds indicate hypoventilation. Decreased sounds may be due to minimal air movement (decreased tidal volume) because of asthma, respiratory depression, or respiratory failure from a variety of causes. Localized areas of absent or decreased sounds can be due to pneumonia, atelectasis, pneumothorax, or hemothorax.

Gurgling is most commonly caused by fluid accumulation in the upper airway of a patient who is breathing or being ventilated. If the patient is not capable of clearing his own airway, use positioning and suctioning to remove fluid from the airway.

Crackles (rales) are caused by fluid in the alveoli and smaller airways. The sound is similar to the fizzing sound that accompanies pouring a carbonated drink. Crackles (rales) indicate an increased diffusion distance for gases crossing the respiratory membrane. CPAP may be helpful in some cases of pulmonary edema resulting in crackles (rales).

Rhonchi are caused by an accumulation of fluid or mucus in larger airways in the lungs, which often occurs in pneumonia and bronchitis, but also can occur when pulmonary edema progresses beyond the smaller airways or in patients who have aspirated fluids (blood, emesis).

Snoring is a rumbling sound associated with tissue vibration caused by a partial obstruction of the upper airway by the tongue and soft tissues. Use manual airway maneuvers and basic adjuncts to relieve snoring.

Stridor is associated with significant partial obstruction of the upper airway, such as from edema or a foreign body. If obstruction is from swelling due to anaphylaxis, epinephrine may be indicated. The patient with stridor requires prompt transport or ALS response.

Wheezing is caused by constriction of the bronchioles, which may occur due to asthma, COPD, anaphylaxis, or inhalation of smoke or other irritants. Wheezing is typically heard on expiration, but in severe cases it also can be heard on inspiration. Depending on the cause, sympathetic beta$_2$ agonists can help reverse smooth muscle spasm in the bronchioles to improve airflow.

16.12   Identify the different presentations and needs of pediatric and geriatric patients with regard to airway, ventilation, and oxygenation.

Pediatric patients have relatively large tongues that can contribute to airway obstruction. The trachea is flexible and narrow, with its narrowest point at the cricoid cartilage. Those features allow the trachea to be easily obstructed. The large occiput of the pediatric head may cause hyperflexion of the neck and airway obstruction. A folded towel or thin blanket under the shoulders can assist in maintaining a neutral alignment of airway structures. The respiratory rate of pediatric patients is higher and the tidal volume is smaller, necessitating changes in ventilation techniques and equipment. Although it is now rare in children due to widespread haemophilus influenza B vaccination, epiglottitis is a bacterial infection that has long been considered a childhood illness.

Geriatric patients may suffer airway problems due to decreased cough and gag reflexes. Efficiency of ventilation and gas exchange decrease with age, making it more difficult for elderly patients to compensate when there is a need for increased ventilation. Lack of dentition or missing dentures can create difficulty in maintaining a seal with the mask of a bag-valve-mask device. Kyphosis can make positioning the airway difficult.

16.13   Take immediate action to correct impaired airway, breathing, and oxygenation.

Refer to the skill checklists at the end of this workbook chapter.

16.14   Utilize manual positioning and suction (portable and fixed devices) to keep the airway clear.

Refer to the skill checklists at the end of this workbook chapter. See Scans 16-1 and 16-2 in the textbook.

16.15   Given a variety of scenarios, select and insert an oropharyngeal or nasopharyngeal airway.

Refer to the skill checklists at the end of this workbook chapter. See Scans 16-3 and 16-4 in the textbook.

16.16   Given a variety of scenarios, select and insert an appropriate advanced airway device (Combitube or supraglottic airway).

Refer to the skill checklists at the end of this workbook chapter.

16.17   Administer supplemental oxygen via devices suited to individual patients' needs, including nasal cannula, nonrebreather mask, partial rebreather mask, simple face mask, tracheostomy mask, and Venturi mask.

Refer to the skill checklists at the end of this workbook chapter. See Scan 16-5 in the textbook.

16.18   Describe the concept of positive end expiratory pressure (PEEP).

At the end of normal expiration, the pressure in the airway is approximately equal to that of atmospheric pressure. PEEP mechanisms (such as CPAP or a mechanical ventilator) provide resistance to expiration, which maintains a slightly positive pressure in the airways at the end of expiration. PEEP can prevent atelectasis, reduce pulmonary edema, and decrease the work of breathing in severe respiratory distress.

16.19   Ventilate or assist the 9 ventilations of patients using the following devices, as appropriate to various situations: automatic transport ventilators, bag-valve-mask device, Combitube, continuous positive airway pressure (CPAP), laryngeal mask airway (LMA), manually triggered ventilation devices, mouth-to-mask, supraglottic airway devices, such as the King LTD or Cobra.

Refer to the skills checklists at the end of this workbook chapter for selected skills.

16.20 Employ appropriate safety precautions when handling, transporting, and administering oxygen.

Oxygen enhances combustion when exposed to fire. Avoid open flame or sparks when administering it. Medical oxygen is stored in pressurized metal cylinders. A crack or break in a pressurized metal cylinder can cause the cylinder to become a deadly missile. See Scan 16-5 in the text.

16.21 Properly utilize oxygen cylinders and regulators to ensure adequate patient oxygenation.

Specially designed regulators and flow meters are used to decrease the pressure of medical oxygen to a safe level for administration and to adjust the amount of oxygen being delivered. You must properly attach and secure the regulator flow meter for safe oxygen administration. See Scan 16-5 in the textbook.

16.22 Modify techniques of managing airway, ventilation, and oxygenation for the following situations: patients with abnormal facial structure and dental appliances, patients with facial trauma, patients with foreign body airway obstruction, patients with potential cervical-spine injuries, patients with stomas and tracheostomies, and pediatric and geriatric patients.

- *Patients with abnormal facial structure and dental appliances:* In general, dentures help provide structure to the face to allow a good seal between the mask and face. However, if dentures are loose, they may need to be removed.
- *Patients with facial trauma:* Instability of the face may make use of a bag-valve-mask device difficult. Consider using an advanced airway. Avoid using a nasopharyngeal airway in patients with trauma to the midface.
- *Patients with foreign body airway obstruction:* Use abdominal thrusts for patients with a pulse and chest thrusts for pulseless patients to relieve complete airway obstruction. Remove fluids with suction.
- *Patients with potential cervical-spine injuries:* Use the modified jaw-thrust maneuver to prevent hyperextension of the neck. Maintain inline manual stabilization of the head and neck and apply a cervical collar as soon as feasible, followed by restriction of spinal movement by immobilizing the patient to a long backboard.
- *Patients with stomas and tracheostomies:* Ventilate through a tracheostomy tube, if present. If there is no tracheostomy tube, place a ventilation mask over the stoma and ensure an adequate seal.
- *Pediatric and geriatric patients:* In pediatric patients, place the airway in a neutral position by padding under the shoulders. In geriatric patients with kyphosis, pad beneath the head.

16.23 Discuss the physiologic differences, including complications, of artificial ventilation.

The use of positive pressure, especially when excessive pressures are used, increases intrathoracic pressure, which impairs blood return to the heart, decreasing cardiac output. The problem is exacerbated in conditions in which blood pressure is decreased, such as in shock or during CPR. In a low perfusion state, such as shock or during CPR, any decrease in cardiac output is a serious problem. Excessive ventilation pressures may force air into the esophagus and stomach, leading to gastric distention. Gastric distention can interfere with ventilation and may result in regurgitation and aspiration of stomach contents. Excessive ventilation pressures can also lead to trauma to the trachea, bronchi, and lung parenchyma.

16.24 Suction the airway of an intubated patient.

Refer to the skill checklists at the end of this workbook chapter.

Resource Central

Resource Central offers extra practice and review materials in a variety of media. To access it, follow the directions on the Student Access Card provided with the Student Textbook. If there is no card, go to www.bradybooks.com and follow the Resource Central link to Buy Access.

Vocabulary and Concept Review

Exercise 1

Write a term from the following list to complete each sentence. (Visit Resource Central for more vocabulary practice.)

bronchoconstriction	tracheostomy	French (Fr.)	hypercapnea
capnography	hypoxia	laryngospasm	hypocapnea
capnometry	ventilation	Yankauer	spirometry
continuous positive flow rate	pulse oximetry	pulmonary edema	peak expiratory flow rate

1. Involuntary closure of the glottic opening is called _____.

2. Decreased oxygen at the cellular level is called _____.

3. The maximal rate at which air can be forcefully exhaled from the lungs, measured in liters per minute, is called the _____.

4. Increased interstitial fluid in the lungs that affects the respiratory membrane is called _____.

5. A surgical opening into the trachea to establish an airway is called a(n) _____.

6. Another name for a rigid suction tip is a(n) _____.

7. Narrowing of the bronchioles, such as by smooth muscle spasm, is called _____.

8. The term for measurement of carbon dioxide in exhaled air is called _____. When the measurement is represented as a waveform, it is called _____.

9. A unit of measure for diameter in which each unit is equal to 0.33 mm is called a(n) _____ unit.

10. An increased level of carbon dioxide in the blood is called _____, while a decreased level of carbon dioxide in the blood is called _____.

11. A mechanism that delivers an even level of increased air pressure to the upper airway through a mask sealed tightly to the face is called _____.

12. A mechanism used to measure the amount of hemoglobin that is bound to oxygen is called _____.

13. The process used to measure various lung volumes and flow rates is called _____.

14. The mechanical process of moving air into and out of the lungs is called _____.

Exercise 2

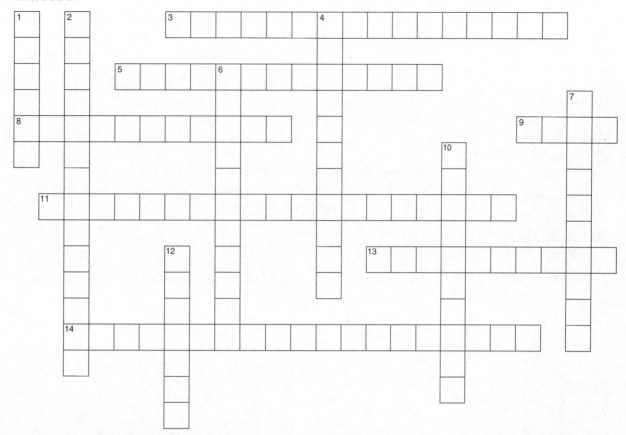

Across

3. Artificial ventilation by forcing air into the airway.

5. Airway adjunct inserted into the mouth to prevent the tongue from occluding the airway.

8. Measurement and graphic representation over time of the level of carbon dioxide in an exhaled air sample.

9. Device that delivers a constant level of air pressure to the airway through a mask sealed tightly on the face. Hint: Abbreviation.

11. Narrowing of a bronchiole passageway.

13. Decreased level of carbon dioxide in the blood.

14. Volume of air that actually reaches the alveoli each minute.

Down

1. Units of measure for the diameter of suction catheters.

2. Airway adjunct inserted through the nose to prevent the tongue from occluding the airway.

4. Movement of air into and out of the lungs.

6. Increased level of carbon dioxide in the blood.

7. Measurement of the level of carbon dioxide in an exhaled air sample.

10. Measurement of various lung volumes and flow rates.

12. Decreased level of oxygen at the cellular level.

Patient Assessment Review

Fill in the following patient assessment flowcharts to describe what steps you would take to manage the airway, ventilation, and oxygenation for each type of patient. Include the decisions you must make in the primary assessment of each patient.

Scenario 1

Scene Size-Up

- Operational aspects: Identify hazards, number of patients, and need for additional resources.
- Clinical aspects: Determine nature of illness/mechanism of injury; and general appearance including age, sex, and whether the patient is responsive or apparently unresponsive.

  Responsive Patient, No Obvious Distress.

Primary Assessment

Scenario 2

Scene Size-Up

- Operational aspects: Identify hazards, number of patients, and need for additional resources.
- Clinical aspects: Determine nature of illness/mechanism of injury and general appearance, including age, sex, and whether the patient is responsive or apparently unresponsive.
  Responsive Patient, Apparent Respiratory Distress.

Primary Assessment

Scenario 3

Scene Size-Up

- Operational aspects: Identify hazards, number of patients, and need for additional resources.
- Clinical aspects: Determine nature of illness/mechanism of injury and general appearance including age, sex, and whether the patient is responsive or apparently unresponsive.

  Apparent Decreased Level of Responsiveness, Breathing.

Primary Assessment

Scenario 4

Scene Size-Up

- Operational aspects: Identify hazards, number of patients, and need for additional resources.
- Clinical aspects: Determine nature of illness/mechanism of injury and general appearance, including age, sex, and whether the patient is responsive or apparently unresponsive.
  Apparently Unresponsive, Breathing.

Primary Assessment

Scenario 5

Scene Size-Up

- Operational aspects: Identify hazards, number of patients, and need for additional resources.
- Clinical aspects: Determine nature of illness/mechanism of injury and general appearance, including age, sex, and whether the patient is responsive or apparently unresponsive.
  Apparently Unresponsive, Not Breathing/Abnormal Breathing.

Primary Assessment

Check Your Recall and Apply Concepts

Select the best possible choice for each of the following questions.

_____ 1. Hypoxia is a condition in which there is _____ at the cellular level.
a. decreased carbon dioxide
b. decreased oxygen
c. increased carbon dioxide
d. increased oxygen

_____ 2. Which one of the following statements most accurately describes ventilation?
a. Gas exchange in the lungs
b. Transport of oxygen in the blood
c. Movement of air in and out of the lungs
d. Gas exchange at the cellular level

_____ 3. Which one of the following structures is part of the upper airway?
a. Nasopharynx
b. Carina
c. Respiratory membrane
d. Trachea

_____ 4. Which one of the following structures is part of the lower airway?
a. Hypopharynx
b. Oropharynx
c. Bronchi
d. Turbinates

_____ 5. Minute volume of ventilation is best defined as the:
a. amount of air that is not available to participate in gas exchange.
b. respiratory rate times tidal volume.
c. amount of air that reaches the alveoli with each breath.
d. maximum amount of air that can be inhaled and then exhaled in a single breath.

_____ 6. A patient who has a history of chronic obstructive pulmonary disease (COPD) presents in tripod position, but is barely aware of your presence. Despite increased respiratory effort, he is moving very little air. He has cyanosis of his lips and looks exhausted. You should identify this patient as suffering from:
a. apnea.
b. respiratory distress.
c. agonal respirations.
d. respiratory failure.

_____ 7. You were dispatched for a possible overdose and have just entered a residence where there is an adult patient lying supine in bed. You can hear him snoring loudly. He fails to respond when you shake his shoulder and loudly ask if he can hear you. The first action you should take is to:
a. perform a head-tilt/chin-lift maneuver.
b. perform a tongue-jaw lift.
c. insert a nasopharyngeal airway.
d. insert an oropharyngeal airway.

_____ 8. You have just entered a residence where a two-year-old child is being held by his mother. The child is anxious and you hear a high-pitched noise with each of his inspiratory efforts. The mother states that the child has not been sick but suddenly started having trouble breathing while playing on the floor. The most likely cause of the patient's problem is:
a. swelling of the lower airways.
b. complete airway obstruction by a foreign body.
c. partial obstruction of the upper airway by a foreign body.
d. upper airway edema.

_____ 9. You have just arrived on the scene of a reported sick person in a liquor store. There is a man lying on the floor. He is not moving and looks cyanotic. He is taking shallow, irregular, gasping breaths. The first thing you should do is:
a. check his pulse.
b. start chest compressions.
c. perform a head-tilt/chin-lift maneuver.
d. start bag-valve-mask ventilations.

_____ 10. You have just responded to a patient who has fallen from a second-story balcony onto the ground below. You hear him taking gurgling breaths as you approach and you can see blood in his nose and mouth. Which one of the following should you do first?
   a. Begin bag-valve-mask ventilations.   c. Apply a cervical collar.
   b. Perform oropharyngeal suctioning.   d. Insert an oropharyngeal airway.

_____ 11. Your patient is a 27-year-old man who was ejected from a vehicle in a high-speed crash. He is unresponsive and has massive head and facial injuries and some obviously fractured extremities. The patient cannot maintain his own airway and is breathing shallowly at 8 times per minute. You have performed a modified jaw-thrust maneuver, but it has not been effective in maintaining the patient's airway. The patient has a gag reflex and cannot tolerate an oropharyngeal airway. You should:
   a. insert a Combitube.
   b. insert a nasopharyngeal airway.
   c. perform a head-tilt/chin-lift maneuver.
   d. continue with the modified jaw-thrust maneuver.

_____ 12. The approximate tidal volume for an average, 70-kg adult is _____ mL.
   a. 350   c. 750
   b. 500   d. 1000

_____ 13. You have performed several abdominal thrusts on an adult patient who is choking on some food when he becomes unresponsive. The next thing you should do is:
   a. place the patient in a supine position and continue abdominal thrusts.
   b. check the carotid pulse.
   c. perform a finger sweep in an attempt to dislodge the food.
   d. place the patient in a supine position and perform chest compressions, just as you would for a patient in cardiac arrest.

_____ 14. You have performed several abdominal thrusts on a four-year-old child who is choking on a piece of hot dog when he becomes unresponsive. The first thing you should do is:
   a. place the patient in a supine position and continue abdominal thrusts.
   b. check the carotid pulse.
   c. attempt to deliver ventilations.
   d. place the patient in a supine position and perform 30 chest compressions.

_____ 15. In which one of the following patients would a combination of back blows and chest thrusts be used to relieve foreign body airway obstruction?
   a. Responsive infant with partial obstruction
   b. Unresponsive infant with complete obstruction
   c. Responsive infant with complete obstruction
   d. Responsive infants and children with partial obstruction

_____ 16. The typical soft suction catheter used to suction the trachea of an adult patient with an endotracheal tube in place is _____ Fr.
   a. 12   c. 14
   b. 13   d. 15

_____ 17. When suctioning is nonemergent (there is no immediate risk of aspiration of blood or vomit), each suction attempt should take no more than _____ seconds.
   a. 5   c. 15
   b. 10   d. 20

_____ 18. To properly size an oropharyngeal airway, measure it from the angle of the patient's jaw to the:
   a. earlobe.   c. closest nare.
   b. corner of the mouth.   d. clavicle.

_____19. A nasopharyngeal airway is a good alternative to an oropharyngeal airway in a patient who has:
  a. a gag reflex.
  b. nasal trauma.
  c. midfacial trauma.
  d. epistaxis.

_____20. In which one of the following cases should you use a Combitube?
  a. 8-year-old child who is unresponsive from a traumatic brain injury and who is having seizures and vomiting
  b. 40-year-old man who is vomiting copious amounts of fresh blood and becomes unresponsive
  c. 55-year-old woman with a suspected overdose of multiple prescription drugs who is unresponsive and in whom you are unable to maintain an airway with an oropharyngeal airway
  d. 12-year-old child in cardiac arrest from drowning in whom an oropharyngeal airway is allowing adequate ventilation.

_____21. In which one of the following patients would an LMA be a good choice for airway management?
  a. 25-year-old diabetic who is unresponsive and has a blood glucose level of 32 mg/dL
  b. 70-year-old woman who was trapped in a burning building and appears to have airway burns and soot in the airway
  c. 7-year-old child in cardiac arrest following a drowning that occurred 35 miles from the closest emergency department
  d. 82-year-old man who is awake, but exhausted from respiratory distress due to pulmonary edema.

_____22. An appropriate ventilation rate when using a bag-valve-mask device for an adult in respiratory arrest is _____ breaths per minute.
  a. 8
  b. 12
  c. 16
  d. 20

_____23. An advantage to automatic transport ventilators is:
  a. decreased chances of overventilation and underventilation as compared to bag-valve-mask devices.
  b. industry standards mandate that all units operate in the same way, regardless of manufacturer.
  c. they allow better sensation of lung compliance as compared to bag-valve-mask devices.
  d. they are ideal for patients with pneumothorax and other lung injuries.

_____24. A disadvantage to CPAP is it:
  a. can only be used with 100 percent oxygen.
  b. is not suited to patients with pulmonary edema.
  c. can only be used in responsive patients who can follow commands.
  d. cannot prevent atelectasis.

_____25. Your patient is a 42-year-old woman who suffered a sudden onset of severe dyspnea accompanied by sharp chest pain. She is awake and anxious, with a respiratory rate of 24 breaths per minute and an SpO_2 of 90 percent on room air. She has clear and equal breath sounds bilaterally. The best choice of oxygen delivery device for this patient is a:
  a. nonrebreather mask.
  b. nasal cannula.
  c. Venturi mask.
  d. simple face mask.

Clinical Reasoning

CASE STUDY: AN INTERFACILITY TRANSFER

Your unit is dispatched for an interfacility transfer from a small emergency department to a regional hospital 75 minutes away. The dispatcher tells you that you are taking a patient in respiratory distress directly to the intensive care unit. When you arrive, you begin to assess your patient while your partner gets a report and paperwork from the nursing staff.

Your patient is a 60-year-old man, Mr. Thompson, with COPD and a 90-pack-year history of smoking. You notice that Mr. Thompson appears sleepy and it takes him a few seconds to register your questions. He gives one- or two-word answers. Mr. Thompson is on oxygen by nasal cannula at 4 L/min. His respirations are currently 24 per minute, and his pulse is 120 beats per minute and irregular. He has wheezes and rhonchi scattered throughout all lung fields and you see prominent use of his sternocleidomastoid muscles with breathing. Mr. Thompsons's SpO_2 is 89 percent. His skin is hot and dry.

Your partner returns from getting a report and tells you that Mr. Thompson's wife drove him to the emergency department after his two-day history of increasing shortness of breath dramatically worsened. He has not received treatment other than oxygen by nasal cannula. There are no physician's orders accompanying the paperwork you received.

1. How would you describe your level of concern about Mr. Thompson's respiratory status?

   _____

   _____

   _____

   _____

   _____

2. How do you anticipate Mr. Thompson's condition will change during transport?

   _____

   _____

   _____

   _____

   _____

3. As an Advanced EMT, do you have the tools and training to manage Mr. Thompson's condition?

_____

_____

_____

_____

_____

4. Describe how you should handle this situation.

_____

_____

_____

_____

_____

Project-Based Learning

You have been asked to help teach a lab in an EMT class. Create a presentation to describe the various airway management, oxygen delivery devices, and ventilatory support devices that you have at your disposal to treat patients. Include a description of the device, what its uses are, what its limitations are, and how to use it.

The EMS Professional In Practice

You have arrived on the scene of a patient with difficulty breathing at a nursing home. The patient, a 92-year-old woman, is sitting up in bed and has obvious signs of respiratory distress. A licensed practical nurse (LPN) tells you she put the patient on oxygen by nasal cannula at a flow rate of 2 L/min. How should you handle this situation? Jot down your thoughts in a notebook or journal for discussion in class and in your study group.

Skills Checklists

These skill checklists cover the major steps of selected skills from Chapter 16. Review the skill checklists prior to your laboratory classes. Practice skills only after they have been demonstrated for you in class and only under the supervision of an authorized instructor or clinical preceptor.

Advanced EMT Skill Checklist: *Inserting an Oropharyngeal Airway*		
Skill Stimulus: Primary assessment indicates that the patient is unresponsive and cannot maintain his airway.		
Step	**Performed**	**Not Performed**
Open the airway using a head-tilt/chin-lift or modified jaw-thrust maneuver.		
If not already done, put on gloves and eye protection.		
Select an oropharyngeal airway and measure to make sure it is equal to the length from the angle of the patient's jaw to the corner of his mouth on the same side.		
If necessary, use the cross-finger technique to open the patient's mouth.		
Insert the airway with the tip pointed toward the palate (roof of the mouth).		
Advance the airway toward the oropharynx while rotating it 180 degrees.		
Advance the airway until the flange rests against the patient's lips.		
Assist with ventilations and apply oxygen as indicated by the patient's condition.		
Skill Completion: The airway has been inserted until the flange rests against the patient's lips, and the procedure did not activate the gag reflex.		

Advanced EMT Skill Checklist: *Inserting a Nasopharyngeal Airway*		
Skill Stimulus: Primary assessment indicates that the patient cannot maintain his airway.		
Step	**Performed**	**Not Performed**
Open the airway using a head-tilt/chin-lift or modified jaw-thrust maneuver.		
If not already done, put on gloves and eye protection.		
Select a nasopharyngeal airway and measure to make sure it is equal to the length from the angle of the patient's jaw to the nare on the same side.		
Lubricate the tip of the airway with water-soluble lubricant.		
Insert the airway with the bevel toward the nasal septum.		
Advance the airway until the flange rests against the patient's nostril.		
Assist with ventilations and apply oxygen as indicated by the patient's condition.		
Skill Completion: The airway has been inserted until the flange rests against the patient's lips, and the patient is able to tolerate the presence of the device.		

Advanced EMT Skill Checklist: *Administering Oxygen*

Skill Stimulus: The patient has indications for the administration of oxygen, and the Six Rights of Medication Administration have been confirmed. The oxygen cylinder has the appropriate regulator/flow meter attached.

Step	Performed	Not Performed
Explain the need for oxygen to the patient (for conscious patients).		
Use the oxygen cylinder wrench to turn the main cylinder valve counterclockwise to open it.		
Attach the tubing from the selected delivery device (nasal cannula, mask, or bag-valve-mask device).		
Adjust the flow meter to the flow rate appropriate to the chosen delivery device. If using a device with a reservoir (bag-valve mask or nonrebreather mask), allow the reservoir to fill with air before applying the device.		
Place the device on the patient.		

Skill Completion: Oxygen is being administered and patient has been reassessed.

Advanced EMT Skill Checklist: *Oral Suctioning*

Skill Stimulus: Excess fluid is noted in the oropharynx.

Step	Performed	Not Performed
Place patient in the left lateral recumbent position.		
Make sure the suction unit is assembled with a rigid suction tip attached and is generating adequate suction.		
If not already done, put on examination gloves and eye protection.		
Measure the suction tip from the angle of the jaw (or the earlobe) to the corner of the patient's mouth on the same side.		
Use the cross-finger technique to open the patient's mouth.		
Without applying suction, insert the rigid suction tip to the premeasured depth.		
Cover the side port on the suction tip to generate suction at the end of the rigid suction catheter.		
Suction fluids as you withdraw the suction tip from the oropharynx.		
Limit suction to 10 seconds (ideally) or the minimum time needed to clear the airway if there are copious amounts of fluid.		
Oxygenate and, if necessary, ventilate the patient.		

Skill Completion: Fluids that can be aspirated are cleared from the airway 9 and the patient is being oxygenated and, if necessary, ventilated. The airway is being monitored for the need for additional suctioning.

Advanced EMT Skill Checklist: *Tracheal Suctioning of an Intubated Patient*

Skill Stimulus: The patient has an endotracheal tube in place and secretions that must be removed from the tube and trachea for effective ventilation. SpO$_2$ and (if permitted) cardiac rhythm are being monitored.

Step	Performed	Not Performed
If the patient is nonemergent, preoxygenate the patient. If copious secretions are interfering with ventilation, skip this step.		
Assemble and check the suction unit. Attach the sterile suction catheter to the suction tubing, but keep the part of the catheter that will be placed in the endotracheal tube covered by the sterile packaging and do not allow it to become contaminated.		
Maintaining the sterility of the catheter, measure it from the earlobe, around the ear, and down the neck to the sternal notch.		
If not already done, put on eye protection.		
Put on sterile gloves, do not contaminate the gloves by touching nonsterile surfaces, and handle the suction catheter only with sterile gloves.		
Without applying suction, insert the suction catheter into the endotracheal tube to the premeasured depth.		
Cover the side port to generate suction and suction secretions while slowly withdrawing the catheter and using a slight twirling motion to rotate the catheter from side to side.		
Limit suctioning to 15 seconds (ideally, 10 seconds).		
Ensure that the patient is being ventilated and oxygenated.		
If suctioning is to be repeated, suction sterile water through the catheter to rinse it.		
Dispose of the used suction catheter by wrapping it around your gloved hand and removing the glove over it and dispose of the glove and catheter in a biohazard bag.		

Skill Completion: Fluids have been cleared from the trachea and endotracheal tube, the patient is being ventilated and oxygenated, and the patient is being monitored for the need for additional suctioning.

Advanced EMT Skill Checklist: *Bag-Valve-Mask Ventilation*

Skill Stimulus: Primary assessment reveals a patient who is not breathing or who is not breathing adequately and needs assisted ventilations. The airway has been opened with a manual maneuver and, if needed, an airway adjunct is in place.

Step	Performed	Not Performed
Put on gloves and eye protection.		
Select a mask and bag suited to the patient's size.		
Attach oxygen tubing and inflate the reservoir bag.		
Achieve a good seal using two hands (two-person technique) or the E-C grip.		
Slowly and smoothly squeeze the bag to deliver the volume of air appropriate to the patient's size.		
Release the bag.		
Deliver ventilations at the rate appropriate to the patient's age.		

Skill Completion: Airflow into the lungs is confirmed by watching chest rise and fall, listening to breath sounds, and monitoring pulse oximetry. Effectiveness of ventilation is being monitored by capnography, if available. Patient is being monitored for signs of over- and underventilation.

Advanced EMT Skill Checklist: *Insertion of a Combitube*

Skill Stimulus: Use of more basic airway management techniques is ineffective or there is a need for prolonged ventilation. Patient is unresponsive and does not have contraindications to the use of a Combitube.

Step	Performed	Not Performed
Put on gloves and eye protection.		
If the airway is patient and bag-valve-mask ventilations are adequate, ventilate and oxygenate the patient for at least 2 minutes prior to the procedure.		
Check the device by inflating the cuffs with the syringes provided.		
Deflate the cuffs and leave the syringes attached with air contained to the appropriate marking for each cuff.		
Place the patient's head in a neutral position.		
Use a tongue-jaw lift to displace the mandible anteriorly and open the mouth.		
Holding the Combitube with a pencil grip, insert it into the oropharynx by orienting it in a caudally (inferiorly), not posteriorly. Insert the Combitube until the patient's front teeth (or gums, if teeth are absent) are between the two black lines on the tube.		
Inflate the pharyngeal cuff with 100 mL of air.		
Inflate the distal cuff with 15 mL of air.		
Attach a ventilation bag and ventilate through the esophageal (blue) tube while checking placement (look for chest rise, auscultate for breath sounds, check for absence of gurgling over the epigastric region).		
If the chest does not rise, breath sounds are not heard, or there is gurgling over the epigastric region, ventilate through the tracheal (clear) tube while checking for placement. (Observe for chest rise, auscultate breath sounds and epigastric region.)		

Skill Completion: Placement and effective ventilation have been confirmed, and patient is being ventilated and continually monitored for signs of over- or underventilation.

Advanced EMT Skill Checklist: *Insertion of a Laryngeal Mask Airway (LMA)*		

Skill Stimulus: Basic airway management techniques are inadequate or there is a need for prolonged ventilation.

Step	Performed	Not Performed
Put on gloves and eye protection.		
If the airway is patient and bag-valve-mask ventilations are adequate, ventilate and oxygenate the patient for at least 2 minutes prior to the procedure.		
Check the device, inflate and then deflate the cuff.		
Lubricate the distal end of the device with water-soluble lubricant.		
Hyperextend the neck slightly to place the head in a "sniffing" position.		
Holding the tube between the thumb and last three fingers, place your index finger between the edge of the cuff and the tube.		
Orient the side of the mask from which the tube protrudes toward the roof of the mouth so that the open side of the mask is toward the patient's tongue.		
Insert your opposite thumb into the patient's mouth to push the mandible inferiorly to open the mouth.		
Slide the LMA along the roof of the patient's mouth and into the pharynx until the tip of the mask is seated in the hypopharynx.		
Inflate the cuff with the amount of air that is indicated for the size of the LMA.		
Attach a ventilation bag and ventilate while assessing the effectiveness of ventilations.		

Skill Completion: Placement and effective ventilation have been confirmed, and patient is being ventilated and continually monitored for signs of over- or underventilation.

Advanced EMT Skill Checklist: *Relieving Complete Foreign Body Airway Obstruction—Conscious Adult or Child*

Skill Stimulus: A conscious adult or child patient exhibits signs of complete foreign body airway obstruction, such as the universal choking sign (grasps the throat with both hands) and sudden inability to speak, cough, or breathe; or has severe partial airway obstruction with inadequate breathing.

Step	Performed	Not Performed
Stand behind the patient and reach around him with both arms.		
Place the thumb side of one fist against the patient's abdomen below the diaphragm. Cup your other hand over your fist.		
Deliver a series of firm inward, upward thrusts.		
Continue until the obstruction is relieved or the patient becomes unresponsive.		
Skill Completion: Obstruction is relieved or patient becomes unresponsive.		

Advanced EMT Skill Checklist: *Relieving Foreign Body Airway Obstruction—Unresponsive Adult or Child*

Skill Stimulus: An unresponsive adult or child patient exhibits signs of complete foreign body airway obstruction, such as apnea and inability to provide artificial ventilation despite manual airway maneuvers, and there is no history that would indicate another cause of obstruction, such as edema from anaphylaxis or airway burns.

Step	Performed	Not Performed
Place the patient supine on a firm surface.		
Perform 30 chest compressions.		
Open the airway in preparation for delivering ventilations and inspect for the presence of the foreign body in the mouth.		
If the foreign body is seen, remove it with a finger sweep.		
Attempt to deliver 2 ventilations.		
Continue a cycle of 30 chest compressions to 2 ventilations.		

Skill Completion: The airway obstruction has been relieved as evidenced by the ability to deliver ventilations, or advanced life support personnel are available to use additional measures to establish an airway and ventilation.

Advanced EMT Skill Checklist: *Relieving Foreign Body Airway Obstruction—Conscious Infant*

Skill Stimulus: A conscious infant patient exhibits signs of complete foreign body airway obstruction, such as sudden inability to speak, cough, or breathe; or has severe partial airway obstruction with inadequate breathing.

Step	Performed	Not Performed
Place the patient prone along your forearm so that you are supporting the upper chest with your hand and the patient's legs are straddling your arm. The patient's head should be slightly lower than his body.		
Perform five back blows.		
Sandwich the patient by placing your other arm over his back, supporting the head with your hand 9, and turn him prone while supporting him with the arm placed on his back.		
Perform five chest thrusts.		
Repeat the series of five back blows and five chest thrusts until the obstruction is relieved or the patient becomes unresponsive.		

Skill Completion: Airway obstruction is relieved or the patient becomes unresponsive.

Advanced EMT Skill Checklist: *Relieving Foreign Body Airway Obstruction—Unresponsive Infant*

Skill Stimulus: An unresponsive infant exhibits signs of complete foreign body airway obstruction, such as apnea and inability to provide artificial ventilation despite manual airway maneuvers; and there is no history that would indicate another cause of obstruction, such as edema from anaphylaxis or airway burns.

Step	Performed	Not Performed
Cradle the infant in a football hold or lay him supine on a firm surface.		
Perform 30 chest thrusts.		
Open the airway in preparation for delivering ventilations and inspect for the presence of the foreign body in the mouth.		
If a foreign body is seen, remove it with a finger sweep.		
Attempt 2 ventilations.		
Continue the cycle of 30 chest compressions to 2 ventilations.		

Skill Completion: The airway obstruction has been relieved as evidenced by the ability to deliver ventilations, or advanced life support personnel are available to use additional measures to establish an airway and ventilation.

Resuscitation: Managing Shock and Cardiac Arrest

Content Area

- Assessment

Advanced EMT Education Standard

- Applies fundamental knowledge of the causes, pathophysiology and management of shock, respiratory failure or arrest, cardiac failure or arrest, and postresuscitation management.

Summary of Objectives

17.1 Define key terms introduced in this chapter.

Knowing and being able to apply the key terms in each chapter is critical to understanding chapter concepts. Write the list of key terms. Then write the definition of each one in your own words. Check your understanding by confirming the definitions in the textbook glossary. Correct any misunderstandings. Create a study aid by writing each key term on the front of an index card and the definition on the back. Use the cards to quiz yourself or to have someone quiz you. The exercises under Vocabulary and Concept Review below will give you additional practice.

17.2 Identify situations in which you should withhold resuscitative attempts.

Always consult your protocols when making decisions about withholding or terminating resuscitative measures. However, in general, resuscitative efforts are not begun for patients who have rigor mortis, dependent lividity, obvious decomposition, or other injuries incompatible with life (such as decapitation or transection of the torso). Also, some terminally ill patients have do not resuscitate (DNR) orders.

17.3 Explain each of the links in the chain of survival of cardiac arrest.

Immediate recognition of cardiac arrest by bystanders and activation of the emergency response system is the first link. Resuscitation from cardiac arrest is most likely to be successful if defibrillation is performed in the first 5 minutes following collapse.

Early CPR with emphasis on chest compressions is next. When sudden cardiac arrest occurs, a certain amount of oxygen is in the blood and in the lungs. Immediate chest compressions help to make the remaining oxygen and blood start circulating.

Rapid defibrillation follows. Early defibrillation is critical for patients presenting with a pulseless ventricular rhythm. The greater the interval between arrest and defibrillation, the poorer the patient's chances of survival.

Early advanced life support is the next link. Certain advanced airway procedures and medications can be beneficial in cardiac arrest.

Integrated post–cardiac arrest care is the final link. The efforts of prehospital, emergency department, cardiology, intensive care, and other personnel are all critical in optimizing the patient's chances of recovery.

17.4 Explain the importance of early defibrillation in cardiac arrest.

Defibrillation terminates the chaotic electrical activity associated with ventricular fibrillation. If the conduction system of the heart is still functional, it will resume coordinated electrical function and, hopefully, mechanical contraction. However, the greater the interval between cardiac arrest and defibrillation, the less likely defibrillation is to be successful.

17.5 Explain the rationale for the "push hard and push fast" approach to CPR.

Compressions should be to a depth of 2 inches and then allow the chest to fully recoil. Adequate compression followed by complete recoil maximizes pressure changes within the chest to allow blood circulation. Compress at a rate of at least 100 compressions per minute in a pattern of 30 compressions followed by 2 ventilations until an advanced airway is placed. This rate builds up pressure within the cardiovascular system to allow perfusion.

17.6 Describe the features, functions, advantages, disadvantages, and precautions in the use of automated external defibrillators (AEDs).

Semiautomatic external defibrillators (SAEDs) require some input from the user, who may have to push a button to begin analysis of the cardiac rhythm or to deliver a shock once the machine indicates a shock is indicated. A fully automatic external defibrillator (AED), once the pads are in place and it is powered on, does not require additional input from the user to function. It analyzes the rhythm and delivers a shock, if indicated, on its own. Often, both AEDs and SAEDs are lumped together under the term *AED*, but you must know how your particular unit works and what steps you must perform to accomplish rhythm analysis and, if indicated, deliver a shock.

The pads of the defibrillator serve to direct a certain amount of electrical energy through the heart, either in one direction (monophasic) or for half the period of defibrillation in one direction and then in the other direction (biphasic). The purpose of the energy is to uniformly depolarize chaotically depolarizing cells, allowing them to receive and respond to a normal stimulus from the sinoatrial node, if it is able to resume function.

Defibrillation is the only way to restore normal heart function in patients with ventricular fibrillation or pulseless ventricular tachycardia. The most up-to-date AEDs are lightweight and can be made widely available in public places to decrease the time to defibrillation in many cases. Defibrillation can result in minor burns to the chest and poses a potential risk of transferring electrical energy to anyone in contact with the patient when the shock is delivered.

17.7 Compare and contrast ventricular fibrillation, ventricular tachycardia, asystole, and pulseless electrical activity.

All of those dysrhythmias can occur in cardiac arrest. Ventricular fibrillation, asystole, and pulseless electrical activity are always accompanied by pulselessness. Ventricular tachycardia can occur with or without a pulse. Ventricular fibrillation and ventricular tachycardia are the most common initial dysrhythmias in sudden cardiac death, and can be treated with defibrillation. Pulseless electrical activity generally has an underlying cause, which is sometimes correctable (such as hypovolemia, hypothermia, hypoxia, and other causes). Asystole is a complete absence of electrical activity in the heart and carries a grave prognosis for return of spontaneous circulation.

17.8 **Describe the safety precautions to be taken to protect yourself, other EMS providers, the patient, and bystanders in resuscitation situations.**

Safety is of paramount concern on every EMS call. Resuscitation situations create stress for all involved. Pay careful attention to family, friends, or bystanders. Anger may be directed at EMS providers. Use appropriate personal protective equipment and, although the patient deserves your focus, be sure to observe the area for any hazards. Also pay attention to safety concerns such as dealing with sharps and safe use of a defibrillator.

17.9 **Given a series of cardiac arrest scenarios involving infants, children, and adults, demonstrate appropriate assessment and resuscitative techniques, including the integrated use of CPR, AEDs, airway management, and ventilation.**

Refer to the skill checklists at the end of this workbook chapter.

17.10 **Explain the purpose and procedure for reassessing patients in shock and cardiac arrest.**

In a cardiac arrest situation, if the patient's spontaneous circulation returns, resuscitative efforts must shift from CPR to maximizing oxygenation and perfusion and preventing secondary brain and organ damage. Periodically assess the patient's pulse for return of spontaneous circulation. Any attempts to breathe spontaneously or response to stimuli should prompt reassessment. When capnometry is used, detection of CO_2 is an indication of return of spontaneous circulation.

17.11 **Given a cardiac arrest scenario, make decisions regarding transport and requesting advanced life support (ALS) backup.**

Initiate transport as soon as logistically possible in the course of a cardiac arrest call, without sacrificing the quality of CPR or delaying defibrillation. The goal for any field unit is definitive care, in the form of a hospital emergency department. For transport of more than a few minutes' duration, request ALS to the scene or request an intercept, if available.

17.12 **Demonstrate assessment and management of a postcardiac arrest patient with return of spontaneous circulation (ROSC).**

Assessment focuses on evaluating and supporting perfusion in the post–cardiac arrest patient. The goal is adequate cerebral and myocardial perfusion so that the heart and brain can return to a functioning state. Management focuses on airway management, ventilation, and oxygenation. Intravenous fluids can help improve perfusion status in some cases. Therapeutic hypothermia is a promising intervention for the post–cardiac arrest patient.

17.13 **Explain the importance of AED maintenance, Advanced EMT training and skills maintenance, medical direction, and continuous quality improvement in the chain of survival of cardiac arrest.**

AED maintenance is an essential element to the chain of survival because it allows for rapid defibrillation. Advanced EMT training is fundamental to all the links. Proper training and continued skills maintenance allows the Advanced EMT a greater knowledge and skill base to call upon in the performance of early CPR/rapid defibrillation/early access to advanced life support/ integrated postarrest care. Also, the Advanced EMT's training can prepare him to train bystanders for the first link: immediate recognition of cardiac arrest. Medical direction provides a means of communication between the licensed health care provider and the field practitioner, further increasing the knowledge-sharing capacity. Continuous quality improvement allows recognition of specific weaknesses in any system so that they can be addressed through education and operational changes.

17.14 Discuss special considerations in the use of an AED in patients with cardiac pacemakers and implanted cardioverter–defibrillators.

Do not place pads over an implanted device to avoid interference with rhythm analysis and damage to the implanted device.

17.15 Discuss the use of mechanical CPR devices.

Mechanical CPR devices can be a useful tool in the case of prolonged CPR or in situations in which extra assistance is scarce. The efficacy of CPR delivered by the devices seems to be equivalent to that of manual compressions, but research is still limited.

17.16 Demonstrate effective mechanisms for controlling external hemorrhage.

Techniques include direct pressure, topical hemostatic agents, and tourniquets. Although there currently is no research to support the use of arterial pressure points and elevation, those techniques have not been proven ineffective, and may be included in some protocols. Immobilization is also an important step in minimizing bleeding.

17.17 Discuss indications, contraindications, complications, and administration of fluids to patients in cardiac arrest and hemorrhagic shock.

Carefully weigh intravenous fluid administration for the patient in hemorrhagic shock, and recall that the blood must maintain specific concentrations of plasma proteins, electrolytes, and formed elements to do its job. Plasma is not simply water. In general, the current practice is to differentiate between patients in whom hemorrhage is ongoing and those in whom hemorrhage has been controlled. In cases of ongoing hemorrhage, permissive hypotension (systolic blood pressure of 80 to 90 mmHg) is considered a prudent way of increasing perfusion but minimizing the increase in bleeding and hemodilution that can occur with aggressive fluid replacement. In cardiac arrest and post–cardiac arrest, fluids can improve perfusion, but can also exacerbate heart failure.

17.18 Discuss the use of the pneumatic antishock garment (PASG) in patients with hemorrhagic shock.

Pneumatic antishock garments are trousers with inflatable compartments. The device was originally thought to work by forcing blood from the legs and pelvis to the upper body, resulting in an autotransfusion of blood. Although most providers who used a PASG saw an initial increase in the patient's blood pressure, research indicated that PASGs do not improve survival. As a result, the use of PASGs has largely fallen out of favor.

17.19 Discuss current trends and research in resuscitation and shock management.

Research has led to changes in the thinking on the amount of intravenous fluids considered to be beneficial, de-emphasis on PASG, emphasis on chest compressions as the first step in CPR, and emphasis on ventilation (while avoiding overventilation) and oxygenation in asphyxial arrest, shock, and return of spontaneous circulation. Use of topical hemostatic agents, tourniquets, and therapeutic hypothermia following cardiac arrest also are supported by research.

Resource Central

Resource Central offers extra practice and review materials in a variety of media. To access it, follow the directions on the Student Access Card provided with the Student Textbook. If there is no card, go to www.bradybooks.com and follow the Resource Central link to Buy Access.

Vocabulary and Concept Review

Exercise 1

Write the letter of the correct definition in the blank next to the term. (See Resource Central for more vocabulary review.)

1. _____ acute respiratory distress syndrome

2. _____ cardiac tamponade

3. _____ defibrillation

4. _____ disseminated intravascular coagulation (DIC)

5. _____ dysrhythmia

6. _____ ischemia

7. _____ permissive hypotension

8. _____ resuscitation

9. _____ sudden cardiac arrest

10. _____ therapeutic hypothermia

a. Maintaining a hemorrhagic shock patient's systolic blood pressure between 80 and 90 mmHg to avoid an increase in bleeding

b. Severely diminished or absent blood flow to tissues

c. Complication of shock and other critical illnesses that result in damage to the lungs, which allows leakage of fluid into the lung parenchyma

d. Complication of shock in which there is systemic activation of the clotting cascade, resulting in both abnormal blood clotting and consumption of clotting factors, which leads to increased bleeding

e. Collection of blood or fluid between the heart and fibrous pericardium, resulting in compression of the heart and reduced preload

f. Electrical current passed through the heart between two pads or paddles that are placed on the chest to terminate lethal ventricular dysrhythmia

g. Heart rhythm that may be irregular, too slow, too fast, or arise from a site other than the sinoatrial node

h. Intervention to actively lower the body temperature following return of spontaneous circulation after cardiac arrest

i. Coordinated medical interventions to stabilize the condition of a critically ill patient, such as one in respiratory failure or arrest, shock, and cardiac arrest

j. Abrupt, unexpected cessation of heart function that often occurs outside the hospital setting

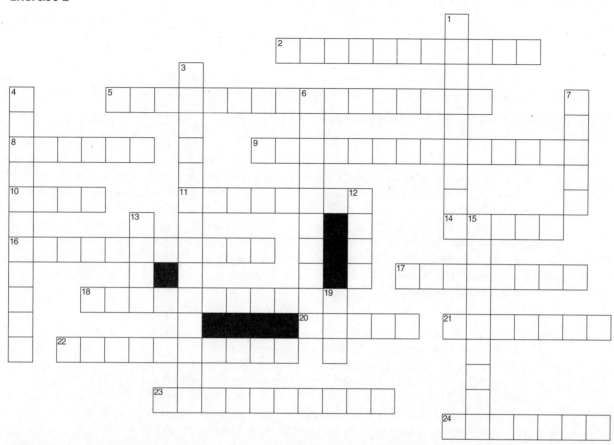

Across

2. A stage of shock that may be difficult to detect because the blood pressure is normal.

5. First step in the response to laceration of a blood vessel.

8. Type of shock that occurs from overwhelming infection.

9. Method that is effective in controlling most external bleeding.

10. Abbreviation that means the pulse has come back in a patient who was in cardiac arrest.

11. State of decreased or absent blood flow to tissues.

14. For CPR purposes, a patient between one and eight years old.

16. Type of shock that occurs when the heart fails.

17. Absence of electrical activity in the heart.

18. Abnormal heart beat.

20. State in which perfusion is inadequate to meet the demands of cellular metabolism.

21. Phase of shock in which micro-emboli are released from the capillary beds.

22. Device for stopping severe, uncontrollable bleeding in an extremity.

23. Process of stopping bleeding.

24. Injectable anticoagulant that can result in excessive bleeding.

Down

1. Way to describe the mechanism behind distributive shock.

3. An adrenal medullary hormone.

4. Tension pneumothorax is a cause of this kind of shock.

6. One of the "Five Ts" that can be an underlying cause of cardiac arrest.

7. What you must instruct all personnel to do before delivering a defibrillation shock to a patient.

12. Abbreviation for a condition of noncardiogenic pulmonary edema.

13. Abbreviation for a complication of shock in which several body systems are damaged and fail.

15. Primary cheminal mediator of anaphylactic reactions that causes vasodilation.

19. Abbreviation for the organization that establishes national guidelines for CPR and emergency cardiac care.

Check Your Recall and Apply Concepts

Select the best possible choice for each of the following questions.

_____ **1.** Hypovolemic shock results from:
  a. decreased fluid in the vascular space.
  b. vasodilation.
  c. obstruction of blood flow.
  d. heart failure.

_____ **2.** Cardiac output is the product of the heart rate and the _____ volume.
  a. minute
  b. tidal
  c. stroke
  d. end-diastolic

_____ **3.** A 14-year-old child has a gunshot wound to his right thigh, just above the knee. He is awake and breathing spontaneously at a rate of 20 breaths/min with slightly increased depth. He is pale, cool, and sweaty; anxious and combative; and has a weak, thready radial pulse. Bleeding from the wound is substantial, and attempts to control it using direct pressure have been ineffective. Of the following, your next action should be:
  a. starting a large-bore IV of lactated Ringer's solution.
  b. splinting the extremity.
  c. applying a tourniquet.
  d. elevating the extremity and applying firm pressure to the femoral artery.

_____ **4.** A 73-year-old patient complains of nausea, vomiting, and diarrhea for three days. She says the vomit has just been "bile" and the diarrhea is "watery and yellow-green." She is lethargic and weak; has cool, pale, dry skin; has poor skin turgor; and states she has not urinated in almost a day. Her radial pulse is weak and thready at a rate of 124, blood pressure 102/64, respirations 20, SpO_2 97 percent on room air, and blood glucose level is 74 mg/dL. Based on this description, the patient's most pressing need is for:
  a. intravenous infusion of isotonic crystalloid solution.
  b. infusion of packed red blood cells.
  c. high-flow oxygen by nonrebreather mask.
  d. intravenous 50 percent dextrose.

_____ **5.** As a rule of thumb, pediatric patients in shock are given an initial intravenous fluid bolus of _____ mL/kg of body weight.
  a. 10
  b. 20
  c. 40
  d. 60

_____ **6.** Which one of the following is the most common cause of cardiac arrest in pediatric patients?
  a. Sepsis
  b. Cardiac dysrhythmia
  c. Hypoxia
  d. Pulmonary embolism

_____ **7.** When an advanced airway, such as a Combitube or an endotracheal tube, has been placed in a patient in cardiac arrest, the relationship between chest compressions and ventilations is:
  a. a ratio of 30:2.
  b. a ratio of 15:1.
  c. a ratio of 5:1.
  d. asynchronous.

_____ **8.** In the initial stages of significant blood loss, which one of the following happens at the level of the peripheral microvasculature?
  a. Both the precapillary and postcapillary sphincters constrict.
  b. The precapillary sphincter constricts and the postcapillary sphincter relaxes.
  c. The precapillary sphincter relaxes and the postcapillary sphincter constricts.
  d. Both the precapillary and postcapillary sphincters relax.

_____ 9. Which one of the following is a cause of distributive shock?
   a. Pulmonary embolism
   c. Overwhelming infection
   b. Pericardial tamponade
   d. Acute myocardial infarction

_____ 10. An early sign of shock is:
   a. unresponsiveness.
   c. bradycardia.
   b. low blood pressure.
   d. anxiety.

_____ 11. You are walking quickly through the airport terminal with just minutes left before the final boarding call for your flight. A man several feet in front of you suddenly stops walking and collapses, appearing to have a few seconds of seizure activity. You reach him in a few steps and see that he is cyanotic and has gasping, irregular breaths. Your first step should be to:
   a. run back and grab the AED you saw about 25 yards away.
   b. open the airway and give two rescue breaths.
   c. designate a specific person to call for help and another to fetch the AED.
   d. perform 15 chest compressions, pushing hard and fast.

_____ 12. The optimum energy level for biphasic defibrillation is:
   a. not yet determined.
   c. 200 joules.
   b. 120 joules.
   d. 360 joules.

_____ 13. Infant CPR is performed at a rate of at least _____ compressions per minute.
   a. 80
   c. 120
   b. 100
   d. 150

Clinical Reasoning

CASE STUDY: TROUBLE IN THE MEADOW

You and your partner, Kent, are dispatched for an allergic reaction to a bee sting. The scene is about 15 miles from your station and nearly 30 miles to the nearest hospital.

1. What is the worst-case scenario in this situation?

_____

_____

_____

_____

When you arrive on the scene you learn that the patient, 38-year-old Pat Shaffer, was mowing in a meadow when he struck a wasps' nest with the mower. He was stung in four different places. He called his wife to tell her what had happened and, while talking with her on the phone, his throat began to itch and he started wheezing and feeling lightheaded. "This is crazy," he told his wife, "I am not allergic to bees but I think I am having an allergic reaction!" His wife, Jordana, called 911 and drove to the area where Mr. Shaffer was mowing. When she arrived she found him sitting on the ground next to the mower. When you get there, Mr. Shaffer is lying on the ground. He is pale, cool, and sweaty, and you can hear him wheezing. He is able to speak and says he feels weak and dizzy and his throat itches. He has a very weak radial pulse of 126 per minute.

2. Explain both the cause and the consequences of Mr. Shaffer's signs and symptoms.

_____

_____

_____

_____

3. Outline your treatment steps and give a rationale for each intervention.

_____

_____

_____

_____

_____

Project-Based Learning

Visit five public locations in your community and look for public-access defibrillation programs. Some places to look include high schools (particularly in the areas for physical education and sports), large department stores or malls, airports, college campuses, and event centers (stadiums, arenas, amphitheaters). If you find AEDs, are they noticeable and accessible? If you do not find AEDs, research how to promote public access defibrillation programs in your community.

The EMS Professional in Practice

You are the team leader on a call for a cardiac arrest. The patient is a 62-year-old man. CPR is continuing as you prepare the patient for transport. What should you say to the patient's family? Jot down your thoughts in a notebook or journal for discussion in class or in your study group.

Skills Checklists

The following skill checklists cover the major steps of selected skills from Chapter 17. Review them prior to your laboratory classes. Practice skills only after they have been demonstrated for you in class and only under the supervision of an authorized instructor or clinical preceptor.

Advanced EMT Skill Checklist: *Adult CPR*		
Skill Stimulus: An adult patient is apparently unresponsive and not breathing or not breathing normally.		
Step	**Performed**	**Not Performed**
If you are off duty, call 911 or designate someone to call 911 and to retrieve an AED if you are in a facility with a public-access defibrillation program.		
Check for a carotid pulse.		
If no pulse is detected within 10 seconds and an AED is not immediately available, perform 30 chest compressions with one hand over the top of the other over the lower half of the sternum. Depress the chest 2 inches. Allow complete recoil.		
If an AED is immediately available, apply the pads, clear all contact with the patient, and turn on the machine.		
If an AED is not immediately available, open the airway and deliver 2 ventilations (if you are off duty and do not have the proper equipment, you may perform hands-only CPR).		
If a defibrillator is not available or following defibrillation, perform CPR with a ratio of chest compressions to ventilations of 30:2 at a compression rate of at least 100 per minute.		
Keep interruptions in compressions to a minimum.		
Periodically check for return of spontaneous circulation.		
Skill Completion: Patient has return of spontaneous circulation or resuscitative efforts are terminated by physician order.		

Advanced EMT Skill Checklist: *Child CPR*		
Skill Stimulus: A child patient is apparently unresponsive and not breathing or not breathing normally.		
Step	**Performed**	**Not Performed**
If you are off duty and alone, perform 2 minutes of CPR before calling 911. If someone else is present, designate a person to call 911 and to retrieve an AED if you are in a facility with a public-access defibrillation program.		
Check a carotid pulse.		
If no pulse is detected within 10 seconds or the pulse is less than 60 per minute and the patient has poor perfusion, and an AED is not immediately available, perform 30 chest compressions.		
Use one or two hands (depending on the size of the child) over the lower half of the sternum. Depress the chest 2 inches or one-third the anterior–posterior dimension of the chest. Allow complete recoil of the chest between compressions.		
If an AED is immediately available, apply the pads, clear all contact with the patient, and turn on the machine.		
If an AED is not immediately available, open the airway and deliver 2 ventilations (if you are off duty and do not have the proper equipment, you may perform hands-only CPR).		
If a defibrillator is not available or following defibrillation, perform CPR with a ratio of chest compressions to ventilations of 30:2 at a compression rate of at least 100 per minute. If two rescuers are performing CPR, the ratio is 15:2.		
Keep interruptions in compressions to a minimum.		
Periodically check for return of spontaneous circulation.		
Skill Completion: Patient has return of spontaneous circulation or resuscitative efforts are terminated by physician order.		

Advanced EMT Skill Checklist: *Infant CPR*		
Skill Stimulus: An infant is apparently unresponsive and not breathing or not breathing normally.		
Step	Performed	Not Performed
If you are off duty and alone, perform 2 minutes of CPR before calling 911. If someone else is present, designate a person to call 911 and to retrieve an AED if you are in a facility with a public-access defibrillation program.		
Check for a brachial pulse.		
If no pulse is detected within 10 seconds or the pulse is below 60 per minute and the patient has poor perfusion, and an AED is not immediately available, perform 30 chest compressions. Use two fingers over the sternum just below the intermammary line, or encircle the chest with the hands and place thumbs over the sternum.		
If an AED is immediately available, apply the pads, clear all contact with the patient, and turn on the machine.		
If an AED is not immediately available, open the airway and deliver 2 ventilations (if you are off duty and do not have the proper equipment, you may perform hands-only CPR).		
If a defibrillator is not available or following defibrillation, perform CPR with a ratio of chest compressions to ventilations of 30:2 at a compression rate of at least 100 per minute. If two rescuers are present, the ratio is 15:2.		
Keep interruptions in compressions to a minimum.		
Periodically check for return of spontaneous circulation.		
Skill Completion: Patient has return of spontaneous circulation or resuscitative efforts are terminated by physician order.		

Advanced EMT Skill Checklist: *AED Use—Adult*		
Skill Stimulus: Cardiac arrest is confirmed in an adult patient by unresponsiveness, absent or abnormal breathing, and absence of a carotid pulse.		
Step	Performed	Not Performed
If you are off duty, call 911 or designate someone to call 911 and to retrieve an AED if you are in a facility with a public-access defibrillation program.		
If available, direct a second rescuer to perform CPR, while you place the defibrillator pads and prepare the machine.		
With the machine turned on, direct everyone to clear the patient.		
Allow the machine to analyze (AED) or push the button to analyze the cardiac rhythm (SAED).		
Allow the machine to shock, or push the button to shock if the machine establishes that a shock is indicated.		
Resume CPR.		
Periodically check the rhythm and for return of spontaneous circulation.		
Skill Completion: Patient has return of spontaneous circulation or resuscitative efforts are terminated by physician order.		

Vital Signs and Monitoring Devices

Content Area

- Assessment

Advanced EMT Education Standard

- Applies scene information and patient assessment findings (scene size-up, primary and secondary assessments, patient history, and reassessment) to guide emergency management.

Summary of Objectives

18.1   Define key terms introduced in this chapter.

Knowing and being able to apply the key terms in each chapter is critical to understanding chapter concepts. Write the list of key terms. Then write the definition of each one in your own words. Check your understanding by confirming the definitions in the textbook glossary. Correct any misunderstandings. Create a study aid by writing each key term on the front of an index card and the definition on the back. Use the cards to quiz yourself or to have someone quiz you. The exercises under Vocabulary and Concept Review below will give you additional practice.

18.2   Discuss the importance of accurate assessment and documentation of vital signs over the course of contact with the patient to identify problems and changes in the patient's condition.

The information available from vital signs, assessment of the skin and pupils, and monitoring devices is useful only if it is relevant and integrated into an overall impression of the patient's condition. A single finding in isolation from the patient's other signs and symptoms is not useful and may result in misguided patient care decisions. The key is to properly prioritize the task of collecting vital signs in relation to the patient's condition, anticipated treatment, and other tasks that you must complete.

18.3   Perform the steps required to assess the patient's breathing, pulse, skin, pupils, blood pressure, and oxygen saturation.

Refer to the skill checklists at the end of the workbook chapter.

18.4 Consider a patient's overall presentation when interpreting the meaning of vital sign findings.

A full set of baseline vital signs is obtained as soon as possible for all patients. For a critical trauma patient, this may mean after the patient is packaged and loaded into the ambulance for transport. For a patient whose medical condition is critical, this may mean having your partner get vital signs while you start an IV at the scene. For a patient whose condition is noncritical, you may take vital signs while your partner takes a history, writes down a list of medications, or talks to a family member.

18.5 Differentiate between normal and abnormal findings when assessing a patient's breathing to include the respiratory rate, depth of respirations, rhythm of respiration, and signs that indicate respiratory distress or respiratory failure.

Evaluation of ventilations begins in the primary assessment. Early on in your assessment, you can identify accessory muscle use, "tripoding," and abnormal breathing sounds (stridor, coughing, gurgling, wheezing, crackles [rales], rhonchi, snoring). Increased and decreased respiratory rate and depth are signs that can indicate respiratory distress or respiratory failure. An adult patient with respirations below 8 per minute or greater than 30 per minute often requires ventilatory assistance. An increased level of CO_2 and decreased SpO_2 are also signs of inadequate breathing. Cyanosis and changes in mental status are indications of respiratory failure.

18.6 Differentiate among normal respiratory rates for adults, children, infants, and newborns.

- Adults and adolescents: 12 to 20 per minute
- School age: 18 to 30 per minute
- Preschooler: 22 to 34 per minute
- Toddler: 24 to 30 per minute
- Infant: 25 to 40 per minute
- Newborn: 30 to 60 per minute

18.7 Evaluate the need to administer treatment based on assessment of a patient's breathing.

Base the decisions to administer oxygen and assist ventilations on the patient's general appearance, mental status, skin color, respiratory effort, respiratory rate, respiratory depth, respiratory pattern, and presence of abnormal respiratory noises.

18.8 Auscultate breath sounds to determine the presence of breath sounds, equality of breath sounds, and the presence of abnormal breath sounds.

Lung sounds are auscultated using a stethoscope to listen for normal air movement and for extra, abnormal sounds. Place the diaphragm of the stethoscope directly on the chest wall with gentle pressure and listen to inspiration and expiration. Compare sounds from one side to the other at each level, listening at the apices, middle areas, and bases of the lungs.

18.9 Identify abnormal sounds associated with breathing as the likely underlying cause, including snoring, gurgling, stridor, wheezing, crackles (rales), and rhonchi.

Snoring is caused by partial occlusion of the upper airway by the tongue. It is easily corrected by manual positioning. Gurgling is an indication of fluid in the airway. You must clear the airway by suctioning to prevent aspiration. Stridor is a high-pitched inspiratory sound caused by partial obstruction of the larynx or trachea, such as by edema or a foreign body. Wheezing is a high-pitched whistling sound heard during expiration (and during inspiration in severe distress) caused by a constriction of the bronchioles, such as in asthma and COPD. Crackles (rales) are fine, popping sounds typically heard during inspiration caused by fluid in the terminal bronchioles and alveoli as seen in collapsed alveoli and pulmonary edema, including pulmonary edema due to left-sided heart failure. Rhonchi are lower-pitched, coarse rumbling sounds associated with a buildup of secretions in the larger airways as seen with COPD, bronchitis, and pneumonia.

18.10 Assess the pulse at each of the following pulse points: carotid, femoral, radial, brachial, popliteal, posterior tibial, and dorsalis pedis.

- *Carotid pulse:* It is on either side of the anterior neck in the groove between the thyroid cartilage and sternocleidomastoid muscle.
- *Femoral pulse:* It is in the groin, anteriorly, in the crease of the hip joint, about halfway between the medial tendon and the bony prominence of the ilium.
- *Radial pulse:* It is on the anterior wrist at the base of the thumb, between the radial styloid (bony prominence) and tendon.
- *Brachial pulse:* In infants, it is along the medial arm over the humerus; in older children and adults, it is on the medial aspect of the antecubital fossa.
- *Popliteal pulse:* It is on the posterior aspect of the knee.
- *Posterior tibial pulse:* It is on the medial side of the ankle behind the bony prominence of the tibia (medial malleolus).
- *Dorsalis pedis pulse:* It is on the top (dorsal surface) of the foot, toward the medial side.

18.11 Consider the patient's age and level of responsiveness when selecting a site to palpate the pulse.

In responsive adults, the radial pulse in the wrist is assessed. In unresponsive adult patients, the carotid pulse in the neck is palpated. During resuscitation efforts and in critical unresponsive patients without a radial pulse, you can assess the femoral pulse as well. In children, you can palpate the brachial pulse in the antecubital fossa. In infants, the brachial pulse along the medial humerus is palpated.

18.12 Differentiate between normal and abnormal findings when assessing a patient's pulse to include the pulse rate, quality of the pulse, and rhythm of the pulse.

Assessing the patient's pulse begins in the primary assessment. The rate will vary depending upon the patient's age and level of exertion. The quality should be regular, strong, and full, and the rhythm should be regular. You should further evaluate an abnormally fast or abnormally slow or irregular pulse to detect any subtle changes and possible underlying causes.

18.13 Differentiate between normal heart rates for adults, children, infants, and newborns.

- Adults: 60 to 100 per minute
- Adolescents: 60 to 105 per minute
- School age: 70 to 110 per minute
- Preschooler: 80 to 120 per minute
- Toddler: 80 to 130 per minute
- Infant: 100 to 160 per minute
- Newborn: 100 to 180 per minute

18.14 Associate abnormalities in the assessment of pulses with possible underlying causes.

Tachycardia can be caused by anxiety, fear, pain, blood loss, dehydration, fever, hypoxia, or stimulants. Some cardiac dysrhythmias also can be tachycardia. Bradycardia can be caused by a problem with the cardiac conduction system, excess stimulation of the vagus nerve, or as a reflex to hypertension. Some medications or the patient's well-maintained physical fitness may lower the resting heart rate. An irregular pulse can be caused by either extra heart beats or by a greater-than-normal delay between some heart beats.

18.15 Describe pulsus alternans and pulsus paradoxus.

Pulsus alternans is an alternating pulse specifically due to left ventricular failure. Pulsus paradoxus is a drop in systolic blood pressure of greater than 10 mmHg during inspiration. There is a normal drop in systolic pressure during inspiration because of the increased pressure within the chest cavity decreasing cardiac output.

18.16 Recognize normal and abnormal findings in the assessment of skin and mucous membrane color, skin temperature and condition, and capillary refill time.

Pallor may be generalized and easily noted or can sometimes be noted by checking the mucous membranes of the mouth and inner lining of the lower eyelid. Cyanosis may be present generally, or in the lips, ears, and nail beds. Jaundice may be seen first in the sclera of the eye, but can become generalized. Redness may be generalized from a hot environment, fever, or exertion. Excessive dryness can have several causes, the most frequent of which is dehydration. Excessive sweating is an indication of exertion, a hot environment, or increased sympathetic nervous system activity, possibly due to shock, myocardial infarction, or other serious conditions. Capillary refill time is the most useful tool to assess perfusion in the pediatric patient younger than three years of age. A normal return of blood flow occurs within 2 seconds of pressing and then releasing pressure from the nail bed.

18.17 Associate abnormal findings in skin color, temperature, and condition with potential underlying causes.

Pallor and mottling represent a decrease in circulation to the skin, which can occur when the patient is cold or in shock. Cyanosis means that cellular oxygenation is poor. Jaundice results from liver disease. Redness may be due to exertion or fever when generalized or may be localized to an area of injury or inflammation. Hot skin can be due to a heat-related emergency, fever, or exertion. Cool skin may be due to hypothermia or shock.

18.18 Explain factors that can affect capillary refill time.

A delay in capillary refill is an indication of poor perfusion to the peripheral tissues. This can be an indication of shock, but also can mean that the patient's hands are cold. Capillary refill time is less reliable in adults as an indication of perfusion status. Pre-existing circulatory disease, cigarette smoking, and other factors can cause a delay in capillary refill in adults.

18.19 Differentiate among normal, dilated, and constricted pupils.

Normal pupil size varies according to light levels, distance from objects being viewed, and the degree of stimulation of the sympathetic and parasympathetic nervous systems. Dilated pupils are unusually large in diameter without a cause such as low ambient light levels, while constricted pupils are unusually small in diameter.

18.20 Recognize anisocoria (inequality of pupils) greater than 2 mm.

The pupils should be equal in size. Anisocoria of 2 mm or greater is of concern. Unequal pupils can be a result of injury to one eye, or a sign of increased ICP.

18.21 Assess the pupils for size, equality, and reactivity to light.

Under normal circumstances, the pupils dilate in dim light and constrict in bright light. The pupils react consensually, which means that when you shine a light into one eye, both pupils constrict at the same time.

18.22 Associate abnormal pupil findings with potential underlying causes.

Complete relaxation of the iris occurs in cerebral hypoxia and death, resulting in the pupils being dilated and nonreactive to light (fixed). Drugs that block the parasympathetic nervous system prevent the pupils from constricting and allow the sympathetic nervous system to control pupil size. Eye drops containing medications that block the parasympathetic nervous system are used to dilate the pupils to allow examination of the retina in the back of the eye. Bright light, some narcotic drugs, and substances that stimulate the parasympathetic nervous system cause pupil constriction. One group of substances that stimulates the parasympathetic nervous system is organophosphate pesticides, which are also potential terrorist weapons. Epinephrine and atropine, two drugs used in cardiac resuscitation, also dilate the pupils, making examination of the pupils unreliable in patients who have received them.

18.23 Explain the underlying physiological processes being evaluated by measuring systolic and diastolic blood pressure.

Blood pressure is the amount of force exerted against the walls of the arteries by the blood flowing through them. A certain amount of pressure is necessary for blood to circulate from the heart, through the miles of blood vessels in the body and back to the heart again. Systolic blood pressure corresponds to the higher pressure associated with ventricular contraction and the diastolic blood pressure corresponds to the lower pressure associated with ventricular relaxation, or diastole.

18.24 Demonstrate the proper techniques of obtaining blood pressure by auscultation, palpation, and noninvasive blood pressure monitoring.

Refer to the skills checklists at the end of the workbook chapter.

18.25 Relate the methods, techniques, and equipment for obtaining a blood pressure measurement to differences in findings and potential errors in blood pressure measurement.

You can obtain blood pressure manually by auscultation or palpation, or you can use an automatic blood pressure cuff. The cuff size must be the proper size for the patient to prevent errors in measurement, and you must palpate the radial pulse while manually inflating the cuff to avoid missing the first of the Korotkoff sounds.

18.26 Determine whether a blood pressure value is consistent with expected values for the patient's age and gender.

Normal blood pressure in females is often lower than in males. Blood pressure is not routinely measured in patients younger than three years old. The normal range of systolic blood pressure for patients in various age groups is as follows:

- Adults: less than 120 mmHg
- Adolescents: 88 to 120 mmHg
- School age: 80 to 115 mmHg
- Preschooler: 78 to 105 mmHg
- Toddler: 72 to 100 mmHg
- Infant: 70 to 90 mmHg
- Newborn: 70 to 90 mmHg

18.27 Use the blood pressure value to find the patient's pulse pressure and mean arterial pressure (MAP).

Pulse pressure is calculated by subtracting the diastolic pressure value from the systolic pressure. Mean arterial pressure (MAP) is the average amount of pressure in the arterial system. A common way of estimating MAP is to add one third of the pulse pressure to the diastolic pressure.

18.28 List potential causes of abnormal findings or changes in blood pressure and pulse pressure.

Blood pressure can be affected by a number of natural processes and by medications. Pain, anxiety, fear, and fever can raise the blood pressure. Conversely, blood pressure can be lowered in a response to blood loss, dehydration, nervous system dysfunction, poor cardiac output, or other mechanisms that cause shock. Some medications can lower blood pressure, both intentionally in the case of chronic hypertension and unintentionally as in the case of medication side effects, interactions, and overdoses.

18.29 Explain the concept of orthostatic (postural) hypotension.

Orthostatic hypotension can occur when a person moves from a supine to a sitting or standing position or when he moves from a sitting to a standing position if the patient's vascular tone or vascular volume is too low to compensate for the effects of gravity (which causes blood to move toward the lower extremities). To take orthostatic vital signs, a patient must be lying in a supine position for 3 minutes before measuring the blood pressure and heart rate. After the patient stands for 3 minutes, the blood pressure and heart rate are checked again. Orthostatic hypotension is defined as a drop in systolic blood pressure of 20 mmHg or an increase in the heart rate of 20 per minute

18.30 Given a patient scenario, determine the frequency with which vital signs should be reassessed.

The frequency with which vital signs and information from monitoring devices is reassessed depends on your determination of how critical the patient is and the treatments you are providing. Assess the critical patient's vital signs every 5 minutes, or sooner. Assess–the vital signs of a patient whose condition is noncritical every 15 minutes or at least once after obtaining the baseline. If you work in an area where some transports are only 5 to 10 minutes long, it may be sufficient to obtain baseline vital signs and one additional set of vital signs.

18.31 Explain what is being measured when pulse oximetry is used.

Pulse oximetry is a measure of the level of saturation of hemoglobin in red blood cells. While it is presumed that the hemoglobin is saturated with oxygen, it also can be saturated with carbon monoxide, resulting in falsely high readings. Pulse oximetry passes light through an area of tissue, such as the finger or earlobe, and compares the wavelength of light emitted by the device to the wavelength of light received by a sensor to measure how much light was absorbed. The normal value for a pulse oximetry reading is 95 to 99 percent.

18.32 Describe factors and limitations that should be taken into consideration when interpreting the meaning of pulse oximetry findings.

Carbon monoxide can bind with hemoglobin in the same way that oxygen does. This will produce a false value because the oximeter probe cannot differentiate what the hemoglobin is saturated with. High-intensity ambient lighting also can affect pulse oximetry readings by interfering with the light source being passed from the probe.

18.33 Explain what is being measured when capnography is used.

Capnography is a display of the measurements of exhaled carbon dioxide represented as waveforms.

18.34 Describe factors and limitations that should be taken into consideration when interpreting the meaning of capnography findings.

Circulation is required for the metabolism that produces carbon dioxide. Therefore, a low carbon dioxide reading can be an indication of inadequate circulation. Increased carbon dioxide readings can indicate hypoventilation.

18.35 Explain what is being measured when a glucometer is used.

A glucometer measures the amount of glucose in a small blood sample. The normal blood glucose level is 70 to 110 mg/dL but can be slightly higher in healthy individuals following a meal.

18.36 Use glucometry values as an adjunct in determining the need for supplemental glucose/ dextrose administration.

Glucose or dextrose should be administered to symptomatic patients with a blood glucose level less than normal (70 mg/dL, or the level specified in your protocols).

18.37 Describe factors and limitations that should be taken into consideration when interpreting the meaning of glucometry findings.

Some diabetics can be symptomatic (of hypoglycemia) despite having what appears to be a "normal" blood glucose level.

18.38 Describe the value of continuous ECG monitoring.

Looking at electrical activity in a single lead allows you to observe the heart rate, rhythm, pacemaker site, and the presence of delays or blocks in electrical conduction.

18.39 Obtain a lead II ECG rhythm.

The lead wires are attached to electrodes placed on the chest. Lead II is obtained by detecting the flow of electricity between an electrode on the right arm or shoulder and one on the lower left side of the chest (representing the left leg). Once the electrodes are placed (three to five of them, depending on the cardiac monitor model), designate lead II on the monitor and observe the screen. If a printout is desired, activate the printer to obtain a hard copy of the rhythm strip.

Resource Central

Resource Central offers extra practice and review materials in a variety of media. To access it, follow the directions on the Student Access Card provided with the Student Textbook. If there is no card, go to www.bradybooks.com and follow the Resource Central link to Buy Access.

Vocabulary and Concept Review

Exercise 1

Write the correct term in the blank that follows each definition. Note that there are more terms than definitions. (See Resource Central for more vocabulary review.)

anisocoria	cyanosis	hypotension	palpate
antecubital fossa	diastolic blood pressure	hypothermia	pyrexia
auscultate		icterus	rhonchi
bradycardia	electrocardiogram	mean arterial pressure	sphygmomanometer
capillary refill time	fever		systolic blood pressure
	hyperglycemia	palpate	
capnography	hyperpyrexia	pulse oximetry	tachycardia
capnometry	hypertension	pulse pressure	tympanic
crackles (rales)	hyperthermia	pulsus alternans	wheezes
Cushing reflex	hypoglycemia	pulsus paradoxus	vital signs

1. Mechanism of checking skin perfusion that is more reliable in children than in adults. _____

2. Increased body temperature due to infection. _____

3. Pulse, respirations, blood pressure, and temperature. _____

4. Force of blood against the arterial walls during ventricular contraction. _____

5. Unequal pupils. _____

6. High body temperature due to exertion or high environmental temperature. _____

7. Extremely high temperature, above 106°F. _____

8. Low blood sugar. _____

9. Blood pressure cuff. _____

10. What is being checked when a fold of skin is pinched up from the underlying tissues. _____

11. Flattened area over the front of the elbow. _____

12. To listen to sounds within the body. _____

13. Measuring carbon dioxide in exhaled air. _____

14. A change in skin color that indicates hypoxemia. _____

15. To use your hands to feel for signs of illness or injury. _____

16. Technique of measuring the degree of saturation of hemoglobin. _____

17. Drop in the systolic blood pressure of 10 mmHg or more on inspiration. _____

18. Type of thermometer that measures the body temperature of the eardrum. _____

19. Yellow discoloration of the sclera. _____

20. Decrease in heart rate accompanying an increase in blood pressure, particularly when intracranial pressure is increased. _____

21. Visual representation of the electrical activity of the heart. _____

22. High blood pressure. _____

23. Systolic blood pressure minus diastolic blood pressure. _____

24. Fine popping or bubbling sound heard in the lungs; an indication of fluid in the alveoli. _____

25. Heart rate greater than 100 beats per minute in an adult. _____

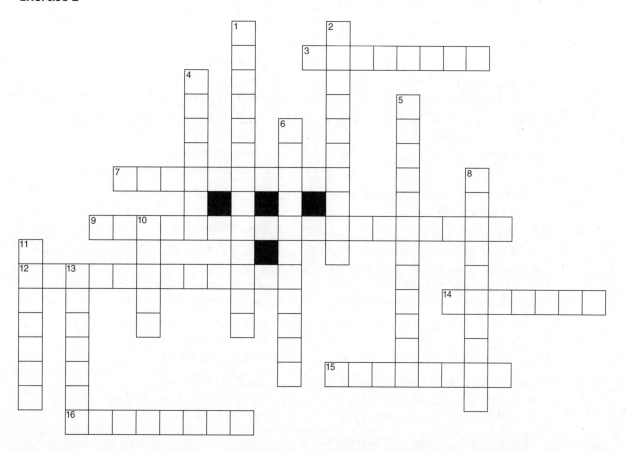

Across

3. Yellow discoloration of the skin resulting from liver disease.

7. Listening to sounds inside the body, usually wih the aid of a stethoscope.

9. An abnormality in the electrical activity of the heart in which it departs from the rules that define normal sinus rhythm.

12. Blood glucose level that is lower than normal.

14. Yellow discolration of the sclera of the eye resulting from the liver disease.

15. Bluish or purplish discoloration of the skin and tissues when there is an increased amount of desaturated hemoglobin in the blood.

16. The amount of CO_2 in exhaled air at the end of expiration.

Down

1. A higher-than-normal blood glucose level.

2. Measurement of CO_2 in expired air.

4. Coarse, rumbling sounds heard on auscultation, indicating the presence of secretions in the bronchi.

5. High blood pressure.

6. A slower than normal heart rate, which is a heart rate less than 60 per minute in adults.

8. A condition in which the pupils are unequal.

10. Fine crackling, popping sounds ausculated on inspiration, indicating fluid at the level of the terminal bronchioles and alveoli.

11. High-pitched whistling sounds that can be heard on exhalation when the bronchioles are constricted.

13. A physical examination in which the examiner uses his hands to feel for signs of illness or injury or to obtain the pulse.

Check Your Recall and Apply Concepts

Select the best possible choice for each of the following questions.

_____ 1. Which one of the following is included in assessment of the vital signs?
   a. Capnography
   b. Pulse oximetry
   c. Respiratory rate
   d. Blood glucose level

_____ 2. Which one of the following vital signs is NOT usually obtained in most patients in the prehospital setting?
   a. Blood pressure
   b. Heart rate
   c. Respiratory rate
   d. Temperature

_____ 3. An example of a central pulse is the _____ pulse.
   a. dorsalis pedis
   b. popliteal
   c. femoral
   d. posterior tibial

_____ 4. A 52-year-old patient has a strong, full, but irregular radial pulse. To most accurately obtain his heart rate, you should count the pulsations in:
   a. 10 seconds and multiply by six.
   b. 15 seconds and multiply four.
   c. 30 seconds and multiply by two.
   d. 60 seconds.

_____ 5. A patient tells you he has atrial fibrillation. You should anticipate a pulse that is:
   a. irregular.
   b. slower than normal.
   c. faster than normal.
   d. weak and thready.

_____ 6. The units in which blood pressure is measured are called:
   a. pounds per square inch (psi).
   b. centimeters of water (cmH$_2$O).
   c. millimeters of mercury (mmHg).
   d. kiloPascals (kPa).

_____ 7. Mean arterial pressure is represented by:
   a. systolic blood pressure minus diastolic blood pressure.
   b. cardiac output times systemic vascular resistance.
   c. diastolic blood pressure plus one third of the pulse pressure.
   d. stroke volume minus end-diastolic volume.

_____ 8. According to the National Heart, Lung, and Blood Institute, adult systolic blood pressure should be less than _____ mmHg.
   a. 160
   b. 140
   c. 130
   d. 120

_____ 9. When taking a blood pressure, you should inflate the blood pressure cuff to:
   a. 20 mmHg past the point where the radial pulse can no longer be palpated.
   b. 200 mmHg.
   c. the point where the Velcro starts to release.
   d. the point where no more air can be forced into the cuff.

_____ 10. The normal body temperature is about _____ degrees Celsius.
   a. 40
   b. 39
   c. 37
   d. 35

_____ 11. Of the following signs, which one is the most specific for a problem with the liver?
   a. Poor skin turgor
   b. Jaundice
   c. Diaphoresis
   d. Mottled skin

_____ 12. A patient is considered severely hypoxic when the pulse oximetry reading is _____ percent or less.
   a. 95
   b. 92
   c. 89
   d. 85

_____ 13. The normal range of end-tidal CO$_2$ is _____ mmHg.
  a. 25 to 35   c. 35 to 45
  b. 30 to 40   d. 40 to 50

_____ 14. When caring for a patient whose condition is noncritical, you should reassess him at
         intervals of no greater than _____ minutes.
  a. 5   c. 15
  b. 10   d. 30

_____ 15. Your patient is a conscious 18-year-old. Which arterial pulse point should you use to
         assess his pulse?
  a. Brachial   c. Carotid
  b. Radial   d. Popliteal

_____ 16. The normal pulse in an adult ranges from _____ beats per minute.
  a. 60 to 100   c. 60 to 80
  b. 80 to 120   d. 70 to 110

_____ 17. Which one of the following terms is best defined as the amount of force exerted against
         the walls of the arteries by the blood flowing through them?
  a. Heart rate   c. Cardiac output
  b. Pulse rate   d. Blood pressure

_____ 18. With all other physiological factors unchanged, which one of the following will result
         from increased systemic vascular resistance?
  a. Increased blood pressure   c. Increased heart rate
  b. Decreased blood pressure   d. Decreased heart rate

_____ 19. Which one of the following statements best describes the pulse pressure?
  a. Mean arterial pressure plus one third of the diastolic blood pressure
  b. Systolic blood pressure minus diastolic blood pressure
  c. Mean arterial pressure times systemic vascular resistance
  d. Diastolic blood pressure divided by mean arterial pressure

_____ 20. The exchange of oxygen and carbon dioxide between tissue cells and capillaries
         describes the process of:
  a. external respiration.   c. internal ventilation.
  b. internal respiration.   d. external ventilation.

_____ 21. The normal respiratory rate for newborns is _____ breaths per minute.
  a. 30 to 60   c. 30 to 50
  b. 20 to 40   d. 40 to 70

_____ 22. The high-pitched inspiratory sound that indicates a partial obstruction of the upper
         airway is called:
  a. stridor.   c. rhonchi.
  b. crackles (rales).   d. wheezing.

_____ 23. A lower-than-normal body temperature is called:
  a. hyperthermia.   c. hypoglycemia.
  b. hyperglycemia.   d. hypothermia.

Clinical Reasoning

CASE STUDY: A TOUCH OF LIGHTHEADEDNESS

Your unit is dispatched to the home of Mrs. Gail Hebert, who called 911 when she nearly lost consciousness after getting out of bed. When you arrive, you find the 29-year-old woman lying on her left side in bed. She looks pale, but her skin is dry and warm. She says that she has "had the flu or something" for the past day and a half, with vomiting and diarrhea. She says she was not too worried about it until she "nearly passed out," when she tried to get out of bed.

1. What do you anticipate about Mrs. Hebert's vital sign values?

_____

_____

_____

_____

_____

2. What are the considerations in whether you should assess orthostatic vital signs?

_____

_____

_____

_____

_____

3. What other monitoring devices and assessment findings would be helpful in determining Mrs. Hebert's condition?

_____

_____

_____

_____

_____

Project-Based Learning

Exercise 1

Utilize your creative and artistic talents and draw a model of the human body. Label the sites where you can assess pulses, using the name of the artery associated with each site.

Exercise 2

Draw the pattern of each one of the following respiratory patterns: eupnea, tachypnea, bradypnea, apnea, hypernea, Cheyne-Stokes, Biot's, Kussmaul's, and apneustic.

The EMS Professional In Practice

You have just taken Mr. Walker's blood pressure and obtained a reading of 182/102. Mr. Walker asks, "Well, what is my pressure today?" How should you answer? Jot down your thoughts in a notebook or journal for discussion in class or in your study group.

Skills Checklists

The following skill checklists cover the major steps of selected skills from Chapter 18. Review them prior to your laboratory classes. Practice skills only after they have been demonstrated for you in class and only under the supervision of an authorized instructor or clinical preceptor.

Advanced EMT Skill Checklist: *Auscultating a Blood Pressure*		
Skill Stimulus: The proper sequence for assessing the patient and obtaining vital signs have been established through the scene size-up and primary assessment, as well as the resources available. You have informed the patient that you are going to take his blood pressure.		
Step	**Performed**	**Not Performed**
Position the blood pressure cuff around the patient's arm with its bottom edge 1 inch above the crease of the elbow. The cuff should be snug, and the marker on the cuff should be in line with the brachial artery.		
Locate the radial pulse and keep your fingers on it. Close the valve on the inflation bulb.		
Inflate the cuff by squeezing the bulb several times quickly and firmly while watching the needle on the gauge. Inflate the cuff 20 mmHg past the point where the radial pulse disappears.		
With the earpieces of the stethoscope in your ears, place the diaphragm of the stethoscope over the patient's brachial artery.		
Listen and watch the gauge while slowly opening the valve on the inflation valve to deflate the cuff at a rate of 5 to 10 mmHg per second while listening for the Korotkoff sounds.		
Quickly release the remaining air from the cuff.		
Record the systolic and diastolic blood pressure.		
Skill Completion: The systolic and diastolic blood pressures have been obtained and recorded.		

Advanced EMT Skill Checklist: *Palpating a Blood Pressure*

Skill Stimulus: The proper sequence for assessing the patient and obtaining vital signs have been established through the scene size-up and primary assessment, as well as the resources available. You have been unable to obtain a blood pressure by auscultation.

Step	Performed	Not Performed
Position the blood pressure cuff around the patient's arm with its bottom edge 1 inch above the crease of the elbow. The cuff should be snug, and the marker on the cuff should be in line with the brachial artery.		
Locate the radial pulse and keep your fingers on it. Close the valve on the inflation bulb.		
Inflate the cuff by squeezing the bulb several times quickly and firmly while watching the needle on the gauge. Inflate the cuff 20 mmHg past the point where the radial pulse disappears.		
Keeping your fingers over the site where you last palpated the radial pulse, watch the gauge while slowly opening the valve on the inflation valve to deflate the cuff at a rate of 5 to 10 mmHg per second. Note the location of the needle on the gauge when the radial pulse reappears.		
Quickly release the remaining air from the cuff.		
Record the systolic blood pressure, noting that the reading was obtained by palpation.		

Skill Completion: The systolic blood pressure has been obtained and recorded.

History Taking, Secondary Assessment, and Reassessment

Content Area

- Assessment

Advanced EMT Education Standard

- Applies scene information and patient assessment findings (scene size-up, primary and secondary assessments, patient history, and reassessment) to guide emergency management.

Summary of Objectives

19.1   Define key terms introduced in this chapter.

Knowing and being able to apply the key terms in each chapter is critical to understanding chapter concepts. Write the list of key terms. Then write the definition of each one in your own words. Check your understanding by confirming the definitions in the textbook glossary. Correct any misunderstandings. Create a study aid by writing each key term on the front of an index card and the definition on the back. Use the cards to quiz yourself-or to have someone quiz you. The exercises under Vocabulary and Concept Review below will give you additional practice.

19.2   Determine a patient's chief complaint.

The patient's chief complaint is his statement, in his own words, of the reason he is requesting medical help.

19.3   Given a scenario, efficiently elicit an adequate patient history using both closed and open-ended questions, as well as active listening techniques.

Work from the patient's presenting problem or chief complaint to obtain a history. Open-ended questions allow the patient to reveal information in his own way, allowing you to get a greater depth and breadth of information. Closed questions help direct the patient toward particular topics so that you can get specific answers. Active listening techniques, such as listening for meaning and clarification, help improve communication.

19.4 Use the mnemonics SAMPLE and OPQRST to ensure that a complete prehospital patient history has been obtained.

SAMPLE serves as a useful checklist to make sure you have obtained a complete history. The letters stand for symptoms, allergies, medications, past medical history, last oral intake, and events leading to the problem. OPQRST provides a framework for asking about the patient's chief complaint. It stands for onset, provocation, quality, radiation, severity, and time.

19.5 React appropriately when confronted with the need to ask questions about sensitive topics or when caring for patients who present special challenges to the history-taking and assessment processes.

Use discretion in when and how you ask questions that could be of a sensitive or personal nature, such as questions about drug abuse, alcohol use, or sexual activity. Those questions are best asked in private, and you must ask them objectively and respond to them nonjudgmentally. Pay attention to the patient's reactions to the questions. Be alert to indications of language barriers and sensory impairments, or changes in mental status that can present challenges to communication.

19.6 Differentiate between relevant and less relevant patient history questions in the prehospital setting.

Relevant questions focus on the patient's chief complaint and the need to elaborate portions of the history that are related to the chief complaint. Knowledge of anatomy, physiology, and pathophysiology serves as a guide to the relevance of your line of questioning. An exhaustive or "shotgun" approach to history taking uses valuable time and can interfere with putting together related details.

19.7 Given a variety of patient scenarios, adapt your approach to the secondary assessment to meet the demands of the situation.

Secondary assessments focus on the physical examination, medical history, and vital signs. The process is altered depending upon the nature of the problem (trauma or medical) and the severity of the patient's condition (critical or noncritical). In general, the history is the key to determining the problem in medical patients and is performed first, after immediate threats to life are addressed in the primary assessment. A rapid physical examination is performed for critical trauma and medical patients to identify immediately life-threatening problems that were not detected in the primary assessment. Critical trauma patients receive a head-to-toe physical examination, while noncritical trauma patients and medical patients usually require only a focused physical examination.

19.8 Given a variety of patient scenarios, differentiate between normal and abnormal findings in the secondary assessment.

Understanding anatomy, physiology, and pathophysiology are important in being able to differentiate between normal and abnormal findings. Experience in assessing a variety of healthy and sick patients helps you refine the ability to differentiate between normal and abnormal findings.

19.9 Provide possible explanations for abnormal secondary assessment findings.

Specific findings are often highly associated with certain conditions. When certain findings are noted, they should prompt further focused investigation. For example, jaundice is highly associated with liver disease; pale, cool, diaphoretic skin is an indication of shock; and fever is often an indication of infection.

19.10 Recognize critical findings in the secondary assessments of medical and trauma patients.

Critical findings include altered mental status or other neurological deficits, and any indication of a problem with the airway, breathing, and circulation. For example, a bruise on the chest wall is an indication of internal injury that can interfere with breathing or be a source of internal bleeding. Abdominal pain and tenderness are often indications of serious underlying illness or injury.

19.11 Explain the anatomical and body system approaches to secondary assessment.

The anatomical approach to a secondary assessment proceeds from head to toe, focusing on each anatomical region of the body. The approach is best used when the patient's problem is unknown or there is a potential for multiple systems to be involved. A body systems approach focuses on assessment of the body system or systems that are related to the patient's chief complaint. For example, in a medical patient with a chief complaint of difficulty breathing, your assessment will focus on the respiratory and cardiovascular systems, which are the two systems most likely to be involved in the pathophysiology of difficulty breathing.

19.12 Compare and contrast the approaches to the secondary assessment in medical and trauma patients.

For a critical trauma patient, the secondary assessment begins with a rapid trauma examination, which focuses on the head, neck, torso (chest, abdomen, back), pelvis, and major extremity trauma. Vital signs and history are integrated according to the resources available. A set of baseline vital signs is obtained, and vital signs are reassessed every 5 minutes, or sooner, if needed. A thorough head-to-toe examination is also called for, but you must not delay on the scene to perform it. It is often best done en route to the hospital. Integrate the use of monitoring devices, such as blood glucose monitoring and pulse oximetry, according to the patient's condition and the resources available.

For a noncritical trauma patient, the secondary assessment is focused on the patient's chief complaint. That is, you perform a focused physical examination. For those patients, also obtain a medical history and vital signs. Reassess the patient every 15 minutes, or sooner, if needed.

For critical medical patients, the approach depends on whether the problem is known or unknown. The history is very often the key to determining the problem in medical patients. You should perform a rapid medical examination to identify any immediately life-threatening problems in all critical medical patients and obtain baseline and repeat (every 5 minutes or sooner) vital signs. If the patient is conscious, the chief complaint (such as chest pain, headache, or difficulty breathing) should guide the assessment. A thorough head-to-toe examination may be useful if the nature of the problem has not been identified through the history and rapid medical examination. Integrate the use of monitoring devices, such as blood glucose determination and pulse oximetry, as indicated by the patient's condition and resources available.

For noncritical medical patients, obtain a history and vital signs and perform a focused physical examination. Reassess the patient every 15 minutes, or sooner, if needed.

19.13 Compare primary and secondary assessment findings with reassessment findings to identify changes in the patient's condition.

Reassessment is a process of repeating tests and examinations performed as part of the primary and secondary assessments and of evaluating the effects of treatment. The goal is to detect the trends of the patient's condition, to determine if he is improving, deteriorating, or stable. Reassessment also may reveal new concerns that were overlooked in the first assessment.

19.14 Integrate history taking into the patient assessment process.

The patient's medical history is always relevant, but the point at which it is obtained and the focus of the history can vary, depending on the patient's condition and chief complaint. For example, a routine history based on the mnemonics SAMPLE and OPQRST will most likely be sufficient in the patient who is complaining of knee pain after tripping on the sidewalk and falling. However, in a patient who is anxious, cool, pale, diaphoretic, and complaining of chest pressure, attempt to collect more information about cardiovascular disease risk factors. A thorough history can be the key to revealing the problem in medical patients. In both medical and trauma patients, the history helps predict potential complications.

19.15 Integrate findings of the scene size-up, primary and secondary assessments, and patient history to formulate an overall impression of the patient's condition and make transport decisions.

You will make an initial decision about what you should do on the scene to treat your patient and how quickly you should initiate transport based on information from the scene size-up and primary assessment. The patient's priority for transport can change, based on treatment or changes in his condition. Always be prepared to revise your initial decision about transport priority. Decision making at this phase of patient care also includes considering the need for advanced life support (ALS) response or intercept, the need for air medical transportation, and the best destination for the patient. In selecting the mode of transport and destination, you must weigh the capabilities of the resources against the time needed to reach them (or for the resources to reach the patient) and the likely consequences to the patient's condition.

19.16 Communicate pertinent patient assessment findings to other health care providers orally and in writing.

You must communicate vital information concisely and clearly to obtain orders, to allow the receiving hospital to properly prepare, and to safely transfer the patient's care to another health care provider. Radio reports, hand-off reports, and the patient care report are all ways to communicate patient information, including the patient's basic demographic information, chief complaint or presenting problem, pertinent positive and negative findings in the assessment and history, treatment provided, and results of reassessment.

Resource Central

Resource Central offers extra practice and review materials in a variety of media. To access it, follow the directions on the Student Access Card provided with the Student Textbook. If there is no card, go to www.bradybooks.com and follow the Resource Central link to Buy Access.

Vocabulary and Concept Review

Exercise 1

Write the letter of the correct definition in the blank next to the term. (See Resource Central for more vocabulary review.)

1. _____ crepitus

    a. Pain that occurs after the pressure of palpation is released

2. _____ ecchymosis

    b. Blue, purple, or black discoloration under the skin from bleeding; a bruise

3. _____ field impression

    c. Sign or symptom that is expected to accompany a particular problem, but is not present

4. _____ incontinence

    d. Indication of illness or injury that can be objectively observed

5. _____ paradoxical movement

    e. Loss of bladder control

6. _____ pertinent negative

    f. Crackling or grating sound within the body, such as bone fragments rubbing together

7. _____ pronator drift

    g. Pain that occurs in another part of the body instead of the part in which the problem originates

8. _____ radiation

    h. Movement of a segment of the chest wall in the opposite direction of the rest of the chest wall during inspiration and expiration

9. _____ rebound tenderness

    i. EMS provider's provisional diagnosis of a patient's medical problem on which the medical treatment plan is based

10. _____ referred pain

    j. Extension of pain from its origin to include other areas of the body

11. _____ sign

    k. Subjective sensation of an abnormality of body function

12. _____ symptom

    l. Involuntary pronation of the hand when the patient's arms are held out in front of him due to weakness of muscles that oppose pronation

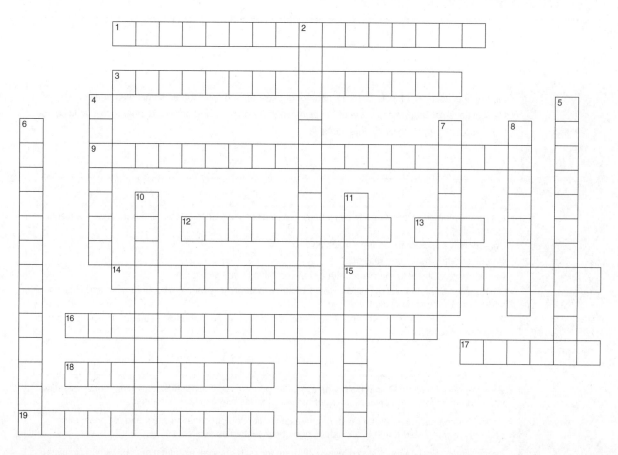

Across

1. They are reassessed every 5 minutes.
3. Understanding of the patient's immediate problems, used to make patient care decisions.
9. What you should suspect in an extremity that has the five Ps: pain, paralysis, pallor, paresthesia, and pulselessness.
12. Type of pain that arises in one location and travels to another, secondary, location.
13. An elaboration of the events surrounding the patient's current problem.
14. A heart condition that should be suspected when the jugular veins are distended.
15. Tingling sensation.
16. Assessment tool that assigns a numerical score to the patient's level of responsiveness.
17. Mnemonic used as a checklist to ensure you have obtained a thorough medical history.
18. What can happen to the trachea when there is a tension pneumothorax.
19. Periumbilical ecchymosis.

Down

2. When a patient with an injury to his head says he did not lose consciousness, you document that information as a(n)_____.
4. A collection of fluid in the abdominal cavity.
5. Type of movement in which the chest wall moves in the opposite direction than expected.
6. A sign that is so characteristic of a certain disorder that it is considered diagnostic.
7. Involuntary penile erection that can indicate spinal cord injury.
8. Type of pain that arises somewhere other than the location of the underlying problem.
10. Pain in the calf with dorsiflexion of the foot; an indication of deep vein thrombosis.
11. Visualizing the body or a part of it to look for signs of illness or injury.

Patient Assessment Review

Scene Size-Up
- Operational aspects: Identify hazards, number of patients, and need for additional resources.
- Clinical aspects: Determine nature of illness/mechanism of injury and general appearance, including age, sex, responsive or apparently unresponsive.

Primary Assessment
- Apparently unresponsive: Quickly confirm level of responsiveness and determine presence or absence of breathing.
- Unresponsive and not breathing: Check pulse.
- No pulse: Start chest compressions.
- Pulse present: Check for problems with airway, breathing, and circulation.
- Responsive: Confirm level of responsiveness; check for problems with airway, breathing, and circulation; and determine chief complaint.
- Perform interventions for airway, breathing, and circulation; and determine whether patient 's condition is critical or noncritical.

Secondary Assessment
- Critical medical patient: Obtain history as available, perform rapid medical examination, obtain baseline vitals and use monitoring devices, and perform head-to-toe examination as needed.
- Critical trauma patient: Perform rapid trauma examination, obtain baseline vitals and use monitoring devices, perform head-to-toe examination, and obtain history as available.
- Noncritical medical patient: Obtain history, perform focused physical examination, and obtain baseline vitals and use monitoring devices.
- Noncritical trauma patient: Perform focused physical examination, obtain baseline vitals and use monitoring devices, and obtain history.

Reassessment
- Primary assessment (level of responsiveness, airway, breathing, and circulation)
- Vital signs and monitoring devices
- Aspects of physical examination
- Changes in complaints
- Specific effects of treatment

FIGURE 19-1 Overview of the Patient Assessment Process.

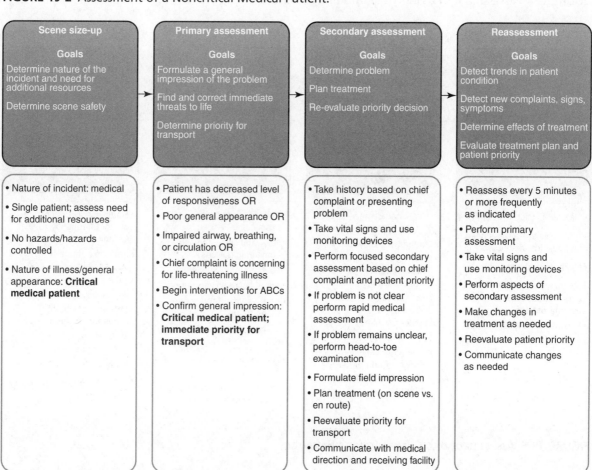

FIGURE 19-2 Assessment of a Noncritical Medical Patient.

Figure 19-2: Assessment of a Noncritical Medical Patient

Scene size-up

Goals
Determine nature of the incident and need for additional resources

Determine scene safety

- Nature of incident: medical
- Single patient; assess need for additional resources
- No hazards/hazards controlled
- Nature of illness/general appearance: **Noncritical medical patient**

Primary assessment

Goals
Formulate a general impression of the problem

Find and correct immediate threats to life

Determine priority for transport

- Patient is alert AND
- Has good general appearance AND
- No impairment of airway, breathing, or circulation AND
- Chief complaint is not concerning for life-threatening illness
- Confirm general impression: **Noncritical medical patient; transport may be delayed for further assessment and treatment**

Secondary assessment

Goals
Determine problem

Plan treatment

Re-evaluate priority decision

- Take history based on chief complaint or presenting problem
- Take vital signs and use monitoring devices
- Perform focused secondary assessment based on chief complaint and patient priority
- Formulate field impression
- Plan treatment and transport
- Reevaluate priority for transport
- Communicate with medical direction and receiving facility as needed

Reassessment

Goals
Detect trends in patient condition

Detect new complaints, signs, symptoms

Determine effects of treatment

Evaluate treatment plan and patient priority

- Reassess every 15 minutes or more frequently as indicated
- Perform primary assessment
- Take vital signs and use monitoring devices
- Perform aspects of secondary assessment
- Make changes in treatment as needed
- Reevaluate patient priority
- Communicate changes as needed

Figure 19-3: Assessment of a Critical Medical Patient

Scene size-up

Goals
Determine nature of the incident and need for additional resources

Determine scene safety

- Nature of incident: medical
- Single patient; assess need for additional resources
- No hazards/hazards controlled
- Nature of illness/general appearance: **Critical medical patient**

Primary assessment

Goals
Formulate a general impression of the problem

Find and correct immediate threats to life

Determine priority for transport

- Patient has decreased level of responsiveness OR
- Poor general appearance OR
- Impaired airway, breathing, or circulation OR
- Chief complaint is concerning for life-threatening illness
- Begin interventions for ABCs
- Confirm general impression: **Critical medical patient; immediate priority for transport**

Secondary assessment

Goals
Determine problem

Plan treatment

Re-evaluate priority decision

- Take history based on chief complaint or presenting problem
- Take vital signs and use monitoring devices
- Perform focused secondary assessment based on chief complaint and patient priority
- If problem is not clear perform rapid medical assessment
- If problem remains unclear, perform head-to-toe examination
- Formulate field impression
- Plan treatment (on scene vs. en route)
- Reevaluate priority for transport
- Communicate with medical direction and receiving facility

Reassessment

Goals
Detect trends in patient condition

Detect new complaints, signs, symptoms

Determine effects of treatment

Evaluate treatment plan and patient priority

- Reassess every 5 minutes or more frequently as indicated
- Perform primary assessment
- Take vital signs and use monitoring devices
- Perform aspects of secondary assessment
- Make changes in treatment as needed
- Reevaluate patient priority
- Communicate changes as needed

FIGURE 19-3 Assessment of a Critical Medical Patient.

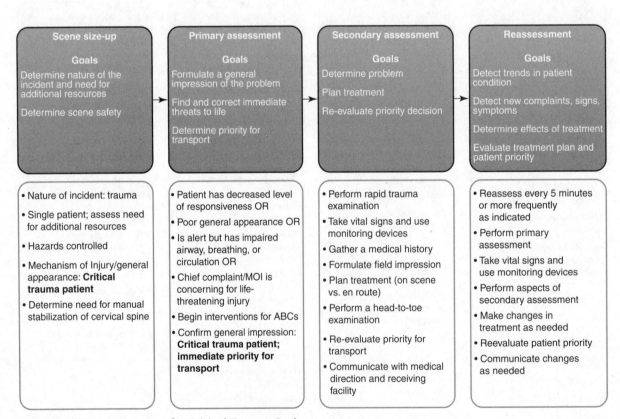

Scene size-up	Primary assessment	Secondary assessment	Reassessment
Goals Determine nature of the incident and need for additional resources Determine scene safety	**Goals** Formulate a general impression of the problem Find and correct immediate threats to life Determine priority for transport	**Goals** Determine problem Plan treatment Re-evaluate priority decision	**Goals** Detect trends in patient condition Detect new complaints, signs, symptoms Determine effects of treatment Evaluate treatment plan and patient priority
• Nature of incident: trauma • Single patient; assess need for additional resources • No hazards/hazards controlled • Mechanism of Injury/general appearance: **Noncritical trauma patient**	• Patient is alert AND • Has good general appearance AND • No impairment of airway, breathing, or circulation AND • Chief complaint/MOI is not concerning for life-threatening injury • Confirm general impression: **Noncritical trauma patient; transport may be delayed for further assessment and treatment**	• Perform a focused examination based on chief complaint or presenting problem • Take vital signs and use monitoring devices • Gather a medical history • Formulate field impression • Plan treatment and transport • Reevaluate priority for transport • Communicate with medical direction and receiving facility as needed	• Reassess every 15 minutes or more frequently as indicated • Perform primary assessment • Take vital signs and use monitoring devices • Perform aspects of secondary assessment • Make changes in treatment as needed • Reevaluate patient priority • Communicate changes as needed

FIGURE 19-4 Assessment of a Noncritical Trauma Patient.

Scene size-up	Primary assessment	Secondary assessment	Reassessment
Goals Determine nature of the incident and need for additional resources Determine scene safety	**Goals** Formulate a general impression of the problem Find and correct immediate threats to life Determine priority for transport	**Goals** Determine problem Plan treatment Re-evaluate priority decision	**Goals** Detect trends in patient condition Detect new complaints, signs, symptoms Determine effects of treatment Evaluate treatment plan and patient priority
• Nature of incident: trauma • Single patient; assess need for additional resources • Hazards controlled • Mechanism of Injury/general appearance: **Critical trauma patient** • Determine need for manual stabilization of cervical spine	• Patient has decreased level of responsiveness OR • Poor general appearance OR • Is alert but has impaired airway, breathing, or circulation OR • Chief complaint/MOI is concerning for life-threatening injury • Begin interventions for ABCs • Confirm general impression: **Critical trauma patient; immediate priority for transport**	• Perform rapid trauma examination • Take vital signs and use monitoring devices • Gather a medical history • Formulate field impression • Plan treatment (on scene vs. en route) • Perform a head-to-toe examination • Re-evaluate priority for transport • Communicate with medical direction and receiving facility	• Reassess every 5 minutes or more frequently as indicated • Perform primary assessment • Take vital signs and use monitoring devices • Perform aspects of secondary assessment • Make changes in treatment as needed • Reevaluate patient priority • Communicate changes as needed

FIGURE 19-5 Assessment of a Critical Trauma Patient.

Check Your Recall and Apply Concepts

Select the best possible choice for each of the following questions.

_____ 1. A 52-year-old patient is complaining of heaviness in his chest and difficulty breathing. He was using a handsaw to cut down a small tree in his yard when the discomfort began. He is pale and sweating profusely. This patient should be initially classified as:
   a. noncritical, medical.
   b. critical, medical.
   c. noncritical, trauma.
   d. critical, trauma.

_____ 2. A 21-year-old woman was the unrestrained driver of a vehicle that was struck by another vehicle on the freeway and then struck the concrete divider on the highway. The patient was ejected through the windshield and landed on the pavement. Your primary assessment found that she responds to pain with rigid extension of the extremities, that she has blood in her airway despite repeated suctioning by the first-responding EMTs, irregular respirations, and a strong carotid pulse of 58 beats per minute. Which one of the following should you direct your team to do next?
   a. Apply a cervical collar and immobilize the patient to a long backboard.
   b. Apply a nonrebreather mask with oxygen at 15 L/min and keep suctioning.
   c. Insert a Combitube or supraglottic airway device and ventilate the patient.
   d. Perform a rapid trauma examination.

_____ 3. A 41-year-old woman became disoriented at work and started behaving strangely. When you arrive, her coworker tells you the patient is a diabetic. The patient is awake, but disoriented to person, place, and time. She is pale with cool, moist skin. Her respirations are 20 breaths per minute and regular, and her radial pulse is thready and rapid. Which one of the following should you do first?
   a. Get a complete medical history.
   b. Obtain baseline vital signs.
   c. Perform a rapid medical examination.
   d. Obtain a blood glucose level.

_____ 4. A 6-year-old child jumped out of a swing from a height of about 4 feet off the ground and landed on his outstretched hands. He has an obvious deformity of his right forearm. He is awake and crying. His skin is warm and moist, and his color is normal. His radial pulse on the uninjured side is strong and regular at a rate of 112 beats per minute. There are no other obvious signs of injury. Which one of the following should you do first?
   a. Obtain the patient's chief complaint.
   b. Perform a rapid trauma examination.
   c. Perform a head-to-toe examination.
   d. Obtain a set of baseline vital signs.

_____ 5. Which one of the following is a symptom?
   a. Deformity of the ankle
   b. Falling from a balcony
   c. Back pain
   d. Laceration on the hand

_____ 6. Which one of the following is the best example of an open-ended question?
   a. What is bothering you today?
   b. Does it hurt when I push on your belly?
   c. On a scale from zero to ten, with zero being no pain and 10 being the worst pain, how badly does your hip hurt?
   d. Is the pain in your side sharp or dull?

_____ 7. A patient states that her back pain is better when she is up and walking around. With respect to the patient's back pain, walking is considered a(n) _____ factor.
   a. provoking
   b. palliating
   c. pertinent negative
   d. pathognomonic

_____ 8. A patient is found prone on the sidewalk with a gunshot wound to his forehead. He is unresponsive and in respiratory arrest. In your patient care report, you should document the gunshot wound as the patient's:
   a. chief complaint.
   b. past medical history.
   c. diagnosis.
   d. presenting problem.

_____ 9. Which one of the following could you find using the examination technique of inspection?
   a. Musty body odor
   b. Icterus
   c. Crackles (rales)
   d. Crepitus

_____ 10. Jugular vein distention is of concern if it is noted when the patient is positioned:
   a. sitting at a 45-degree angle or higher.
   b. lying supine.
   c. sitting at a 30-degree angle or lower.
   d. in the recovery position.

_____ 11. All of the following should be considered with a finding of jugular vein distention EXCEPT:
   a. hypovolemic shock.
   b. pericardial tamponade.
   c. tension pneumothorax.
   d. heart failure.

_____ 12. You press on the lower right quadrant of your patient's abdomen. When you release the pressure, the patient winces and says, "Oh man! It didn't hurt when you pressed down but it hurt like heck when you let up." You should document this finding as:
   a. referred pain.
   b. radiating pain.
   c. voluntary guarding.
   d. rebound tenderness.

_____ 13. You ask a patient to close her eyes and hold her arms straight out in front of her, palms up. What are you checking for?
   a. Glasgow Coma Scale score
   b. Pronator drift
   c. Homan's sign
   d. Paresthesia

_____ 14. Which one of the following adult patients has a critical mechanism of injury?
   a. Involved in a rollover motor vehicle collision
   b. Stab wound to the hand
   c. Fell from a 5-foot deck onto the ground
   d. Hit a barrier with a motorcycle at a speed of 10 mph and fell off the motorcycle

_____ 15. Pain that is intense and well localized, often described as "sharp," is most consistent with _____ pain.
   a. visceral
   b. colicky
   c. somatic
   d. neuropathic

_____ 16. Your partner asks a 15-year-old girl complaining of lower right quadrant abdominal pain to stand on her tip-toes and then drop sharply onto her heels. Your partner is checking for:
   a. the patient's ability to follow directions.
   b. a possible blood clot in the leg.
   c. inflammation of the peritoneum.
   d. signs of stroke.

_____ 17. While assessing a patient's breathing, you find that he has a fecal odor to his breath. That finding should increase your suspicion that the patient is suffering from:
   a. gangrene.
   b. diabetic ketoacidosis.
   c. cyanide poisoning.
   d. a bowel obstruction.

_____ 18. A finding of pupils that are unequal with 2 mm or greater difference in size should make you suspect:
   a. narcotic overdose.
   b. hypoxia.
   c. traumatic brain injury.
   d. organophosphate exposure.

Clinical Reasoning

CASE STUDY: 49-YEAR-OLD MAN WITH CHEST PAIN

You and your partner, Tiffany, have just arrived on the scene for a report of chest pain. The location is a residence and your patient is 49-year-old Marvin Knight. It is a quiet residential street with no traffic as you pull up to the curb. There are no bystanders, unusual noises, or other indications of danger at the scene. Once you are on the porch, you see that the door is open and you see Mr. Knight sitting on a chair in the living room, looking worried and uncomfortable. He is rubbing the center of his chest and tells you he thinks he has bad indigestion, but he wants you to check him out, just to be sure.

1. What are the initial considerations in determining whether Mr. Knight is critical or noncritical?

_____

_____

_____

_____

_____

2. How does your decision about whether the patient's condition is critical or noncritical affect the priorities and sequence of your history and physical examination?

_____

_____

_____

_____

_____

_____

Project-Based Learning

Create a table to compare and contrast the approach to each part of the patient assessment process in critical and noncritical medical patients and critical and noncritical trauma patients. In each row of the table, be sure to show the similarities and differences among the four categories of patients.

The EMS Professional in Practice

Upon arriving at a movie theater for a report of a sick person, you and your partner are directed to the ladies restroom. Your patient is a 20-year-old woman who is lying on a bench. There is a middle-aged woman patting her hand and telling her she will be alright. There are several other women in the restroom looking to see what is going on. The patient is awake, but is pale and shaking and is complaining of lower abdominal pain. She seems hesitant to answer questions. What will you do to gain the patient's confidence and encourage her to be more forthcoming? Jot down your thoughts in a notebook or journal for discussion in class or in your study group.

Skills Checklists

The following skill checklists cover the major steps of selected skills from Chapter 19. Review them prior to your laboratory classes. Practice skills only after they have been demonstrated for you in class and only under the supervision of an authorized instructor or clinical preceptor.

Advanced EMT Skill Checklist: *Assessment—Noncritical Medical Patient*		
Skill Stimulus: Scene size-up and primary assessment establish that the patient is a noncritical medical patient.		
Step	**Performed**	**Not Performed**
Obtain a history based on chief complaint or presenting problem.		
Assess vital signs.		
Use monitoring devices as appropriate to the situation.		
Perform a focused secondary assessment.		
Skill Completion: A field impression and treatment plan are established.		

Advanced EMT Skill Checklist: *Assessment—Critical Medical Patient*		
Skill Stimulus: Scene size-up and primary assessment establish that the patient is a critical medical patient.		
Step	**Performed**	**Not Performed**
Obtain a history based on chief complaint or presenting problem.		
Assess vital signs.		
Use monitoring devices as appropriate to the situation.		
Perform a focused secondary assessment.		
If the problem is not clear, perform a rapid medical examination.		
If the problem remains unclear, perform a head-to-toe examination.		
Skill Completion: A field impression and treatment plan are established.		

Advanced EMT Skill Checklist: *Assessment—Noncritical Trauma Patient*		
Skill Stimulus: Scene size-up and primary assessment establish that the patient is a noncritical trauma patient.		
Step	Performed	Not Performed
Perform a focused secondary assessment based on the chief complaint or presenting problem.		
Take vital signs and use monitoring devices as appropriate to the situation.		
Gather a medical history.		
Skill Completion: **A field impression and treatment plan are established.**		

Advanced EMT Skill Checklist: *Assessment—Critical Trauma Patient*		
Skill Stimulus: Scene size-up and primary assessment establish that the patient is a critical trauma patient.		
Step	**Performed**	**Not Performed**
Perform a rapid trauma examination.		
Take vital signs and use monitoring devices as appropriate to the situation.		
Perform a head-to-toe examination (en route to hospital)		
Skill Completion: A field impression and treatment plan are established.		

Advanced EMT Skill Checklist: *Assessment—Head-to-Toe Exam*		
Skill Stimulus: Patient is a critical trauma patient or critical medical patient in whom the problem has not been established.		
Step	**Performed**	**Not Performed**
Inspect and palpate the patient's head.		
Inspect and palpate the patient's face.		
Inspect the ears.		
Inspect the mouth.		
Inspect and palpate the neck.		
Inspect and palpate the chest.		
Auscultate the breath sounds		
Inspect and palpate the abdomen.		
Inspect and gently compress the pelvis.		
Inspect and palpate the upper extremities.		
Assess the upper extremities for distal pulse, motor function, and sensation.		
Inspect and palpate the lower extremities.		
Assess the lower extremities for distal pulse, motor function, and sensation.		
Skill Completion: All signs of injury have been identified.		

Advanced EMT Skill Checklist: *Assessment—Rapid Physical Exam*		
Skill Stimulus: Scene size-up and primary assessment establish that the patient is a critical trauma patient or a critical medical patient in whom the problem has not been identified.		
Step	**Performed**	**Not Performed**
Expose the patient by removing or cutting clothing as needed; cover each area after it is examined to preserve patient warmth.		
Inspect and palpate the head and face.		
Inspect and palpate the patient's neck.		
Inspect, palpate, and auscultate the chest.		
Inspect and palpate the abdomen.		
Inspect and gently compress the pelvis.		
Quickly palpate and inspect the lower extremities.		
Logroll the patient and check the posterior body.		
Skill Completion: Potentially life-threatening injuries have been identified.		

20 Respiratory Disorders

Content Area

- Medicine

Advanced EMT Education Standard

- Applies fundamental knowledge to provide basic and selected advanced emergency care and transportation based on assessment findings for an acutely ill patient.

Summary of Objectives

20.1 Define key terms introduced in this chapter.

Knowing and being able to apply the key terms in each chapter is critical to understanding chapter concepts. Write the list of key terms. Then write the definition of each one in your own words. Check your understanding by confirming the definitions in the textbook glossary. Correct any misunderstandings. Create a study aid by writing each key term on the front of an index card and the definition on the back. Use the cards to quiz yourself or to have someone quiz you. The exercises under Vocabulary and Concept Review below will give you additional practice.

20.2 Explain the importance of being able to quickly recognize and treat patients with respiratory emergencies.

Patients who present in respiratory distress can deteriorate rapidly into respiratory failure and respiratory arrest. No matter what the underlying cause, death follows quickly unless measures are taken to restore ventilation and oxygenation.

20.3 Obtain an appropriate history for a patient with a respiratory problem.

The history may prompt you to check for additional signs and symptoms that provide information about the underlying cause of the problem. The patient's medications yield important clues. Regardless of whether the patient has a history of respiratory disease, heart disease, allergic reactions, recent surgery, or other medical problems play a crucial role in clinical reasoning.

20.4 Conduct an appropriate examination for a patient with a respiratory problem.

In the primary assessment, ensure that the patient has an open airway. Use manual positioning, suction, and basic adjuncts as needed. Assess the adequacy of breathing, checking for adequate air movement. In the secondary assessment, focus on things that will provide you with the most relevant information first. That includes auscultation of breath sounds, vital signs, pulse oximetry, capnometry and cardiac monitoring if available, and the patient's medical history.

20.5 Explain the relationship between dyspnea and hypoxia.

Dyspnea is an indication of a problem with breathing, which can lead to inadequate oxygenation. Hypoxia is an inadequate oxygenation of the tissues. Dyspnea is a sign of possible hypoxia.

20.6 Describe the pathophysiology by which each of the following conditions leads to inadequate oxygenation: asthma, cystic fibrosis, hyperventilation syndrome, lung cancer, obstructive pulmonary diseases, pneumonia, poisonous/toxic exposure, pulmonary edema, pulmonary embolism, spontaneous pneumothorax, and viral respiratory infections.

- *Asthma:* Causes increased inflammation, leading to swelling of the bronchioles and increased mucus production, and smooth muscle constriction of the bronchioles.
- *Cystic fibrosis:* A genetic disease that results in the production of extremely viscous mucus. In the respiratory tract, the thick secretions can obstruct the airways and lead to life-threatening infection.
- *Hyperventilation syndrome:* A condition in which the patient's minute ventilation exceeds his metabolic demands, which can lead to a drop in arterial pCO_2, which, in turn, can lead to vasospasm, including coronary vasospasm, and impaired offloading of oxygen at the cellular level.
- *Lung cancer:* Signs and symptoms depend on the disease progression, and the patient also may have respiratory depression and hypotension from high doses of narcotic medications.
- *Obstructive pulmonary diseases:* Chronic bronchitis causes production of more mucus than normal, which can impair ventilation and oxygenation. Emphysema causes extensive destruction of the walls of the alveoli, resulting in reduced surface area for gas exchange.
- *Pneumonia:* A condition in which infectious material consolidates in affected areas, preventing ventilation of part of the lung and a VQ mismatch.
- *Poisonous/toxic exposures:* Effects may be immediate, from airway obstruction, swelling, bronchospasm, inflammation, and noncardiac pulmonary edema, or can be delayed. Both ventilation and gas exchange can be impaired.
- *Pulmonary edema:* Occurs when there is an increase in interstitial fluid that increases the distance of gas diffusion between alveoli and pulmonary capillaries. Noncardiogenic pulmonary edema is caused by acute respiratory distress syndrome (ARDS) and delayed toxin-induced lung injury. Ventilation and gas exchange are affected.
- *Pulmonary embolism:* A condition in which the pulmonary arterial system is obstructed by a blood clot. This means that a portion of the lung is ventilated, but is not able to participate in gas exchange.
- *Spontaneous pneumothorax:* A condition in which air has accumulated within the pleural cavity, outside the lung, interfering with the ability of the lung to expand during inspiration. The degree of impaired ventilation and hypoxia depend on how much air has accumulated within the pleural space.
- *Viral respiratory infections:* Infections in the upper airway are rarely life threatening, but can result in obstruction. Lower airway infections can impair gas exchange.

20.7 Use patient histories and clinical presentations to differentiate among causes of respiratory emergencies.

An important consideration is the presence of pre-existing respiratory problems. Understanding the pathophysiology and risk factors for respiratory emergencies is critical in differentiating the causes of signs and symptoms.

20.8 Engage in effective clinical reasoning in order to recognize indications for the following interventions in patients with respiratory complaints/emergencies: establishing an airway, administration of oxygen, positive pressure ventilation, administration/assistance with self-administration of an inhaled beta₂ agonist, expediting transport, and ALS backup.

- *Establishing an airway:* You must be able to differentiate between adequate and inadequate air movement and respond to inadequate air movement with appropriate manual maneuvers, basic airway adjuncts, and advanced airways.
- *Administration of oxygen:* Administer oxygen to those presenting in respiratory distress and with an SpO_2 of less than 95 percent.
- *Positive pressure ventilation:* You must be able to differentiate between adequate and inadequate ventilation and be able to assist patients in severe respiratory distress, respiratory failure, and respiratory arrest with bag-valve mask ventilations.
- *Administration/assistance with self-administration of an inhaled beta₂ agonist:* Inhaled beta₂ agonists, such as albuterol, are indicated in respiratory distress due to constriction of bronchiolar smooth muscle. You must understand how a small-volume nebulizer and metered-dose inhaler work to efficiently and effectively deliver the medication when it is indicated.
- *Expediting transport:* Transport is expedited for critical patients (those who have a life-threatening problem with their airway, breathing, or circulation).
- *ALS backup:* Consider advanced life support response and transport when transport times are prolonged and when you cannot correct the underlying problem, such as an upper airway obstruction; or when advanced life support personnel can offer additional treatment to correct the underlying problem.

20.9 Given a list of patient medications, recognize medications that are associated with respiratory disease.

Medications that can indicate respiratory disease include antibiotics, anti-inflammatories (steroids, mast cell stabilizers, leukotriene inhibitors), long-acting and short-acting bronchodilators (beta₂ agonists, anticholinergics, and xanthines), cough suppressants, expectorant/mucolytics, pancreatic enzymes (may indicate cystic fibrosis), and oxygen.

20.10 Differentiate between short-acting beta₂ agonists appropriate for prehospital use and respiratory medications that are not intended for emergency use.

Short-acting medications (such as the beta₂ agonist albuterol) are administered for their immediate onset of action and short duration in the acute phase of bronchospasm. Anticholinergics, corticosteroids, anti-inflammatories, and long-acting bronchodilators often have a longer onset of action, making them ineffective in the acute phase of respiratory distress. Those medications are better suited to preventing acute exacerbations and treating the underlying inflammatory reaction.

20.11 Use reassessment to identify responses to treatment and changes in the conditions of patients presenting with respiratory complaints and emergencies.

Reassess patients whose condition is critical every 5 minutes or sooner, and reassess patient's whose condition is noncritical every 15 minutes or sooner. Reassess the mental status, airway, breathing, and circulation. Also reassess complaints, lung sounds, and vital signs, as well as other relevant aspects of the secondary assessment. Look for signs of improvement, effects of treatments, and indications of deterioration that can change your clinical impression and treatment.

Resource Central

Resource Central offers extra practice and review materials in a variety of media. To access it, follow the directions on the Student Access Card provided with the Student Textbook. If there is no card, go to www.bradybooks.com and follow the Resource Central link to Buy Access.

Vocabulary and Concept Review

Exercise 1

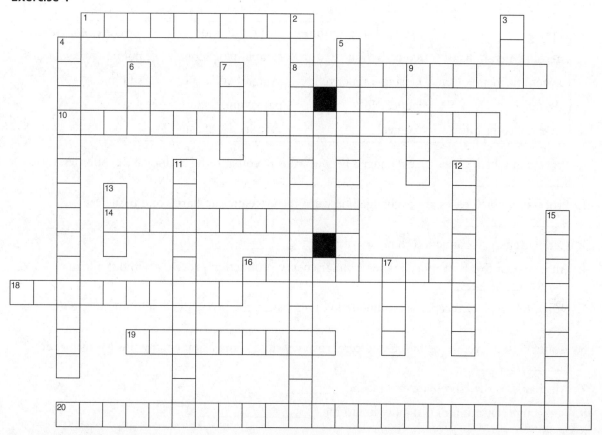

Across

1. Inflammation of the voice box, resulting in hoarseness or loss of voice.
8. Collapsed alveoli.
10. Lung collapse with progressive accumulation of air under pressure in the thoracic cavity.
14. Sore throat.
16. Impairment of either ventilation or circulation to the lung, resulting in hypoxia.
18. Its chronic form results from smoking and causes increased mucus production.
19. Type of chest pain that is often sharp in nature and worsened by inspiration.
20. Collapse of the lung in the absence of trauma.

Down

2. Severe, prolonged bronchospasm that cannot be broken with repeated doses of beta$_2$ agonsists.
3. A cold is one type.
4. Genetic disease in which mucus is thick and sticky, which can affect the lungs and gastrointestinal tract.
5. Coughing up blood.
6. Condition in which minute volume of respiration exceeds metabolic needs.
7. Condition that encompasses three types of long-standing lung disease that results in poor ventilation and gas exchange.
9. Laryngotracheobronchitis.
11. Tingling sensation.
12. Expectoration.
13. Severe lung and organ failure, often fatal, resulting from contact with infected excrement of deer mice.
15. Progressive lung disease characterized by loss of elasticity of the airways and destruction of alveoli.
17. Noncardiogenic pulmonary edema from lung injury.

Exercise 2

Write the term from the table beside its correct definition. Note that there are more terms than there are definitions.

apnea	external respiration	carbon dioxide	tension pneumothorax
aerobic metabolism	exacerbation	sympathetic alpha$_1$	pulmonary embolism
anaerobic metabolism	Hering–Breuer reflex	sympathetic beta$_2$	smoking
dyspnea	lactic acid	parasympathetic	genetics
internal respiration	oxygen	carpopedal spasm	

1. Process in which gases are exchanged between the alveoli and the pulmonary capillaries. _____

2. Process in which gases are exchanged between the systemic capillaries and tissue cells. _____

3. Cellular energy production that uses oxygen. _____

4. An excess of this is produced when cellular energy production proceeds without adequate oxygen. _____

5. When this type of receptor is stimulated in lung tissue, the bronchiolar smooth muscle relaxes. _____

6. An increased level in the blood and cerebrospinal fluid is the primary stimulus for inspiration. _____

7. Mechanisms that stimulate expiration. _____

8. Subjective sensation of difficulty breathing. _____

9. Absence of breathing. _____

10. The most common cause of emphysema and chronic bronchitis. _____

11. Sudden worsening of a chronic condition. _____

12. A blood clot that obstructs the circulation in the lungs. _____

13. Sign associated with hyperventilation syndrome. _____

Patient Assessment Review

Your patient is in respiratory distress and has signs of hypoxia. In the following table, write the features (such as signs, symptoms, typical characteristics) that help you determine whether each condition is more or less likely. This exercise is designed to help you differentiate among causes of respiratory emergencies.

Problem	Common Features
Pneumonia	
Cardiogenic pulmonary edema	
Asthma	
Pulmonary embolism	
Simple pneumothorax	
Tension pneumothorax	

Check Your Recall and Apply Concepts

Select the best possible choice for each of the following questions.

_____ 1. The tiny, hairlike cellular projections in the respiratory tract that help move foreign material trapped in mucus up and out of the airway are called:
   a. mucins.
   b. alveoli.
   c. cilia.
   d. villi.

_____ 2. The inspiratory center in the brain could be affected if there was an injury or stroke involving the:
   a. cerebral cortex.
   b. medulla oblongata.
   c. occipital lobes.
   d. cerebellum.

_____ 3. You have a patient who is 6 feet, 5 inches tall and weighs 320 pounds. What should you anticipate is his normal tidal volume?
   a. 750 to 1,000 mL
   b. 500 mL
   c. 1,000 to 1,500 mL
   d. 650 mL

_____ 4. A 65-year-old patient presents with an altered mental status. (He is awake and sitting up, but he does not speak to you or acknowledge your presence.) He also has obvious dyspnea with use of accessory muscles; cyanosis of the lips, earlobes, and nail beds; and profuse diaphoresis. He is thin and barrel chested. His respiratory rate is 30 breaths per minute, but his tidal volume is shallow. When you auscultate the chest, you can barely detect air movement. Of the following actions, which one should you do first?
   a. Assist his ventilations with a bag-valve-mask and supplemental oxygen.
   b. Determine his SpO_2 on room air.
   c. Get a history to determine the underlying problem.
   d. Apply a nonrebreather mask with oxygen at 15 L/min.

_____ 5. The cause of most cases of COPD (emphysema and chronic bronchitis) is:
   a. idiopathic.
   b. smoking.
   c. genetic.
   d. environmental.

_____ 6. In addition to oxygen administration, the primary prehospital treatment for acute exacerbation of COPD is:
   a. sympathetic $beta_2$ agonists.
   b. parasympatholytics.
   c. corticosteroids.
   d. leukotriene inhibitors.

_____ 7. The oxygen delivery device that provides very specific flow rates of oxygen and sometimes is used to treat COPD patients during prolonged transport is called a:
   a. nasal catheter.
   b. CPAP.
   c. flow-restricted oxygen-powered ventilation device.
   d. Venturi mask.

_____ 8. Your patient is a 15-year-old child with a history of asthma who began wheezing and having dyspnea while skateboarding at the park. He used a rescue inhaler repeatedly, which initially helped, but his wheezing and dyspnea have been getting progressively worse over the past 6 hours. By the time you arrive, the patient is responsive only to painful stimuli and there is no appreciable air movement at the mouth and nose, despite respiratory effort. Which one of the following should you do first?
   a. Administer 2.5 mg of albuterol by small-volume nebulizer.
   b. Apply CPAP.
   c. Insert a supraglottic airway.
   d. Begin bag-valve-mask ventilations.

_____ 9. A 28-year-old woman presents with a sudden onset of confusion and agitation. Other symptoms include cyanosis; pale, cool, diaphoretic skin; tachypnea; and a weak, rapid radial pulse. You are unable to obtain any history about the patient. Although you are anticipating abnormal lung sounds, you are surprised to hear clear, equal breath sounds. Of the following disorders, which one is most consistent with the limited information you have about the patient?

   a. Pneumonia
   b. Spontaneous pneumothorax
   c. Pulmonary embolism
   d. Status asthmaticus

_____ 10. Which one of the following would be appropriate in the treatment of a patient with suspected spontaneous pneumothorax?

   a. Nitrous oxide
   b. Oxygen by nonrebreather mask
   c. CPAP
   d. Bolus of isotonic IV fluids

_____ 11. Your patient is a 42-year-old woman who is alert, anxious, and breathing 30 times per minute with adequate tidal volume. She says she cannot catch her breath. Her skin is warm and moist with good color, her breath sounds are clear and equal bilaterally, and her SpO_2 is 100 percent on room air. She complains of sharp chest pain, lightheadedness, weakness, and tingling in her hands and around her mouth. The best initial treatment for this patient, while obtaining more information, is:

   a. starting an IV.
   b. having the patient breathe into a paper bag.
   c. reassurance.
   d. sublingual nitroglycerin.

_____ 12. Which one of the following statements concerning epiglottitis is true?

   a. Its incidence is increasing among children.
   b. It is caused by respiratory syncytial virus.
   c. It also is known as _croup_.
   d. There is an effective vaccine to prevent it.

_____ 13. Your patient is a 62-year-old man with a history of chronic bronchitis, atrial fibrillation, hypertension, and heart failure. He began taking an antibiotic two days ago for an exacerbation of chronic bronchitis. His difficulty breathing has become increasingly worse despite taking the antibiotic. He appears to be in moderate respiratory distress, using accessory muscles to breathe. His room air SpO_2 is 89 percent. You hear scattered rhonchi and wheezing throughout his lung fields. His skin is warm and moist, and his color is slightly dusky, with mild cyanosis of the lips and nail beds. He has moderate edema of both lower extremities. Which one of the following is the highest priority in the management of this patient?

   a. Administer albuterol by small-volume nebulizer.
   b. Administer oxygen by nonrebreather mask.
   c. Start an IV and give a fluid bolus.
   d. Give 0.4 mg of nitroglycerin sublingually.

Clinical Reasoning

CASE STUDY: DIFFICULTY BREATHING AT A NURSING HOME

You and your partner, Bart, are dispatched to a nursing home for difficulty breathing. When you arrive, you are directed to the room of Mr. Brian Maloney, an 82-year-old man who suffers from dementia and is paralyzed on the right side following a stroke 6 months ago. His nurse tells you that his confusion is much worse this evening and he has become progressively short of breath over the past 4 hours. Mr. Maloney has a productive cough with yellow sputum. His skin is hot and moist. His breath sounds have crackles (rales) in the lower right fields and rhonchi and wheezing on the lower left side. You notice moderate bilateral pedal edema. His vital signs are: pulse 124 and irregular, respirations 28, and blood pressure 132/88. His SpO_2 on the 4 L/min of oxygen administered by nursing home staff is 91 percent.

1. What are your hypotheses about Mr. Maloney's problem?

_____

_____

_____

_____

_____

2. What additional information will help you in your decision making?

_____

_____

_____

_____

_____

3. What are your treatment goals for this patient?

_____

_____

_____

_____

_____

Project-Based Learning

Select one respiratory disease you would like to learn more about. Write three questions about the disease. Make sure they are questions to which you would really like to find answers. For example: What is the most current research about the disease? What programs exist to help patients with the disease? What treatments are available beyond the ones discussed in this textbook?

Visit the websites of the American Lung Association (http://www.lungusa.org) and the National Heart, Lung, and Blood Institute (http://www.nhlbi.nih.gov) as a starting place for your answers. Then write the answers to the following questions in your journal or notebook:

1. What is the most interesting or useful thing you learned about the disease?

2. What are you interested in learning more about?

The EMS Professional in Practice

Examine your feelings about the role of smoking as a cause of disease. How does it affect your empathy for patients with smoking-related diseases? What is your role as a health care provider in promoting smoking cessation? How should the topic of smoking cessation be approached with patients? Jot down notes in your notebook or journal so that you are prepared to discuss the issues in class or in your study group, or consider starting a blog about it on your class learning management system.

21 Cardiovascular Emergencies

Content Area

• Medicine

Advanced EMT Education Standard

• Applies fundamental knowledge to provide basic and selected advanced emergency care and transportation based on assessment findings for an acutely ill patient.

Summary of Objectives

21.1 Define key terms introduced in this chapter.

Knowing and being able to apply the key terms in each chapter is critical to understanding chapter concepts. Write the list of key terms. Then write the definition of each one in your own words. Check your understanding by confirming the definitions in the textbook glossary. Correct any misunderstandings. Create a study aid by writing each key term on the front of an index card and the definition on the back. Use the cards to quiz yourself or to have someone quiz you. The exercises under Vocabulary and Concept Review below will give you additional practice.

21.2 Explain the relationship between electrical and mechanical events in the heart.

The electrical activity of the heart is designed to lead to mechanical contraction of the cardiac muscle. An electrical stimulus is generated in a pacemaker cell conducted to contractile cells, resulting in mechanical contraction. Calcium in the electrical cycle of the heart activates the contractile fiber system of cardiac cells, transforming the electrical activity into mechanical activity.

21.3 Describe the processes of depolarization, repolarization, and the flow of electricity through the cardiac conduction system.

Depolarization occurs when positively charged ions flow to a less positively charged area until the electrical difference between the two areas becomes zero. In repolarization, the difference in the charges is restored. Because ions must move against the typical direction of electrical flow, active cellular mechanisms (the sodium/potassium pump) that use energy in the form of ATP are required for repolarization and to maintain the polarized state (the resting potential) until the next depolarization.

21.4   Relate the waves and intervals of a normal lead-II ECG to the physiological events they represent.

The P wave represents atrial depolarization. The P-R interval is the length of time for the depolarization wave to travel through the atria and AV node. The QRS complex represents ventricular depolarization. Finally, the T wave represents ventricular repolarization. There is a small amount of energy involved in atrial repolarization, but it is covered by the waves that represent ventricular depolarization.

21.5   Discuss the relationship among hypoxia, damage to the cardiac conduction system, premature ventricular contractions, ventricular tachycardia, and ventricular fibrillation.

When higher portions of the cardiac conduction system are impaired, such as by ischemia in acute coronary syndrome, they do not function normally to initiate and conduct electrical impulses. As a compensatory mechanism, the lower areas of the cardiac conduction system are capable of initiating electrical impulses, although at a much slower than normal rate. Hypoxic cells in the ventricles can become irritable and may depolarize at random. When these ectopic pacemakers fire occasionally, it is called a premature ventricular contraction. Sometimes one or more ectopic ventricular pacemakers will fire in rapid succession in a dysrhythmia called ventricular tachycardia, which can have a pulse or be pulseless. When multiple cells in the ventricles become ectopic pacemakers, the result is chaotic electrical activity that cannot produce effective contraction of the heart, causing ventricular fibrillation.

21.6   Describe the roles of the heart and blood vessels in maintaining normal blood pressure, including the concepts of cardiac output and systemic vascular resistance.

Perfusion to the cells of the body depends on adequate blood pressure. Adequate blood pressure, in turn, depends on the volume of blood available, the output of blood from the heart, and the capacity of the blood vessels. The cardiac output is the volume of blood leaving the heart every minute, as determined by multiplying the volume of blood that leaves the heart with each contraction (stroke volume) by the number of times the heart contracts each minute (heart rate). Systemic vascular resistance is based on the diameter of small blood vessels at any given time. The more constricted the blood vessels, the smaller the diameter, which in turn means more resistance to blood flow. Mean arterial pressure is determined by the cardiac output multiplied by the systemic vascular resistance.

21.7   Explain the importance of early recognition of signs and symptoms and early treatment of patients with cardiac emergencies.

The concept behind early recognition and management of cardiac emergencies, particularly in acute coronary syndrome (ACS), is that time equals muscle. The longer a portion of the myocardium goes without adequate perfusion, the more damage that is done to the heart. In any case in which the function of the heart is impaired, systemic perfusion is decreased. The patient needs timely interventions to restore perfusion. Delays in treatment of cardiac emergencies can lead to heart failure, dysrhythmias, and out-of-hospital sudden cardiac death.

21.8   Explain the pathophysiology of the following: acute coronary syndrome including classic and unstable angina pectoris and myocardial infarction, aortic aneurysm and dissection, atherosclerosis, cardiac arrest, hypertension, left- and right-sided heart failure, and cardiogenic shock.

- *Acute coronary syndrome:* The underlying cause of ACS is usually narrowing or obstruction of a coronary artery from atherosclerotic disease. Coronary vasospasm also can result in myocardial ischemia. In ACS there is insufficient blood flow to the myocardium to meet the heart's need for oxygen. With prolonged ischemia, myocardial cells die, resulting in myocardial infarction.
- *Aortic aneurysm and dissection:* The aortic tissue can weaken as a result of long-standing hypertension and atherosclerotic disease. The pressure within the aorta causes the weakened

area to dilate. When the diameter of the aorta increases by 50 percent or more, by definition, an aortic aneurysm has developed. Dissection occurs when there is a tear in the tunica intima of the arterial wall. Blood enters the tear and creates a false lumen.

- *Atherosclerosis:* The first event in atherosclerosis development is damage of the endothelium of the tunica intima, preventing it from acting as an effective barrier between blood components and the elastic lamina and tunica media beneath it. In the second step, the damaged endothelial layer allows lipids from the bloodstream to enter and accumulate in the tissues beneath the intima. This causes lipids to be deposited into tissues, where they would normally not be, and are seen as invaders and attacked by white blood cells. The result of their interaction is foam cell deposits. The resulting plaque narrows the lumen of the artery and may rupture, causing coronary artery obstruction.

- *Cardiac arrest:* Cardiac arrest occurs when there is no cardiac output. The underlying cause may be electrical, such as a dysrhythmia that does not produce mechanical contraction, or mechanical, such as a ruptured ventricle or pericardial tamponade. Dysrhythmias implicated in sudden cardiac arrest are ventricular fibrillation, pulseless ventricular tachycardia, and asystole. Pulseless electrical activity can also occur. The result of any cause of cardiac arrest is absence of tissue perfusion. Tissues with high ischemic sensitivity, such as the brain and heart, suffer damage almost immediately and cells begin to die in as little as 4 minutes without perfusion. CPR and defibrillation are the primary treatments to restore perfusion.

- *Hypertension:* The exact mechanism of most cases of hypertension is not well understood, but problems with vascular tone and fluid and electrolyte balance contribute. Renal disease may also result in hypertension. Hypertension is one cause of damage to the endothelium of blood vessels, making it a risk factor for ACS, aortic aneurysm, and stroke.

- *Left- and right-sided heart failure and cardiogenic shock:* Right-sided heart failure can be caused by pulmonary disease and by left-sided heart failure. In chronic lung disease, there is increased resistance to pulmonary blood flow, increasing the workload of the right side of the heart. Failure of the left side of the heart, often caused by hypertension or myocardial infarction, results in pulmonary congestion, which then increases the workload of the right side of the heart. In left-sided heart failure, the increased pressure in the pulmonary circulation can result in pulmonary edema. In right-sided heart failure, ascites and pedal edema are common. When the weakened heart is no longer able to maintain adequate cardiac output and tissue perfusion is impaired, the patient is in cardiogenic shock.

21.9   Recognize cardiac emergency patients with both typical and atypical presentations.

The typical presentation includes complaints of chest pain or discomfort; pain or discomfort in the arms, shoulders, neck, or jaw; difficulty breathing; weakness; palpitations; syncope; altered mental status; nausea; vomiting; or possibly just cardiac arrest. A typical presentations include the possibility of pain or discomfort in the back, arms, jaw, or upper abdomen; a sensation of indigestion; or general weakness without the presence of the chest pain.

21.10   Differentiate between patients with adequate perfusion and patients with inadequate perfusion.

Signs of inadequate perfusion include changes in mental status, such as confusion, anxiety, or decreased responsiveness; skin that is pale or mottled and cool; diaphoresis; hypotension; and tachycardia or bradycardia. Signs of adequate perfusion include warm, dry skin that is normal in color. Normal vital signs do not rule out hypoperfusion. The body's compensatory mechanisms allow the blood pressure to remain normal despite decreased cardiac output.

21.11   Explain the importance of managing airway, breathing, and circulation and administering oxygen to patients with cardiac problems.

You must correct any problems with the airway, breathing, and circulation to improve the patient's perfusion. Poor perfusion can lead to unresponsiveness, inability to maintain the airway, and apnea. Hypoxia further impairs cardiac function and may prevent treatment for cardiac arrest, such as defibrillation, from being effective. Patients in cardiac arrest require CPR to perfuse vital organs and correction of underlying causes, such as ventricular fibrillation.

21.12 Explain the indications, contraindications, mechanism of action, side effects, dosage, and administration of the following: aspirin, nitroglycerin, nitrous oxide, and oxygen.

- Aspirin is indicated in the initial treatment of ACS and contraindicated in the presence of an allergy or sensitivity to aspirin. It works by reducing platelet aggregation, which helps prevent further clotting at the site of the plaque rupture. The dosage is 81 to 325 mg by mouth.
- Nitroglycerin is indicated in the initial and continued treatment of ACS and contraindicated in the presence of hypotension or recent use of certain medications such as those used for erectile dysfunction. It works by dilating arteries, including coronary arteries, to improve myocardial perfusion. The dosage is up to three doses of 0.4 mg spaced 3 to 5 minutes apart, sublingually, as long as the patient's systolic blood pressure is 90 mmHg or higher.
- Nitrous oxide is indicated for the treatment of chest pain and contraindicated in patients who cannot follow instructions or who are intoxicated. It is a self-administered analgesic gas, which is given by having the patient hold the mask over his face and inhaling.
- Oxygen is indicated for any situation in which ischemia or hypoxia may be present to maintain an SpO_2 of 95 percent or higher. There are no absolute contraindications in the prehospital setting, but do not administer it if there are no indications for it. Increasing the alveolar pO_2 helps with onloading of oxygen onto hemoglobin in order to increase hemoglobin saturation and increase oxygen delivery to the tissues. The dosage is 2 to 15 liters per minute, using a delivery device appropriate to the flow rate.

21.13 Given a variety of scenarios, demonstrate the assessment-based management of a variety of patients with cardiovascular emergencies, including the following: angina pectoris, aortic aneurysm or dissection, cardiac arrest (including CPR and AED use), cardiogenic shock, congestive heart failure, hypertensive emergencies, and myocardial infarction.

- Angina pectoris is a form of acute coronary syndrome (ACS) often relieved by rest or nitroglycerin. Treat chest pain that persists until EMS arrives according to your protocols for ACS, which will include aspirin and nitroglycerin as long as there are no contraindications. Patients with an SpO_2 of less than 95 percent should receive oxygen to maintain an SpO_2 of at least 95 percent. There is no evidence that oxygen benefits patients with uncomplicated ACS (those who are alert, breathing normally, and have good perfusion). Most protocols include starting an IV in patients with ACS.
- Aortic aneurysm or dissection management is rapid transport to a facility capable of surgical treatment. Administer oxygen to maintain an SpO_2 of 95 percent or above. Start at least one large-bore IV but unless profound hypotension is present, administer fluid at a keep-open rate to reduce the chance of increasing the vascular pressure and risking rupture.
- Cardiac arrest (including CPR and AED use) resuscitation follows the most current American Heart Association guidelines as outlined in your protocols. Early recognition, immediate EMS activation, high-quality chest compressions with minimal interruptions, and immediate defibrillation are the initial treatment. CPR is performed with a ratio of 30 chest compressions to 2 ventilations. IV access and insertion of advanced airways are considerations in resuscitation. You also should look for and correct possible underlying causes, such as hypoxia, shock, and hypoglycemia.
- Congestive heart failure is treated by maintaining a patent airway and ensuring adequate oxygenation and ventilation. Depending on the patient's condition, treatment may include oxygen by nonrebreather mask, CPAP, and assisting ventilations with a bag-valve-mask device or ventilating through an advanced airway. IV fluids are restricted to prevent worsening of pulmonary edema. Some EMS systems allow Advanced EMTs to administer nitroglycerin to cause vasodilation and reduce the workload of the heart.
- Hypertensive emergencies are managed by reducing the patient's anxiety and ensuring an adequate airway, breathing, and oxygenation. IV access is indicated. Transport the patient without delay for definitive management.

- Myocardial infarction is a form of ACS that can present with chest pain. Treat chest pain that you suspect is ACS with aspirin and nitroglycerin as long as there are no contraindications. Patients with an SpO_2 less than 95 percent should receive oxygen to maintain an SpO_2 of at least 95 percent. There is no evidence that oxygen benefits patients with uncomplicated ACS (those who are alert, breathing normally, and have good perfusion). Most protocols include starting an IV in patients with ACS. Advanced EMTs might also administer nitrous oxide as an analgesic if chest pain persists despite administration of nitroglycerin.

21.14 Discuss the purpose of fibrinolytic therapy and percutaneous coronary interventions (PCIs) in patients with cardiac emergencies.

Definitive treatment for ACS is reopening obstructed coronary arteries. Fibrinolytic therapy and percutaneous coronary interventions, or cardiac catheterizations, accomplish this if they are initiated within a narrow window of opportunity. Reperfusion helps to restore blood flow to the affected tissue and may save the muscle that would have otherwise died. Fibrinolytics are powerful medications that break down fibrin clots. Cardiac catheterization is a mechanical intervention in which a catheter is threaded through the femoral artery and into the central circulation until the tip of the catheter enters the affected coronary artery.

21.15 Discuss considerations in the use of advanced life support personnel to transport patients with cardiovascular emergencies.

In some cases, particularly when transport times are prolonged, paramedics can give additional medications that can benefit patients with cardiac emergencies. They may give diuretics, antidysrhythmics, other medications, and electrical therapies (synchronized cardioversion, transcutaneous pacing) and perform endotracheal intubation. However, definitive treatment takes place in the hospital setting and you must weigh the time needed for ALS to arrive against potential delays in transport.

21.16 Describe the purpose of using CPAP in patients with pulmonary edema.

CPAP helps by improving ventilation and oxygenation in patients with pulmonary edema. The positive end-expiratory pressure provided by CPAP can reduce the amount of fluid that can cross into the alveoli.

Resource Central

Resource Central offers extra practice and review materials in a variety of media. To access it, follow the directions on the Student Access Card provided with the Student Textbook. If there is no card, go to www.bradybooks.com and follow the Resource Central link to Buy Access.

Vocabulary and Concept Review

Exercise 1

Write the letter of the correct definition in the blank next to the term. (See Resource Central for more vocabulary review.)

1. _____ afterload

    a. Substances that promote the excretion of water through the kidneys

2. _____ angina pectoris

    b. Amount of resistance provided by the systemic vasculature, which the heart must overcome to effectively pump blood from the left ventricle

3. _____ aortic dissection

    c. Sensation of feeling the heart beat within the chest

4. _____ asystole

    d. Collection of conductive cells at the junction of the atria and ventricles; part of the cardiac conduction system

5. _____ atrioventricular (AV) node

    e. Sudden loss of consciousness resulting from a temporary decrease in cerebral perfusion

6. _____ diuretics

    f. Condition in which blood enters through a tear in the tunica intima of the aorta and is forced between the layers of the aorta

7. _____ ejection fraction

    g. Substance that breaks down blood clots by initiating the body's normal mechanism for dissolving blood clots

8. _____ fibrinolytic

    h. Collection of pacemaker cells in the upper right atrium that serve as the primary pacemaker of the heart

9. _____ palpitations

    i. Chest pain that results from ischemia of the heart muscle, usually from coronary artery disease

10. _____ preload

    j. Amount of blood in the left ventricle at the end of diastole

11. _____ sinoatrial (SA) node

    k. Proportion of blood in the left ventricle at the end of diastole that is ejected during systole, expressed as a percentage

12. _____ syncope

    l. Absence of electrical activity in the heart, resulting in cardiac standstill

Exercise 2

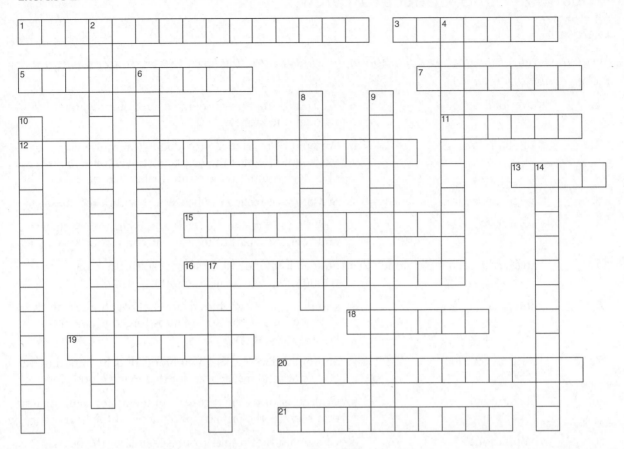

Across

1. Unhealthy condition of the arteries in which plaque narrows the lumen of the vessel.
3. Fainting, sometimes because of dysrhythmia.
5. Smallest of the arteries.
7. End-diastolic volume.
11. One of the two upper chambers of the heart.
12. Sign or symptom, other than chest pain, that represents myocardial ischemia.
13. Treatment that produces PEEP to improve ventilation and oxygenation in pulmonary edema.
15. Lethal ventricular dysrhythmia.
16. Subjective sensation of the heart beating in the chest.
18. Fluid transport medium for blood cells.
19. Heart valve that is also called the mitral valve.
20. Medication given in suspected ACS to relax vascular smooth muscle.
21. Condition in which blood separates the layers of the aorta.

Down

2. Stroke volume expressed as a portion of the end-diastolic volume.
4. Rhythm seen on the ECG when the heart is healthy and has a properly functioning electrical system.
6. Tissue death due to ischemia.
8. When activated, they clump together at the site of injury in a blood vessel.
9. Heart's primary pacemaker.
10. Stroke volume times heart rate.
14. Tough, fibrous sac that surrounds the heart.
17. Medication given in suspected ACS to reduce platelet aggregation.

Patient Assessment Review

Exercise 1

You have been dispatched for a "possible heart attack." Using the summary of the following patient assessment process as a structure, answer the questions to elaborate your clinical reasoning at each step of the process.

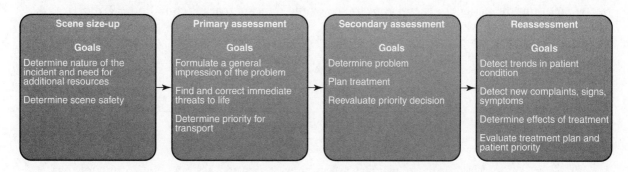

1. What about the scene size-up would give an indication that the patient has a cardiac emergency?

_____

_____

_____

_____

2. What hazards could be present at the scene of a medical emergency?

_____

_____

_____

_____

3. Are there any hazards specific to cardiac emergencies?

_____

_____

_____

4. How would you control any hazards at the scene?

_____

_____

_____

_____

5. Under what circumstances might you need additional resources?

_____

_____

_____

_____

6. What about the patient's general appearance would indicate that his condition is critical?

_____

_____

_____

_____

Exercise 2

1. What are you looking for in the primary assessment of a patient with a chief complaint that could be related to a cardiac emergency?

_____

_____

_____

2. What might give you a clue to a cardiac problem as you complete the primary assessment?

_____

_____

_____

3. What interventions are required in the primary assessment?

_____

_____

_____

4. What are some special considerations in the primary assessment interventions for a patient with a cardiac emergency?

_____

_____

_____

5. What information will influence your decision about the patient's priority for transport?

_____

_____

_____

Exercise 3

1. What are the important questions to ask when obtaining the medical history of a patient with a possible cardiac problem?

    _____

    _____

    _____

2. What can the vital signs tell you about the patient's condition?

    _____

    _____

    _____

3. What monitoring devices can provide important information about a potential cardiac patient?

    _____

    _____

    _____

4. What is the role of physical examination in cardiac patients?

    _____

    _____

    _____

5. Summarize findings that would make you suspect acute coronary syndrome.

    _____

    _____

    _____

6. Summarize findings that would make you suspect heart failure with pulmonary edema.

    _____

    _____

    _____

Exercise 4

1. Describe considerations in the reassessment process of a patient with ACS.

    _____

    _____

    _____

    _____

    _____

Check Your Recall and Apply Concepts

Exercise 1

Select the best possible choice for each of the following questions.

_____ 1. Perfusion of the coronary arteries requires an adequate period of:
   a. atrial systole.
   b. atrial diastole.
   c. ventricular systole.
   d. ventricular diastole.

_____ 2. The lung tissue is perfused by the _____ arteries.
   a. bronchial
   b. portal
   c. mediastinal
   d. pulmonary

_____ 3. Which one of the following best represents mean arterial pressure?
   a. Systolic blood pressure minus diastolic blood pressure
   b. Diastolic blood pressure plus one third of the pulse pressure
   c. Systolic blood pressure minus one third of the pulse pressure
   d. Diastolic blood pressure plus one third of the systolic blood pressure

_____ 4. When the flow of ions from a more positively charged area to a less positively charged area equalizes the charges across the cell membrane, it is known as:
   a. polarization.
   b. depolarization.
   c. resting potential.
   d. repolarization.

_____ 5. The QRS complex of the ECG represents:
   a. atrial depolarization.
   b. a delay in conduction at the atrioventricular node.
   c. ventricular depolarization.
   d. ventricular repolarization.

_____ 6. Recurrent chest pain that comes on during exertion or stress and is relieved by rest is called:
   a. myocardial infarction.
   b. stable angina.
   c. unstable angina.
   d. acute coronary vasospasm.

_____ 7. Your patient is a 49-year-old man whose chief complaint is severe pressure in his chest. The pain began while he was working in his garage at home. The pain has been continuous since it started and the patient feels weak and nauseated. He rates the pain as a 9 out of a possible 10. He is pale and diaphoretic. His pulse is 84 and regular, his blood pressure is 88/56, respirations are 20, and SpO_2 is 97 percent on room air. His lungs sounds are clear and equal bilaterally and there is no pedal edema. Which one of the following will benefit the patient the most?
   a. Obtain IV access.
   b. Apply oxygen by nonrebreather mask.
   c. Give 0.4 mg of nitroglycerin sublingually.
   d. Give 325 mg of chewable aspirin by mouth.

_____ 8. Your patient is a 61-year-old man who began having chest pain as soon as he got out of bed this morning. He has a history of atherosclerosis, angina, hyperlipidemia, chronic bronchitis, and hypertension and is a type 2 diabetic. Among other medications for his conditions, he takes nitroglycerin. He took one nitroglycerin tablet before your arrival with no relief from his chest pain. He describes the pain as "dull and heavy," and rates it a 6 out of a possible 10. The patient is obese and has moderate pedal edema. He is alert and anxious, but oriented, and his vital signs are heart rate 88, blood pressure 154/92, respirations 20, and SpO$_2$ 96 percent on room air. His skin is moist but his color is good. He has some scattered rhonchi in his lungs bilaterally. Which one of the following should you do first in the care of this patient?

   a. Check his blood glucose level.
   b. Administer 0.4 mg nitroglycerin sublingually.
   c. Administer 2.5 mg albuterol by small-volume nebulizer.
   d. Place him on the stretcher in Fowler's position and prepare for transport.

_____ 9. Your patient is a 71-year-old woman who awoke at 0130 hours with severe dyspnea. She is sitting up on a chair when you arrive and is in a tripod position. You can hear crackling breath sounds as you approach the patient. She has cyanosis of her lips, earlobes, and nail beds and is diaphoretic. She is using accessory muscles to assist with breathing and cannot speak more than two to three words without a breath. Of the following choices, which one should you do first?

   a. Set up CPAP and explain it to the patient.
   b. Give 0.4 mg nitroglycerin sublingually.
   c. Give 2.5 mg albuterol by small-volume nebulizer.
   d. Insert a nasopharyngeal airway and ventilate by bag-valve mask.

_____ 10. Medical direction may order sublingual nitroglycerin for patients with severe pulmonary edema because it may help in which one of the following ways in the management of left-sided heart failure?

   a. Increases perfusion pressure
   b. Relaxes bronchiolar smooth muscle
   c. Decreases afterload
   d. Causes mild diuresis

_____ 11. Your patient is a 31-year-old woman with a chief complaint of lightheadness and a sensation that her heart is "fluttering" in her chest. She is pale and diaphoretic and slightly dyspneic. Her radial pulse is weak and too rapid to get an accurate count. When you apply the pulse oximeter, it gives a reading of 95 percent and indicates a heart rate of 174 per minute. Her lung sounds are clear and equal bilaterally. According to the friend with her, she has no known past medical history. They were shopping and doing errands when the patient suddenly became lightheaded. Which one of the following conditions is most consistent with the patient's presentation?

   a. Aortic aneurysm with hypovolemia
   b. Paroxysmal supraventricular tachycardia
   c. Acute coronary syndrome
   d. Left-sided heart failure

_____12. Continuing with the scenario in the previous question, your patient is a 31-year-old woman with a chief complaint of lightheadness and a sensation that her heart is "fluttering" in her chest. She is pale and diaphoretic and slightly dyspneic. Her radial pulse is weak and too rapid to get an accurate count. When you apply the pulse oximeter, it gives a reading of 95 percent and indicates a heart rate of 174 per minute. Her lung sounds are clear and equal bilaterally. According to the friend with her, she has no known past medical history. They were shopping and doing errands when the patient suddenly became lightheaded. You have a 25-minute transport time. Which one of the following orders do you anticipate from medical direction?

   a. Administer two large-bore IVs and a 500-mL fluid bolus.
   b. Administer 0.4 mg of nitroglycerin sublingually.
   c. Apply CPAP.
   d. Ask the patient to bear down as if she is having a bowel movement.

Exercise 2

For the following statements, write a T in the blank if the statement is true and an F in the blank if the statement is false. If the statement is false, rewrite it so that it is correct.

1. _____There is normally fluid in the pericardial sac.

   _____

2. _____The aortic valve opens when the left ventricle contracts.

   _____

3. _____In the average adult, cardiac output is approximately 8.5 L/min.

   _____

4. _____The most common event that leads to myocardial infarction is rupture of an atherosclerotic plaque.

   _____

5. _____A patient must have a systolic blood pressure of at least 120 mmHg to receive nitroglycerin for chest pain.

   _____

6. _____The pain associated with myocardial infarction is usually relieved by rest, oxygen, and nitroglycerin.

   _____

7. _____The most common initial rhythm in sudden cardiac arrest is asystole.

   _____

8. _____Cor pulmonale is a severe form of left-sided heart failure.

   _____

9. _____The Advanced EMT treatment for left-sided heart failure is an intravenous fluid bolus.

   _____

10. _____Aortic dissection is a ballooning out of a weakened area of the aorta.

   _____

Clinical Reasoning

CASE STUDY: 80-YEAR-OLD MAN WITH DIFFICULTY BREATHING

You and your partner are dispatched to a nursing home in the late hours of the night for an 80-year-old man who is complaining of difficulty breathing. Your partner, Tonya, leaves the ambulance first and grabs your equipment bags and you grab the defibrillator, just in case. You find the patient, Mr. Phillips, in his room, perched on the edge of his bed in a tripod position and showing signs of mild respiratory distress. He is alert, but confused. The nursing staff tells you he has Alzheimer's disease and that his level of confusion is about the same as always. However, he is able tell you that he woke up with shortness of breath and the nursing staff confirms that. You auscultate his breath sounds and hear crackles (rales) in the lung bases bilaterally. You ask him to take a couple of deep breaths and listen again. The crackles remain. Mr. Phillips' vital signs are pulse 92 and irregular, blood pressure 132/84, respirations 24 and slightly labored. His SpO$_2$ on room air is 91 percent. The nursing staff reports from his chart that the day shift noted that Mr. Phillips slept more than usual and complained of "not feeling well," but could not give any specific complaints. Mr. Phillips' skin is warm and moist and his color appears normal. He has mild bilateral pedal edema.

1. What is your field impression for the patient and how did you come to that conclusion?

    _____

    _____

    _____

    _____

    _____

2. What treatments will be beneficial and why are they indicated?

    _____

    _____

    _____

    _____

    _____

3. What is another possibility for Mr. Phillips' problem? Why do you believe it is less likely than the field impression you chose?

    _____

    _____

    _____

    _____

    _____

Project-Based Learning

Exercise 1

Visit the American Heart Association website to learn more about preventing cardiovascular disease. Go to: http://www.heart.org/HEARTORG/ and click on the tab "Getting Healthy." Jot down in your journal or notebook three goals for reducing your personal risk of heart disease.

Exercise 2

Check into resources in your community through which you can obtain an intact beef heart. You may be able to obtain one from a butcher or meat locker, although some groceries stores sell them. A beef heart is similar to (although much larger than) a human heart. Identify the chambers of the heart, the pulmonary vein, pulmonary artery, vena cava, aorta, heart valves, chordae tendonae, papillary muscles, and coronary arteries.

The EMS Professional in Practice

What is your role, as a health care professional, in educating your family, friends, and the public about reducing the risk of cardiovascular disease? What are some specific things you can do? Jot down your thoughts in a notebook or journal for discussion in class or in your study group.

Neurologic Disorders

Content Area

• Medicine

Advanced EMT Education Standard

• Applies fundamental knowledge to provide basic and selected advanced emergency care and transportation based on assessment findings for an acutely ill patient.

Summary of Objectives

22.1 Define key terms introduced in this chapter.

Knowing and being able to apply the key terms in each chapter is critical to understanding chapter concepts. Write the list of key terms. Then write the definition of each one in your own words. Check your understanding by confirming the definitions in the textbook glossary. Correct any misunderstandings. Create a study aid by writing each key term on the front of an index card and the definition on the back. Use the cards to quiz yourself or to have someone quiz you. The exercises under Vocabulary and Concept Review below will give you additional practice.

22.2 Recognize complaints that may indicate a neurologic problem.

The patient may present with complaints of altered mental status (sometimes reported by family or caregivers), behavioral changes, sensory impairment, headache, or weakness or paralysis to one or more sections or sides of the body.

22.3 List possible underlying causes of altered mental status, neurologic deficit, headache, seizures, and syncope.

Underlying causes of altered mental status can be any number of disorders from each of the body's physiologic processes. Syncope results from an inadequate brain perfusion, often from cardiac dysrhythmia, volume depletion, or vasoconstriction from a rapid change in position. A neurologic deficit, or stroke, often can result from atherosclerosis of cerebral arteries or of the internal carotid arteries that supply blood to the brain. Seizures are often idiopathic in nature, and diagnosed as epilepsy. Toxins, drugs, metabolic disorders, head trauma, and stroke also can cause an acute onset of seizures. Headaches are caused by a pressure or tension on pain-sensitive structures surrounding the brain or from abnormal nerve transmissions. Often a stroke will present its first symptom to be headache. Use of the mnemonic AEIOU-TIPS is useful in all the listed conditions.

22.4   Explain the importance of airway assessment and management in patients with altered mental status and neurologic deficit.

Treatment for all conditions that are neurologic in origin include managing the airway, breathing, and circulation and searching for possible underlying causes. The patient is extremely vulnerable and may have lost the gag or cough reflex or have respiratory depression.

22.5   Obtain information in the patient history that is focused on the evaluation of altered mental status, neurologic deficit, headache, seizure, or syncope.

Neurologic conditions, such as those listed, create a high potential that the patient will not be able to give an adequate history. Your knowledge of medication uses will be vital because you can piece together a history based upon the prescribed medications. Also, your knowledge of pathophysiology will be vital to understanding how certain conditions can precipitate others. For instance, a stroke can cause a headache, syncope, and seizures. You will need to utilize diagnostic tools at your disposal (such as a glucometer) as well in the diagnosis of the unresponsive patient.

22.6   Given a scenario with a patient with altered mental status, neurologic deficit, headache, seizure, or syncope, perform a physical examination that is focused on relevant findings and anticipated consequences.

Your physical examination of the neurologic patient should include vital signs but should also routinely include the check of blood glucose, cardiac monitoring, and exhaled carbon dioxide. Blood glucose can be low in the patient with diabetes and is easily correctable upon detection. Cardiac monitoring ensures that a declining mental status or syncope is not related to a potentially fatal dysrhythmia. Exhaled carbon dioxide acquisition is essential in the detection of hypercapnea, or too much carbon dioxide, and this again can lead to corrective measures in the prehospital environment.

22.7   Integrate scene size-up information, the patient's history, vital signs, and physical examination findings with knowledge of anatomy, physiology, and pathophysiology to identify more likely causes of the patient's condition.

Underlying causes of altered mental status can be any number of disorders from any of the body's physiologic processes. Use the mnemonic AEIOU-TIPS (alcohol, environment, insulin, overdose, uremia [renal failure], trauma, infection, psychosis or poisoning, and stroke) to ensure you consider all common causes of altered mental status. Your assessment of the scene and recognition of scene clues will allow you to detect alcohol use, environmental causes, possibly overdose if containers are present, trauma, or poisoning. Your primary assessment will allow you to detect altered mental status potentially from hypoglycemia or stroke. In all instances, the patient's history will be the greatest information possible to "connect the clues."

22.8   Determine the need for the following interventions in patients with a neurologic emergency: interventions to open and maintain the airway, manual spinal stabilization, oxygenation, and ventilation.

- *Interventions to open and maintain the airway:* Patients with a neurologic emergency may be at risk of losing their gag reflex and preventing aspiration. Any patient without this ability should have some form of manual airway placed.
- *Manual spinal stabilization:* Unresponsive patients or those appearing to have suffered some type of trauma should have spinal stabilization held to prevent further, potentially deadly, injury.

- *Oxygenation:* Hypoxia can cause symptoms much like neurological emergencies. In addition, patients will generally benefit from a superior level of available oxygen.
- *Ventilation:* Any patient, regardless of suspected cause, who has inadequate breathing, should be manually ventilated by the EMS provider.

22.9   Identify the signs and symptoms of stroke.

The signs and symptoms of stroke can be subtle. They include confusion, difficulty with speaking or vision, and loss of coordination. Headache is often the first recognized symptom for the patient. Other signs and symptoms include sudden numbness or weakness of the face, arm, or leg (especially on one side of the body) or an inability to control one's emotions.

22.10   Describe the pathophysiology of stroke.

Ischemic stroke, or a stroke caused by a blood clot blocking arterial blood flow, is often the result of atherosclerosis of cerebral arteries or the internal carotid arteries that supply the blood to the brain. Hemorrhagic strokes can occur due to rupture of an aneurysm in the brain or from arteriovenous malformation (AVM). The high demand of oxygen and glucose by the brain means that dysfunction of the affected areas occurs immediately and neurologic damage and death can begin to occur within 4 minutes. The initial signs and symptoms of stroke reflect the area of the brain deprived of perfusion.

22.11   Explain the importance of early recognition of stroke signs and symptoms by patients, family or bystanders, and EMS personnel.

Early recognition will lead to faster treatment. As many as 1.9 million neurons and 14 billion synapses can die for each minute a portion of the brain is without perfusion. The best outcomes are seen in patients who are treated within a 2-hour timeframe from the onset of symptoms.

22.12   Describe the relationship between stroke and transient ischemic attack.

A transient ischemic attack (TIA) presents with similar, and often the same, symptoms as a stroke but will resolve itself within 24 hours without intervention. Treatment should still be sought upon detection of signs and symptoms because a TIA is only diagnosed after the fact; it should not be seen as a "wait and see" diagnosis. A TIA places the patient at high risk for strokes.

22.13   Assess the patient with possible stroke for neurologic deficits, including use of a stroke scale: Cincinnati Prehospital Stroke Scale and Los Angeles Prehospital Stroke Scale.

The Cincinnati Prehospital Stroke Scale includes use of three detection parameters: facial droop, arm drift, and abnormal speech. Facial symmetry is the norm. In contrast, one side of the face drooping or not moving at the same interval is an abnormal finding. Both arms should have symmetrical movement. In contrast, one arm drifting downward is an abnormal finding. Speech should be clear with the correct phrase repeated without slurring.

The Los Angeles Prehospital Stroke Scale includes many factors to recognize presenting symptoms. Scene size-up can reveal certain risk factors, including age greater than 45 years, duration of symptoms less than 24 hours, patient's status as being either wheelchair bound or bedridden. Further assessment will reveal the presence of a history of seizures or epilepsy and a blood glucose level between 60 and 400 mg/dL. Those are all Yes/No/Unknown findings. Further testing for the scale includes having the patient look up, smile with teeth showing (to assess symmetry), comparing grip strength in the upper extremities (to assess symmetrical movement ability), and assessing arm strength for drift or weakness (to assess pronation or muscle weakness).

22.14   Discuss the role of blood glucose determination in the assessment of patients with altered mental status, neurologic deficits, and seizures.

Blood glucose measurement has become a quick and relatively accurate measurement and if found to be inadequate, can be resolved quickly with pharmacologic intervention. The further depleted a patient's circulating glucose becomes, the greater the risk of seizure, stroke, and death.

22.15 Describe ways of communicating with patients who have difficulty speaking.

Patients with difficulty speaking do not necessarily have difficulty understanding what you are saying. To allow communication, they may be able to write their response to your questions or you may be able to write a selection of responses for the patient to point to and choose. In the latter instance, questions should be closed ended and direct to minimize the interaction and frustration of the patient.

22.16 Recognize indications that a headache may have a potentially life-threatening underlying cause, such as toxic exposure, hypertension, infectious disease, or hemorrhagic stroke.

The key to differentiating between a non–life-threatening and life-threatening headache is the history. Your assessment needs to focus on the progression of symptoms and whether the headache is its own condition or a sign of another underlying condition. A subarachnoid hemorrhage occurs when there is bleeding that accumulates between the brain and the arachnoid layer of the meninges. There is typically a sudden onset of a severe headache, unlike any other headache experienced by the patient.

22.17 Describe measures that you can take to improve the comfort level of the patient suffering from a headache.

Many headaches will have accompanied photophobia or otophobia. You can easily limit the amount of light exposure or noise exposure of the patient by using a towel when extricating the patient from the scene and reducing the amount of light in your ambulance. You can minimize personnel interacting with the patient so that noise is minimal.

22.18 Explain the importance of reassessment of the patient with altered mental status, neurologic deficit, headache, seizure, or syncope.

Reassessment, as with other patient complaints, should repeat the primary assessment to identify new or changing immediate threats to life in the form of inadequate airway, breathing, or circulation. The mental status must be continually reassessed to track changes over the period of your contact with the patient. In addition, changes as a result of any interventions performed need to be reassessed to ensure they were useful.

22.19 Describe the various ways that seizures can present.

Generalized seizures are subcategorized as tonic–clonic or absent. Tonic–clonic seizures are motor seizures involving the entire body. Absence seizures present most often in children and involve a loss of awareness but no change in muscle tone. Partial seizures are subcategorized as focal, simple, or complex. Focal seizures are localized to one area of the brain. Simple partial seizures often maintain consciousness unless there is secondary generalization of the seizure activity. Complex partial seizures may be accompanied by an aura and involve impairment of awareness associate with stereotyped movements.

22.20 Discuss possible underlying causes of seizures.

Seizures can be caused by toxins, drugs, metabolic disturbances, trauma, stroke, tumors, and fever. Toxins and drugs are generally self-administered but can sometimes be accidentally ingested. Metabolic disturbances can result from a breakdown of the pathophysiologic processes of the body resulting in a reduced ability to excrete the normal by-products. Trauma to the head can cause seizures. Stoke and tumors generally result in increased intracranial pressure, impose pressure on the brain, and reduce its ability to function normally. Finally, fever can be the by-product of an infection and the root infection can affect the brain and alter its ability to function chemically.

22.21 Explain the concerns associated with prolonged or successive seizures.

Prolonged and successive seizures, by definition status epilepticus, can cause cerebral edema, hypoxia in the hippocampus, sclerosis of the amygdala, neurogenic pulmonary edema, fibrosis of the cardiac conduction system, or liver congestion, all not recognizable until autopsy. Obstructive apnea and cardiac dysrhythmias may be implicated.

22.22 Describe the assessment and emergency medical care of patients with tonic–clonic, simple partial, complex partial, febrile, and absence seizures, and patients in a postictal state.

Treat patients in the various forms of seizures and in the postictal state with oxygen, and if appropriate, bag-valve mask ventilations, and search for a cause of the seizure. Once the patient is postictal, you may need to suction secretions from the airway. Hypoglycemia is easily identifiable by blood glucometry and rectified by glucose administration. For those in active seizures, an anticonvulsant agent may be indicated, if it is within your protocol.

22.23 Anticipate bystander reactions to patients having seizures and measures needed to stop any unnecessary or inappropriate interventions.

In the instance of children, the family or caregiver may be able to provide direct insight into the care of a patient with a chronic seizure condition. Except for that instance, limit bystanders from access to the patient because they become a risk to be injured if the patient's convulsions cause muscle jerking and flailing. The most well-meaning bystanders can cause further injury if they are not familiar with proper emergency care, regardless of the problem at hand.

22.24 Differentiate between features of dementia and delirium.

Dementia is a progressive condition in which intellectual function is severely impaired and that may be accompanied by emotional and behavioral changes. Delirium is an acute state of confusion that occurs from an underlying problem, such as infection, metabolic disturbances, toxins, or medications. Thus, dementia is generally a long-term, chronic illness. The elderly may suffer delirium during acute illness, but delirium also can affect younger patients in acute illness and in a particular form of delirium called excited delirium syndrome, which is associated with cocaine and methamphetamine usage.

22.25 Describe basic information about various neurologic disorders, such as Bell's palsy, vertigo, Parkinson's disease, Wernicke-Korsakoff syndrome, multiple sclerosis, normal pressure hydrocephalus, and others that may affect the assessment and management of patients.

Bell's palsy is a temporary weakness or paralysis of the facial nerve (cranial nerve VII). Vertigo is a subjective sensation of movement when there is none, often described by patients as dizziness. Vertigo can be accompanied by nausea, vomiting, and abnormal eye movements (nystagmus), and may be precipitated by sudden movement of the head. Vertigo can be caused by problems with the structures of the inner ear, the eighth cranial nerve, or the brainstem. Normal pressure hydrocephalus (NPH) occurs when the CSF produced in the ventricles of the brain cannot be properly reabsorbed or drained, allowing it to collect in abnormal amounts. The condition occurs most commonly in patients over the age of 55, and often there is a history of subarachnoid hemorrhage, traumatic brain injury, infection, or a tumor. Parkinson's disease typically occurs in patients over the age of 50, but can occur early. The mechanism is a loss of dopamine-producing cells in the brain, resulting in movement disorder. Multiple sclerosis is an autoimmune disease in which the myelin sheath of nerves is destroyed, resulting in problems with nerve conduction. The onset of the disease is generally first noticed between the ages of 20 and 40. Wernicke-Korsakoff syndrome is a spectrum of degenerative neurologic disorders that includes Wernicke's encephalopathy and Korsakoff's amnesic syndrome. Both are caused by thiamine (vitamin B_1) deficiency, which is common in alcoholics, those with eating disorders, and patients who are malnourished.

Resource Central

Resource Central offers extra practice and review materials in a variety of media. To access it, follow the directions on the Student Access Card provided with the Student Textbook. If there is no card, go to www.bradybooks.com and follow the Resource Central link to Buy Access.

Vocabulary and Concept Review

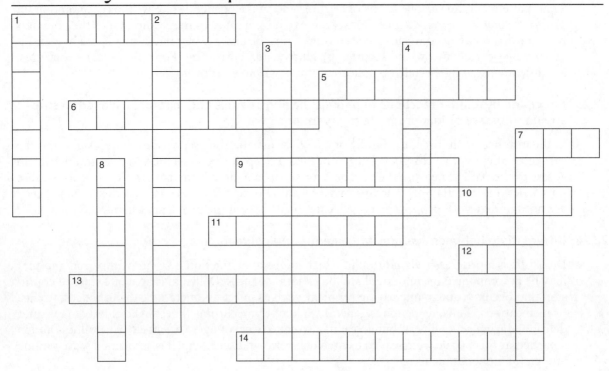

Across

1. Condition in which there are recurrent seizuers.
5. Subjective sensation of spinning or moving while stationary; dissiness.
6. Period of altered mental status following a seizure.
7. Abbreviation of transient ischemic attack.
9. Lack of blood flow to an area of tissue, such as in the brain.
10. Abnormal sensation that precedes some seizures and migraine headaches.
11. Point where two nerve cells communicate with each other.
12. Abbreviation of arteriovenous malformatin.
13. Motor activity produced by a generalized seizure.
14. Signs reflective of inflammation of the meninges.

Down

1. Mass, which may be a blood clot or other matter, that moves through the bloodstream and may cause an obstruction.
2. Hypersensitivity of the eyes to light.
3. Almost fainting.
4. Loss of coordination, often presenting as difficulty walking.
7. Blood clot that causes obstruction of a blood vessel at the site where it forms.
8. Consider a low level of this important cellular nutrient as a cause of altered mental status.

Patient Assessment Review

Exercise 1

Practice assessing a patient with a suspected stroke. Complete the table to demonstrate your knowledge of the Cincinnati Prehospital Stroke Scale.

Sign of Stroke	Patient Activity	Interpretation
Facial droop		
Arm drift		
Abnormal speech		

Check Your Recall and Apply Concepts

Select the best possible choice for each of the following questions.

_____ 1. What type of stroke is caused by a ruptured aneurysm?
  a. Ischemic
  b. Microvascular
  c. Hemorrhagic
  d. Cardiovascular

_____ 2. What type of seizure is characterized by a rapid rise in the patient's temperature?
  a. Tonic–clonic
  b. Febrile
  c. Focal
  d. Complex partial

_____ 3. A series of seizures or a continued seizure lasting more than 5 minutes is:
  a. status epilepticus
  b. febrile seizures
  c. hypoglycemia
  d. arteriovenous malformation

_____ 4. A sensitivity to light and noise characterizes what type of neurologic condition, which represents the most common emergency room visit?
  a. Seizure
  b. Stroke
  c. Cerebral palsy
  d. Headache

_____ 5. Alzheimer's disease is characterized by the presence of amyloid deposits in the brain and degeneration of the microtubules of cerebral neurons. In what category of neurologic disorder is Alzheimer's disease?
  a. Dementia
  b. Delirium
  c. Convulsion
  d. Stroke

Clinical Reasoning

CASE STUDY: A SHAKING FEELING

You are dispatched for a report of a person seizing in the park. You arrive to find a woman in her 20s in a tonic–clonic seizure next to a park bench. Bystanders have gathered around her but no one offers themselves as a family.

1. What is the most important principle for you in your assessment of this patient? Why?

   _____

   _____

   _____

   _____

2. What other things can you assess to gain a better understanding of the patient's condition?

   _____

   _____

   _____

   _____

3. Your patient stops seizing but is now not responding to you. Is this normal? Explain your answer.

   _____

   _____

   _____

   _____

Project-Based Learning

Create a diagram displaying the common characteristics of the neurologic conditions presented in this chapter. Be sure to include signs and symptoms so that a new provider could reference your project to gain a better understanding of neurologic emergencies.

The EMS Professional in Practice

A sudden onset of neurologic deficit can be very distressing for a patient and his family. What can you say to give the patient reassurance without being misleading? Jot down your thoughts in a notebook or journal for discussion in class or in your study group.

Endocrine Disorders

Content Area

• Medicine

Advanced EMT Education Standard

• Applies fundamental knowledge to provide basic and selected advanced emergency care and transportation based on assessment findings for an acutely ill patient.

Summary of Objectives

23.1 Define key terms introduced in this chapter.

Knowing and being able to apply the key terms in each chapter is critical to understanding chapter concepts. Write the list of key terms. Then write the definition of each one in your own words. Check your understanding by confirming the definitions in the textbook glossary. Correct any misunderstandings. Create a study aid by writing each key term on the front of an index card and the definition on the back. Use the cards to quiz yourself or to have someone quiz you. The exercises under Vocabulary and Concept Review below will give you additional practice.

23.2 Describe the pathophysiology of diabetes mellitus to include differences from normal glucose metabolism, roles of insulin and glucagon, consequences to cellular metabolism and water balance of insufficient insulin, similarities and differences between type 1 and type 2 diabetes mellitus, mechanisms by which the classic signs and symptoms of untreated diabetes mellitus are produced, and events leading to hypoglycemia.

• *Differences from normal glucose metabolism:* Normal cell metabolism requires a steady source of glucose. Simple carbohydrates such as glucose are rapidly absorbed from the digestive tract to provide a source of fuel. In diabetes mellitus, there is insufficient insulin present to facilitate the movement of glucose into the cells. Cells must rely on alternative fuel sources, such as fats, which leads to production of toxic by-products (ketones).

• *Roles of insulin and glucagon:* When the blood glucose level (BGL) is low, alpha cells in the pancreas secrete glucagon, a hormone that increases the glucose level by promoting breakdown of glycogen in the liver. When the glucose level is high, glucagon levels drop and beta cells in the pancreas secrete insulin, which facilitates use and storage of glucose, which allows blood glucose levels to drop to normal. In diabetes, either there is no insulin or the cellular sensitivity to insulin has decreased, preventing glucose from entering cells in sufficient quantities.

- *Consequences to cellular metabolism and water balance of insufficient insulin:* Insufficient insulin prevents the glucose molecules from moving into the cells; consequently, the glucose stays in the circulatory system. The higher concentration of glucose molecules cannot be reabsorbed from the filtrate in the kidneys. That causes the movement of more water into the filtrate (osmosis). The result is glucose in the urine and osmotic diuresis, the loss of large amounts of urine. The loss of excess water leads to dehydration and thirst. Because glucose cannot be used for cellular metabolism, cells use fats for energy, resulting in accumulation of the waste products called ketones.

- *Similarities and differences between type 1 and type 2 diabetes mellitus:* Type 1 diabetes is also known as juvenile diabetes or insulin-dependent diabetes mellitus (IDDM). Type 1 patients do not secrete any insulin; consequently, they must inject insulin to maintain adequate BGLs. Those patients are usually thin because fats are used in metabolism and are not stored to a significant degree. Type 2 diabetes is also known as non–insulin-dependent diabetes mellitus (NIDDM) or adult-onset diabetes. Type 2 patients usually make some insulin, but their cells become insulin resistant. They initially control their disease with diet and oral medications, but may progress to needing insulin injections. Adult onset diabetes usually occurs in middle age in overweight people. In untreated disease, both types of diabetes present with high blood glucose due to insufficient insulin or ineffective use of insulin by the cells.

- *Mechanisms by which the classic signs and symptoms of untreated diabetes mellitus are produced:* When the blood glucose level is excessive, the excess glucose cannot be reabsorbed from the filtrate in the kidney during urine production. The high osmolarity of the filtrate causes additional water to be pulled into the filtrate, producing large volumes of urine (polyuria). The loss of large volumes of urine results in dehydration and thirst (polydipsia). Despite the presence of high blood glucose levels, the glucose cannot enter the cells. The use of fats for energy is not efficient, resulting in insufficient cellular energy and a starvation metabolism, resulting in excessive hunger (polyphagia).

- *Events leading to hypoglycemia:* The blood glucose level of a patient with diabetes may drop below normal if he has taken too much insulin or other medications to reduce blood glucose levels in relation to the amount of calories he has consumed. An increase above normal physical activity may deplete glucose as well.

23.3 Given a patient's blood glucose level, determine whether it is within normal limits.

Normal BGLs are between 70 and 110 mg/dL. Hypoglycemic patients require treatment when their BGL is less than 60 mg/dL. Hyperglycemia exists when the BGL is more than 140 mg/dL.

23.4 Recognize the brain's particular sensitivity to decreased blood glucose levels.

The brain is particularly sensitive to hypoglycemia, because it needs a constant supply of glucose and cannot readily use other sources of energy. Hypoglycemia can lead to damage and death of brain cells and must be detected and treated immediately. Because the brain is so acutely affected by hypoglycemia, seizures may occur.

23.5 Predict the consequences of insufficient glycogen stores.

The primary storage reservoir for glycogen is the liver. As glucose levels start to decrease, glycogen is broken down into glucose. Without a sufficient supply of glycogen, there is no reserve glucose to supply the body's energy needs. Glucose is used up very rapidly, so the body depends on its stores of glycogen between meals. Without sufficient glycogen stores, life-threatening hypoglycemia may occur very quickly.

23.6 Compare and contrast the speed of onset and signs and symptoms of hypoglycemia and hyperglycemia.

The onset of hypoglycemia is rapid because insulin acts quickly to facilitate entry of glucose into the cells, where it is quickly metabolized. Without glucose, brain cells dysfunction and can begin to die in a short period of time. Most of the effects of hypoglycemia are due to the lack of glucose delivered to the brain cells and activation of the sympathetic nervous system. Altered mental status; pale, cool, sweaty skin; and tachycardia are common signs. Hyperglycemia occurs over a period of hours to days because even without insulin, a small amount of glucose is able to get into the cells for metabolism, and signs and symptoms usually do not occur until the blood glucose level is significantly elevated and the patient has become dehydrated from osmotic diuresis. In type 1 diabetes, the use of fats as an energy source results in ketoacidosis. In an attempt to buffer the acidosis, the respiratory rate and volume increases to rid the body of excess carbon dioxide. There is a gradual onset of altered mental status with dry, often flushed, skin and signs of volume depletion.

23.7   Compare and contrast diabetic ketoacidosis (DKA) and nonketotic hyperosmolar coma (NKHC).

Both conditions lead to dehydration through osmotic diuresis. Electrolytes (particularly potassium) are lost through the diuresis. Dehydration and electrolyte abnormalities lead to altered mental status and increase the risk of cardiac dysrhythmia. In DKA, the use of fats for energy results in ketone production, lowering the blood pH. Dehydration, acidosis, and electrolyte abnormalities lead to altered mental status and increase the risk of cardiac dysrhythmias. Kussmaul's respirations are an attempt to compensate for metabolic acidosis. NKHC leads to dehydration through osmotic diuresis. In NKHC, ketoacidosis does not occur because the cells can use enough glucose to prevent fat metabolism.

23.8   Describe how to direct history taking and assessment to obtain information relevant to the patient with a diabetic emergency.

Recognizing signs and symptoms of endocrine disorders when the history is unknown requires a process of inductive reasoning, from the collection of signs and symptoms to their potential causes. To do this effectively, you must understand the basic functions of some of the glands most often involved in endocrine emergencies. You may note some early indications that the problem may be endocrine related. Patients with hypoglycemia can be agitated, confused, and combative. Look for clues such as a hypoglycemic patient who may have been in the process of trying to unwrap a candy bar or buy a soda. Many patients with endocrine disorders have already been diagnosed, so examining their medications can provide vital clues. Family and friends can be invaluable in determining diabetes as a factor.

23.9   List common complications of diabetes.

Complications include cardiovascular disease, stroke, blindness, amputations, nonhealing wounds, peripheral neuropathy, peripheral vascular disease, and kidney failure. The risk for AMI and stroke are also increased.

23.10   Given a scenario with a patient suffering a diabetic emergency, provide emergency medical care for the patient.

A specific Advanced EMT treatment for DKA is to administer large volumes of isotonic crystalloid IV fluids to begin treatment of dehydration. Start one or two IVs, preferably with at least 18-gauge catheters and administer fluids at the rate prescribed by your medical director or in consultation with on-line medical direction. Generally, a bolus of fluid (1 to 2 L) is followed by an infusion at a prescribed rate. Treatment for hypoglycemic patients who are awake and able to control their airways is to offer a concentrated form of sugar to eat or drink. Sucrose (table sugar), fructose (from fruits and juices and added to many sweets), and dextrose are similar in chemical structure to glucose and can be used by the body for energy. Never give anything by mouth to patients with a decreased level of responsiveness. The most effective way of increasing the BGL in those patients is to start an IV and administer a solution of 50 percent dextrose. When you cannot start an IV, administer 1 mg of glucagon intramuscularly.

23.11 Identify indications and contraindications to the administration of oral glucose, intravenous dextrose, and intramuscular glucagon.

Oral glucose is indicated for a conscious and alert patient with low blood sugar. It is contraindicated for patients with a decreased level of responsiveness. IV dextrose is indicated for hypoglycemic patients with a decreased level of responsiveness. Do not push dextrose through an IV that is not flowing freely or that has infiltrated. You can administer IM glucagon to adult hypoglycemic patients who have a decreased level of responsiveness and in whom you cannot establish an IV. Glucagon has a much slower onset, and its effectiveness relies on the patient having adequate liver glycogen stores.

23.12 Describe the reassessment of a patient with a diabetic emergency.

Reassess critical patients every 5 minutes, including the primary assessment, vital signs, complaints, and relevant aspects of the secondary assessment. Perform reassessment more frequently, if warranted. Reassess noncritical patients every 15 minutes. If you have given oral glucose, 50 percent dextrose, or glucagon to treat hypoglycemia, you must re-evaluate the patient's blood glucose level.

23.13 Document the assessment and management of a patient with a diabetic emergency.

Documentation includes details of the primary assessment, the results of the secondary assessment, vital signs, and BGL. Document the patient's response to treatment, including the mental status and BGL after treatment. In the event a hypoglycemia patient refuses transport after treatment, be sure to document your full assessment and treatment. Document all steps you took to ensure the patient has eaten or will eat and has adequate supervision. Include a description of your attempts to persuade the patient to consent to transport and his responses.

23.14 Give a brief overview of the pathophysiology and the signs and symptoms of hyperthyroidism and hypothyroidism.

Thyroid disorders arise from secreting either too much or too little thyroid hormone. Hyperthyroidism results in increased metabolism, which leads to weight loss, heat intolerance, and other problems. Hypothyroidism results in weight gain, cold intolerance, and in severe cases, coma.

23.15 Give a brief overview of the pathophysiology and the signs and symptoms of disorders of the adrenal glands, including Cushing's syndrome and Addison disease.

In Addison disease, adrenal cortical hormones are insufficient. Addison disease results from damage to the adrenal cortex, which may occur as a result of autoimmune disease, infection, or hypoperfusion. Adrenal cortical insufficiency also can occur because of sudden withdrawal of long-term steroid therapy. Signs and symptoms can include a decreased BGL and electrolyte abnormalities resulting in cardiac dysrhythmias. The inability to fight infection can lead to sepsis.

A common cause of Cushing's syndrome is long-term administration of steroids to treat a medical condition such as COPD, asthma, and autoimmune diseases and to prevent rejection of transplanted organs and tissues. Complications of Cushing's syndrome include osteoporosis (with increased risk of fractures), hypertension, diabetes, muscle wasting, and susceptibility to infection. The skin of patients with Cushing's syndrome is thin and easily injured. Patients with Cushing's syndrome may present with a "moon face" appearance, appear obese around the trunk but thin in the extremities, and have an accumulation of excess fat in the upper back.

Resource Central

Resource Central offers extra practice and review materials in a variety of media. To access it, follow the directions on the Student Access Card provided with the Student Textbook. If there is no card, go to www.bradybooks.com and follow the Resource Central link to Buy Access.

Vocabulary and Concept Review

Exercise 1

Write the letter of the correct definition in the blank next to the term. (See Resource Central for more vocabulary review.)

1. _____ Addison's disease

2. _____ adrenal crisis

3. _____ antihyperglycemic agent

4. _____ Cushing's syndrome

5. _____ diabetes mellitus

6. _____ diabetic ketoacidosis

7. _____ glucagon

8. _____ gluconeogenesis

9. _____ glycogenolysis

10. _____ goiter

11. _____ Graves' disease

12. _____ hyperglycemia

13. _____ hyperthyroidism

14. _____ hypoglycemia

15. _____ hypothyroidism

16. _____ insulin

a. Hormone secreted by alpha cells of the pancreas in response to low blood glucose levels

b. Medication taken by patients with type 2 diabetes to lower blood glucose levels through a variety of mechanisms

c. Hormone secreted by the beta cells of the pancreas in response to increased blood glucose levels

d. Form of hyperthyroidism

e. Severe, life-threatening form of decreased metabolism resulting from hypothyroidism

f. Form of diabetes with onset at a younger age that requires insulin replacement therapy because of autoimmune destruction of pancreatic beta cells

g. Complication of type 2 diabetes in which the blood glucose level may reach 1,000 mg/dL, resulting in diuresis, dehydration, thirst, and electrolyte disorders without ketoacidosis

h. Failure of the adrenal cortices to produce adequate amounts of adrenal cortical hormones, which affects carbohydrate and protein metabolism and electrolyte and water balance

i. Hyperglycemic diabetic emergency in which the patient suffers from dehydration, acidosis, and electrolyte imbalance

j. Breakdown of glycogen stores into glucose

k. Complication of Addison disease in which the body cannot maintain homeostasis because of a lack of adrenal cortical hormones

l. Doughy edema of the tissues in hypothyroid conditions; often associated with coarseness of the skin

m. Acidic substances that accumulate in the blood when fats are used for energy in large quantities

n. Condition of low blood glucose, less than 70 mg/dL

o. Enlargement of the thyroid gland, which may be associated with both hypothyroid and hyperthyroid conditions

p. Form of diabetes with typical onset in middle-aged, obese individuals; usually controlled by diet, exercise, weight loss, and oral medications

(continued on the next page)

17. _____ ketones

q. Class of oral antihyperglycemic agents that act by stimulating the pancreas to increase insulin production

18. _____ Kussmaul's respirations

r. Disorder caused by oversecretion of adrenal cortical hormones or by long-term corticosteroid therapy

19. _____ myxedema

s. Synthesis (creation) of glucose from amino and fatty acids

20. _____ myxedema coma

t. Regular, deep, rapid respirations that reflect the body's attempt to compensate for metabolic acidosis in diabetic ketoacidosis (DKA)

21. _____ nonketotic hyperosmolar coma

u. Extreme, life-threatening form of hyperthyroidism that includes tachycardia, hyperthermia, and altered mental status

22. _____ sulfonylurea

v. Oversecretion of thyroid hormones, leading to signs and symptoms associated with increased metabolic rate

23. _____ thyrotoxicosis

w. Disorder of glucose metabolism resulting from insufficient insulin

24. _____ tropic hormone

x. Hormones secreted by one endocrine gland that stimulate another endocrine gland

25. _____ type 1 diabetes

y. Condition in which insufficient amount of thyroid hormones are secreted, resulting in signs and symptoms that reflect slowed metabolism

26. _____ type 2 diabetes

z. High level of glucose in the blood, greater than 140 mg/dL

Exercise 2

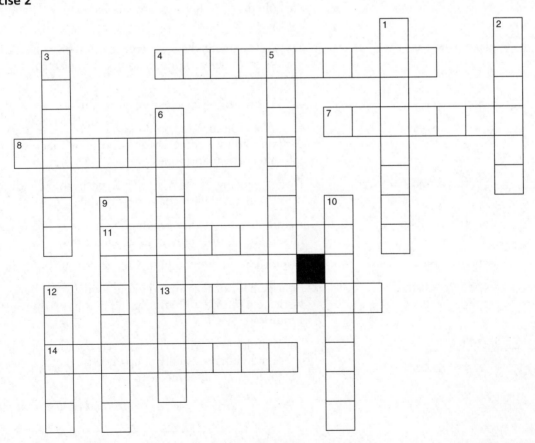

Across

4. Excessive hunger.
7. Chemical messenger of the endocrine system.
8. A 50% solution of this is administered intravenously to unresponsive hypoglycemic patients.
11. System of ductless glands.
13. Secretes insulin, glucagon, and somatostatin.
14. Two-part endocrine gland that communicates with the hypothalamus.

Down

1. Effect on the kidneys when the blood glucose level is extremely high.
2. Clumps of endocrine tissue in the pancreas.
3. Glands that secrete epinephrine and norepinephrine.
5. This part of the pituitary gland releases antidiuretic hormone and oxytocin.
6. Excessive thirst.
9. Site on a cell that is selective for a specific hormone.
10. This type of feedback mechanism works like a thermostat.
12. Pancreas cells that secrete glucagon.

Patient Assessment Review

You have been dispatched for a "sick person with diabetes." Using the summary of the following patient assessment process as a structure, answer the questions to elaborate on your clinical reasoning at each step of the process.

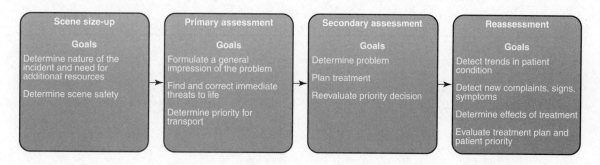

Scene size-up	Primary assessment	Secondary assessment	Reassessment
Goals	**Goals**	**Goals**	**Goals**
Determine nature of the incident and need for additional resources	Formulate a general impression of the problem	Determine problem	Detect trends in patient condition
Determine scene safety	Find and correct immediate threats to life	Plan treatment	Detect new complaints, signs, symptoms
	Determine priority for transport	Reevaluate priority decision	Determine effects of treatment
			Evaluate treatment plan and patient priority

Scene Size-Up

1. What about the scene size-up would give an indication that the patient has a diabetic emergency?

   _____

   _____

   _____

2. What hazards could be present at the scene of a medical emergency?

   _____

   _____

   _____

3. Are there any hazards specific to diabetic emergencies? If so, what are they?

   _____

   _____

   _____

4. How would you control any hazards at the scene?

   _____

   _____

   _____

5. Under what circumstances might you need additional resources?

   _____

   _____

   _____

6. What about the patient's general appearance would indicate that he is a critical patient?

   _____

   _____

   _____

Primary Assessment

7. What are you looking for in the primary assessment of a patient with diabetes?

   _____

   _____

   _____

8. What might give you a clue to a diabetic emergency as you complete the primary assessment?

   _____

   _____

   _____

9. What interventions are required in the primary assessment?

   _____

   _____

   _____

10. What are some special considerations in the primary assessment interventions for a patient with diabetes?

_____

_____

_____

11. What information will influence your decision about the patient's priority for transport?

_____

_____

_____

Secondary Assessment

12. What are the important questions to ask when obtaining the medical history of a patient who potentially has diabetes?

_____

_____

_____

13. What can the vital signs tell you about the patient's condition?

_____

_____

_____

14. What monitoring devices can provide important information about a patient who potentially has diabetes?

_____

_____

_____

15. What is the role of physical examination in patients with diabetes?

_____

_____

_____

16. Summarize findings that would make you suspect a hyperglycemic emergency.

_____

_____

_____

17. Summarize findings that would make you suspect a hypoglycemic emergency.

_____

_____

_____

Reassessment

18. Describe considerations in the reassessment process of a patient with diabetes.

_____

_____

_____

Check Your Recall and Apply Concepts

Exercise 1

For the following statements, write a T in the blank if the statement is true or an F if the statement is false.

1. _____ Glucagon should not be given with along with D50.

2. _____ Only cells with a receptor for specific hormone molecules are affected by the presence of the hormone.

3. _____ Hormonal secretion is regulated by negative feedback.

4. _____ There are no contraindications for oral glucose for a patient with hypoglycemia.

5. _____ The first treatment for a patient with hyperglycemia is oral glucose.

6. _____ When the glucose level is low, glucagon levels drop and other pancreas cells secrete insulin.

7. _____ The hypothalamus controls the pituitary gland.

8. _____ The suffix –tropic (or –tropin) means "to stimulate."

9. _____ Hormonal secretion is regulated by negative feedback.

10. _____ Glucose that is not used right away is converted to glucagon.

11. _____ Thyroid gland hormones control the rate of energy metabolism by cells.

12. _____ The adrenal glands sit atop the medulla oblongata.

13. _____ Gestational diabetes occurs only during pregnancy.

14. _____ Patients with type 1 diabetes are insulin resistant.

15. _____ Type 1 diabetes is associated with nonketotic hyperosmolar coma (NKHC).

Exercise 2

Place a check mark in the appropriate column to identify which sign or symptom is associated with hypoglycemia and which is associated with hyperglycemia. Some signs or symptoms may accompany both or neither.

Presentation	Hypoglycemia	Hyperglycemia
Acetone breath		
High insulin level		
Thirst		
Seizure		
Dehydration		
Acute onset		
Dry, warm skin		
Bizarre behavior		
Diaphoretic skin		

Clinical Reasoning

CASE STUDY: PATIENT WITH DIABETES

Your crew is called to care for a patient with a possible diabetic emergency. You arrive to find a 28-year-old woman with slow, snoring respirations. Her roommate tells you the patient has a type 1 diabetes but she has not been eating well since she has been sick. You check her blood sugar and determine it to be 45 mg/dL.

1. What do you think is the cause of this patient's diabetic emergency?

_____

_____

_____

_____

2. Should you place a supraglottic airway to secure her airway? Why or why not?

_____

_____

_____

_____

_____

3. What should be your first treatment for this patient?

_____

_____

_____

_____

_____

_____

Project-Based Learning

Locate a family member or friend who has diabetes and interview him regarding the impact the illness has had on his lifestyle. This will help you understand diabetes and the lifestyle changes that go along with it, from the patient's personal perspective. Diabetes is so common these days, so it should not be too difficult to find a person who has diabetes to talk to.

The EMS Professional in Practice

You are called for an older man who has had his leg amputated above the knee due to circulatory problems secondary to diabetes. He has fallen from his wheelchair and is unable to right himself. Your service responds to public assist calls, so your unit has responded. Due to his handicap, it is obvious that he is unable to work, but he also lives in substandard housing. How do calls of this nature make you feel? What can you or your service do to help this man? Jot down your thoughts in a notebook or journal for discussion in class or in your study group.

Abdominal Pain and Gastrointestinal Disorders

Content Area

• Medicine

Advanced EMT Education Standard

• Applies fundamental knowledge to provide basic and selected advanced emergency care and transportation based on assessment findings for an acutely ill patient.

Summary of Objectives

24.1 Define terms introduced in this chapter.

Knowing and being able to apply the key terms in each chapter is critical to understanding chapter concepts. Write the list of key terms. Then write the definition of each one in your own words. Check your understanding by confirming the definitions in the textbook glossary. Correct any misunderstandings. Create a study aid by writing each key term on the front of an index card and the definition on the back. Use the cards to quiz yourself or to have someone quiz you. The exercises under Vocabulary and Concept Review below will give you additional practice.

24.2 Compare and contrast the general characteristics of hollow and solid abdominal organs.

Solid organs are inelastic and covered by a fibrous capsule. They are dense and highly vascular. Examples of solid organs include the liver, spleen, pancreas, and kidneys (retroperitoneal). Hollow organs are tube-like structures that serve to transport and store substances. Hollow organs have a coat of smooth muscle that allows them to contract to propel their contents forward or release them from the body. Examples of hollow organs include the stomach, intestines, gallbladder, ureters, and urinary bladder.

24.3 List the general mechanisms and types of abdominal pain.

The general causes of abdominal pain are inflammation or infection, stretching of tissues from distention or traction, and ischemia. Stretching mechanisms affect the hollow organs and the capsules surrounding solid organs. Rapid distention is especially painful. A crampy or colicky pain is usually caused by distention, infection, obstruction, or inflammation of a hollow organ.

Increased peristalsis and pain can occur in gastroenteritis, bowel obstruction with proximal distention of the intestine, intestinal gas, a kidney stone passing through a ureter, and urinary tract infection.

Visceral pain arises from the organs in the abdominal cavity and is difficult for the patient to localize. The diffuse nature of the pain is due to the sparse supply of sensory nerves to the organs.

Parietal (somatic) pain arises from inflammation of the peritoneum that lines the abdominal cavity (parietal peritoneum). The pain is generally intense, constant, and often described as sharp. The pain is well localized, meaning that the patient is able to point to the exact area that hurts.

Referred pain is experienced at a site remote from the affected organ. The sensation is often felt in the skin or deeper tissues and is well localized. It arises when the area shares a sensory nerve pathway with the affected organ.

24.4 Describe the pathophysiology, risk factors, assessment, and management of patients with emergencies related to hepatic diseases, including viral hepatitis, cirrhosis, and hepatic encephalopathy.

Hepatitis has both infectious and noninfectious causes. Most infectious causes are viral. Noninfectious causes include medications and toxins, such as an acetaminophen overdose. Some types of hepatitis are asymptomatic, and some can become chronic, eventually resulting in liver failure. Acute hepatitis can present with pain in the upper right quadrant of the abdomen, nausea, malaise, and fever. Jaundice occurs when the inflamed liver cannot rid the body of bilirubin. Chronic hepatitis can lead to liver cancer, cirrhosis, and portal hypertension.

Cirrhosis is a progressive disease caused by chronic inflammation of the liver causing scar tissue. Common causes of cirrhosis are chronic alcohol abuse, fatty liver, and chronic hepatitis. In cirrhosis, the liver cannot metabolize drugs, vitamins, and other substances, rid the body of the pigments from red blood cell breakdown, effectively store glycogen, or produce the albumin, clotting factors, and other substances it normally produces. As a result, levels of ammonia, bilirubin, and other toxins increase, and blood clotting is impaired.

The resistance to blood flow through the diseased liver results in portal vein hypertension. The increased hydrostatic pressure in the portal system, coupled with low albumin, results in an accumulation of fluid in the abdomen called ascites. Ascites can result in abdominal distention and interferes with diaphragmatic movement. When ammonia levels become high from progressive liver failure, hepatic encephalopathy can occur.

Management will focus on maintaining an adequate airway, ventilation, oxygenation, and circulation. Vomiting is always an issue with patients with abdominal pain. Allow the patient to assume a position of comfort, which typically will be lying on his side with the legs drawn up. Consider administration of fluids if the patient is dehydrated. Administer pain medications as indicated.

24.5 Explain the pathophysiology, assessment, and management of the following abdominal and gastrointestinal disorders: abdominal aortic aneurysm or dissection, appendicitis, bowel obstruction, cholecystitis, constipation, diarrhea, esophageal varices, gastroenteritis, hernia, inflammatory disorders of the bowel, pancreatitis, peritonitis, and upper and lower gastrointestinal bleeding.

Abdominal emergencies have several general causes, including atherosclerotic disease, which can lead to abdominal aortic aneurysm or dissection and infarction of the organs. Hemorrhage, including hemorrhage from rupture aneurysm, esophageal varies, gastritis or ulcers, gastrointestinal cancer, and ruptured diverticula can be life-threatening. The obstruction of hollow structures, such as the bowel or bile duct, can lead to pain and complications related to the obstruction of substances moving through the lumen of the structure, including ischemia of the structure and rupture. Inflammatory disorders, such as pancreatitis and Crohn's disease and other inflammatory bowel diseases, can lead to significant pain and dysfunction. Pancreatitis is highly associated with alcohol abuse but has other causes. Constipation is uncomfortable and can result in bowel obstruction, while diarrhea can lead to dehydration. Infection or inflammation of the appendix can lead to appendicitis.

Identify problems with the airway, breathing, and circulation in the primary assessment. Vomiting and reduced level of responsiveness can lead to airway obstruction. Abdominal pain and distention can impair breathing and oxygenation. Patients with abdominal emergencies may be hypovolemic. Use manual maneuvers, suction, and airway adjuncts as needed to maintain the airway. Provide oxygen, if needed, to maintain an SpO_2 of 95 percent or higher and assist ventilations as needed.

The history is important in determining the potential causes of abdominal disorders, including obtaining associated complaints and exploring the nature of the chief complaint. For women, it is often useful to obtain an obstetric and gynecological history when the chief complaint is abdominal pain. During the secondary exam, inspection and palpation of the abdomen can be useful, as well as checking for Murphy's sign and checking for pain with a heel drop. If a mass is palpated, determine whether it is pulsating, which can indicate aortic aneurysm. If aneurysm or dissection is suspected, check the circulation in the lower extremities.

Obtain IV access, if needed, to treat hypovolemia and provide a route for medication administration. The use of nitrous oxide for analgesia is contraindicated in patients with potential bowel obstruction. If indicated and permitted in your system, treat nausea and vomiting with antiemetics. Allow the patient to assume a position of greatest comfort for transport, unless contraindicated for airway management or treatment of hypovolemia.

24.6 Develop an effective line of questioning for patients presenting with abdominal pain and gastrointestinal complaints.

Using the mnemonics SAMPLE and OPQRST, you must follow up on your patient's chief complaint. The patient's answers to questions should lead you to other questions that help you find out relevant information about the patient's condition.

24.7 Effectively communicate the assessment findings, history, and treatment of patients with gastrointestinal complaints and abdominal pain orally and in writing.

A good summary distinguishes between relevant and irrelevant information and paints a picture that helps other health care providers understand the evolution of the illness and the patient's current condition.

Resource Central

Resource Central offers extra practice and review materials in a variety of media. To access it, follow the directions on the Student Access Card provided with the Student Textbook. If there is no card, go to www.bradybooks.com and follow the Resource Central link to Buy Access.

Vocabulary and Concept Review

Write the letter of the correct definition in the blank next to the term. (See Resource Central for more vocabulary review.)

1. _____ anorexia

    a. Fibrotic scarring of the liver from chronic liver disease such as hepatitis or alcohol abuse

2. _____ bile

    b. Laceration of the esophageal mucosa at the junction of the stomach and esophagus, usually due to forceful vomiting

3. _____ cholecystitis

    c. Inflammation of the liver, either infectious or noninfectious

4. _____ chyme

    d. Opening on the surface of the abdomen that connects the cut end of the colon to outside of the body

5. _____ cirrhosis

    e. Increased pressure throughout the portal venous system of the digestive tract as a result of liver disease

6. _____ colostomy

    f. Powerful digestive enzyme in the stomach that breaks down proteins

7. _____ diverticulitis

    g. Black, tarry stool due to the presence of blood exposed to digestive juices

8. _____ emesis

    h. Distended, varicose veins in the esophagus due to portal vein hypertension

9. _____ esophageal varices

    i. Inflammation of the gallbladder

10. _____ hematemesis

    j. Condition in which the stomach slides through the diaphragmatic hiatus

11. _____ hematochezia

    k. Loss of appetite

12. _____ hepatitis

    l. Hidden; not obvious

13. _____ hiatal hernia

    m. Twisting of a loop of bowel around itself, cutting off circulation to the affected area

14. _____ intussusception

    n. Erosion of the gastric or duodenal mucosa

15. _____ jaundice

    o. Vomit

16. _____ Mallory-Weiss tear

    p. Telescoping of part of the bowel over itself

17. _____ melena

    q. Inflammation of the parietal peritoneum

18. _____ occult

    r. Digestive fluid excreted from the liver into the duodenum to emulsify fats

19. _____ pepsin

    s. Bloody stool

20. _____ peptic ulcer

    t. Infection and inflammation of a diverticulum

21. _____ peristalsis

    u. Yellow pigmentation of the skin from deposition of excess bilirubin

22. _____ peritonitis

    v. Mixture of partially digested food and digestive fluids that leaves the stomach and enters the duodenum

23. _____ portal hypertension

    w. Rhythmic smooth muscle contractions that propel the contents of hollow, tubular organs forward

24. _____ volvulus

    x. Vomiting blood, either fresh or partially digested

Patient Assessment Review

Fill in the following table with the possible sources of complaints of abdominal pain.

Abdominal Region	Organs	Sources of Referred Pain
Right upper quadrant		
Epigastric region		
Left upper quadrant		
Umbilical and hypogastric		
Right lower quadrant		
Left lower quadrant		

Check Your Recall and Apply Concepts

Exercise 1

Select the best possible choice for each of the following questions.

_____ 1. Which one of the following is considered a hollow organ?
   a. Liver
   b. Spleen
   c. Gallbladder
   d. Kidneys

_____ 2. The dividing line between the thoracic cavity and the abdominal cavity is the:
   a. umbilicus.
   b. rib cage.
   c. diaphragm.
   d. liver.

_____ 3. Accessory organs of the digestive system include the:
   a. appendix.
   b. pancreas.
   c. cecum.
   d. duodenum.

_____ 4. An enzyme in saliva that breaks down complex carbohydrates into simple sugars is:
   a. amylase.
   b. albumin.
   c. bile.
   d. bilirubin.

_____ 5. Ecchymosis of the flanks is known as:
   a. Battle's sign.
   b. Cullen's sign.
   c. Murphy's sign.
   d. Grey-Turner's sign.

Exercise 2

Complete each statement by filling in the missing term.

1. Patients with pancreatitis have intense pain in the _____ region.

2. Noninfectious causes of _____ include medications and toxins, such as acetaminophen overdose.

3. Jaundice occurs when the inflamed liver cannot rid the body of _____.

4. _____ can cause referred pain to the upper quadrant of the abdomen on the affected side.

5. Intense, tearing pain in the lower back or abdomen and pain that radiate down one or both legs suggests _____.

6. The posterior portion of parietal peritoneum separates the abdominal organs from the _____ organs, which lie between the peritoneum and the posterior body wall.

7. Another term for colostomy is _____.

8. Certain medications, such as NSAIDs, corticosteroids, some herbal supplements, and excessive alcohol ingestion can increase the risk of _____ bleeding.

9. A crampy or colicky pain is usually caused by distention, infection, obstruction, or inflammation of a(n) _____ organ.

10. _____ pain arises from the organs in the abdominal cavity and is difficult for the patient to localize.

Clinical Reasoning

CASE STUDY: FAST FOOD FIASCO

Your crew is called to a residence for a woman with abdominal pain. The patient is doubled over with her knees drawn up and she is holding her stomach. She states she ate a hamburger and French fries from a fast food drive-through about an hour ago. In answer to your questions, she tells you that the pain is in her right shoulder as well as on the right side under her rib cage.

1. What do you suspect is wrong with the patient?

_____

_____

_____

_____

_____

2. What would be one of the most important questions to ask her?

_____

_____

_____

_____

_____

3. What treatment will you provide for her?

_____

_____

_____

_____

_____

Project-Based Learning

Practice assessing a patient with abdominal pain. Imagine: You are called to a patient complaining of abdominal pain for 2 hours. She was seated at her desk at work and began to feel nauseated. Make a list of at eight questions that you need to ask the patient that relates directly to her abdominal pain.

The EMS Professional in Practice

Abdominal pain is one of those chief complaints for which you have to take your patient's word. Just because you cannot verify that your patient is actually sick, should you treat the patient any differently than a patient with an obvious broken bone? Is it more difficult to be empathetic for a patient who could be faking it? Jot down your thoughts in a notebook or journal for discussion in class or in your study group.

Chapter 25

Renal, Genitourinary, and Gynecologic Disorders

Content Area

- Medicine
- Trauma

Advanced EMT Education Standards

- Applies fundamental knowledge to provide basic and selected advanced emergency care and transportation based on assessment findings for an acutely ill patient.
- Applies fundamental knowledge to provide basic and selected advanced emergency care and transportation based on assessment findings for an acutely injured patient.

Summary of Objectives

25.1 Define terms introduced in this section.

Knowing and being able to apply the key terms in each chapter is critical to understanding chapter concepts. Write the list of key terms. Then write the definition of each one in your own words. Check your understanding by confirming the definitions in the textbook glossary. Correct any misunderstandings. Create a study aid by writing each key term on the front of an index card and the definition on the back. Use the cards to quiz yourself or to have someone quiz you. The exercises under Vocabulary and Concept Review below will give you additional practice.

25.2 Describe the pathophysiology of acute and chronic renal failure.

Acute renal failure (ARF) is a loss of renal function over hours to days with the accumulation of nitrogen-containing wastes in the blood. The causes of acute renal failure are classified by whether the underlying problem occurs outside the urinary system, in the kidney (intrinsic renal failure), or after urine leaves the kidney.

Prerenal renal failure is caused by issues or disease elsewhere in the body (such as hypotension) that affects the kidney's ability to produce urine. Intrinsic renal failure, such as loss of nephrons, is caused by diseases in the kidneys.

Postrenal failure occurs after urine leaves the kidney and is commonly due to obstruction of a ureter.

Chronic renal failure (CRF) is defined as irreversible kidney dysfunction with increased urea in the blood for greater than three months. Any type of renal failure can leave the patient without functioning kidneys, which leads to chronic renal failure requiring dialysis. CRF is often caused by diabetes or hypertension.

25.3 Discuss the complications of end-stage renal disease.

End-stage renal disease requires kidney transplant or dialysis and results from long-standing problems with diabetes and hypertension. Complications involving central lines and dialysis shunts may occur as a result of treatment for end-stage renal disease. Graft complications include thrombosis and stenosis and can become infected. CRF patients have poorly functional platelets, which can lead to bleeding issues. Attachment to a machine as a lifeline can become a psychologic burden that can lead to medical problems including malnutrition, hypertension, hyperlipidemia, pruritus, and skin rashes.

25.4 Explain the assessment and management of patients with emergencies related to renal failure and dialysis.

To assess these patients, you must determine how well the patient is doing. Is he making it to his dialysis appointments? What is his nutritional status? Is his blood pressure controlled? Does he have bone disease that requires rehabilitation? What is his level of functioning? Those are all important questions in understanding the status of that individual.

Keys to managing ARF patients are to remove any offending agents and to maintain their fluid status as close to normal as possible. Because their kidneys are not functioning well, large fluid boluses, even in the face of hypotension, can be devastating. Patients with crackles (rales) should not receive large amounts of saline regardless of blood pressure. Instead, intravenous medications that raise the blood pressure through vasoconstriction are indicated.

25.5 Explain the processes of hemodialysis and peritoneal dialysis.

Long-term hemodialysis patients will have a catheter placed in the subclavian area and a shunt graft placed in one arm. The subclavian line is used for temporary dialysis access while the graft heals, or "matures." In the hemodialysis machine, the patient's blood circulates on one side of a synthetic semipermeable membrane while a solution called dialysate circulates on the other. The difference in the concentration of substances across the membrane allows wastes to be removed from the blood. The blood then flows from the dialysis machine through tubing that returns it to the venous circulation. To accomplish this task, the graft shunt, which is a small section of tubing, surgically connects an artery and vein.

Peritoneal dialysis (PD) uses the peritoneal membrane of the abdominal cavity to remove wastes from the blood. At varying times during the day, PD patients place large quantities of fluid in their abdomen and wait for the toxins in the blood to equilibrate by osmosis with this fluid before they remove it again. In this manner, they remove many of the toxins without having to be hooked up to an expensive dialysis machine and avoid the required travel to the dialysis center. The machine for peritoneal dialysis is portable and small in comparison with hemodialysis machines.

25.6 Discuss the pathophysiology, assessment, and management of patients with urinary retention.

Urinary retention is a common complication of benign prostatic hypertrophy though it also can be caused by nerve dysfunction, constipation, infection, or medications. Spine injuries or bladder obstruction can block the passage of urine and lead to urine retention.

A physical examination may show a large nontympanic (dull to percussion, indicating the presence of fluid) mass in the lower abdomen, which is the enlarged bladder. Urine not only backs up into the bladder, but also backs up through the ureters into the kidney.

Relieving the obstruction is done with a Foley catheter in the hospital emergency department. In many cases, the patient requires surgery to prevent future re-obstruction. Giving a bolus of IV fluid can worsen the patient's condition. Transport in the position of comfort is indicated.

25.7 Discuss the pathophysiology, assessment, and management of patients with urinary system infections (UTIs).

UTIs are more common in female than in male patients because of their shorter urethra, which allows bacteria to reach the bladder before being eliminated from the urethra during urination. It is also common in patients with indwelling Foley catheters or who are catheterizing themselves, and patients with spinal-cord disease or trauma.

Signs of UTI include abdominal or pelvic pain, hematuria, foul or strong odor to the urine, frequent urination or urge to urinate, and pain on urination or intercourse.

Treatment is the same as for other renal disorders—oxygen if indicated, position of comfort, and limited fluids.

25.8 Identify complications associated with catheterization of the urinary bladder.

Introduction of bacteria is a major concern with urinary catheterization. Pulling on the inflated balloon can cause internal trauma and lead to infections. You must take care to maintain the urine bag below the level of the patient to allow the free flow of urine into the bag. Positioning the bag above patient level can lead to backflow of urine.

25.9 Discuss the pathophysiology, assessment, and management of patients with renal calculi.

Metabolic problems can result in the production of small stones in the kidney (renal calculi), usually no bigger than grains of sand. They can normally pass through the lower urinary tract as long as they are less than 6 mm in size.

Assessment reveals constant, severe flank pain, often radiating to the groin, or lower abdominal pain, tenderness over the costovertebral angle, and nausea. The patient usually moves about trying to find a comfortable position. He typically will be pale and diaphoretic and may complain of blood in the urine. Many times, there is a family or personal history of kidney stones.

Treatment includes allowing the patient to find his most comfortable position. Start an IV, because a bolus of fluid could help flush out the stone and alleviate the pain. You may consider the administration of analgesics, in consultation with medical direction.

25.10 Discuss the pathophysiology, assessment, and management of patients with trauma to the male genitourinary system.

Males' genital organs are mostly external to the body cavity, which can lead to significant tears, lacerations, and other injuries to the scrotum or penis. Trauma may be accidental, self-induced, or a result of sexual assault.

Injuries to the genitalia may distract both you and the patient from noticing other, potentially life-threatening injuries. Despite the situation, always conduct a physical examination appropriate to the mechanism of injury and the patient's overall presentation.

Treat problems involving the airway, ventilation, oxygenation, and sources of significant external bleeding first. Cover open wounds with a sterile dressing, apply gentle pressure to control bleeding, and use a wrapped ice pack to reduce swelling. Make the patient as comfortable as possible and transport.

25.11 Discuss the pathophysiology, assessment, and management of patients with epididymitis, orchitis, and Fournier gangrene.

Epididymitis is defined as an inflammation of the epididymis at the posterior pole of the testicle. It is a common finding in young males who have sexually transmitted infections (STIs), and elderly men. It presents much like testicular torsion, a surgical emergency, and therefore is important not to misdiagnose. Ice and elevation of the testicles will help a case of epididymitis; however, elevation of a torsed testicle will worsen the condition.

Orchitis is inflammation of the testicle itself. On examination, the testicle will be tender, but the epididymis will be normal and nontender. Occurrence of orchitis is relatively rare; treatment is if indicated, position of comfort, and ice.

Fournier's gangrene is a bacterial infection of the skin that affects both the genitals and the perineum, usually developing from a wound or abrasion to the skin. Presentation includes a small scab or lesion on the surface, but the infection is deeply seated in the pelvis. Symptoms include crepitus of the area around the scrotum and perineum (a spongy feeling with crackling under the skin), pus weeping from a small gray-colored lesion, a foul odor in the area, severe swelling of the scrotum and penis, and a patient who is lethargic and febrile. This is a true emergency. Field management is comfort and establishment of an IV for further access in the emergency department. If the patient is hypotensive, fluid replacement is important.

25.12 Describe the basic anatomy and physiology of the female reproductive system.

The internal organs of the female reproductive system are the vagina, uterus, ovaries, and fallopian tubes. The vagina functions as the birth canal during childbirth, receives the penis during sexual intercourse, and serves as a passageway for menstrual flow. The ovaries are the primary sex gland and are located on each side of the uterus. They develop and release eggs necessary for reproduction. The fallopian tubes transmit the fertilized ovum for implantation in the uterus. If implantation does not occur, the endometrium sloughs off during menses.

25.13 Obtain a relevant history from patients with a suspected gynecologic problem.

The history will be crucial in developing differential diagnoses. However, your approach to the history will determine how comfortable the patient feels in sharing information with you. If you appear uncaring, uncomfortable, or unknowledgeable concerning the history or potential problems, the patient is not likely to share information with you. When a patient complains of abdominal pain, one of the most frequent complaints associated with gynecologic disorders, anticipate the direction your history may take and provide the patient with privacy. If you believe a patient's complaint may be caused by a gynecologic problem, questions about her menstrual and reproductive history can add important information to your understanding of her problem.

25.14 Describe signs and symptoms associated with common gynecologic and female genitourinary system causes of acute abdominal pain, including dysmenorrhea, endometriosis, endometritis, ovarian cyst, pelvic inflammatory disease, sexually transmitted infections, and urinary tract infection.

- Dysmenorrhea is painful menstruation and may be felt as strong abdominal cramps.
- Endometriosis presents with abdominopelvic or lower back pain, which may radiate down the legs. Changes in pain level are often cyclical, accompanying changes in the menstrual cycle.
- Endometritis most often occurs after childbirth or uterine surgery or instrumentation in patients complaining of abdominal pain with fever and abnormal vaginal discharge, or a history of recent childbirth and gynecologic procedures, including abortion and dilation and curettage.
- An ovarian cyst, if ruptured, can cause a small amount of bleeding and release of the follicular fluid. This causes irritation of the peritoneum. The cyst may leak, rather than suddenly rupture, leading to a longer period of peritoneal irritation.
- Pelvic inflammatory disease (PID) is inflammation of the peritoneum resulting in intense pelvic pain. When the patient walks, each heel strike transmits vibration to the peritoneum, resulting in severe pain. For this reason, patients with PID may walk with a shuffling gait to avoid lifting the feet and striking the heel against the floor.
- Sexually transmitted infections cause symptoms that may be localized, such as complaints of an ulceration on the genitals, or they may include generalized symptoms, such as seen in disseminated gonorrhea.
- Urinary tract infection involves urethral discharge, which is common if the patient has an infection of the urethra or prostate. If the infection is in the bladder, the usual complaint is painful, frequent, cloudy, and malodorous urine. Painful urination, and the frequent urge to urinate are common symptoms.

25.15 Describe special considerations in the assessment and management of patients with sexual assault and vaginal bleeding.

Sexual assault injuries to the genitalia are generally quite concerning to patients and may distract both you and the patient from noticing other, potentially life-threatening, injuries. Despite the situation, always conduct a physical examination appropriate to the mechanism of injury and the patient's overall presentation. Management is largely supportive. Administer oxygen if needed, and control external bleeding from traumatic injury. Allow the patient to assume a position of comfort and provide empathetic and nonjudgmental care.

Vaginal bleeding care depends on your approach to the patient's history. It will determine how comfortable the patient feels in sharing information with you. If you appear uncaring, uncomfortable, or unknowledgeable concerning the history or potential problems, the patient is not likely to share information with you. Care is mainly supportive other than providing oxygen and controlling bleeding. With excessive bleeding, treat for shock.

25.16 Effectively communicate assessment findings for patients with gynecologic and genitourinary/renal complaints to other health care providers, orally and in writing.

Provide a full oral report to the next health care provider, while being sensitive to the patient's need for privacy. When writing your patient care report, you must fully document all patient history obtained and results of a full assessment. You must record all care provided and patient outcomes from treatment.

Resource Central

Resource Central offers extra practice and review materials in a variety of media. To access it, follow the directions on the Student Access Card provided with the Student Textbook. If there is no card, go to www.bradybooks.com and follow the Resource Central link to Buy Access.

Vocabulary and Concept Review

Exercise 1

Write the letter of the correct definition in the blank next to the term. (See Resource Central for more vocabulary review.)

1. _____ acute renal failure (ARF)

2. _____ benign prostatic hypertrophy (BPH)

3. _____ chronic renal failure (CRF)

4. _____ dialysis

5. _____ dysmenorrhea

6. _____ dysuria

7. _____ ectopic pregnancy

8. _____ end-stage renal disease

9. _____ endometriosis

a. Noncancerous enlargement of the prostate gland

b. Presence of endometrium outside the uterine cavity

c. Painful menstruation

d. Implantation of a fertilized ovum outside the uterus, usually in the fallopian tube

e. Inflammation of the epididymis

f. Painful urination

g. Progressive loss of kidney function over time

h. Benign tumor of the uterus

i. Process of placing blood in contact with a semipermeable membrane (synthetic or peritoneum) that separates it from a dialysate to remove wastes from the blood

(continued on the next page)

10. _____ epididymitis

11. _____ Foley catheter

12. _____ hematuria

13. _____ paraphimosis

14. _____ polycystic renal disease

15. _____ priapism

16. _____ shunt graft

17. _____ uremia

18. _____ uremic encephalopathy

19. _____ uremic frost

20. _____ uterine fibroid

j. Altered mental status caused by uremia

k. Irreversible kidney damage requiring dialysis or transplant

l. Flaky deposits of urea on the skin of severely uremic patients

m. Short-term inability of the kidney to produce urine, measured by levels of creatinine and blood urea nitrogen

n. Constriction of the foreskin behind the glans penis, causing restriction in lymphatic drainage and circulation, resulting in pain, swelling, and potential necrosis of the glans

o. Blood in the urine

p. Clear plastic tube passed through the urethra and anchored in the bladder with an inflatable balloon to allow urine to drain into an external collection bag

q. Artificial tube connecting an artery and vein in the arm to allow for hemodialysis

r. Condition including signs and symptoms of renal failure with an increase in blood urea nitrogen (BUN) and creatinine, which would normally be excreted by the kidneys

s. Hereditary disease in which cysts form within the kidney, eventually destroying the nephrons

t. Painful erection of the penis lasting more than 4 hours

Exercise 2

Fill in the blank with the correct term that matches the definition.

1. Kidney failure caused by problems within the kidney, such as damage to the nephrons. _____

2. Serious infection of the subcutaneous tissues of the peritoneum. _____

3. An autoimmune disease that affects many tissues, including the kidneys. _____

4. Kidney failure caused by a problem outside the urinary system, such as hypotension resulting from shock or heart failure. _____

5. A serious condition resulting from toxins of *E. coli* strain 0157:H7. Manifestations include renal failure, pulmonary edema, and anemia. _____

6. The number of times a woman has given birth. _____

7. A stone formed in the kidney. _____

8. Kidney failure caused by urinary obstruction, such as that from BPH or renal calculi. _____

9. Pain along the length of the ureter associated with renal calculi. _____

10. The total number of times a woman has been pregnant, regardless of the outcome. _____

11. Frequent urination after going to bed. _____

12. Condition in which the foreskin is constricted and cannot be retracted from the glans penis. _____

13. Inflammation of the kidneys. _____

Exercise 3

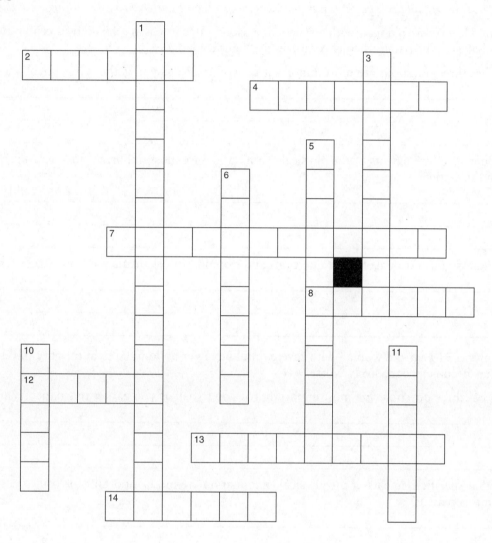

Across

2. Complication of renal failure due to decreased erythropoietin production
4. Microscopic unit of the kidney that produces urine
7. Physician who specializes in treating kidney diseases.
8. Type of pregnancy that is implanted outside of the uterine cavity.
12. Autoimmune disease that can affect the kidneys.
13. Cause of pelvic inflammatory disease.
14. Life-threatening complication of an untreated urinary tract infection.

Down

1. Most common non traumatic cause of priapism.
3. Physician who specializes in treating problems of the male genitalia.
5. Tissue that is shed during menstruation.
6. Area of skin between the genitals and anus.
9. Outer layer of the kidney.
10. Where the pain associated with a kidney stone is often experienced.
11. What you will feel if you lightly palpate a properly functioning shunt graft in a hemodialysis patient.

Patient Assessment Review

Write at least three aspects of the history and physical examination that are particularly important for each patient. Do not list everything you would do or ask, just the three that are most important. Then explain how your choices would help find out what is wrong with the patient and determine what treatment is required. The status of all three patients is noncritical (no problems with airway, breathing, or circulation).

1. Patient #1: 41-year-old man with a syncopal episode as he is leaving the dialysis center after hemodialysis. The patient's chief complaint is "lightheadedness."

   a. What three questions are most important for you to ask as you gather this patient's history?

   _____

   _____

   _____

   b. What specific elements of the physical examination are most important for you to perform on this patient?

   _____

   _____

   _____

   c. What is your rationale for the questions and examination elements you chose to list earlier?

   _____

   _____

   _____

2. Patient #2: 31-year-old woman with severe, midline lower abdominal pain that began yesterday and has become progressively worse.

   a. What three questions are most important for you to ask as you gather this patient's history?

   _____

   _____

   _____

   b. What specific elements of the physical examination are most important for you to perform on this patient?

   _____

   _____

   _____

   c. What is your rationale for the questions and examination elements you chose to list earlier?

   _____

   _____

   _____

3. Patient #3: 56-year-old male patient who complains that he has not been able to empty his bladder for 24 hours. He complains of bladder fullness and discomfort, but says he cannot produce a full urine stream to relieve his bladder.

    a. What three questions are most important for you to ask as you gather this patient's history?

       _____

       _____

       _____

    b. What specific elements of the physical examination are most important for you to perform on this patient?

       _____

       _____

       _____

    c. What is your rationale for the questions and examination elements you chose to list earlier?

       _____

       _____

       _____

       _____

Check Your Recall and Apply Concepts

Exercise 1

Complete the following sentences by filling in the missing words.

1. The renal system refers to the part of the urinary system composed of the _____

2. The kidneys lie in the retroperitoneum at their respective costovertebral angles, at the _____ pair of ribs, which articulates with T12.

3. The _____ is the basic functional unit of the kidney.

4. The normal rate of urine production is typically between _____ and _____ mL/hour.

5. The prostate gland is located on the inferior aspect of the _____.

6. The _____ is a tube that carries testicular secretions from the epididymis to the prostate.

7. Erection occurs when the _____ nervous system causes vasodilation of the penile arterial supply.

8. The _____ is the lining of the uterus.

9. The uppermost portion of the uterus is the _____ and the lowest portion is the _____.

10. Hypotension may also occur as a result of _____ in patients with an overwhelming UTI.

Exercise 2

Write a T in the blank provided if the statement is true and an F if the statement is false.

1. _____ In patients with renal disease, if dehydration or other volume loss is suspected, you should check orthostatic vital signs.

2. _____ Kidney failure can lead to many complications and can prevent patients from compensating for other illnesses and injuries.

3. _____ The presence of a Foley catheter indicates the patient has a serious UTI.

4. _____ Anemia is a frequent complication of benign prostatic hypertrophy.

5. _____ Spine injuries can disrupt the nervous control over the urethral outflow of urine.

6. _____ Renal calculi affect women more often than men.

7. _____ UTIs are more common in female than in male individuals.

8. _____ Hemodialysis is more effective than peritoneal dialysis.

9. _____ After acute renal failure, kidney function may return to reasonably normal function.

10. _____ If the kidney produces too little urine, it is called *polyuria*.

Clinical Reasoning

CASE STUDY: CALL TO A LOCAL MIDDLE SCHOOL

Your crew has been dispatched to Central Baldwin Middle School for a 14-year-old female patient complaining of acute onset of abdominal pain. When you arrive, you find her in the nurse's office on a cot in left lateral recumbent position.

1. What possible diagnoses immediately cross your mind?

_____

_____

_____

_____

_____

The patient is cool, pale, and diaphoretic, and states that she gets dizzy when she stands up. She rates her pain as a 10 on the 10-point scale as she continues to hold her abdomen and cry.

2. What assessments and treatments should you consider for this patient?

_____

_____

_____

_____

_____

En route, you complete a full assessment and examination. Your patient tells you that she feels nauseated and proceeds to vomit.

3. How does this information influence your differential diagnoses?

_____

_____

_____

_____

_____

Project-Based Learning

To help you understand the results of renal disease, call your local dialysis center and make an appointment to take a tour of the facility. The staff there should be more than glad to help you understand the care they provide. Write in your journal or notebook the two things that surprise you most about your visit.

The EMS Professional in Practice

Patients on dialysis have chronic, debilitating disease. Much of our interaction with, and care for, patients with dialysis is one of support. Describe things you can do or say that demonstrate your empathy for your patient. Jot down your thoughts in a notebook or journal for discussion in class or in your study group.

Content Area

• Medicine

Advanced EMT Education Standard

• Applies fundamental knowledge to provide basic and selected advanced emergency care and transportation based on assessment findings for an acutely ill patient.

Summary of Objectives

26.1 Define terms introduced in this chapter.

Knowing and being able to apply the key terms in each chapter is critical to understanding chapter concepts. Write the list of key terms. Then write the definition of each one in your own words. Check your understanding by confirming the definitions in the textbook glossary. Correct any misunderstandings. Create a study aid by writing each key term on the front of an index card and the definition on the back. Use the cards to quiz yourself or to have someone quiz you. The exercises under Vocabulary and Concept Review below will give you additional practice.

26.2 Describe the anatomy and physiology of the hematologic system.

Blood consists of a liquid transport medium, plasma, and formed elements with specific functions. The formed elements of the blood are erythrocytes, leukocytes, and thrombocytes. Plasma is about 55 percent of the blood volume and contains about 92 percent water, comprising a large proportion of the body's extracellular fluid. Many of the proteins that comprise the remainder of plasma volume are manufactured in the liver. The formed elements comprise about 45 percent of the blood volume and arise from stem cells in the bone marrow in adults, and from the bone marrow, spleen, liver, thymus, and lymph nodes during fetal development. The liver, spleen, and bone marrow play roles in eliminating aged and damaged blood cells. The kidneys, and to a smaller degree, the liver, secrete the hormone that stimulates RBC production: erythropoietin.

26.3 Describe the pathophysiology and complications of sickle cell disease.

Sickle cell disease is a genetic disorder more common in people of African, Mediterranean, Middle Eastern, Caribbean, and South and Central American origin or descent. Those patients have an abnormal form of hemoglobin that causes RBCs to take on an abnormal curved (sickle-shaped) appearance when oxygen dissociates from them in the tissues. It can regain its normal shape when re-oxygenated, but the changes in shape of the cell damage it, decreasing its life span from the normal 120 days to only 10 to 20 days. The abnormal shape of sickle cells makes it difficult for them to move through capillaries, and they are more prone to clumping. The tissues supplied by the obstructed capillaries become ischemic, resulting in pain and microinfarction of tissues.

26.4 Recognize the signs and symptoms of vaso-occlusive crisis.

During a vaso-occlusive crisis, the tissues supplied by the obstructed capillaries become ischemic, resulting in pain and microinfarction of tissues. Vaso-occlusive crises can result in priapism in males. The intensity of crises varies, but they can be excruciatingly painful, requiring narcotic analgesia.

Blood can pool in the spleen, resulting in painful enlargement of the spleen and a decrease in circulating blood volume. Patients are at risk for stroke, blindness, leg ulcers, and renal failure, and the excessive amount of bilirubin from hemolysis can lead to gallstones and cholecystitis.

26.5 Describe the etiologies and pathophysiology of anemias.

The three causes of anemia are decreased production of RBCs, increased destruction of RBCs, or a loss of RBCs (hemorrhage), each of which decreases the oxygen-carrying capacity of the blood. As a result, the cells do not receive enough oxygen for energy production.

Causes of decreased RBC production include aplastic anemia, iron-deficiency anemia, and pernicious anemia.

Anemia from increased destruction of RBCs is called hemolytic anemia. Sickle cell disease is one cause of premature RBC destruction but other causes include genetic and autoimmune problems and exposure to toxic chemicals or drugs.

The loss of red blood cells occurs mainly through hemorrhage.

26.6 Explain the etiology and pathophysiology of diseases of the white blood cells, including leukemias and lymphomas.

Diseases of white blood cells present with either an increase or decrease in the number of WBCs. Leukemia is a cancer that causes the bone marrow to rapidly produce large numbers of abnormal WBCs. The abnormal cells can crowd out normal cells, resulting in anemia, bleeding, and infection. Some types of leukemia, such as acute lymphoblastic leukemia and acute myelogenous leukemia, occur in children and adults, while others, such as chronic lymphocytic leukemia and chronic myelogenous leukemia, occur primarily in adults.

Lymphomas are cancers of lymphocytes, either B lymphocytes or T lymphocytes, that are localized to the lymph nodes. Lymphomas may either be Hodgkin's lymphoma or non-Hodgkin's lymphoma. Hodgkin's lymphoma involves specific types of B lymphocytes and non-Hodgkin's lymphoma can involve abnormal B lymphocytes or T lymphocytes.

Multiple myeloma is a cancer of cells in the bone marrow in which abnormal cells multiply and crowd out normal cells. This results in decreased production of blood cells, and can result in pathologic fracture of the affected bone.

26.7 Describe the etiology and pathophysiology of disorders of coagulation and hemostasis, including disseminated intravascular coagulation (DIC) and hemophilia.

Coagulation or clotting disorders are collectively known as coagulopathies. The underlying problem can involve platelets or the clotting cascade. Impaired hemostasis can occur from a low number of platelets or altered platelet function.

Hemophilia is an inherited disease that leads to deficiencies in certain clotting factors. Patients with hemophilia and deficiencies of other clotting factors can have mild to severe impairment in blood clotting.

DIC results from systemic overactivation of clotting mechanisms resulting from blood transfusion reactions, sepsis, surgery, and severe trauma. Small blood clots form that cause infarcts of affected organs, including the brain, liver, and kidneys. Because of the excess clotting,

clotting factors are consumed and subsequent bleeding cannot be stopped. At this point, the patient has bleeding from multiple sites.

26.8 Discuss the risk factors, signs and symptoms, and consequences of deep vein thrombosis.

Risk factors for deep vein thrombosis (DVT) include fractures, abdominal surgery, immobilization (including sitting for long periods, especially with the legs crossed), pregnancy, hormones used for birth control or hormone replacement therapy after menopause, cancer, and heart and lung disease. Signs and symptoms include a warm, painful, swollen lower extremity. If the DVT is in lower leg, pain may increase in the calf with dorsiflexion of the foot. If a DVT breaks loose, it can travel to right side of the heart and into the pulmonary circulation, causing a pulmonary embolism. Upper extremity DVTs are very rare, usually seen only in IV drug users, but their ability to cause pulmonary emboli is similar to that of lower extremity DVT.

26.9 Develop a list of differential diagnoses for patients presenting with signs and symptoms of hematologic disorders.

Patients presenting with signs and symptoms of hematologic disorders may have any of the following: anemia, hemophilia, sickle cell disorder, disseminated intravascular coagulation, leukemia, polycythemia, Hodgkin's or non-Hodgkin's lymphoma, multiple myeloma, deep vein thrombosis, and disseminated intravascular coagulation.

26.10 Provide prehospital treatment appropriate to the needs of patients with a variety of hematologic disorders.

In the general management of patients with hematologic disorders, consider the need for oxygen, intravenous fluids, and analgesia. Before providing analgesia, you should perform bleeding control and suctioning if bleeding has compromised the airway. Sickle cell disease patients will need administration of oxygen and fluids along with analgesia. You should manage other hematologic disorders based on presentation and management is usually supportive in nature.

Resource Central

Resource Central offers extra practice and review materials in a variety of media. To access it, follow the directions on the Student Access Card provided with the Student Textbook. If there is no card, go to www.bradybooks.com and follow the Resource Central link to Buy Access.

Vocabulary and Concept Review

Exercise 1

Write the letter of the correct definition in the blank next to the term. (See Resource Central for more vocabulary review.)

1. _____ anemia

   a. Hormone released, primarily from the kidneys, in response to hypoxia to stimulate bone marrow to increase red blood cell production

2. _____ coagulopathies

   b. Pinpoint hemorrhages in the skin

3. _____ clotting cascade

   c. Defects in blood clotting with either inadequate or excessive blood clotting

4. _____ epistaxis

   d. Predisposition toward excessive or uncontrolled bleeding

5. _____ erythropoietin

   e. Decreased number of red blood cells

6. _____ fibrin

7. _____ hematoma

8. _____ hemophilia

9. _____ lymphadenopathy

10. _____ pathologic fracture

11. _____ petechiae

12. _____ purpura

f. Small, blotchy areas of hemorrhage (greater than 3 mm in diameter) in the skin

g. Collection of blood in the tissues causing swelling

h. Complex series of events by which proteins in the blood are activated, leading to formation of a fibrin blood clot

i. Fracture produced with little force because of a diseased state of the bone

j. Nosebleed

k. Insoluble protein fibers that form the structure of blood clots

l. Swelling of the lymph nodes

Exercise 2

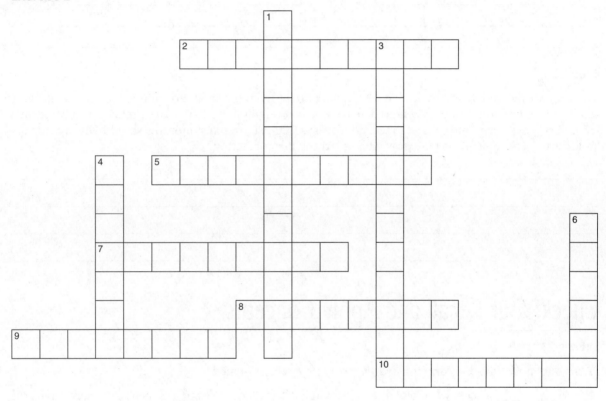

Across

2. Percentage of blood by volume that is composed of formed elements.

5. Disease in which hemoglobin takes on an abnormal shape in low-oxygen conditions.

7. Microhemorrhages.

8. Source of histamine and heparin.

9. Nutrient that is important in blood clotting.

10. Bone marrow cancer in which large numbers of abnormal white blood cells are produced.

Down

1. Type of fracture that occurs due to a disease process that weakens the bone.

3. Lacks a nucleus when mature; contains hemoglobin.

4. Blotchy, hemorrhagic rash.

6. Liquid part of blood.

Patient Assessment Review

Exercise 1

Your patient is a seven-year-old boy with leukemia. What signs and symptoms should you specifically look for? List the signs and symptoms on the left. Then to the right of each one, write the possible significance of the finding.

Signs and Symptoms   Significance of Finding

_____   _____

_____   _____

_____   _____

_____   _____

_____   _____

_____   _____

Exercise 2

You are transporting a 31-year-old male trauma patient from the small hospital where he was initially stabilized to a regional trauma center. The patient is receiving blood. You are preparing to perform a secondary assessment and obtain a medical history. What signs and symptoms should you specifically look for to determine if the patient is having a transfusion reaction?

_____

_____

_____

_____

Check Your Recall and Apply Concepts

Exercise 1

Fill in the blank with the correct word that completes the statement.

1. _____ occurs when blood clots form in the deep, large veins of legs, pelvis, or more rarely, the arms.

2. Systemic overactivation of clotting mechanisms, blood transfusion reactions, sepsis, surgery, and severe trauma is called _____.

3. _____ is a cancer of cells in the bone marrow in which abnormal cells multiply and crowd out normal cells.

4. Chronic hypoxia from living at a high altitude results in _____.

5. Type _____ blood is the universal recipient type because the individual does not have anti-A, anti-B, or anti-Rh antibodies.

6. Rh-negative women are given an injection of _____, an antibody that destroys any fetal Rh-positive blood cells that enter her blood before she can produce antibodies against them.

7. Patients suffering from a sickle cell crisis may benefit from administration of _____ for pain relief.

8. Consider _____ in a patient of Mediterranean descent who complains of severe pain in his joints.

9. A patient with severe anemia may present with very _____ skin and heart rate that is _____.

10. _____ anemia is due to a genetic deficiency in the ability of the stomach lining to produce intrinsic factor.

11. The blood disorder that can present with profuse, abnormal night sweats is _____.

Exercise 2

1. List three causes of decreased red blood cell production.

_____

_____

_____

_____

2. Describe what causes the pain experienced by a patient with sickle cell crisis.

_____

_____

_____

_____

3. Explain why the red blood cells of a sickle cell patient have such a short life span compared to normal red blood cells.

_____

_____

_____

_____

4. Name four types of leukemia.

_____

_____

_____

_____

5. List four complications of thrombocytopenia.

_____

_____

_____

_____

Clinical Reasoning

CASE STUDY: AIR TRAVEL

You and your partner, along with an engine crew from the fire department, are called to the airport for a patient who became ill during flight. The plane, en route from New York City, had to divert before reaching its intended destination of Denver. The patient is a 62-year-old woman, Phoebe Ross, who is complaining of shortness of breath. She says she suddenly had trouble catching her breath about an hour into the flight. She says she has no health problems and does not take any medications regularly. Her breath sounds are clear, but her SpO_2 is 91 percent on room air. She has no fever or cough. During your assessment, you see that she is wearing a splint on her left ankle, which is still healing from a recent fracture.

1. What are your initial hypotheses about the patient's problem?

2. What questions and assessments will help you test your hypotheses?

3. What prehospital treatments make sense for this patient?

Project-Based Learning

Prepare an information sheet to be handed out at civic organizations detailing the risk factors and signs and symptoms of DVT. Many people are unaware of this information and do not realize DVT can happen to otherwise healthy people. You may even prepare a short presentation to give at local organization meetings.

The EMS Professional in Practice

When you think about patients with blood disorders, your first thought might be concern about AIDS. How can that concern and concern about other bloodborne pathogens affect your attitude toward patients with hematologic disease? What can you do to not let your fears interfere with providing your patients with the very best care? Jot down your thoughts in a notebook or journal for discussion in class or in your study group.

27 Immunologic Disorders

Content Area

• Medicine

Advanced EMT Education Standard

• Applies fundamental knowledge to provide basic and selected advanced emergency care and transportation based on assessment findings for an acutely ill patient.

Summary of Objectives

27.1 Define key terms introduced in this chapter.

Knowing and being able to apply the key terms in each chapter is critical to understanding chapter concepts. Write the list of key terms. Then write the definition of each one in your own words. Check your understanding by confirming the definitions in the textbook glossary. Correct any misunderstandings. Create a study aid by writing each key term on the front of an index card and the definition on the back. Use the cards to quiz yourself or to have someone quiz you. The exercises under Vocabulary and Concept Review below will give you additional practice

27.2 Explain the importance of being able to recognize and treat anaphylactic reactions.

Quick recognition of, and intervention for, problems with the airway, breathing, and circulation are the highest priorities for all patients, and can truly make the difference between life and death for patients with anaphylaxis.

27.3 Describe the pathophysiologic process by which exposure to an antigen results in anaphylaxis.

The body is exposed to an antigen that normally does not provoke an immune response, and develops immunologic memory. On subsequent exposure, there is a rapid response to the antigen, called a secondary response. There may be a delayed cell-mediated hypersensitivity reaction or a more acute immediate hypersensitivity response. In the acute response, the body overestimates the danger from the allergen and over-reacts.

27.4 Recognize the signs, symptoms, and history associated with anaphylaxis.

Patients who have an anaphylactic reaction have been exposed to the allergen in the past and may not have been aware of it. The patient likely has a history of increased response to a particular allergen. Signs and symptoms include airway edema and respiratory distress, hoarseness, and wheezes. Circulatory collapse that presents as hypotension can occur. Other signs include uticaria.

27.5 Explain the life-threatening mechanisms of anaphylaxis, including airway compromise, impaired ventilation and oxygenation, and impaired perfusion.

The vasodilation and increased vascular permeability results in itching, hives, edema, distributive shock, and hypovolemic shock. Edema in the airway can cause varying degrees of airway obstruction, resulting in hoarseness, stridor, or complete obstruction. The smooth muscle constriction results in bronchospasm with restriction to airflow and wheezing and sometimes in abdominal cramping and diarrhea.

27.6 Describe the effects of excessive histamine release on the body.

The exaggerated response to the foreign antigen causes an excessive histamine release from the white blood cells. This response triggers widespread vasodilation and increases vascular permeability, which causes the respiratory and circulatory problems seen in anaphylaxis.

27.7 Describe the difference between an anaphylactic and an anaphylactoid reaction.

In an anaphylactic response, the patient has had a previous exposure to the antigen. In an anaphylactoid reaction, the exaggerated response occurs on initial exposure to the antigen, in that no sensitization is required. The antigen itself causes the release of histamine.

27.8 Apply knowledge of substances that commonly cause anaphylactic and anaphylactoid reactions to develop an appropriate index of suspicion for those conditions.

The most common offenders causing anaphylaxis are medications. Among them are antibiotics such as penicillin, sulfa antibiotics, and cephalosporin antibiotics; aspirin; opiates; and local anesthetics such as lidocaine, novocaine and procaine. Foods—such as peanuts, shellfish, eggs, and milk—also can cause anaphylactic reactions. Bees, wasps, hornets, fire ants, and other insects are known to cause severe allergic reactions. Pollen and latex also can cause anaphylactic reactions.

Anaphylactoid reactions usually occur from exposure to dyes used in radiology procedures.

As a general rule, the more rapid the onset, the more severe the reaction, so you can often gauge the potential severity based on the speed of onset. Also, knowing which allergens typically cause the most acute reaction will help you project the likely course.

27.9 Discuss each of the ways that an antigen can be introduced into the body.

Antigens can enter the body through injection, which includes bites, stings, needles, and infusions. The patient can ingest or inhale the antigen. Some antigens, such as poison ivy, can be absorbed through contact with the skin.

27.10 Differentiate between patients who require prehospital treatment with epinephrine and those who do not.

Patients who present with obvious signs of anaphylaxis such as respiratory compromise or hypotension are candidates for epinephrine. Other ominous signs include altered mental status and uticaria. Less serious signs and symptoms, which would not likely require epinephrine, are localized reactions such as swelling and itching without respiratory distress or blood pressure problems.

27.11 Explain the importance of limiting exposure to the antigen as a step in the treatment of the patient with an allergic or anaphylactic reaction.

If the patient is still exposed to the allergen, the reaction will continue. When possible, it is important to be sure that the offending agent is no longer in contact with the patient.

27.12 Describe the roles of airway management, fluid administration, and medications in the treatment of allergic and anaphylactic reactions.

The course of anaphylaxis can progress very rapidly, leading to airway compromise due to bronchoconstriction and edema. You must prepare to maintain the airway. One of the responses in anaphylaxis is widespread vasodilation and fluid loss. IV fluid boluses are a necessary treatment combined with epinephrine to facilitate vasoconstriction as well as to relax the smooth muscle in the bronchi.

27.13 Given a variety of scenarios of patients with allergic and anaphylactic reactions, implement an appropriate treatment plan for each.

Monitor patients with no airway or circulatory compromise to manage any escalation of the reaction. There may be some localized swelling, itching, and hives, but the patient should have no alteration in mental status. You can consider diphenhydramine to prevent additional histamine from binding with histamine receptors.

Moderate reactions may include some wheezing, present with more widespread hives, and the patient may show early signs of respiratory distress and possibly hypotension. Mild to moderate reactions may benefit from diphenhydramine and albuterol.

Severe anaphylactic reactions require aggressive airway management and fluid resuscitation. To reverse the effects of the exposure, the patient will require epinephrine. The usual dosage of epinephrine is 0.3 to 0.5 mg of 1:1,000 for adults. Epinephrine can be very effective, but its duration of action is short—about 10 to 20 minutes when given intramuscularly; therefore, patients may require an additional dose of epinephrine.

27.14 Explain the necessity of ongoing evaluation of the patient having, or at risk for, an anaphylactic reaction.

Patients with anaphylaxis are dynamic. Initially, a patient may appear to be having only a mild reaction but may have a delayed response, so ongoing evaluation is crucial. A patient having a more serious reaction may have a rebound reaction after the initial dose of epinephrine wears off. Additionally, medications given to manage anaphylaxis—epinephrine and albuterol—could cause adverse side effects. The more serious ones (such as tachycardia) can be harmful to patients with cardiac disease. This is why continued monitoring is critical.

27.15 Recognize conditions that compromise immunity.

A number of diseases can temporarily or permanently impair immune function. The human immunodeficiency virus (HIV), which causes acquired immune deficiency syndrome (AIDS), is perhaps the most well known. Autoimmune diseases include rheumatoid arthritis, psoriasis, systemic lupus erythematosus (SLE), Grave's disease (hyperthyroidism), Crohn's disease, multiple sclerosis (MS), and many others.

27.16 Describe the basic pathophysiology of common autoimmune/collagen vascular diseases.

Normally, the immune system effectively distinguishes molecules as being either "self" or "nonself." Nonself molecules are attacked by the immune system and self molecules are not. In autoimmune diseases, the immune system fails to recognize certain molecules in the body as "self" and destroys them, affecting the function of the tissues involved. Often, the treatment for autoimmune diseases involves suppressing the immune system. The unfortunate side effect is that the person is also left less able to fight infectious diseases and cancers.

27.17 Describe considerations for patients living with transplanted organs or tissues.

Patients who have received organ transplants take medications that suppress the immune response to prevent rejection of the donor organ. Unfortunately, immune suppression is not highly selective and the patient is placed at increased risk of infection. Medications taken for other reasons, such as corticosteroids, also suppress the immune system.

Resource Central

Resource Central offers extra practice and review materials in a variety of media. To access it, follow the directions on the Student Access Card provided with the Student Textbook. If there is no card, go to www.bradybooks.com and follow the Resource Central link to Buy Access.

Vocabulary and Concept Review

Exercise 1

Write the letter of the correct definition in the blank next to the term. (See Resource Central for more vocabulary review.)

1. _____ anaphylactoid reaction

2. _____ anaphylaxis

3. _____ angioedema

4. _____ antibody

5. _____ antigen

6. _____ autoimmune disease

7. _____ urticaria

a. Swelling of blood vessels within the tissues that produces edema

b. Life-threatening reaction to a substance that presents with signs and symptoms similar to anaphylaxis, but is not mediated by IgE

c. Red, raised areas on the skin caused by swelling of and release of fluid from blood vessels in the skin in response to an allergic reaction

d. Foreign material that provokes an immune response

e. Life-threatening allergic reaction that produces shock through vasodilation and fluid shifts, with the potential for asphyxia

f. Immunoglobulin; a substance that recognizes foreign material in the body to promote an immune response

g. Disease in which the immune system fails to recognize some of the body's molecules as its own, resulting in an immune response against the body's own tissues

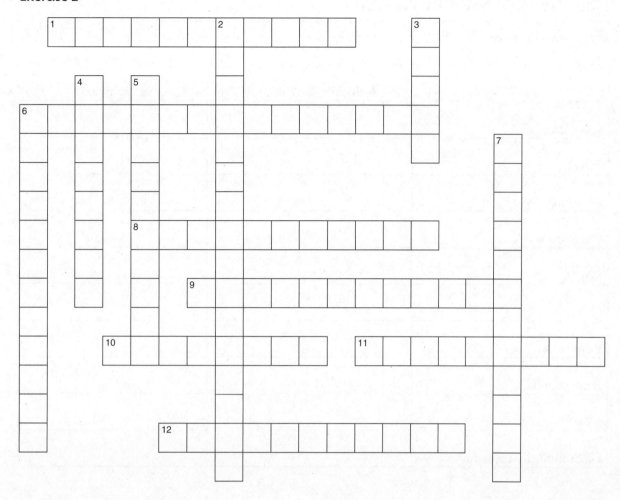

Across

1. White blood cells that carry out the immune response.
6. Antibody that plays a role in allergic reactions.
8. Drug that is indicated in the treatment of anaphylactic shock.
9. Cause of hypotension in anaphylaxis.
10. Basophil that has migrated into the tissues.
11. Suitable medication for a patient with an allergic reaction who is wheezing but who does not have severe respiratory distress or hypotension.
12. Life-threatening allergic reaction.

Down

2. Systemic lupus erythematosus and rheumatoid arthritis are in this classification of autoimmune diseases.
3. Common name for urticaria.
4. Ability for the body to defend itself against specific antigens.
5. Response to certain medications that can present as anaphylaxis.
6. Nonspecific response to tissue injuries and antigens.
7. Check to see if a patient with a history of anaphylaxis carries one of these.

Patient Assessment Review

Fill in the table to compare the assessment findings of a mild allergic reaction to those of anaphylaxis.

	Mild Allergic Reaction	Anaphylaxis
Speed of onset		
Airway		
Breathing		
Circulation		
Skin		
Pulse		
Respiratory rate		
Lung sounds		
Blood pressure		
Gastrointestinal system		

Check Your Recall and Apply Concepts

Exercise 1

Fill in the blanks with the best word to complete the sentence.

1. Cellular ingestion of foreign material and debris is called _____.

2. Specific resistance to disease is called _____.

3. The functions of the immune system are carried out by white blood cells called _____.

4. Both types of lymphocytes have surface proteins that act as _____ receptors.

5. One way in which immunologic memory works is through the creation of specific _____ that recognize specific antigens.

6. The antibody involved in allergic and anaphylactic reactions is _____, abbreviated IgE.

7. The onset of anaphylaxis usually begins within _____ to _____ _____ after exposure to the antigen.

8. The actions of _____ can help reduce airway edema, dilate bronchiolar smooth muscle, and constrict the peripheral vasculature.

9. The duration of action of epinephrine is short, at about _____ to _____ minutes, when given intramuscularly.

10. Both allergic reactions and anaphylactic reactions are known as _____ reactions.

1. Name four common side effects of epinephrine administration.

   _____   _____

   _____   _____

2. List four signs and symptoms of anaphylaxis.

   _____   _____

   _____   _____

3. Name the four ways that an antigen can enter the body.

   _____   _____

   _____   _____

4. Name four autoimmune diseases.

   _____   _____

   _____   _____

5. Name four of the most common food allergens that cause anaphylaxis.

   _____   _____

   _____   _____

Clinical Reasoning

CASE STUDY: DISPATCH FOR RESPIRATORY DISTRESS

Your crew is called for a woman having difficulty breathing. When you arrive you find a 35-year-old with obvious wheezing and stridor. She is awake, sitting upright, and is able to speak four to five words at a time. You notice that her skin appears to be flushed and moist. You immediately place her on oxygen by nonrebreather mask while you try to gather some history.

1. What are your initial hypotheses about the problem based on the little bit of information you have?

   _____

   _____

   _____

   _____

2. What questions should you begin with to obtain the history? What is the importance of each of the questions you will ask?

   _____

   _____

   _____

   _____

The patient's husband tells you she has "spring allergies" that evolved into a sinus infection, for which she began taking amoxicillin two days ago. She does not have a history of asthma, chronic obstructive pulmonary disease (COPD), or other lower respiratory problems. The patient also takes birth control pills and citalopram (Celexa) for depression. The patient has no known medication or food allergies. She last had food and drink about 2 hours ago at lunch. After returning home from lunch, the patient started complaining of itching on her hands, arms, and back; then she started complaining of a "tickle in her throat." While the team is debating what to do, she begins wheezing and having a feeling of tightness in her throat.

You continue your assessment and notice that the patient has urticaria on her upper arms, neck, and back. Your partner has gotten an initial set of vital signs as follows: respirations 24, pulse 116, blood pressure 96/62. Her SpO_2 is 94 percent after 2 minutes of oxygen by nonrebreather mask. Expiratory wheezing is present in all lung fields.

3. What care should you consider as the history unfolds? How should you prioritize care?

_____

_____

_____

_____

_____

Project-Based Learning

You have learned about the most common causes of allergic reaction. Make a list of all of the foods that are the most likely offenders. Go to the pantry in your home and look at all of the canned food and packaged or boxed foods to see how many of them contain items that can cause allergic reactions. Jot down your findings in your notebook or journal.

The EMS Professional in Practice

When you get that first anaphylactic patient, you will have to make a decision regarding whether to administer epinephrine. Your indecision can have fatal consequences to your patient with severe anaphylaxis. On the other hand, epinephrine is a powerful drug and has some significant side effects. Sometimes "pulling the trigger" can be one of the hardest parts of being an Advanced EMT. How can you prepare yourself to be sure you will make the correct decision and follow through with it? Jot down your thoughts in a notebook or journal for discussion in class or in your study group.

28 Infectious Illnesses

Content Area

- Medicine

Advanced EMT Education Standard

- Applies fundamental knowledge to provide basic and selected advanced emergency care and transportation based on assessment findings for an acutely ill patient.

Summary of Objectives

28.1 Define key terms introduced in this chapter.

Knowing and being able to apply the key terms in each chapter is critical to understanding chapter concepts. Write the list of key terms. Then write the definition of each one in your own words. Check your understanding by confirming the definitions in the textbook glossary. Correct any misunderstandings. Create a study aid by writing each key term on the front of an index card and the definition on the back. Use the cards to quiz yourself or to have someone quiz you. The exercises under Vocabulary and Concept Review below will give you additional practice.

28.2 Describe the body's defenses against infectious illnesses.

The body has many mechanisms to protect against infectious illness. The skin and mucous membranes provide a barrier between the external environment and the internal environment of the body. Body fluids contain antimicrobial substances, and some white blood cells recognize foreign material, even without prior exposure, and defend the body against it. Inflammation and fever are also responses that fight infectious disease. The body even uses micro-organisms to prevent disease in the body.

28.3 Explain the actions health care providers must take to prevent the spread of communicable illnesses to themselves and others.

Health care providers are responsible for their own safety, including protecting themselves from infectious disease through the use of Standard Precautions, hand washing, cleaning and disinfecting equipment and the work environment, immunizations, and maintaining general good health. Health care personnel also have an obligation to protect patients from exposure to infectious diseases.

28.4   Describe the routes of transmission of infectious illnesses.

Infectious diseases can be transmitted through direct contact, through the air, through sexual contact, through contact with infected blood, and through the gastrointestinal system.

28.5   Discuss what constitutes a significant exposure to a communicable illness.

A significant exposure occurs when there is contact between a patient's blood or body fluids and your nonintact skin or mucous membranes

28.6   Describe the stages of infectious illnesses.

Once a pathogen gains access to the body, it has been exposed to the pathogen. The host must be exposed to the disease before he can acquire it. The incubation period occurs between exposure and the onset of signs and symptoms. The window phase is the period between exposure and the production of enough antibodies to be detected in the blood. The disease period is the period of time in which the patient has signs and symptoms. The disease period ends when the signs and symptoms resolve or if the patient dies from the disease.

28.7   Identify the general signs and symptoms of infectious illnesses.

General signs and symptoms include fatigue, malaise, headache, muscle or joint pain, fever, chills, swollen lymph nodes, nausea, vomiting, and rash.

28.8   Describe the nature of agents of infectious illnesses, including bacteria, viruses, fungi, helminths, protozoa, and external parasites.

Bacteria are single-celled organisms that are capable of reproduction. Bacteria can cause damage to the tissues directly or produce toxins that cause detrimental effects.

Viruses contain either DNA or RNA, but not both. They must gain access to a host's cell, where they use the cell's genetic material to replicate themselves, essentially turning the infected cell into a virus factory. Viral illnesses often result in immunologic memory, conferring lifelong immunity.

Fungi are simple plants, such as yeasts, that can live and reproduce in the body and exist in the normal flora. When the immune system is compromised or body conditions otherwise provide a favorable environment, such as a decrease in normal bacterial flora, fungi can reproduce at a greater rate, causing opportunistic infection.

Protozoa are single-celled animals with the ability to move. The protozoa cryptosporidium and *Giardia lamblia* are found in contaminated water, and can cause gastrointestinal illness.

Internal parasites include helminths (worms), such as pinworms, hookworms, trichinella (the cause of trichinosis from eating undercooked pork or bear meat), and tapeworms. External parasites include scabies and lice.

28.9   Discuss the causative agents, pathophysiology, routes of transmission, methods of prevention, and management of the following: bacterial and viral meningitis; gastroenteritis and foodborne illnesses; hantavirus pulmonary syndrome (sin nombre); hepatitis types A, B, C, D, E, and G; HIV/AIDS; influenza; measles and rubella; mononucleosis; mumps; parasites and vectorborne illnesses, including scabies, lice, Lyme disease, viral encephalitis; pneumonia; rabies; sexually transmitted infections, including chlamydia, gonorrhea, and syphilis; staphylococcal infections, including MRSA; streptococcal infections, and vancomycin-resistant enterococcus (VRE); tetanus; tuberculosis; upper respiratory infections; varicella and herpes infections.

Meningitis can be viral or bacterial and is an inflammation and swelling of the meninges that surround the central nervous system. Viral meningitis tends to be less severe, while bacterial meningitis can be fatal. The meningococcal bacterium, under certain circumstances, gains access to the cerebrospinal fluid, causing meningitis. Meningococcal bacteria can enter the blood, causing damage to blood vessels with bleeding into the organs and skin. Bacterial meningitis is transmitted through contact with nasal and oral secretions and generally requires close contact with the infected person. All health care workers who were in significant contact with the patient must take prophylactic antibiotics. Treatment is based on symptoms, recognizing the potential for hypoxia, sepsis, and hypotension in severe cases.

Many gastrointestinal illnesses are caused by foodborne or waterborne pathogens or through the oral–fecal route of transmission. Causes include salmonella, *Eshcerichia coli*, norovirus, and staphylococcal bacteria, among others. Occasionally, outbreaks can be traced to a specific source, which may be local, regional, or national. In *E. coli* infection, red blood cells are destroyed, resulting in kidney failure. Cholera is a severe form of gastroenteritis that can occur following disasters that have an impact on water sanitation, but is rare in the United States. Prevention revolves around ensuring sanitation of food and water sources. Treatment is mostly supportive with severe cases requiring IV fluids for dehydration.

Hantavirus pulmonary syndrome (sin nombre) is carried by deer mice in the U.S. Southwest and by rice and cotton rats in the U.S. Southeast. However, nearly all documented cases have occurred in the area common to Utah, Colorado, New Mexico, and Arizona. Hantavirus is transmitted through the airborne route from the dried excrement of infected mice. It begins with flu-like signs and symptoms but progresses to a cardiopulmonary stage with hypotension, acute respiratory distress syndrome (ARDS), and multiple organ failure.

Hepatitis types are A, B, C, D, E, and G. All but hepatitis types A and E are transmitted through infected blood and body fluids. A and E spread through the gastrointestinal tract. Hepatitis C can become chronic, and patients may live many years with the infection. In some cases, for example, in patients with hepatitis B, the patient is a carrier who remains capable of transmitting the disease, though signs and symptoms have resolved or perhaps were never present. Hepatitis primarily affects the liver.

The human immunodeficiency virus (HIV) is a bloodborne pathogen that infects T lymphocytes by combining with a molecule on the cell surface so that it can gain entry. The virus uses the cell to replicate itself, producing thousands of copies of itself. In the process, the affected lymphocytes are damaged and their number decreases, resulting in immune suppression called acquired immunodeficiency syndrome (AIDS), which is called HIV/AIDS. HIV is capable of mutating frequently so that the immune system cannot recognize and destroy it. The mutations also make strains of HIV less susceptible to the effects of drugs intended to limit their replication (antiretroviral drugs). As a result, patients with HIV/AIDS are prone to numerous infections and cancers, including opportunistic infections and rare cancers, and the central nervous system is eventually affected as well (AIDS dementia complex). Prevention is targeted at preventing contact with blood products of infected persons.

Influenza, or the flu, occurs from infection with one of several influenza viruses through the airborne route. Flu viruses are highly contagious and some have a significant mortality rate from complications. Complications include dehydration, pneumonia, and encephalitis. Influenza vaccines for the strains expected to infect patients in the United States are available each year at the start of the influenza season and they are suggested for health care workers and high-risk populations such as children and the elderly and chronically ill, immunocompromised, and pregnant patients. Antiviral drugs are available and can be effective in some types of flu early in the illness, but some flu strains have become resistant to antiviral medications.

Measles and rubella are viral illnesses that cause fever and rash. Both are usually mild, but rubella can cause severe birth defects when contracted by pregnant women in the first 20 weeks of pregnancy. All health care providers should be vaccinated against them. The illnesses themselves require no particular prehospital treatment. Notify the receiving facility that you are transporting patients suspected of having these illnesses.

Mononucleosis is a viral infection (Epstein-Barr virus). It causes fever and fatigue and affects the upper respiratory system, resulting in sore throat, swollen tonsils, and enlarged painful lymph nodes. The phagocytes in the spleen are affected, resulting in an enlarged spleen in many patients. It is transmitted through direct contact with saliva. By adulthood, about 95 percent of the population has been infected and developed antibodies.

Mumps is a viral infection that affects glandular tissue, particularly the parotid salivary glands, causing painful swelling.

Scabies, lice, and ringworm can all present with intense itching and skin lesions. Both scabies and lice are external parasites. Scabies is caused by a mite that burrows under the skin and lays eggs, which causes a rash with intense itching. Scabies is transmitted through direct skin-to-skin contact with an infected person and is more common under crowded conditions, such as institutional settings. A particularly severe form of scabies, Norwegian scabies, can affect the elderly and immunocompromised. This type of scabies also can be transmitted by contact with contaminated linens, clothing, and other items. Scabies is treated by application of a topical scabicidal lotion or cream that is available by prescription. Lice are tiny insects that infest the body, using the hair shafts to deposit their eggs. Over-the-counter and prescription preparations are available to treat lice, but some infestations are resistant. Ringworm is a fungus that results in itching, circular lesions on the skin. It is more common in warm, humid environments and in immunocompromised patients. Ringworm is spread through direct contact with an infected person, but can be contracted through contact with contaminated soil or an infected pet. Over-the-counter antifungal medications such as miconazole and clotrimazole are used to treat ringworm. Lyme disease is a bacterial infection transmitted by black-legged ticks. A characteristic sign is a red, circular, "bull's eye" rash that begins at location of the bite. Other signs and symptoms include general signs of infectious illness: fatigue, fever, chills, headache, muscle and joint pain, and swollen lymph nodes. The infection can lead to Bell's palsy, headaches, meningitis, and cardiac dysrhythmia. A majority of patients develop severe arthritis in the months following infection, and a few patients develop chronic neurologic problems. Encephalitis is an inflammation of brain tissue. Common causes are domestic arboviruses, such as West Nile virus, St. Louis encephalitis, and Eastern Equine encephalitis, which are tickborne or mosquitoborne illnesses. Signs and symptoms are similar to those of meningitis.

Pneumonia can be caused by many different infectious agents, including viruses, fungi, and many strains of bacteria. Pneumonia may affect anyone, but the risk is increased in smokers, the elderly, those with chronic illnesses, and in immunocompromised patients. Pneumonia infection and the body's response to it produce purulent material in the lungs. Pneumonia is often localized to one lobe of the lung, resulting in localized crackles (rales) and wheezes from the fluid produced and inflammation of the lung tissue. Accumulated fluid in the alveoli can collapse the affected alveoli and oxygen saturation can be significantly reduced. Provide oxygen and assist ventilation as needed. IV fluids for dehydration and beta$_2$ agonists for patients who are wheezing can be administrated as needed according to protocols.

Rabies is very rare, but fatal in humans, and is contracted through contact with the saliva of infected animals. Bats aerosolize urine in caves where large numbers of bats can result in transmission through mucous membranes. Wild animals are often carriers of rabies. Rabies is a viral disease that attacks the central nervous system causing a number of neurologic signs and symptoms. The rabies virus travels along nerves from the bite to the brain, where the virus multiplies and enters the salivary glands. Immediate treatment with a combination of vaccination and immune globulin injection is highly effective in preventing illness. Thoroughly cleaning the wound in the prehospital setting significantly decreases infection rates.

Sexually transmitted infections include chlamydia, gonorrhea, and syphilis. Gonorrhea is a bacterial infection that causes painful urination and purulent urethral discharge in males, but is often asymptomatic in females. Untreated gonorrhea can lead to infection of other genital structures and is a cause of pelvic inflammatory disease (PID). Untreated gonorrhea can lead to septic arthritis. Syphilis is a bacterial infection that is transmitted sexually, but may be transmitted through other contact with its lesions. Contact with the blood of an infected person, such as through a needle stick, can result in disease transmission, but the risk is low. Untreated infected women can pass the infection to the fetus, resulting in congenital syphilis. Syphilis infection evolves through four stages if it remains untreated. Chlamydia is caused by an organism that has characteristics of bacteria but lives within cells. It can affect the eyes and respiratory system and is spread through transfer of infected secretions and sexual contact. Chlamydia can cause blindness and pneumonia in babies born to infected mothers and is a cause of PID. In the genital system, its signs and symptoms are similar to those of gonorrhea.

Staphylococcal ("staph") infections include methicillin-resistant *Staphylococcus aureus* (MRSA), streptococcal infections, and VRE. Staphylococcus is a primary pathogen that causes disease in humans. Manifestations range from boils to impetigo and include *S. aureus*, a common bacterium, which can produce a toxin that leads to toxic shock syndrome. MRSA is resistant to antibiotics usually used to treat staphylococcal infections, and usually affects the skin. In the community setting, MRSA presents as pustules or boils just like other staph infections, often at the site of an injury or other break in the skin. MRSA in health care settings is a nosocomial infection and can result in serious infections. Some nursing homes may have a high prevalence of MRSA. Use Standard Precautions, including frequent hand-washing to prevent spread of MRSA between patients. Clean equipment, including the stretcher, between patients. VRE is another nosocomial infection of concern. Again, use Standard Precautions, hand washing, and cleaning and disinfection to prevent transmission.

A patient who has not been immunized against tetanus may receive an injection of tetanus immune globulin if he has injury at high risk for tetanus.

Tuberculosis is commonly spread through the respiratory route. It manifests as respiratory disease, but can affect different parts of the body. Tuberculosis occurs at a higher rate among patients with HIV/AIDS and in recent immigrants. Transmission requires repeated, close contact, making it more prevalent in situations in which people are in prolonged, close proximity to each other. Treatment requires antibiotics, but there are multiple drug-resistant strains. A single occupational exposure is very unlikely to result in disease, but still requires the use of Standard Precautions, including an N-95 respirator in cases of known or suspected active pulmonary tuberculosis.

Upper respiratory infections include colds, pharyngitis, and epiglottitis. Some of the illnesses, such as respiratory syncytial virus (RSV) and epiglottitis, are more prevalent in pediatric populations. The goal of management of patients with respiratory infections is to ensure an open airway and adequate breathing and oxygenation.

Chickenpox, or varicella, is a viral disease in the herpes family that causes general malaise and itchy, fluid-filled blisters on the skin that later crust and scab. It is highly contagious and easily spread between infected and nonimmune individuals. After recovery, the virus remains dormant in the body, usually in a dorsal spinal nerve, where it can be reactivated, causing a painful, unilateral rash called shingles. A person with shingles can transmit the virus to someone who has never had chickenpox or been immunized against varicella. Herpes simplex viruses primarily affect the mucous membranes and skin. Infection results in blisters that ulcerate. Herpes simplex type 1 usually affects the oral mucosa, resulting in cold sores. Herpes simplex type 2 usually affects the genitals. General signs and symptoms of infectious disease, including fever and malaise, often accompany primary infection. In both cases, the virus remains dormant between outbreaks, but does not go away. The viruses are spread through direct contact, and lesions may not visible during the contagious period.

28.10 Discuss the significance and prevention of nosocomial infections and antibiotic-resistant infections.

There are antibiotic-resistant strains of bacteria, such as MRSA, VRE, and resistant forms of tuberculosis. The development of antibiotic resistant strains of bacteria is largely due to the overuse of antibiotics. Use antibiotics only when clearly indicated. Nosocomial infections are acquired and spread in the health care setting. The use of Standard Precautions, hand washing, and cleaning and disinfection are necessary to prevent transmission.

28.11 Given various scenarios involving known or suspected infectious disease, obtain relevant history and assessment information, formulate and implement an appropriate treatment plan, and take precautions to prevent disease transmission.

Several chief complaints are associated with infectious disease, including fever, cough, nausea, vomiting, diarrhea, muscle aches, fatigue, general malaise, runny nose, rash, headache, pain, swelling, and stiff neck. It is very important that you perform a good scene size-up before beginning treatment so you can don the appropriate personal protective equipment (PPE). Presentations that could indicate infectious disease include seizure and altered mental status, including confusion, delirium, jaundice, and decreased responsiveness. Use your knowledge of pathophysiology and the patient's responses to develop your line of questioning and adapt your assessment as information emerges. If a patient denies having a cough, ask about other signs and symptoms. If your patient states he has had a cough, follow up with questions about the nature of the cough, and if you have not already done so, listen to breath sounds. It is not possible to definitively diagnose a specific infectious disease in the prehospital setting, but you should be able to recognize if infectious disease is a possibility and what body systems are affected. Treatment depends on the patient's complaints and problems, rather than a specific diagnosis. If the patient has a respiratory compromise, you may consider a beta₂ agonist. If you suspect sepsis, start an IV and administer fluids.

Resource Central

Resource Central offers extra practice and review materials in a variety of media. To access it, follow the directions on the Student Access Card provided with the Student Textbook. If there is no card, go to www.bradybooks.com and follow the Resource Central link to Buy Access.

Vocabulary and Concept Review

Exercise 1

Write the letter of the correct definition in the blank next to the term. (See Resource Central for more vocabulary review.)

1. _____ carrier

2. _____ communicable disease

3. _____ disease period

4. _____ exudate

5. _____ fomite

6. _____ fulminant

7. _____ immunocompromise

8. _____ incubation period

9. _____ latent

10. _____ normal flora

11. _____ nosocomial infection

12. _____ opportunistic infection

13. _____ vector

14. _____ virulent

15. _____ window phase

a. Suppression of immune system function resulting in increased susceptibility to infection and cancers

b. Phase of an infection in which the individual has signs and symptoms

c. Infection acquired in a health care setting

d. Period of time between infectious disease exposure and development of detectable amounts of antibody, during which the disease may be transmissible

e. Infectious illness that can spread from person to person through direct or indirect contact

f. Time from exposure to an infectious disease to the onset of signs and symptoms

g. Animal or insect that can spread diseases from one organism to another

h. Inanimate object that can transfer infectious material, resulting in disease

i. Asymptomatic individual who is infected with and can transmit a communicable disease

j. Strong, able to overcome body defenses

k. Material that has seeped out of injured or inflamed tissues or blood vessels

l. Micro-organisms that normally inhabit the body without producing disease

m. Severe, with a rapid onset

n. Inactive or dormant

o. Disease that occurs from pathogens that are normally destroyed by the immune system or kept in check by normal flora

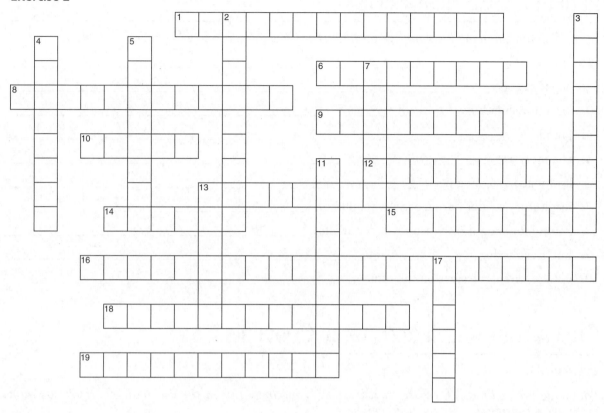

Across

1. Unusual cancer that is seen in immunocompromised patients, such as those with HIV/AIDS.

6. Rare in humans, this disease is highly infectious and carries high morbidity, making it a possible weapon of bioterrorism.

8. Relatively rare infection, reduced due to widespread HiB vaccine, that can cause upper airway obstruction.

9. Usually thought of as a form of food poisoning, it also can cause skin infection, particularly in IV drug abusers.

10. Laryngotracheobronchitis.

12. Type of infection acquired in the health care system.

13. Pathogens that are very strong and able to overcome body defenses.

14. Viral infection, transmitted from animals to humans, that causes hypersalivation and fear of water.

15. Very common sexually transmitted infection.

16. Infection that occurs only under conditions of immune compromise or because antibiotics have altered normal flora.

18. Type of immunity that occurs as a result of having an infectious illness.

19. Infestation with lice.

Down

2. Whooping cough.

3. Virus that can manifest as chickenpox or shingles.

4. Oozing, streptococcal infection of the skin that is more common in children than in adults.

5. Single-celled animals capable of producing disease.

7. Period when disease is present but not causing signs and symptoms.

11. There are at least six different types of this viral illness, some of which are bloodborne and some that spread through the fecal–oral route.

13. Flea that carries the bubonic plague from rodents to humans is one of these.

17. An unsterilized surgical instrument is an example of one.

Patient Assessment Review

For each of the following signs and symptoms, list an infectious illness with which it is highly associated.

1. Stiff neck _____

2. Night sweats _____

3. Oral thrush (adults) _____

4. Jaundice _____

5. Hemoptysis _____

6. Prolonged coughing fits _____

7. Inspiratory stridor during activity (children) _____

8. Painful, unilateral rash (usually older adults) _____

9. Bull's eye rash _____

10. Itching, circular lesions on the skin _____

Check Your Recall and Apply Concepts

Exercise 1

Following are methods of disease transmission. Using the terms in the list, write the most common method of transmission for the following infections.

airborne	food/waterborne	sexually transmitted
vectorborne	bloodborne	direct

1. Tuberculosis _____

2. Hepatitis B _____

3. Influenza _____

4. Hepatitis A _____

5. Herpes simplex type 2 _____

6. Malaria _____

7. Trichinella _____

8. Scabies _____

9. Sudden acute respiratory syndrome (SARS) _____

10. Pertussis _____

11. Hantavirus _____

12. Eastern equine encephalitis _____

13. Bacterial meningitis _____

14. Lyme disease _____

15. Cholera _____

Fill in the blanks with the best word to complete the sentence.

1. _____ is very rare, but fatal in humans, and is contracted through contact with the saliva of infected animals.

2. If your protocols allow, you should consider administering an _____ for severe vomiting.

3. _____ is a deadly bacterium that produces a neurotoxin causing paralysis by blocking the release of acetylcholine in motor neurons.

4. Concern exists over the use of _____ toxin and _____ as agents of bioterrorism.

5. _____ is a painful and itchy rash with fluid-filled vesicles that crust and is more commonly seen in children than adults.

Clinical Reasoning

CASE STUDY: MRSA

Your crew has been called to transport a patient from an acute care hospital to a rehabilitation facility. When you approach the patient's room, you notice a cart outside the door. There is a sign on the door that says "MRSA."

1. What does this mean to your crew?

_____

_____

_____

_____

_____

2. What do you need to know about the patient's MRSA? You notice that a nurse is putting on a mask and gown before entering the patient's room.

_____

_____

_____

_____

_____

3. Does this tell you anything important?

_____

_____

_____

_____

_____

Project-Based Learning

Visit http://wwwnc.cdc.gov/travel/ to see what the federal government recommends regarding immunizations required for travel overseas. Different areas in the world have different health recommendations. Make a list of the illnesses you have learned about in this chapter and match them with their prevalence in the world.

The EMS Professional in Practice

You have learned about nosocomial infections, and you know that they are acquired in the health care setting. Should this weigh heavily on the health care industry? People who are already sick or injured are made sicker due to contact with health care professionals. What can you do as a health care professional to try to prevent nosocomial infections? Jot down your thoughts in a notebook or journal for discussion in class or in your study group.

Chapter 29

Nontraumatic Musculoskeletal and Soft-Tissue Disorders

Content Area

- Medicine

Advanced EMT Education Standard

- Applies fundamental knowledge to provide basic and selected advanced emergency care and transportation based on assessment findings for an acutely ill patient.

Summary of Objectives

29.1 Define key terms introduced in this chapter.

Knowing and being able to apply the key terms in each chapter is critical to understanding chapter concepts. Write the list of key terms. Then write the definition of each one in your own words. Check your understanding by confirming the definitions in the textbook glossary. Correct any misunderstandings. Create a study aid by writing each key term on the front of an index card and the definition on the back. Use the cards to quiz yourself or to have someone quiz you. The exercises under Vocabulary and Concept Review below will give you additional practice.

29.2 Obtain a relevant history from patients presenting with nontraumatic musculoskeletal disorders.

Muscle aches, weakness, rashes, changes in skin color, and other musculoskeletal and soft-tissue complaints can be signs and symptoms of additional health problems, making them parts of a patient's overall medical history and your assessment of the patient's condition. There are specific soft-tissue and musculoskeletal disorders that can result in a request for prehospital treatment and transport. As a health care provider, you need a basic understanding of how those disorders affect patient health. In some cases, that understanding helps you make decisions about transport and special considerations in patient handling to avoid increasing the patient's discomfort.

There may be little you can do in the prehospital setting for patients with nontraumatic musculoskeletal and soft-tissue disorders. However, obtaining a thorough history, including a complete list of medications, paying attention to patient comfort, and recognizing that musculoskeletal and soft-tissue problems can be quite serious are important ways you can help them.

29.3 Describe the pathophysiology of, and concerns for, patients with osteoporosis.

A significant decrease in bone mass occurs in osteoporosis. Osteoporosis predominantly affects the jaws, vertebrae, and epiphyses of bones. It also is more common in women, particularly Caucasian and Asian women of smaller stature. As the bones weaken, pathologic fractures become common. Compression fractures of the vertebrae result in loss of height of the vertebrae. That, along with decreased thickness of intervertebral discs, can result several inches in reduction of height in the elderly. Osteoporosis can increase the likelihood of fractures from even minor traumas.

29.4 List etiologies of nontraumatic back, neck, muscle, and joint pain.

Back pain is sometimes difficult to diagnose and treat. Lumbar strain and disc problems are common causes of low back pain. Nontraumatic back and neck pain can be a result of past injuries and poor posture. Neck stiffness and pain can result from sleeping with the head turned or bent to the side. Lumbar strain, stretching or tearing the muscles in the lumbar area, occurs during activity, such as over-reaching or lifting, and is common in EMS providers. Other causes of low back pain include a herniated (or displaced) disc that impinges on a nerve, resulting in pain. When the sciatic nerve is compressed, the pain can radiate through the buttocks and down the leg, resulting in sciatica.

29.5 Explain considerations in assessing and managing patients with nontraumatic musculoskeletal complaints.

Nontraumatic musculoskeletal complaints can have many underlying causes. Always consider systemic causes, as well as localized problems, in your history and assessment of the patient. Obtain a list of the patient's medications with those complaints, because several problems have been traced to the side effects of specific medications. Although most musculoskeletal complaints are not life threatening, you can play a significant role in patient comfort. Management of patients with non-traumatic musculoskeletal complaints focuses on comfort of the patient. Do not place a patient on a long backboard unless it is indicated for spinal immobilization.

29.6 Describe the pathophysiology of arthritis, including osteoarthritis, septic arthritis, rheumatoid arthritis, and gout.

The most common type of arthritis, osteoarthritis, occurs from wear and tear on joints over time and is more common in middle-aged and older adults. Rheumatoid arthritis is an autoimmune disorder. In osteoarthritis, or degenerative joint disease (DJD), the articular cartilage is damaged and breaks down. Arthritis is common in the hands, spine, and weight-bearing joints, such as the knee and hip, but can occur in any joint. Infection (septic arthritis) and trauma can lead to arthritis. Gout is a form of arthritis that occurs from uric acid crystals being deposited in a joint, often in the foot. The disorder is a result of abnormal uric acid metabolism and is associated with a sudden onset of a hot, painful, swollen joint.

29.7 List various etiologies of myalgia.

The most common causes of myalgia are the overuse or overstretching of a muscle or group of muscles. Muscle aches in addition to other signs and symptoms may indicate other health problems, making them parts of a patient's overall medical history and your assessment of the patient's condition. Fibromyalgia is a chronic inflammatory disease of the musculoskeletal system commonly associated with chronic fatigue syndrome.

29.8 Describe the pathophysiology, progression, and needs of patients with muscular dystrophy.

Muscular dystrophies are genetic diseases that result in abnormalities of structural and functional muscle proteins, causing progressive muscle degeneration and weakness. The most common type of muscular dystrophy is Duchenne's muscular dystrophy, which affects males with onset between 3 and 7 years of age. Most boys with Duchenne's muscular dystrophy are wheelchair bound by 12 years of age, and death often occurs by their early 20s due to respiratory failure. Other types of muscular dystrophies can affect female and elderly patients. Weakness of the respiratory muscles can lead to increased risk of pneumonia, and immobile patients are at risk for decubitus ulcers.

29.9 Describe the pathophysiology and management of rhabdomyolysis.

Rhabdomyolysis is a breakdown of skeletal muscle that results in release of myoglobin and other muscle cell contents, which can enter the blood. Rhabdomyolysis can also be caused by sepsis, seizures (particularly status epilepticus), prolonged exertion (running a marathon), and side effects of some drugs and toxins. The accompanying muscle edema can result in compartment syndrome. One of the primary treatments for rhabdomyolysis is administration of isotonic crystalloid intravenous fluids to promote fluid excretion through the kidneys.

29.10 Discuss various types of soft-tissue infection and inflammation, such as cellulitis, gangrene, and necrotizing fasciitis.

Dry gangrene is the death of tissue due to ischemia, often in patients with poor circulation because of peripheral vascular disease. Wet gangrene occurs as a result of an untreated infection, and the infected area oozes foul-smelling liquid. The infection causes swelling, which decreases capillary perfusion and increases ischemia. Necrotizing fasciitis is a rapidly spreading infection, usually caused by group A hemolytic streptococci. The infection often begins at the site of an injury, which may be minor, or a surgical procedure, or even at the site of an IM or IV injection. In some cases, a history of injury cannot be found but is more likely to occur in the presence of diabetes or alcoholism. A particularly significant complaint is pain that seems out of proportion with the appearance of the affected area. The infection can spread significantly within hours, and gangrene can develop. Cellulitis is an infection of the skin and subcutaneous tissues, resulting in the classic signs of inflammation: redness, swelling, warmth, and pain. It is a localized infection that can progress to necrotizing fasciitis and sepsis.

Resource Central

Resource Central offers extra practice and review materials in a variety of media. To access it, follow the directions on the Student Access Card provided with the Student Textbook. If there is no card, go to www.bradybooks.com and follow the Resource Central link to Buy Access.

Vocabulary and Concept Review

Exercise 1

Match each term on the left with its definition on the right by placing the letter of the definition in the blank next to the term. (See Resource Central for more vocabulary review.)

1. _____ abscess

2. _____ ankylosing spondylosis

3. _____ cellulitis

4. _____ decubitus ulcer

5. _____ fascia

6. _____ gangrene

7. _____ gas gangrene

8. _____ gout

9. _____ kyphosis

a. Abnormal curvature of the upper spine that can cause a hunchback appearance

b. Death of tissue; necrotic tissue

c. Loss of bone density resulting in fragile bones

d. Breakdown of skeletal muscle

e. Form of arthritis, more common in men, in which the affected vertebrae can fuse

f. Gangrene associated with gas-producing bacteria

g. Neuralgia (nerve pain) of the sciatic nerve

h. Rapidly spreading infection of fascia with tissue death and separation of tissues from the fascia

i. Pocket of pus (white blood cells and cellular debris) in the tissues

(continued on the next page)

10. _____ myoglobin

11. _____ necrotizing fasciitis

12. _____ osteoarthritis

13. _____ osteoporosis

14. _____ pathologic fracture

15. _____ rhabdomyolysis

16. _____ sciatica

j. Fracture that occurs with little force in diseased bone

k. Age-related degenerative joint disease with loss of articular cartilage

l. Inflammation of the skin, including the dermis and subcutaneous layers, usually caused by bacterial infection

m. Pigment in the muscle that can bind with oxygen

n. Bedsore; pressure sore

o. Arthritis caused by uric acid crystals deposited in a joint

p. Inelastic fibrous tissue that surrounds each muscle compartment

Exercise 2

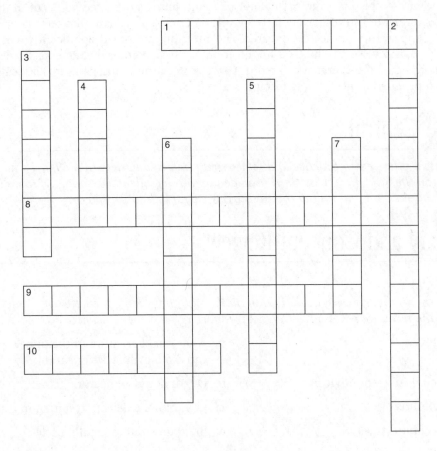

Across

1. Most superficial layer of the skin.
8. Breakdown of muscle tissue with release of muscle cell contents.
9. It is evidenced by tea- or cola-colored urine.
10. Pigment in the skin.

Down

2. Syndrome in which 10 percent or less of total body surface area is affected by epidermal detachment.
3. Decubitis ulcer.
4. Fluid-filled cushion that protects the soft tissues from ligaments and tendons.
5. Decrease in bone mass.
6. Lateral curvature of the spine.
7. Muscle compartment.

Check Your Recall and Apply Concepts

Determine whether the following statements are true or false. Write a "T" for true or an "F" for false in the blank.

1. _____ Rhabdomyolysis can cause renal failure and electrolyte disturbances.

2. _____ The epidermis is very vascular and can bleed heavily when damaged.

3. _____ The neurotransmitter acetylcholine causes shortening of the muscle fiber.

4. _____ Decubitus ulcers result from compromised circulation to the extremities.

5. _____ Clostridia produce a putrid gas, resulting in the condition called *dry gangrene*.

6. _____ Toxic epidermal necrolysis has been linked to NSAIDs and antiretroviral medications.

7. _____ Bursitis is an inflammation of the synovial fluid-filled sacs that protect the soft tissues adjacent to joints.

8. _____ Ewing's sarcoma is one of the most common types of skin cancer.

9. _____ Rhabdomyolysis can also be caused by prolonged exertion such as running a marathon.

10. _____ Scoliosis is an abnormal anterior curvature of the cervical spine.

11. _____ Displaced disc material can place pressure on the sciatic nerve, resulting in pain.

12. _____ When skin is exposed to ultraviolet (UV) radiation from the sun, it synthesizes vitamin D_2.

Clinical Reasoning

CASE STUDY: SPINAL IMMOBILIZATION

Your crew has been called to transport an elderly patient who has been injured in a motor vehicle collision. She is stable, but she complains of neck and upper back pain. As you gather her history, you note that she has kyphosis. The mechanism of injury indicates that she should be spinal immobilized.

1. How should you alter your normal spinal immobilization technique to accommodate the patient who has those musculoskeletal conditions?

   _____

   _____

   _____

   _____

   _____

2. What other steps can you take to protect your patient from prolonged confinement to the long backboard?

   _____

   _____

   _____

   _____

   _____

3. Are there any other pieces of equipment that you might consider?

_____

_____

_____

_____

_____

Project-Based Learning

A patient with severe arthritis may have difficulty performing simple tasks such as holding a pen to write or counting out change. To better appreciate how difficult those types of activities are for some patients, splint all of your fingers together in the extended position. Now, try to hold a pen and sign your name to a run report. Try to dial a phone number on your cell phone. Try to pick up some change that you dropped on the floor. Jot down the thoughts and feelings you experienced during this exercise in your notebook or journal. Then consider how you can apply what you learned to your practice as an Advanced EMT.

The EMS Professional in Practice

You are called into the supervisor's office to discuss a recent patient of yours. She tells you that Mrs. Johnson, whom you recently transported for a diabetic emergency, has contracted necrotizing fasciitis (flesh-eating bacteria) at the site of your IV injection. You remembered that you were extremely busy that day with back-to-back calls and you placed an IV to administer D50. You recall that necrotizing fasciitis is caused by group A hemolytic streptococci.

How does this make you feel? Do you think you might have done something differently if you had it to do over? Jot down your thoughts in a notebook or journal for discussion in class or in your study group.

Chapter 30

Disorders of the Eye, Ear, Nose, Throat, and Oral Cavity

Content Area

- Medicine

Advanced EMT Education Standard

- Applies fundamental knowledge to provide basic and selected advanced emergency care and transportation based on assessment findings for an acutely ill patient.

Summary of Objectives

30.1 Define key terms introduced in this chapter.

Knowing and being able to apply the key terms in each chapter is critical to understanding chapter concepts. Write the list of key terms. Then write the definition of each one in your own words. Check your understanding by confirming the definitions in the textbook glossary. Correct any misunderstandings. Create a study aid by writing each key term on the front of an index card and the definition on the back. Use the cards to quiz yourself or to have someone quiz you. The exercises under Vocabulary and Concept Review below will give you additional practice.

30.2 Describe the etiology and pathophysiology of the following: chalazion, conjunctivitis, glaucoma, hordeolum, orbital cellulitis, and periorbital cellulitis.

Chalazion is a chronic condition that results from granular tissue formation from an unresolved hordeolum. Conjunctivitis is an inflammation of the conjunctiva of the eye, sometimes called "pinkeye," due to the red, bloodshot appearance of the eye. Causes include viruses, bacteria, and allergies. Glaucoma is an increase in intraocular pressure from obstruction of aqueous humor drainage; it leads to blindness if untreated. Hordeolum is an infection of a duct along the margin of the eyelid causing a swollen bump at the base of the eyelashes; it is also called a sty. The usual cause is staphylococcus infection. Orbital cellulitis and periorbital cellulitis are bacterial infections of the tissues around the eye that can be very serious and sometimes occur as a complication of a sinus infection or infection of an insect bite.

30.3 Develop a list of differential diagnoses for patients presenting with eye complaints.

A variety of conditions can cause eye pain and inflammation. The history will help narrow possible causes. Consider a foreign body, conjunctivitis, hordeolum or chalazion, periorbital or orbital cellulitis, and glaucoma. Sudden partial or total vision loss in one or both eyes indicates a very serious problem, such as stroke, retinal artery occlusion, or detached retina.

30.4 Develop a treatment plan for patients presenting with an eye problem in the prehospital setting.

Patients with an eye problem in the prehospital setting require transport. A warm compress over the closed eyes can help in conjunctivitis, hordeolum, or chalazion. You can remove small, nonembedded foreign bodies by irrigation with saline. If eye injury is suspected, cover both eyes to minimize eye movement.

30.5 Describe the etiology and pathophysiology of the following: foreign body in the ear, otitis externa, otitis media, and vertigo.

Foreign body in the ear may include insects or objects placed by a child into his ear canal. Objects can result in soft-tissue damage and infection, and a physician must remove them. Otitis externa is an inflammation of the external auditory canal; swimmer's ear is one form. Otitis media is an inflammation or infection of the middle ear, often associated with an upper respiratory infection. Vertigo is dizziness, which can be caused by labyrinthitis, Ménière disease, a sudden change in position, benign paroxysmal positional vertigo, or stroke.

30.6 Develop a list of differential diagnoses for patients presenting with ear complaints.

Ear pain can be caused by a foreign body in the ear or otitis media or externa. Sudden hearing loss may be due to cerumen impaction, ruptured tympanic membrane, medication side effects, or a blow to the head that disrupts the ossicular chain.

30.7 Develop a treatment plan for patients presenting with ear complaints in the prehospital setting.

In most cases, only transport is indicated. However, keep in mind that some ear problems are associated with dizziness, nausea, and vomiting. If allowed by medical direction, you can place several drops of oil (such as olive oil) in the ear if there is a clear history of an insect entering the ear and its movements are distressing to the patient.

30.8 Describe the etiology and pathophysiology of the following: epistaxis, nasal foreign bodies, and sinusitis.

Epistaxis can be caused by trauma to the nose, including a blow to the nose or inserting a finger or object into the nose; excessively dry or fragile nasal mucosa; sinus infection; anticoagulant medications; and hypertension. Bleeding can usually be controlled, but in some cases, especially with a posterior bleed due to hypertension, bleeding can be severe. Airway obstruction and aspiration of blood are possible.

Nasal foreign bodies usually occur in the pediatric population and can cause infection if not removed, or the patient may aspirate them.

Sinusitis is an inflammation or infection of the sinuses that produces headache, facial pain and pressure, and usually nasal discharge, which can be copious and purulent. Untreated sinus infection can occasionally lead to orbital cellulitis, osteomyelitis, or meningitis.

30.9 Develop a list of differential diagnoses for patients with nasal complaints.

Epistaxis is easily differentiated from other complaints. Signs and symptoms and history are often specific to the problem, such as a sinus infection or foreign body in the nose.

30.10 Describe the etiology and pathophysiology of the following: dentalgia and dental abscess, epiglottitis, and peritonsillar abscess.

Dentalgia and dental abscess produce dental pain caused by caries (cavities), a broken or cracked tooth, gum disease, or a dental abscess (infection). Tooth or jaw pain also can be caused by myocardial infarction, ear infection, or sinus infection. Dental abscesses can extend to the soft tissues of the floor of the oral cavity (Ludwig's angina) and can lead to sepsis if untreated.

Epiglottitis is a bacterial infection of the epiglottis that leads to severe throat pain, difficulty swallowing, and possible airway obstruction.

Peritonsillar abscess is an infection of the capsule around the palatine tonsils, usually involving streptococcal or staphylococcal bacteria. Airway obstruction is a concern.

30.11 Develop a list of differential diagnoses for patients with indications of problems of the throat and oropharynx.

Consider dental problems, sinus infection, ear infection, myocardial infarction, peritonsillar abscess, and epiglottitis in your differential diagnoses.

30.12 Develop a treatment plan for patients presenting with problems of the nose, throat, or oropharynx in the prehospital setting.

Be particularly aware of the possibility of airway obstruction due to bleeding or swelling.

Resource Central

Resource Central offers extra practice and review materials in a variety of media. To access it, follow the directions on the Student Access Card provided with the Student Textbook. If there is no card, go to www.bradybooks.com and follow the Resource Central link to Buy Access.

Vocabulary and Concept Review

Exercise 1

Match each term on the left with its definition on the right by placing the letter of the definition in the blank next to the term. (See Resource Central for more vocabulary review.)

1. _____ chalazion

a. Infection of the mastoid process of the temporal bone

2. _____ conjunctivitis

b. Property by which a substance, such as a drug, can cause temporary or permanent dysfunction in ear function

3. _____ glaucoma

c. Condition of the inner ear leading to tinnitus, vertigo, and hearing loss

4. _____ hordeolum

d. Acute infection of a gland in the eyelid; a sty.

5. _____ labyrinthitis

e. Infection of the external ear canal

6. _____ mastoiditis

f. Chronic cyst in the eyelid

7. _____ Ménière disease

g. Increased intraocular pressure leading to damage of the optic nerve and blindness

8. _____ otitis externa

h. Inflammation of the lining of the maze of canals in the inner ear

9. _____ otitis media

i. Lighted instrument used to inspect the ear canal and tympanic membrane

10. _____ otoscope

j. Infection of the middle ear

11. _____ ototoxic

k. Inflammation of the conjunctiva, the outermost layer of the eye

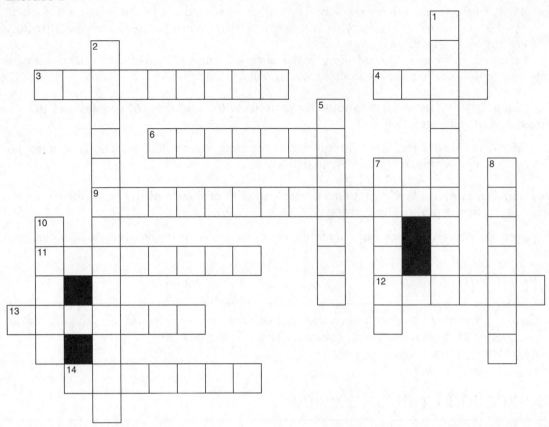

Across

3. Nosebleed.

4. Condition in which dizziness results from head movements.

6. Common name for the tympanic membrane.

9. Location of the visual cortex.

11. Tiny bones of the middle ear.

12. Hard, outer layer of a tooth.

13. Ear wax.

14. Clumps of lymphatic tissue in the pharynx.

Down

1. Bacterial infection that can cause a pseudomembrane in the respiratory tract.

2. Semisolid gel in the posterior chamber of the eye.

5. Enzyme in saliva that breaks down complex carbohydrates.

7. Clear outer layer of the eye that receives oxygen from tears.

8. Common name for conjunctivitis.

10. Color-sensitive pigmented cells in the retina.

Patient Assessment Review

For each of the following patients, list conditions you should specifically investigate further in the history and assessment.

Patient	Conditions to Investigate
1. A 73-year-old woman complains of a severe headache with nausea and vomiting for 12 hours. The pain is focused in her right eye. The eye is very red and hazy looking. She says she is seeing halos around lights.	
2. A 52-year-old man complains of a sudden, painless loss of vision in his right eye. He has no past medical history or other complaints.	
3. A 4-year-old child complains of right ear pain. His father says he has not been ill, and that he started complaining of ear pain 3 hours ago, and that the pain seems to be getting progressively worse. The patient is alert with warm, dry skin and normal color.	
4. A 34-year-old woman complains of a severe sore throat and difficulty swallowing. The pain began 4 hours ago and rapidly worsened.	

Check Your Recall and Apply Concepts

Select the best possible choice for each of the following questions.

_____ 1. Which one of the following is the underlying cause of glaucoma?
   a. A buildup of aqueous humor
   b. Detachment of the retina
   c. Paralysis of the oculomotor nerve
   d. Degeneration of the pigmented cells of the eye

_____ 2. The structure that allows equalization of pressure between the middle ear and the atmosphere is the:
   a. mastoid process.   c. Eustachian tube.
   b. stapes.   d. cochlea.

_____ 3. The narrow band of tissue that attaches each of lips to the gum behind it is the:
   a. lingual tonsil.   c. papilla.
   b. frenulum.   d. cementum.

_____ 4. A 44-year-old female patient complains of burning and a gritty, itchy feeling in her eyes. When you inspect the eyes, you see they are both red and irritated. The findings are most consistent with which one of the following disorders?
   a. Glaucoma   c. Conjunctivitis
   b. Hordeolum   d. Periorbital cellulitis

_____ 5. Inflammation or infection of the inner ear is called:
   a. vertigo.   c. ototoxicity.
   b. Ménière disease.   d. labyrinthitis.

_____ **6.** In the prehospital setting, epistaxis is best treated by:
   a. having the patient sit up, lean forward, and pinch the nostrils.
   b. having the patient tilt his head back and pinch the nostrils.
   c. packing the nares with absorbent gauze.
   d. placing cold packs over the nose.

Clinical Reasoning

CASE STUDY: DENTON BLACKSTONE

You and your partner, Jeff, respond to a call for a sick child. Your patient, four-year-old Denton Blackstone, is sitting on his mother's lap. His skin appears pale, but his cheeks are flushed. He has swelling and discoloration around his left eye and is complaining of eye pain. He is sitting quietly on his mother's lap and clearly does not feel well. His mother says he had a mosquito bite under his eye that he kept scratching. When Denton woke up from his nap, his eye was swollen and he complained that it "hurts to look at things."

1. What problems should you consider in your differential diagnoses?

_____

_____

_____

_____

_____

2. How should you approach your assessment and history?

_____

_____

_____

_____

_____

3. What prehospital treatment does Denton need?

_____

_____

_____

_____

_____

_____

Project-Based Learning

Research current Centers for Disease Control and Prevention recommendations for diphtheria vaccination. What are the differences between recommendations for adults and children? Put together a half- to a full-page fact sheet on diphtheria vaccination recommendations. This information will help you answer questions patients might have about vaccinations.

The EMS Professional in Practice

You are dispatched for a sick person at 2330 hours. When you arrive, you find that your patient is a 32-year-old man complaining of severe tooth pain. He says he is miserable and cannot sleep because of the pain. Your partner is clearly irritated at having to respond to the call. He whispers under his breath, "I am not a freaking dentist." How do you feel about your partner's actions and statement? Jot down your thoughts in a notebook or journal for discussion in class or in your study group.

Chapter 31

Mental Illness and Behavioral Emergencies

Content Area

- Medicine

Advanced EMT Education Standard

- Applies fundamental knowledge to provide basic and selected advanced emergency care and transportation based on assessment findings for an acutely ill patient.

Summary of Objectives

31.1 Define key terms introduced in this chapter.

Knowing and being able to apply the key terms in each chapter is critical to understanding chapter concepts. Write the list of key terms. Then write the definition of each one in your own words. Check your understanding by confirming the definitions in the textbook glossary. Correct any misunderstandings. Create a study aid by writing each key term on the front of an index card and the definition on the back. Use the cards to quiz yourself or to have someone quiz you. The exercises under Vocabulary and Concept Review below will give you additional practice.

31.2 Explain the importance of being able to recognize and respond to patients suffering from behavioral emergencies.

Patients with behavioral emergencies require assistance in coping with an acute situation that has triggered an emergency, or need longer-term treatment for a mental illness. In some cases, a behavioral emergency is the outward manifestation of a physiologic problem, such as hypoglycemia or hypoxia, for which the patient needs emergency care. In some cases, patients with a behavioral emergency may be a danger to themselves or others unless they receive the treatment they need.

31.3 Describe indications of danger associated with response to behavioral emergencies.

A patient with a behavioral emergency may pose a threat of physical violence toward others, including health care providers. A past history of violent behavior, drug or alcohol use, a loud voice, profanity, pacing, possession of a weapon, threats of violence, throwing things, punching inanimate objects, and clenching the fists all are indications of potential violent behavior.

31.4 Discuss the underlying physical and psychologic causes of behavioral emergencies.

Behavioral emergencies due to physical causes could be caused by infection, tumor, neurologic damage, recent or past traumatic brain injury, stroke, seizure, endocrine problems, hypoxia, metabolic disturbances, drugs, toxins, or hypoxia.

31.5 Describe the focus of assessment and history taking for patients experiencing behavioral emergencies.

Be alert to indications of impending violence; assess the airway, breathing, and circulation; consider underlying physiologic causes of behavioral emergencies; and use the assessment and history-taking process as part of the intervention (therapeutic communications).

31.6 Recognize behavioral characteristics of the following conditions: anxiety, bipolar disorder, depression, panic attack, paranoia, phobias, psychosis, and schizophrenia.

Anxiety is a state of worry and fear that interferes with social and occupational functioning. Bipolar disorder is an uncommon mood disorder characterized by periods of depression interspersed with periods of abnormal elation and grandiosity. Depression is a mood disorder in which the patient might have feelings of guilt, sadness, or worthlessness; changes in sleeping and eating behaviors; inability to concentrate; and loss of interest in things once considered pleasurable. Panic attack is a brief period of intense fear, anxiety, and discomfort that is often accompanied by fear of having a heart attack, going crazy, or losing control; and a sensation of unreality. Paranoia is an abnormal suspiciousness that others' behaviors are intended to cause harm, or that one is being followed or spied on. Phobias are intense, unrealistic fears. Psychosis is a mental state in which reality is distorted. Schizophrenia is a psychotic disorder in which the perception of reality is distorted; patients may have delusions, disorganized thoughts, hallucinations, flat affect, and impaired reasoning.

31.7 Describe risk factors associated with violence toward others and suicide.

Suicide is common in many mental illnesses, including depression, schizophrenia, personality disorders, and substance abuse disorders. Feelings of hopelessness, lack of social support, and access to a lethal weapon also are risk factors. Psychosis, some personality disorders, and substance abuse are risk factors for violent behavior.

31.8 Incorporate the basic principles presented in the text into the assessment, communication, and management of patients with behavioral emergencies.

Empathy and respect are essential in the care of patients with behavioral emergencies. Maintain your own safety; ensure an adequate airway, breathing, and circulation; consider physiologic causes of the emergency; treat any injuries noted; and reassure the patient without making false reassurances.

31.9 Prioritize patient care needs in terms of managing physical and behavioral problems.

Maintain your own safety, and that of the patient and bystanders. Look for and treat immediate threats to life, and use therapeutic communication as an essential part of prehospital management of patients with behavioral emergencies.

31.10 Explain the importance of reassessment of patients with behavioral emergencies.

Patients with behavioral emergencies may have initially undetected medical problems and can deteriorate. Frequent reassessment is essential to detecting and managing those problems.

31.11 Evaluate the need for law enforcement and medical direction involvement in a behavioral emergency situation.

Involve law enforcement any time there are concerns about safety and any time there are questions about a patient's capacity to consent. Consult medical direction if there is a question about the appropriateness of restraint.

31.12 Recognize indications for physical restraint of a patient.

Only restrain patients if necessary for their own safety or the safety of others.

31.13 Follow principles of safe physical restraint of patients.

Use four-point restraints (both arms and both legs) and restrain the patient to the stretcher in a supine position. Leather restraints are best, but if necessary, a wide, inelastic material, such as a sheet, can be used. Frequently assess and document the status of the patient's sensation, motor function, and circulation in his restrained extremities and assess and document the patient's level of responsiveness, airway, breathing, circulation, vital signs, and relevant aspects of the secondary assessment.

31.14 Comply with legal and ethical principles when responding to patients with behavioral emergencies.

Treat patients with behavioral emergencies with empathy and respect. Carefully determine the patient's ability to consent to or refuse treatment, and document the patient's mental status. Restrain only if necessary to protect the patient and others. Document the reasons for restraint, methods of restraint, and reassessment following restraint.

31.15 Document all information pertinent to calls involving behavioral emergencies and patient restraint.

Special considerations in documentation of behavioral emergency calls includes documenting the patient's mental status and ability to consent to care or refuse care, the patient's behaviors, physical examination aimed at finding possible underlying medical problems, and if the patient is restrained, document the behavior that led to the decision to restrain, method of restraint, and continued reassessment after restraint.

31.16 Given a number of patient scenarios, assess and manage patients presenting with indications of a psychiatric disorder or behavioral emergency.

Behavioral emergencies can present with a wide range of behaviors. Be prepared to spend time with the patient and use therapeutic communications as part of your management strategy.

31.17 Consider physiologic differential diagnoses for patients presenting with indications of a psychiatric disorder.

Consider hypoxia, hypoglycemia, overdose, poisoning, recent or past traumatic brain injury, stroke, infection, neurologic impairment, seizures, endocrine problems, and metabolic problems.

31.18 Discuss substance abuse as a psychiatric disorder.

Substance abuse and addiction are diagnosable mental illnesses that require professional evaluation and treatment.

31.19 Describe the acute and long-term behavioral and physiologic effects of alcohol abuse and alcohol withdrawal.

Acute alcohol intoxication leads to behavioral changes and CNS depression. Vomiting in combination with decreased responsiveness can lead to aspiration and airway obstruction. Acute alcohol poisoning can be fatal. In the long term, there are many social, psychologic, and physical consequences of alcohol abuse. A person's job, family, and living situation can be affected. The brain, heart, gastrointestinal tract, pancreas, liver, and other organs can be damaged by long-term alcohol abuse. Alcohol is physically addictive, and withdrawal can lead to tremors, headaches, weakness, sweating, seizures, and delirium tremens.

Resource Central

Resource Central offers extra practice and review materials in a variety of media. To access it, follow the directions on the Student Access Card provided with the Student Textbook. If there is no card, go to www.bradybooks.com and follow the Resource Central link to Buy Access.

Vocabulary and Concept Review

Exercise 1

Write the letter of the correct definition in the blank next to the term. Note that there are more definitions than there are terms. (See Resource Central for more vocabulary review.)

1. _____ affect

2. _____ anxiety

3. _____ behavior

4. _____ behavioral emergency

5. _____ bulimia nervosa

6. _____ catatonic

7. _____ delirium

8. _____ delusion

9. _____ dementia

10. _____ ethanol

11. _____ hallucination

12. _____ illusion

13. _____ paranoid

14. _____ phobia

15. _____ somatoform

a. Intense, unrealistic fear

b. One's visible emotional state

c. Eating disorder characterized by binging and purging, such as by vomiting or use of laxatives

d. Type of disorder in which the patient has physical symptoms without apparent physical causes

e. Beverage alcohol

f. Mental state in which reality is distorted

g. A person's observable actions

h. Behavior characterized by rigidity or slackness of the extremities

i. Actions that are intolerable to a person or those around him

j. False belief maintained despite evidence to the contrary

k. Acute confusional state

l. Misinterpretation of actual stimuli

m. Syndrome that occurs due to alcohol withdrawal in a physically dependent person

n. State of excessive worry and fear

o. Progressive, irreversible deterioration in cognitive state

p. Falsely believing that there is a threat to oneself

q. Perception or sensation in the absence of actual stimuli

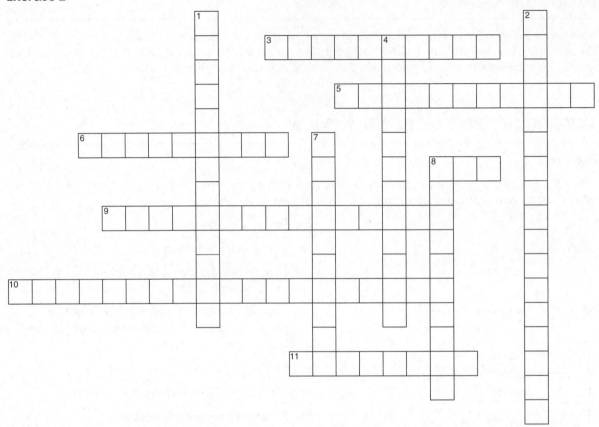

Across

3. This syndrome in self-harm or producing false signs and symptoms is motivated by the desire to assume the sick role; there is no external gain.

5. Disorder involving impulsive stealing.

6. Mental state in which reality is distorted.

8. American Psychological Association guide to identifying mental illnesses.

9. Syndrome that occurs due to withdrawal from alcohol in a person who is physically dependent.

10. Problem characterized by maladaptive ways of perceiving, thinking, and relating to others.

11. Eating disorder characterized by dietary restrictions and severely limited food intake.

Down

1. Psychotic disorder with disordered thinking, often with delusions, hallucinations, and flat affect.

2. Alcoholic syndrome that affects the brain, first reversibly, then irreversibly.

4. An intermediate breakdown product of alcohol.

7. Mood disorder characterized by loss of interest in things, disordered sleep, and feelings of worthlessness or guilt.

8. Patients with this disorder are preoccupied with a physical defect not apparent to others.

Patient Assessment Review

For each phase of the patient assessment process, list possible indications of a behavioral emergency.

1. Scene size-up

   _____

   _____

   _____

2. Primary assessment

   _____

   _____

   _____

3. Secondary assessment

   _____

   _____

   _____

4. Reassessment

   _____

   _____

   _____

Check Your Recall and Apply Concepts

Exercise 1

In the blank next to each item, write "T" to indicate a true statement and "F" to indicate a false statement.

1. _____ Most patients with mental illnesses pose a threat to themselves or others.

2. _____ In general, depressed patients are more likely to require restraints than patients with psychotic disorders.

3. _____ When medical personnel are attacked by hostile patients, it is usually because the health care provider did something to provoke the patient.

4. _____ If you suspect a patient may have harmed himself, you should ask him if has tried to hurt himself.

5. _____ Addiction means a person must take more and more of a substance to get the same effects.

Exercise 2

Select the best possible choice for each of the following questions.

_____ 1. A patient tells you he is nervous and cannot relax and that he feels he must always be alert to the possibility of something going wrong. He is alert and oriented. You observe that he seems tense. Based on the information available, the patient's presentation is most consistent with a(n) _____ disorder.
   a. cognitive
   b. mood
   c. anxiety
   d. psychotic

_____ 2. A patient tells you he is worried about a change in his bowel habits. Despite visits to three different physicians and a negative colonoscopy, the patient's fears persist. The patient's concerns are most consistent with which one of the following disorders?
   a. Hypochondriasis
   b. Munchausen syndrome
   c. Conversion disorder
   d. Body dysmorphic disorder

_____ 3. You have been called to a residential psychiatric treatment facility for juveniles. Your patient is a male 15-year-old who has been diagnosed with pyromania. Pyromania is the inability to control an impulse to:
   a. pull out one's own hair.
   b. cut one's skin.
   c. set fires.
   d. steal others' belongings.

_____ 4. Your patient is a 26-year-old woman whose coworker called 911 because the patient has not been to work or called in for two days in a row and does not answer the phone. Law enforcement arrived before you and found the patient lying on the sofa. The patient looks dejected and moves very slowly and with great effort. She will not make eye contact with you, and has great difficulty answering your questions because she seems to have difficulty processing what you are saying. The patient's current state is most consistent with:
   a. bipolar disorder.
   b. post-traumatic stress disorder.
   c. a cluster B personality disorder.
   d. depression.

_____ 5. Which one of the following is most characteristic of schizophrenia?
   a. Homicidal violence
   b. Disorganized thinking
   c. Self-harm motivated by a desire to assume the sick role
   d. Delirium tremens

_____ 6. When a person experiences acute mental and behavioral changes as a result of taking a substance, he is said to be:
   a. intoxicated.
   b. addicted.
   c. habituated.
   d. dependent.

Clinical Reasoning

CASE STUDY: MANDY PARKER

You and your partner respond to a residence for a behavioral emergency. Law enforcement is on the on the scene when you arrive. One of the officers tells you the patient is a 32-year-old woman named Mandy Parker, who has a history of schizophrenia and who stopped taking her medication. The patient's sister called 911 because the patient has become convinced that she is being spied on and that her medications are intended to make her cooperate with the spies. The patient became very upset with her sister and is now convinced that her sister is part of the conspiracy. The patient has not threatened violence and is not currently behaving in a way that would increase your anticipation of violent behavior.

1. How will you maintain control of the situation?

   _____

   _____

   _____

   _____

   _____

2. Describe your approach to assessing this patient.

   _____

   _____

   _____

   _____

   _____

3. What are the considerations in transporting this patient?

   _____

   _____

   _____

   _____

   _____

Project-Based Learning

What mental health services are available in your community? Research the resources available in your community. If behavioral health clinical rotations are not part of your clinical education requirements, enlist your instructor's help in arranging a shift with a behavioral health service. During your experience, pay attention to how the staff interacts with patients. After observing staff interactions with patients, ask questions about their approach to the patient. Write down in your journal or notebook at least three things you learned that will help you in your interactions with patients experiencing behavioral emergencies.

The EMS Professional in Practice

You are on the scene of a 35-year-old man with a history of depression and alcohol abuse who has ingested 24 500-mg acetaminophen tablets in a suicide attempt. As you approach the patient, a police officer says, "Why don't you guys tell him if he really wants to get the job done, he ought to take something that is going to kill him?" What are your thoughts about the officer's statement? How would you react to this situation? Jot down your thoughts in a notebook or journal for discussion in class or in your study group.

Chapter 32

Toxicologic Emergencies

Content Area

- Medicine

Advanced EMT Education Standard

- Applies fundamental knowledge to provide basic and selected advanced emergency care and transportation based on assessment findings for an acutely ill patient.

Summary of Objectives

32.1 Define key terms introduced in this chapter.

Knowing and being able to apply the key terms in each chapter is critical to understanding chapter concepts. Write the list of key terms. Then write the definition of each one in your own words. Check your understanding by confirming the definitions in the textbook glossary. Correct any misunderstandings. Create a study aid by writing each key term on the front of an index card and the definition on the back. Use the cards to quiz yourself or to have someone quiz you. The exercises under Vocabulary and Concept Review below will give you additional practice.

32.2 Describe the importance of understanding the pathophysiology and assessment-based management of patients with toxicologic, drug, and alcohol emergencies.

Understanding various toxidromes helps you understand what is happening to patients physiologically as a result of exposure to a substance and helps you anticipate problems. Regardless of the underlying toxin, follow some basic principles of assessment and management, including maintaining your own safety and ensuring that the patient has an open airway and adequate breathing and circulation. In some cases, you may be able to take specific actions to counteract the effects the substance.

32.3 Give examples of common substances involved in intentional and unintentional toxicologic emergencies in adults and children.

The substances most frequently involved in fatal exposures include sedative–hypnotics, opioids, cardiovascular drugs, acetaminophen, antidepressants, anticonvulsants, alcohol, stimulants, and street drugs. In the pediatric population, analgesics, batteries, hydrocarbons, plants, cough and cold preparations, and other medications are involved.

32.4 **Describe each of the four routes by which a poison can enter the body: absorption, ingestion, inhalation, and injection.**

Absorption refers to a material that crosses the skin or mucous membranes to enter the body. *Ingestion* refers to a material that enters the body through the gastrointestinal tract. *Inhalation* refers to fumes or gases that are breathed in and enter the body through the respiratory tract. *Injection* refers to a material that is delivered through the skin into the subcutaneous, muscular, or vascular systems.

32.5 **Perform a scene size-up to identify indications that a patient may be suffering from a toxicologic or substance abuse emergency.**

Involvement of more than one patient, unusual odors, the presence of vapors or spills of unknown substances, unresponsive patients, behavioral emergencies, and patients presenting with altered mental status should all increase your suspicion of a toxicologic emergency.

32.6 **Given a scenario involving a patient with a toxicologic-, drug-, or alcohol-related emergency, anticipate special considerations in protecting your safety and that of other personnel, the patient, and bystanders.**

Anticipate the potential for violence and for exposure to toxins. Consider the need for hazardous materials response (e.g., if you suspect you may have responded to a methamphetamine lab or other situation in which toxic chemicals are involved) and patient decontamination.

32.7 **Given a series of scenarios, demonstrate the assessment-based management of patients suffering a variety of toxicologic, drug, and alcohol-related emergencies.**

Assess for and manage immediately life-threatening problems with the airway, breathing, and circulation. Anticipate decreased responsiveness, respiratory depression, vomiting and potential airway compromise, impaired perfusion, and impaired thermoregulation. In cases in which it is appropriate, such as in suspected narcotic overdose, administer the indicated medications as an antidote.

32.8 **Anticipate the effects of various classifications of toxins and commonly abused substances on the respiratory, nervous, cardiovascular, and gastrointestinal systems.**

Stimulants, depressants, hallucinogens, asphyxiants, and other classes of toxins act in different ways on the body. For example, narcotics, barbiturates, and benzodiazepines all have depressant effects and can depress respirations. Stimulants, such as cocaine and methamphetamine, may result in excited delirium, hypertension, and cardiovascular emergencies, such as stroke and heart attack. Organophosphates result in overstimulation of the parasympathetic nervous system, which is accompanied by bronchospasm, increased gastrointestinal activity, and copious secretions.

32.9 **Explain the limited role of specific antidotes in toxicologic emergencies.**

There are no specific antidotes for most toxins. Notable exceptions in the Advanced EMT scope of practice include oxygen for carbon monoxide poisoning, naloxone for narcotic overdose, and atropine and pralidoxime for organophosphate poisoning.

32.10 **Explain the importance of identifying the following historical information for patients who have been exposed to a toxin: substance or substances involved, including ingestion of alcohol with other substances; amount of substance(s) involved; length of time since exposure, and time period over which exposure occurred; any attempted treatment of the poisoning; underlying psychiatric or medical conditions; patient's weight; types of substances available to the patient; and medications.**

- *Substance or substances involved, including ingestion of alcohol with other substances:* You must be able to anticipate the effects of the toxins and understand the potential for interactions and resistance to treatments when multiple substances are involved.

- *Amount of substance(s) involved:* The amount of substances involved can affect treatment plans and anticipated outcomes.
- *Length of time since exposure, and time period over which exposure occurred:* It is important to anticipate whether the levels of the toxin may be continuing to increase in the body.
- *Any attempted treatment of the poisoning:* Attempted home treatments can complicate patient management. For example, inducing vomiting can cause soft-tissue damage in the case of ingested corrosives or result in aspiration in the case of ingested hydrocarbons.
- *Underlying psychiatric or medical conditions:* Underlying psychiatric illnesses may present as suicide attempts by poisoning; the presence of pre-existing medical conditions can lead to additional complications.
- *Patient's weight:* The patient's weight is used to assess the significance of the exposure and to calculate the dosage of some antidotes.
- *Types of substances available to the patient:* The patient may not give a reliable history of exposure, so you must anticipate that substances found at the scene could be involved.
- *Medications:* Toxins can interact with medications a patient is already taking.

32.11 **Anticipate pitfalls in obtaining an accurate and complete history from patients with poisoning, drug abuse, or alcohol-related emergencies.**

Patients may intentionally or unintentionally provide an unreliable history.

32.12 **Describe the indications, contraindications, mechanism of action, side effects, dosage, and administration of activated charcoal.**

Activated charcoal is occasionally given, on the advice of medical direction or poison control, to adsorb ingested toxins in the stomach and prevent their absorption into the body. It is not given to patients who cannot protect their airway and is not effective in adsorbing some toxins. Side effects include nausea and vomiting. Activated charcoal preparations containing sorbitol can lead to diarrhea and fluid loss. The usual dosage is 1 gram per kilogram of body weight, with a minimum of 30 grams administered by mouth. Activated charcoal is a powder that is given as a slurry mixed with water or sorbitol.

32.13 **Describe special considerations in assessing and managing patients with each of the following: carbon monoxide poisoning; CNS stimulants (cocaine, amphetamines, methamphetamines); cyanide poisoning; delirium tremens; ethanol ingestion; ethylene glycol ingestion; exposure to acid or alkali substances; exposure to hydrocarbons; exposure to poisonous plants; food poisoning; hallucinogens; huffing; isopropanol ingestion; methanol ingestion; prescription and over-the-counter medication overdose; and withdrawal syndromes.**

- *Carbon monoxide poisoning:* Suspect carbon monoxide poisoning when there are multiple patients in the same location with a source of exposure. Protect yourself from exposure. Remove patients to fresh air and administer high-flow oxygen, assisting respirations as needed. Consider transport to a facility with a hyperbaric oxygen chamber.
- *CNS stimulants (cocaine, amphetamines, methamphetamine):* Anticipate violent behavior and excited delirium, as well as hypertension, cardiac dysrhythmia, acute coronary syndromes, and the potential for stroke.
- *Cyanide poisoning:* Be aware of the potential for responder exposure and request additional resources as needed. Remove patient to fresh air and administer oxygen, assisting respirations as necessary. Consider requesting ALS transport for administration of an antidote (hydroxocobalamin or a three-part antidote kit).
- *Delirium tremens:* Anticipate the possibility of seizures. Request ALS response if transport is prolonged.
- *Ethanol ingestion:* Death can occur from acute alcohol poisoning. Anticipate vomiting and the patient's inability to control his own airway.
- *Ethylene glycol ingestion:* Contact poison control and request ALS response if the patient's condition warrants it or if transport times are long. Death may occur with even small amounts of ingested ethylene glycol.

- *Exposure to acid or alkali substances:* Do not induce vomiting. Activated charcoal may be ineffective and is not indicated. Anticipate complicated airway control; nonvisualized airway devices are contraindicated in caustic ingestion. Consult with poison control for specific considerations related to each substance.
- *Exposure to hydrocarbons:* Halogenated or aromatic hydrocarbons are especially dangerous. Multiple body systems can be affected.
- *Exposure to poisonous plants:* Find out what part of the plant was ingested. Transport a sample of the plant so that it can be definitively identified.
- *Food poisoning:* Suspect food poisoning if there are multiple patients with similar signs and symptoms and history of exposure to the same food. Treatment is symptomatic. Anticipate dehydration and treat with IV fluids. Consult with medical direction about the use of antiemetics, if allowed in your scope of practice.
- *Hallucinogens:* Anticipate violent behavior, especially with phencyclidine (PCP). These are rarely fatal, but they may be combined with other drugs.
- *Huffing:* Huffing may lead to pneumonitis, dyspnea, and hypoxia. Cardiac dysrhythmias and death can occur.
- *Isopropanol ingestion:* Isopropyl alcohol is sometimes ingested as an ethanol substitute when the patient does not have access to ethanol. Anticipate altered mental status and ataxia. Gastrointestinal irritation and bleeding may occur. Treat for hypotension and hypoperfusion with IV fluids.
- *Methanol ingestion:* Patients may be tachypneic in an attempt to reduce severe metabolic acidosis. Blindness may result. Activated charcoal is not effective. Maintain renal perfusion by administering IV fluids.
- *Prescription and over-the-counter medication overdose:* Do not underestimate the potential toxicity of over-the-counter (OTC) medications. Consider that any medications in the environment (even those that are not the patient's) may be involved in the overdose. Anticipate that multiple substances are involved.
- *Withdrawal syndromes:* Seizures can occur and vital signs may become unstable. Manage the patient's airway, breathing, and circulation.

32.14 Explain the importance of contacting the poison control center with as complete a patient history as possible.

Poison control centers maintain accurate and up-to-date information on many substances and can very quickly give advice on signs, symptoms, anticipated problems, and treatment.

32.15 Explain the importance of careful assessment and conscientious management of patients who have ingested drugs or alcohol.

The effects of drugs and alcohol can make patients less aware of injuries and medical problems, and their judgment may be affected.

32.16 Explain the purpose and process of reassessing patients with a toxicologic-, drug-, or alcohol-related emergency.

Toxin levels may be increasing as you spend time with the patient, and his condition can deteriorate with little warning.

Resource Central

Resource Central offers extra practice and review materials in a variety of media. To access it, follow the directions on the Student Access Card provided with the Student Textbook. If there is no card, go to www.bradybooks.com and follow the Resource Central link to Buy Access.

Vocabulary and Concept Review

Exercise 1

Use the following word list to fill in the blanks in each statement.

ataxic	cardiac glycosides	confabulate
half-life	myoclonus	nystagmus
toxin	toxidrome	scombroid fish poisoning

1. A patient who experiences involuntary twitching or jerking of the muscles is experiencing a phenomenon known as _____.

2. A(n) _____ is any substance that has a negative effect on the body.

3. The signs and symptoms associated with a specific class of poisons are collectively known as a(n) _____.

4. _____ is a phenomenon in which there are rapid lateral, vertical, or oscillating involuntary eye movements.

5. The ingestion of fish in which bacterial compounds have converted compounds in fish tissue into histamine can lead to an illness called _____.

6. A person who lacks motor coordination is said to be _____.

7. Unconsciously filling in gaps in memory with events that could have happened, but did not actually happen, is called _____.

8. Purple foxglove is an example of plants that are classified as _____, which have therapeutic value in the treatment of heart problems, such as atrial fibrillation and heart failure.

9. The time that it takes for the level of a toxin in the body to decrease by 50 percent is the toxin's _____.

Exercise 2

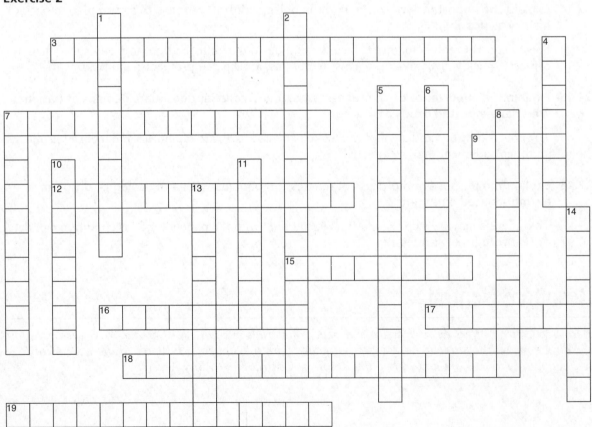

Across

3. One of more than 60 specialized organizations staffed by toxicology experts 24 hours a day, 7 days a week.

7. Class of drugs used to reduce anxiety; diazepam is an example.

9. Common class of antidepressants that includes citalopram and sertraline.

12. Over-the-counter analgesic that causes hepatotoxicity in relatively small doses.

15. Classification to which most poisonous snakes belong.

16. Toxin that accumulates in older fish in some species as a result of them ingesting organisms called dinoflagellates.

17. Most poisonous mushrooms are from this class.

18. Used in some cases of poisoning by ingestion to adsorb toxins to prevent them from being absorbed into the body.

19. Odorless gas produced by incomplete combustion that has a higher affinity for hemoglobin that oxygen does.

Down

1. Plant that can result in anticholinergic signs and symptoms when smoked or ingested as a tea for the purposes of intoxication.

2. Atropine and pralidoxime are antidotes to this kind of poisoning.

4. Toxin found in many forms, including a gas emitted from burning synthetic household items, and acts as a cellular asphyxiant.

5. Medication no longer recommended to induce vomiting in the treatment of poisoning by ingestion, but can still be obtained in small quantities over the counter.

6. Used to reverse respiratory depression associated with narcotic overdose.

7. Shiny, black spider whose venom is a potent neurotoxin.

8. Toxic alcohol found in mouthwash and other readily available products that sometimes is used as an ethanol substitute.

10. Strong acids and alkalis are in this category of toxins.

11. White powder derived from leaves of the coca plant.

13. Route of poison exposure in which toxins enter the body through the respiratory system.

14. Toxic alcohol that is used to manufacture methamphetamine and causes severe metabolic acidosis and blindness when ingested.

Patient Assessment Review

Fill in the following table to describe the assessment findings associated with each toxidrome. For some toxidromes, there are no specific effects on every body system listed.

	Cholinergic	Anticholinergic	Narcotic	Sympathomimetic
Nervous system				
Respiratory system				
Cardiovascular system				
Musculoskeletal system				
Gastrointestinal system				
Skin				

Check Your Recall and Apply Concepts

Exercise 1

Supply a short answer for each of the following items.

1. What is the most common route for toxins to enter the body?

   _____

   _____

   _____

2. To which classification of toxins do organophosphates belong?

   _____

   _____

3. Summarize the signs and symptoms of cholinergic toxins.

   _____

   _____

4. Summarize signs and symptoms of the extrapyramidal toxidrome.

   _____

   _____

5. What makes pulse oximetry unreliable in patients with carbon monoxide poisoning?

   _____

   _____

6. What is the most prevalent source of cyanide poisoning?

   _____

   _____

7. What are some common sources of hydrocarbons?

   _____

   _____

8. What is the most common source of organophosphate poisoning?

   _____

   _____

9. What are some of the long-term effects of alcohol abuse?

_____

_____

_____

10. What signs and symptoms are commonly associated with histamine fish poisoning?

_____

_____

_____

Exercise 2

Select the best possible choice for each of the following questions.

_____ 1. The majority of poisonings occur in patients who are _____ years old.
   a. 35 to 60
   b. 20 to 40
   c. 40 to 49
   d. under 20

_____ 2. The most common route of poisoning is:
   a. inhalation.
   b. absorption.
   c. ingestion.
   d. injection.

_____ 3. The highest priority when responding to any toxicologic emergency is:
   a. airway management.
   b. provider safety.
   c. decontamination.
   d. administering an antidote.

_____ 4. You have arrived on the scene of a reported overdose. As you approach the patient, a man in his 40s, you see that he is not moving and does not appear to be breathing. Your first action should be to:
   a. check the patient's pulse.
   b. attach the AED.
   c. open the patient's airway.
   d. begin bag-valve mask ventilations.

_____ 5. A 15-year-old female has ingested 24 capsules of an over-the-counter medication containing 350 mg of acetaminophen in each capsule 3 hours ago. She is alert and oriented, distraught, and complaining of nausea. Her skin is warm and moist. She has a heart rate of 84 per minute, respiratory rate of 16, blood pressure of 112/78, and her SpO$_2$ is 100 percent on room air. Of the following, which one is the most urgent priority?
   a. Request ALS response.
   b. Administer activated charcoal.
   c. Administer oxygen by nonrebreather mask.
   d. Find out if the patient took any other substances.

_____ 6. During the first chilly weekend of the fall, you are called for a sick person at a residence. An 80-year-old woman tells you that her husband, Kenneth, who is 84 years old, has come down with a bad case of the flu. She says she feels like she is getting the flu as well, and she cannot take care of Kenneth and is worried about him. Both patients complain of severe headaches, nausea, and vomiting. Kenneth is confused and sleepy, which the woman states is unusual. Your first action should be to:
   a. ask both patients if they have received an influenza vaccine this year.
   b. look around for any potential sources of carbon monoxide.
   c. remove both patients from the home.
   d. use a carbon monoxide (CO) oximetry device to assess the patients' oxygen and carbon monoxide levels.

_____ 7. All patients with suspected carbon monoxide poisoning should be treated with:
   a. oxygen.
   b. hydroxocobalamin.
   c. atropine and pralidoxime.
   d. a three-part antidote kit.

_____ 8. In which one of the following ingestions should you suspect cyanide poisoning?
   a. Rhubarb leaves
   b. Green parts of potatoes
   c. Daffodil bulbs
   d. Cherry pits

_____ 9. Which one of the following best describes the mechanism by which cyanide causes harm?
   a. It prevents cellular oxygen use.
   b. It binds with hemoglobin, displacing oxygen and resulting in hypoxia.
   c. It causes severe metabolic acidosis.
   d. It causes severe central nervous system depression and respiratory arrest.

_____ 10. A four-year-old boy accidentally drank from a cup that contained a strong alkali. When you arrive on the scene, he is sitting up and appears very ill. He is having difficulty breathing and swallowing and complains of chest and abdominal pain. He has chemical burns in his mouth. Which one of the following best describes the appropriate management of this patient?
   a. Administer 1 gram per kilogram of body weight of activated charcoal.
   b. Have the patient drink a large amount of milk or water to dilute the substance.
   c. Induce vomiting.
   d. Administer high-flow oxygen and transport immediately.

_____ 11. A 41-year-old woman was found disoriented in an alley behind a convenience store. She has metallic paint smeared around her mouth and nose and on her clothing. There is a red rash around her mouth and nose. She is awake but confused and has moderate dyspnea. When you listen to her lungs, you hear severe wheezing, especially on the right side. Her heart rate is 96, respiratory rate 24, blood pressure 104/74, and SpO_2 is 88 percent on room air. Which one of the following is indicated in the treatment of this patient?
   a. 0.3 mg of epinephrine, IM or SC
   b. Oxygen by nonrebreather mask
   c. Self-administered nitrous oxide
   d. 1 mg of naloxone, IV

_____ 12. Which one of the following best explains the way that organophosphates cause harm?
   a. They cause immediate breakdown of acetylcholine resulting in inhibition of the parasympathetic nervous system.
   b. They inhibit an enzyme needed to break down norepinephrine at the neuroeffector junction.
   c. They inhibit an enzyme that breaks down acetylcholine at the neuroeffector junction.
   d. They cause immediate breakdown of norepinephrine resulting in inhibition of the sympathetic nervous system.

_____ 13. Which one of the following signs is consistent with organophosphate poisoning?
   a. Bradycardia
   b. Urinary retention
   c. Dry mucous membranes
   d. Hyperthermia

_____ 14. Sudden cessation of alcohol intake in a physically dependent person can result in:
   a. Wernicke-Korsakoff syndrome.
   b. acute blindness.
   c. delirium tremens.
   d. renal failure.

_____ 15. A syndrome of paresthesias, reversal of hot and cold sensations, joint and muscle pain, itching, lack of coordination, dizziness, weakness, and tooth pain occurs in _____ poisoning.
   a. Botulism
   b. Ciguatera
   c. _E. coli_
   d. Scombroid fish

_____ 16. A patient states she believes she was bitten by an insect or small animal while she was cleaning out a shed in her yard. The bite was small initially, but has increased in size and become more painful, swollen, and red. The affected area on her arm is now about 5 inches in diameter. This scenario is most consistent with a bite from which one of the following animals?
  a. Brown recluse spider
  b. Black widow spider
  c. Bark scorpion
  d. Coral snake

_____ 17. On a dare, a male 19-year-old picked up a rattlesnake that he and his buddy found while hiking. The snake bit the patient on the back of his left hand. He is very upset. The area around the bite is painful, swollen, and discolored. It continues to seep blood. The best treatment for this patient is to:
  a. elevate the extremity so that the level of the bite is above the heart.
  b. apply ice packs.
  c. place a constricting band proximal to the wound.
  d. immobilize the limb in a neutral position.

_____ 18. An 8-year-old girl was stung by a jellyfish while swimming at the beach. As part of the treatment, you should:
  a. apply ice to the area.
  b. flush the affected area with saline.
  c. scrub the area to remove remaining nematocysts.
  d. elevate the affected area above the heart.

_____ 19. An overdose of which one of the following would result in salicylate poisoning?
  a. Aspirin
  b. Tylenol
  c. Ibuprofen
  d. Diphenhydramine

_____ 20. A 20-year-old male patient has taken several oxycodone tablets. You should consider administering naloxone if which one of the following signs is present?
  a. Pinpoint pupils
  b. Decreased level of responsiveness
  c. Respiratory depression
  d. Tachycardia

_____ 21. An overdose of venlafaxine, sertraline, duloxetine, or escitalopram is most likely to result in:
  a. confusion, hallucinations, seizures, tachycardia, and cardiac dysrhythmias and heart blocks.
  b. hypotension and respiratory depression.
  c. hypertensive crisis.
  d. agitation, excess salivation, goose bumps, flushed skin, hyperthermia, tachycardia, and myoclonus.

_____ 22. You have responded to a high school for a reported overdose. A male 16-year-old has taken several tablets of his friend's medication for ADHD. It is most likely the drug he has taken is a(n):
  a. barbiturate.
  b. narcotic.
  c. amphetamine.
  d. benzodiazepine.

_____ 23. The drug classification of hallucinogens includes:
  a. PCP and LSD.
  b. Ecstasy and marijuana.
  c. cocaine and methamphetamine.
  d. rohypnol and GHB.

Clinical Reasoning

CASE STUDY: MAN DOWN AT THE BUS STOP

You and your partner, Wanda, have just arrived at a city bus stop in front of a grocery store. Your unit responds to this location frequently. Many of the patients you encounter are homeless and have substance abuse problems, in addition to a variety of other health problems. You often respond to injuries from fights and environmental emergencies. As you pull into the grocery store parking lot behind the bus stop, safely out of traffic, you see that law enforcement is on scene. As you approach the patient, one of the police officers tells you to be careful because they found a syringe with a needle attached in the patient's coat pocket.

The patient does not respond to painful stimuli and is snoring, but he is breathing about 10 times per minute. With no obvious mechanism of injury or signs of trauma present, you use a head-tilt/chin-lift maneuver to open the airway and relieve the snoring. His skin is cool and dry, and his pupils are midsized and sluggishly reactive to light. He has a weak radial pulse of 80 per minute. You notice old and new puncture marks on the patient's arms. Meanwhile, the police have found a glass pipe in the patient's belongings.

1. How will you continue with your assessment?

   _____

   _____

   _____

   _____

2. What specific information would be helpful in determining the problem and treatment?

   _____

   _____

   _____

   _____

3. What treatments are required, based on the information you have so far?

   _____

   _____

   _____

   _____

Project-Based Learning

Take an inventory of the plants and trees in your home, yard, garden, or neighborhood. Identify poisonous plants. If you are not sure what some of the plants are, you can identify them using a book from the library or an online resource. Often, the county extension office has an expert who can help identify plants. For each poisonous plant identified, make an index card. Draw an example of the plant and write its name on one side of the card. On the opposite side, list the toxin that makes the plant poisonous and the signs and symptoms induced by the toxin. Use the cards when you study. Compare the cards you developed to those developed by others in your study group and class.

The EMS Professional in Practice

You and your partner have responded to a residence for a report of a poisoning in a two-year-old male child. The mother tells you that this is the third time the ambulance has responded because her son, Charlie Jr., has gotten into substances stored in the basement, garage, and kitchen. On this occasion, she believes that Charlie ate several of her prenatal vitamins. What are your ethical and legal obligations in this case? Jot down your thoughts in a notebook or journal for discussion in class or in your study group.

Trauma Systems and Incident Command

Content Area

- Trauma
- EMS Operations

Advanced EMT Education Standard

- Applies fundamental knowledge to provide basic and selected advanced emergency care and transportation based on assessment findings for an acutely injured patient.
- Applies knowledge of operational roles and responsibilities to ensure patient, public, and personnel safety.

Summary of Objectives

33.1 Define key terms introduced in this chapter.

Knowing and being able to apply the key terms in each chapter is critical to understanding chapter concepts. Write the list of key terms. Then write the definition of each one in your own words. Check your understanding by confirming the definitions in the textbook glossary. Correct any misunderstandings. Create a study aid by writing each key term on the front of an index card and the definition on the back. Use the cards to quiz yourself or to have someone quiz you. The exercises under Vocabulary and Concept Review below will give you additional practic.

33.2 Describe the epidemiology and significance of trauma.

Unintentional injury is the fifth leading cause of death in the United States. Injuries result in more than 40 million emergency department visits.

33.3 Explain the importance and components of injury prevention programs in reducing trauma morbidity and mortality.

Injury prevention programs are important because they can result in a dramatic decrease in injury morbidity and mortality.

33.4 Describe each of the components of a comprehensive trauma care system.

The components of a comprehensive trauma care system are leadership, professional resources, education and advocacy, information management, finances, research, and technology.

33.5 Identify the characteristics of each level of trauma center as designated by the American College of Surgeons Committee on Trauma.

A Level I (regional) trauma center is capable of managing any type of traumatic injury 24 hours a day, 365 days a year. A Level II (area) trauma center is capable of managing most traumatic injuries 24 hours a day, 365 days a year and is capable of stabilizing patients with more severe injuries and arranging for transfer to a Level I trauma center. A Level III (community) trauma center provides some surgical capability and specially trained emergency department (ED) staff to manage trauma. A Level IV trauma facility typically is a smaller hospital located in a remote area and is capable of stabilizing trauma patients for transfer to a higher-level center.

33.6 Explain the importance of having an understanding of how to manage situations in which there are multiple patients.

You must understand how managing scenes with multiple patients differs from managing scenes with a single patient. The priorities of a multiple-casualty incident are slightly different, in that you must provide the best care for the greatest number of patients. That requires that some aspects of the approach are different from those used on single-patient calls.

33.7 Explain the importance of immediately identifying the number of patients at a scene.

Failure to recognize all patients can result in delays in providing emergency care and cause underestimation of the resources needed.

33.8 Compare the needs of an event to the resources available to identify multiple-casualty incidents in a given EMS system.

The scene size-up includes an assessment of the number of patients in order to identify the need for additional resources. The number of patients that constitute a multiple-casualty incident vary according to the resources available in the EMS system.

33.9 Differentiate between the management goals of single-patient and multiple-patient incidents.

In a single-patient incident, once scene safety has been established, the Advanced EMT's focus is on providing emergency care to the patient. In a multiple-patient incident, the Advanced EMT must establish incident command and begin triage to determine which patients have the highest priority for treatment and transport.

33.10 Discuss some common issues with communications in multiple-casualty incidents and disaster situations.

Communications systems can be damaged and inoperable in disaster situations. Radio systems from outside agencies arriving to help may be incompatible with the system in the affected area, and if communication policies are not established and followed, confusion can result.

33.11 Prioritize your actions as the first provider on the scene of a multiple-casualty incident.

You must first identify the nature of the incident, report it, and request additional resources. You must take on the responsibility of incident command until command is assumed according to policy.

33.12 Describe the principles of an incident command system.

Incident command systems ensure common understanding of goals, procedures, and terminology and coordination of efforts when there are multiple agencies responding to an incident. The guiding principle is to prevent duplication of efforts while maximizing resource capabilities.

33.13 Identify the roles and responsibilities that may be assigned to EMS units at a multiple-casualty incident.

EMS units are involved in triage, treatment, and transport of patients during multiple-casualty incidents.

33.14 Describe the principles of a triage system.

Triage is a process of identifying patients' priorities for treatment and transport based on the severity of their injuries.

33.15 Given a scenario with multiple patients, categorize patients according to a color-coded triage system.

Patients categorized as needing immediate treatment and transport receive red tags, patients whose treatment and transport can be delayed receive yellow tags, patients with minor injuries receive green tags, and patients who are unlikely to be salvaged receive black tags, indicating the lowest priority for resources.

33.16 Explain the principles used in the START triage system.

In the START triage system, patients with minor injuries are first separated from those needing further triage by asking them to get up and walk on their own to a designated area. Remaining patients are assessed for the ability to maintain an airway. Those who cannot maintain an airway on their own are tagged as deceased. Those who are able to breathe after the airway is opened are tagged as immediate. Patients who do not require the airway to be opened are tagged immediate if the respiratory rate is greater than 30. Patients who are breathing less than 30 times per minute but who have poor perfusion status also are tagged as immediate. Patients who are breathing less than 30 times per minute, who have adequate perfusion, but who have an altered mental status also are tagged as immediate. Patients who are breathing less than 30 times per minute, have adequate perfusion, and who are able to follow simple commands are tagged as delayed.

33.17 Describe adaptations of START triage to JumpSTART for pediatric patients.

In JumpSTART, patients whose airway must be opened but who have a palpable pulse are provided with five rescue breaths if they are not breathing. If spontaneous breathing does not resume after five rescue breaths, the patient is tagged "deceased." The criteria for being tagged as "immediate" based on respirations are a respiratory rate greater than 45 per minute or less than 15 per minute.

33.18 Perform primary and secondary triage in a multiple-casualty incident.

You should be able to apply the START and JumpSTART criteria, or other criteria used in your EMS service, to identify patient priorities for treatment and transport.

33.19 Use triage tags to document assessment and care of patients in a multiple-casualty incident.

It is not feasible to document patient care in multiple-casualty incidents using a patient care report because of the volume of patients involved and the need to return to service immediately without time for lengthy documentation. The basics of assessment and treatment are summarized on the triage tag to provide a means of communication about patient care.

33.20 Describe considerations in determining the transport destination for patients in a multiple-casualty incident.

Which hospitals patients are transported to depends on the disaster plan and the resources of each community. Often, each hospital will advise how many patients it can accept. Incident command works with the hospitals to ensure that patients receive the care they need without overwhelming one hospital and underutilizing another. It is not desirable to transport all patients to the closest hospital because it can overwhelm the resources of that hospital and create further confusion and delays in patient care.

Resource Central

Resource Central offers extra practice and review materials in a variety of media. To access it, follow the directions on the Student Access Card provided with the Student Textbook. If there is no card, go to www.bradybooks.com and follow the Resource Central link to Buy Access.

Vocabulary and Concept Review

Exercise 1

Use the following word list to fill in the blanks in each statement.

finance/administration	information officer	START triage
incident command system (ICS)	incident commander	primary triage
multiple-casualty incident	planning section	triage
logistics section	unified command	triage tags
JumpSTART triage system	singular command	trauma system
national incident management system (NIMS)	secondary triage	safety officer

1. The first assessment and assignment of patient priority during a multiple-casualty incident is called: _____.

2. The scheme used by any EMS system to coordinate the leadership and various functions that must be carried out in a multiple-casualty incident is called a(n): _____.

3. A standardized approach to assigning treatment and transport priority to pediatric patients in a multiple-casualty incident is: _____.

4. An event in which the number of patients exceeds the available resources is called a(n): _____.

5. The standardized scheme of coordinating the response to large-scale disasters is called the: _____.

(continued on the next page)

6. The person designated to oversee the protection of responders and patients at a multiple-casualty incident is called the: _____.

7. The process during which patients' initial priorities for treatment and transport are re-evaluated is called: _____.

8. The type of coordination used to manage smaller incidents is called: _____.

9. The division of personnel in a multiple-casualty response that is responsible for distributing supplies and equipment is called the: _____.

10. The person who is responsible for communicating with the media during a multiple-casualty incident is the: _____.

Exercise 2

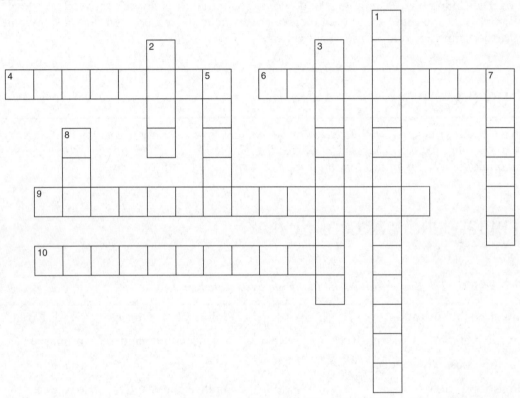

Across

4. Incident command section that analyzes data to improve future responses.
6. Modified triage approach used for pediatric patients.
9. Person who coordinates activities of the incident command system with outside agencies.
10. Strategy for injury prevention that focuses on legislation.

Down

1. Opportunity to practice the implementation of the response to multiple-casualty incidents and use of the incident command system.
2. Organizational structure used to ensure coordination and effective communication among all agencies responding to a disaster.
3. Patient priority denoted by a red triage tag.
5. Triage tag color assigned to the walking wounded.
7. Quick sorting process to establish patient priorities for treatment and transport.
8. Event in which the number of patients exceeds the available resources.

Patient Assessment Review

You are working the triage sector at the scene of a bus crash on the interstate. Assign each of the following patients a triage category (green for minor, yellow for delayed, red for immediate, or black for expectant/deceased).

Patient	Triage Category
1. 21-year-old man, who responds to painful stimuli. He is breathing spontaneously at 30 times per minute, has a weak radial pulse, and his capillary refill time is greater than 2 seconds.	
2. Nine-year-old girl, who is unresponsive and not breathing spontaneously. She begins breathing 8 times per minute after you open the airway. She has a capillary refill time greater than 2 seconds.	
3. 50-year-old woman, who is awake and follows commands, but not able to stand and walk in response to the request for those with minor injuries to do so. She is breathing spontaneously and has a strong radial pulse.	
4. 24-year-old man who is unresponsive and not breathing spontaneously. He does not begin breathing after you open the airway. He has a weak, irregular carotid pulse.	
5. 32-year-old woman who is awake, breathing spontaneously, has a strong radial pulse, and walked to the area designated when requested to do so.	

Check Your Recall and Apply Concepts

Exercise 1

Select the best possible choice for each of the following questions.

_____ **1.** Enacting a law to require all persons under the age of 18 years to wear a helmet when riding recreational vehicles, such as snowmobiles and all-terrain vehicles, is an example of an injury prevention initiative using:
    a. education.   **c.** entitlement.
    b. enforcement.   **d.** engineering.

_____ **2.** The first step in the public health approach to injury prevention is to:
    a. define the problem.   **c.** develop prevention strategies.
    b. identify risk factors.   **d.** evaluate the impact of the program.

_____ **3.** St. John's Hospital has general surgeons and several types of specialty services, such as orthopedic surgery and plastic surgery, available 24 hours a day, but cannot care for patients with severe traumatic brain injury or spinal-cord injury beyond initial stabilization. It most likely would be categorized as a Level _____ trauma center.
    a. I   **c.** III
    b. II   **d.** IV

_____ **4.** Which one of the following best describes a multiple-casualty incident?
    a. Charter bus crash with 15 patients
    b. Seven people affected by fumes in a factory
    c. Any situation in which there are more patients than can be easily managed by available resources
    d. Four critically injured patients from a head-on motor vehicle collision (MVC)

_____ 5. You have arrived on the scene of a situation reported to be an industrial accident and immediately see that scaffolding has collapsed and there are at least eight individuals with what appear to be serious injuries. Which one of the following should you do first?

    a. Notify dispatch that you have at least eight patients who will require transport.

    b. Perform primary triage on all patients.

    c. Treat the most seriously injured patient.

    d. Perform a thorough search of the area to find all patients before notifying dispatch.

_____ 6. As an Advanced EMT, you are most likely to be assigned to the _____ section in a multiple-casualty incident.

    a. logistics   c. planning

    c. finance   d. operations

Clinical Reasoning

CASE STUDY: RUSH HOUR IN THE RAIN

As you and your partner, Craig, finish changing the main oxygen cylinder on your ambulance, your unit, as well as several others, are dispatched to a multiple-vehicle collision on the interstate. Low visibility and flooding of the roadway led to a collision involving at least 14 vehicles. En route, you hear the battalion chief establish incident command and request that all EMS vehicles approach the scene in the southbound lanes from the Morton Street on-ramp. The request requires that you backtrack to get to the on-ramp, but you will be the first-arriving EMS vehicle.

1. Why must you enter from the direction advised by the incident commander?

_____

_____

_____

_____

2. As the first-arriving EMS vehicle, what tasks are you likely to be assigned when you get to the scene?

_____

_____

_____

_____

3. What criteria will you use to determine which patients should be treated and transported first?

_____

_____

_____

_____

_____

Project-Based Learning

Every family should have a disaster plan. Because anyone can be affected by a natural or manmade disaster, you want the peace of mind of knowing that your family is prepared and able to cope while you are fulfilling your obligations as an EMS responder. Visit the Centers for Disease Control and Prevention (http://emergency.cdc.gov/preparedness/) and Federal Emergency Management Agency (http://www.fema.gov/areyouready/) family disaster preparedness websites to obtain guidance on developing a family disaster plan. Put your plan on paper, discuss it with your family, and then take the steps necessary to prepare.

The EMS Professional in Practice

What types of multiple-casualty incidents are likely in your community? Do you live in an area where tornados, high winds, hurricanes, earthquakes, flooding, or severe winter weather can lead to multiple injuries? Are there industries in your area that could result in multiple-casualty incidents if there was a fire, explosion, or other unexpected events? Are there heavily traveled highways, high-rise apartment complexes, or other situations that could lead to multiple-casualty incidents? How can you anticipate scenarios that might occur and be as prepared as possible for a multiple-casualty incident? Jot down your thoughts in a notebook or journal for discussion in class or in your study group.

Mechanisms of Injury, Trauma Assessment, and Trauma Triage Criteria

Content Area

- Trauma

Advanced EMT Education Standard

- Applies fundamental knowledge to provide basic and selected advanced emergency care and transportation based on assessment findings for an acutely injured patient.
- Pathophysiology, assessment, and management of the trauma patient: trauma scoring, rapid transport and destination issues, transport mode.

Summary of Objectives

34.1 Define key terms introduced in this chapter.

Knowing and being able to apply the key terms in each chapter is critical to understanding chapter concepts. Write the list of key terms. Then write the definition of each one in your own words. Check your understanding by confirming the definitions in the textbook glossary. Correct any misunderstandings. Create a study aid by writing each key term on the front of an index card and the definition on the back. Use the cards to quiz yourself or to have someone quiz you. The exercises under Vocabulary and Concept Review below will give you additional practice.

34.2 Describe the purpose and goals of trauma patient assessment.

Trauma patients are assessed to identify and manage immediate threats to life and determine the need to transport the patient to a trauma center for definitive treatment.

34.3 Describe the components of the trauma patient assessment process.

Trauma patient assessment begins with a scene size-up that includes analyzing the mechanism of injury and continues with a primary assessment, secondary assessment, and reassessment.

34.4 Discuss the decisions that must be made during the trauma patient assessment process.

Patient care decisions include determining what should be included in patient treatment, how quickly the patient must be transported, by what means the patient should be transported, and what the transport destination should be.

34.5 Explain the importance of various decision-making and problem-solving approaches in the trauma patient assessment and patient care processes.

Decision making is based on understanding the kinematics of trauma and relating them to the patient's mechanism of injury, presentation, and complaints to develop an index of suspicion for injuries. Trauma patients often present in circumstances that do not allow for easy application of a rigid approach to assessment, packaging, and management. It is sometimes necessary to be innovative to solve problems while adhering to principles of assessment and management.

Resource Central

Resource Central offers extra practice and review materials in a variety of media. To access it, follow the directions on the Student Access Card provided with the Student Textbook. If there is no card, go to www.bradybooks.com and follow the Resource Central link to Buy Access.

Vocabulary and Concept Review

Exercise 1

Write the letter of the correct definition in the blank next to the term. (See Resource Central for more vocabulary review.)

1. _____ crepitus

2. _____ ejection

3. _____ kinetics

4. _____ law of conservation of energy

5. _____ law of inertia

6. _____ mechanism of injury

7. _____ Newton's second law of motion

8. _____ primary blast injury

9. _____ secondary blast injury

10. _____ tertiary blast injury

a. Principle that energy cannot be created or destroyed, only transformed from one type to another

b. Physics of objects in motion

c. Being thrown out of a vehicle during a collision

d. Principle that a body in motion stays in motion and a body at rest stays at rest

e. Grating sensation, such as from bone fragments rubbing together

f. Law represented as: Force = Mass × Acceleration

g. Trauma from the pressure wave of an explosion

h. Trauma produced when the victim of a blast is moved by the pressure of the blast and lands some distance away

i. Type of incident that leads to the application of trauma-producing forces to the body

j. Trauma received in an explosion when the patient is struck by debris

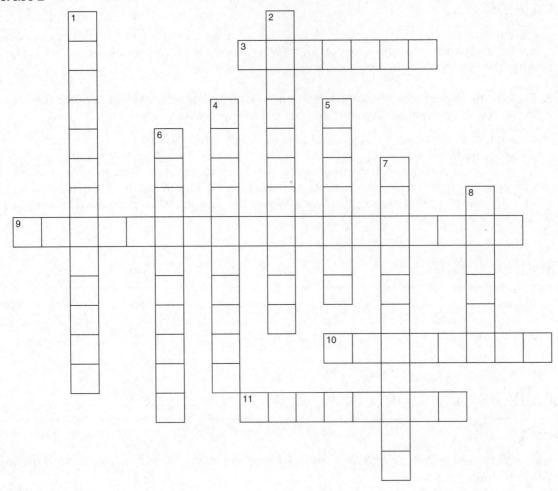

Across

3. Coma scale used to assign a score from 3 to 15 to the patient's neurologic status.

9. Ruptured ear drums from an explosion is an example of this.

10. Severe abrasions obtained in a motorcycle collision caused by friction of the body against the pavement.

11. Factor in kinetic energy commonly represented by the speed of the object.

Down

1. Sometimes called a T-bone collision.

2. Result of being struck by a baseball bat, for example.

4. Assessment term that refers to neurologic deficit, including decreased level of responsiveness.

5. Type of energy possessed by an object in motion.

6. Collision in which a vehicle is struck from behind.

7. Trauma resulting from being impaled by a screwdriver, for example.

8. Injury produced by external forces applied to the body.

Patient Assessment Review

Exercise 1

Apply trauma triage criteria to each of the following situations to evaluate the need for the patient to be transported to a trauma center.

Patient	Trauma Center (Yes or No)
1. Four-year-old boy fell from the top of a 5-foot-tall retaining wall onto the muddy ground. There was no loss of consciousness, but he bit his tongue, which is bleeding, and is complaining of right arm pain. His mother reports that the fall "knocked the wind out of him."	
2. 44-year-old man received a stab wound to his right forearm in a fight. Bleeding was initially profuse, but was controlled with direct pressure. He is awake and alert and has warm, dry skin.	
3. 19-year-old female passenger in a motor vehicle collision complains of pain in both feet and ankles following a frontal collision. She has an abrasion over her right clavicle from her seatbelt and abrasions to her face from the airbag. The driver of the vehicle was declared dead at the scene.	
4. 17-year-old male has a small-caliber gunshot wound to his abdomen. He is awake, but agitated. He has cool, pale, sweaty skin.	

Exercise 2

Document the Glasgow Coma Scale score for each patient in the space provided.

Patient	Glasgow Coma Scale Score
1. 65-year-old man is awake and anxious after being mugged by two assailants. He has a cut above his right eyebrow and abrasions on his hands and elbows. He gives a clear history and cooperates with your examination.	E: V: M: Total:
2. 27-year-old motorcyclist rear-ended a car that stopped in front of her. She was wearing a helmet and suffered no loss of consciousness. She is awake but confused about what happened. She complains of pain in both legs and has an obvious deformity of her right thigh. She is able to move all extremities on your command.	E: V: M: Total:
3. 15-year-old was ejected from his all-terrain vehicle when he hit a large rock. He was not wearing a helmet. He responds to painful stimuli by extending and internally rotating his arms. He is nonverbal and does not open his eyes on command.	E: V: M: Total:
4. 70-year-old woman fell down her basement stairs, striking her head. She responds to verbal stimuli by opening her eyes and gives inappropriate answers to your questions. She moves all of her extremities but does not cooperate with your commands. When you palpate painful areas she tries to push your hand away.	E: V: M: Total:

Check Your Recall and Apply Concepts

Exercise 1

Select the best possible choice for each of the following questions.

_____ 1. A construction worker falls from a second story roof. When his body strikes the ground, his organs continue moving until they impact the inside of the body cavity. Which one of the following principles of physics is best demonstrated by this scenario?
   a. Law of conservation of energy
   b. Relationship between mass, velocity, and kinetic energy
   c. Newton's second law of motion
   d. Law of inertia

_____ 2. A 61-year-old man is struck in the leg by a rock that was propelled from beneath a lawn mower. He has a laceration over his tibia. The laceration is an example of what kind of injury?
   a. Penetrating   c. Indirect
   b. Direct   d. Deceleration

_____ 3. A 37-year-old woman fell backward 10 feet from a stepladder and struck her head on a ceramic tile floor. She is diagnosed with a cerebral contusion. Her injury is an example of what kind of injury?
   a. Direct   c. Penetrating
   b. Deceleration   d. Indirect

_____ 4. Being stabbed with a knife is an example of a(n) _____ velocity penetrating injury.
   a. low   c. high
   b. medium   d. ultra-high

_____ 5. The threshold for considering a frontal-impact motor vehicle collision significant is when the amount that the vehicle exterior is compressed by the damage is _____ inches or more.
   a. 12   c. 24
   b. 18   d. 36

_____ 6. Which one of the following techniques is used to minimize movement of the cervical spine as you begin the primary assessment of a trauma patient?
   a. Manual stabilization
   b. Cervical collar
   c. Towel rolls or commercial head-stabilizing device
   d. Short spinal immobilization device

_____ 7. You have arrived on the scene of a motor vehicle collision in which a patient lost control of his vehicle, resulting in a rollover collision. He was not wearing a seatbelt. According to witnesses, the patient crawled out of the vehicle on his own. The vehicle has substantial damage to all parts of it. The patient is awake, but confused about what happened. His speech is slurred, and you smell an odor of alcohol on his breath. He denies any injuries. Which one of the following approaches to the secondary assessment is most appropriate?
   a. Baseline vital signs, SAMPLE history
   b. Baseline vital signs, SAMPLE history, focused physical examination
   c. Rapid trauma examination, baseline vital signs, SAMPLE history
   d. Rapid trauma examination, baseline vital signs, SAMPLE history, head-to-toe examination

Clinical Reasoning

CASE STUDY: LUCA HANEY

31-year-old Luca Haney is an avid bicyclist. Weather permitting, he bikes 7 miles each way to and from work several times each week. He takes safety seriously and always wears a helmet and reflective clothing. This morning, as he crosses a busy intersection on a green light, an SUV runs the red light and strikes him. It is estimated that the vehicle was traveling 35 mph. Luca and his bicycle are thrown several yards. When you arrive, you see immediately that Luca has several open extremity fractures and is not moving.

1. How can you relate principles of the kinematics of trauma to this situation?

_____

_____

_____

_____

_____

2. Based on the mechanism of injury, what types of injuries do you predict Luca has?

_____

_____

_____

_____

3. What should your first actions be at the scene?

_____

_____

_____

_____

_____

Project-Based Learning

Visit the safecar.gov website at http://www.safercar.gov/Vehicle+Shoppers–Star+Safety+Ratings/1990–2010+Vehicles to research the crash test safety rating of your vehicle. How does your vehicle compare to others in its class? If you could buy any vehicle you wanted based on its safety ratings, what would it be? Jot down your thoughts in a notebook or journal for discussion in class or in your study group.

The EMS Professional in Practice

You are on the scene of a patient who has been severely injured in a fight. He is unresponsive and has an irregular respiratory pattern. As you begin your assessment, his brother becomes upset that you are not moving the patient into the ambulance and speeding toward the hospital, though he is not threatening. Law enforcement is on the scene. How could you quickly summarize what you are doing to defuse the situation? Jot down your thoughts in a notebook or journal for discussion in class or in your study group.

Chapter 35

Soft-Tissue Injuries and Burns

Content Area

- Trauma

Advanced EMT Education Standard

- The Advanced EMT applies fundamental knowledge to provide basic and selected advanced emergency care and transportation based on assessment findings for an acutely injured patient.

Summary of Objectives

35.1 Define key terms introduced in this chapter.

Knowing and being able to apply the key terms in each chapter is critical to understanding chapter concepts. Write the list of key terms. Then write the definition of each one in your own words. Check your understanding by confirming the definitions in the textbook glossary. Correct any misunderstandings. Create a study aid by writing each key term on the front of an index card and the definition on the back. Use the cards to quiz yourself or to have someone quiz you. The exercises under Vocabulary and Concept Review below will give you additional practice.

35.2 Discuss the epidemiology and significance of burns and soft-tissue injuries.

Soft-tissue injuries are extremely common types of injuries. Most are not life threatening, but those that produce significant bleeding can lead to shock and death. About half a million people require medical treatment for burns each year, and about 4,000 people die from burns each year.

35.3 Describe the structure and function of the skin.

The skin is composed of three layers: the epidermis, dermis, and subcutaneous tissue. The skin functions to protect the body from fluid loss and pathogens, plays a role in thermoregulation, and provides sensory input about the environment.

35.4   Describe the consequences of damage to the skin.

Damaged skin allows micro-organisms to enter the body. When large areas are affected, fluid loss and impaired temperature regulation are potential threats to life.

35.5   Describe special considerations in the scene size-up when responding to calls involving burned patients.

Consider the potential for multiple patients and the dangers of smoke inhalation at fire scenes. Chemical burns may occur in situations that turn out to be hazardous materials incidents, requiring specialized response.

35.6   Describe the effects of burns on the circulatory, respiratory, renal, nervous, musculoskeletal, and gastrointestinal systems.

Severe burns can result in massive fluid loss and shock; eschar around the chest, which can restrict breathing; inhalation of heated air, smoke, or steam, which can cause lung injury; patients with severe burns can develop acute respiratory distress syndrome (ARDS); hypoperfusion of the kidneys can lead to renal failure and the complications (such as electrolyte balances and anemia) that accompany it; and hypoperfusion of the gastrointestinal system can occur in shock.

35.7   Identify indications of inhalation injury in the burned patient.

Indications of inhalation injury include being in a confined space in a fire, being unresponsive in a fire, soot in and around the nose and mouth, a sore throat, hoarseness, and shortness of breath.

35.8   Describe the process of stopping the burning process when responding to a burned patient.

Heat is retained in the tissues after a burn, leading to deeper injury. Smoldering or melted clothing also can continue to worsen the burn. Burns are cooled by removing burned clothing and flushing the burn with cold water.

35.9   Given a description or picture of a burn, classify the burn by depth and body surface area involved, for both adult and pediatric patients.

The rule of nines is used to estimate the percent of body surface area involved in adults. It is modified in pediatric patients to reflect the greater proportion of body surface area accounted for by the head. Burns are classified as superficial, partial thickness, or full thickness.

35.10   Consider burn depth and location, body surface area involved, the patient's age, and any pre-existing medical conditions in determining the severity of burn injuries.

Critical burns include any burn accompanied by respiratory involvement or traumatic injury; partial- or full-thickness burns of the face, hands, feet, or genitalia; full-thickness burns involving greater than 10 percent of the total body surface area; partial-thickness burns involving greater than 30 percent of the total body surface area; and circumferential burns.

35.11   Discuss each of the following types of burns: chemical, electrical, inhalation, radiation, and thermal.

- *Chemical:* Strong acids can cause tissue damage by coagulation necrosis, and strong alkalis can cause damage by liquefaction necrosis. Brush dry chemicals away before irrigation; irrigate chemical burns with copious amounts of plain water. Avoid exposure to the chemical involved.

- *Electrical:* Electrical current can pass through the body, causing damage to tissues between the point of entry and point of exit. Rhabdomyolysis and cardiac dysrhythmia may complicate electrical burns.
- *Inhalation:* Inhalation burns may cause immediate airway obstruction and respiratory distress or delayed toxin-induced lung injury can occur. Be prepared to establish an airway and assist ventilations.
- *Radiation:* Evidence of radiation burns may not occur until days after the exposure.
- *Thermal:* Thermal burns are the type of burn most commonly encountered by EMS personnel. Severity depends on several factors, including the depth of the burn and the percentage of total body surface area involved. Complications include infection, fluid loss, and hypothermia.

35.12 Discuss each of the following mechanisms of burn injuries: contact, electrical, flame, flash, gas, scald, and steam.

Contact burns occur from touching a hot surface, such as a stove or clothes iron. Electrical burn sources include lightning and electrical current, such as from household current. Contact with high-voltage power lines is rare but may occur. The extent of an electrical burn is much worse than indicated by the external wounds. Flame burns occur from exposure to an open flame, such as from a lighter or fire. Flash burns occur from being in close proximity to ignition of a flammable gas or liquid that burns very quickly. Gas burns often involve the airway as a result of breathing in superheated gases in smoke. Scald burns are caused by coming into contact with hot liquids. Steam burns can be very severe because steam reaches extremely high temperatures. The heat of steam is not dissipated in the airway like that of dry heat and can cause more severe thermal burns to the airway structures than inhalation of dry heat.

35.13 Describe special considerations in responding to, assessing, and managing patients with chemical and electrical burns.

In addition to the differences in mechanism of injury, both chemical and electrical burns carry special risks to the safety of EMS responders and bystanders.

35.14 Describe the Parkland formula and demonstrate the ability to calculate proper volumes of fluid to be infused into the burn patient.

The Parkland formula is 4 mL of fluid × the patient's weight in kilograms × the percent of body surface area involved for patients with 10 percent body surface area or more of partial-thickness or full-thickness burns.

35.15 Describe each of the following types of soft-tissue injury: abrasions, amputations, avulsions, closed injury, contusion, crush injury, hematoma, impaled objects, incisions and lacerations, open injury, and punctures.

Abrasions are caused by irregular scraping away of the epidermis and varying depths of dermis as a result of friction. An amputation is a separation of a body part from the body. An avulsion is a flap of skin that has been torn away completely or left attached at one edge or by a small strip of skin. In a closed injury, the skin is not broken, but blood vessels below the surface can be damaged. Examples are contusions and hematomas. A contusion is a bruise. A crush injury is caused by extreme forces, such as those that would occur from being trapped beneath a heavy object. Such injuries destroy large masses of cells, which release their contents resulting in complications such as rhabdomyolysis and electrolyte imbalances. A hematoma is a pocket or collection of blood that causes swelling. An impaled object, such as a knife or pencil, remains in the wound after penetrating the tissue and must be stabilized in place. An incision is a smooth-edged wound from a sharp object. A laceration is a jagged wound or splitting of the skin from blunt trauma. An open injury is one in which the integrity of the skin is broken.

A puncture is a wound that is small in diameter and deeper than its diameter, such as would occur from stepping on a nail.

35.16 Describe the pathophysiology and management of the following complications of soft-tissue injuries and burns: bleeding, blood and fluid loss, compartment syndrome, edema, infection, pain, toxic inhalation, and traumatic rhabdomyolysis.

- Bleeding occurs from disruption of blood vessels. You can control most external bleeding with direct pressure. Tourniquets are sometimes needed for severe bleeding from extremity trauma. Internal bleeding may require surgery to stop it.
- Blood and fluid loss from soft-tissue wounds or burns can lead to hypovolemia and shock. Control bleeding and use IV fluids to maintain perfusion.
- Compartment syndrome occurs as a result of swelling within the fascia that surrounds a muscle, increasing the pressure in the compartment to a level that exceeds the perfusion pressure of the tissues. Minimizing swelling is essential to decreasing the chance of compartment syndrome.
- Edema is swelling that occurs from blood loss into the tissues and third-spacing of fluids and increases pain and disability. Elevation and application of cold are ways of minimizing swelling.
- Infection can occur from contamination of open wounds. Cleaning and covering wounds are important to minimizing chances of infection.
- Pain results from tissue damage and can be significant. Consider pain management for significant injuries, particularly burns.
- Toxic inhalation occurs from exposure to the gaseous products of combustion. Respiratory distress can occur immediately or can occur days later. Be prepared to manage the airway and assist breathing. Administer oxygen to maintain an SpO_2 of 95 percent or higher.
- Traumatic rhabdomyolysis is a result of the release of the contents of damaged skeletal muscle cells. Myoglobin released from the cells is toxic to the kidney tubule cells, resulting in renal failure. Hyperkalemia can occur due to the release of potassium from the damaged cells.

35.17 Engage in a process of clinical reasoning to effectively prioritize the steps in management of patients with burns and soft-tissue injuries.

No matter how dramatic the injury or how distraught the patient, the priorities are always scene safety and the patient's airway, breathing, and circulation. Perform a secondary assessment to find all injuries and develop a treatment plan.

35.18 Demonstrate effective methods of controlling bleeding and dressing and bandaging wounds and burns, using a variety of dressing and bandaging materials.

Most external bleeding is controllable with direct pressure. When bleeding from an extremity is severe and cannot be controlled with direct pressure, a tourniquet may be lifesaving. Although there are some basic principles of dressing and bandaging wounds, creativity is sometimes necessary to properly manage specific wounds. Staple supplies in dressing and bandaging include sterile gauze squares for dressings and gauze rolls and tape or self-adherent bandages to secure the dressings in place.

35.19 Describe considerations in retrieving, caring for, and transporting amputated parts.

It is desirable to transport amputated parts with the patient, but you must not delay on the scene to retrieve them. Remove gross debris from the amputated part. Wrap in a sterile saline dressing and place the part in a plastic bag. Keep the part cool, but do not place it directly on ice.

Resource Central

Vocabulary and Concept Review

Exercise 1

Fill in the blank with the most appropriate vocabulary word from the following list.

abrasion	avulsion	crush injury
dressing	epistaxis	hematoma
hemostatic agent	impaled object	rule of nines
traumatic rhabdomyolysis	zone of stasis	

1. A topical substance applied to a wound to stop bleeding is called a(n): _____.

2. A nosebleed is also called: _____.

3. Swelling caused by a collection of blood within the tissues is a(n): _____.

4. An uneven scraping away of the skin from friction produces a wound called a(n): _____.

5. Severe tissue damage from compression of the tissue is a(n): _____.

6. Placed directly onto an open wound to help control bleeding and prevent contamination, this is a(n): _____.

7. When an article creates a penetrating wound and remains in the tissue, it is called a(n): _____.

8. A burn caused by exposure to hot liquids is called a(n): _____.

9. When muscles are damaged resulting in the release of their contents, the condition is called: _____.

10. An injury in which a flap of skin has been separated from the tissue beneath it is called a(n): _____.

11. The area of a burn in which blood flow is compromised but in which the tissue may survive if circulation is restored is called a(n): _____.

12. A method of estimating the extent of the total body surface area affected by burns, especially when larger areas of the body are involved, is called: _____.

Exercise 2

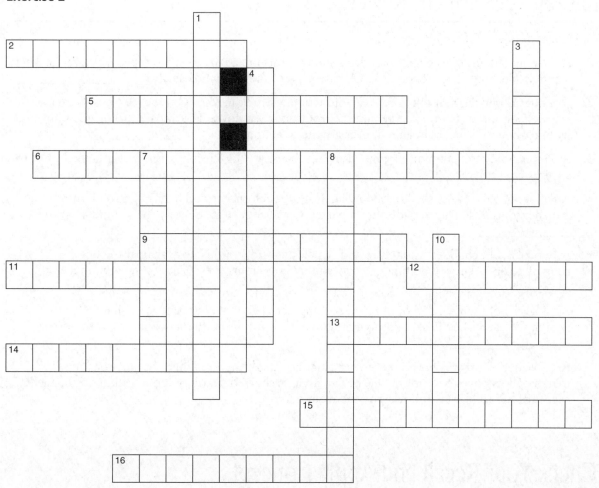

Across

2. Outermost zone of a burn in which there is increased blood flow.

5. Type of necrosis that occurs when tissues are exposed to a strong alkali substance.

6. Increased pressure within the fascia due to swelling, which interferes with perfusion.

9. Type of burn injury that occurs from lightning strike or contact with high-voltage power lines.

11. Thick, inelastic tissue resulting from full-thickness burns.

12. Material that is applied to secure a dressing in place.

13. Condition in which a body part is severed from the body.

14. Source of slow, steady oozing bleeding, usually minor in nature.

15. Type of tissue necrosis produced by exposure to strong acids.

16. Outermost layer of the skin.

Down

1. Compressing the tissues as a method of controlling bleeding.

3. Contusions and hematomas are examples of this type of soft-tissue injury.

4. Cut or tear in the skin.

7. Source of bright red bleeding under pressure.

8. Deepest layer of the skin, in which adipose tissue predominates.

10. Sometimes called a second-degree burn, this thickness of burn presents with blisters, redness, and pain.

Patient Assessment Review

Classify each of the following wounds.

1. A 10-year-old girl crashed her bicycle as she was turning a corner and scraped both knees. There is minor bleeding from each injury. Classify each of these wounds as a(n): _____.

2. In a lateral-impact collision, a 32-year-old woman struck her head on the "B" post of her vehicle (support structure just behind the front door window). The impact produced an open wound about 1.5 inches in length. Classify the wound as a(n): _____.

3. A 51-year-old man cut himself while using a table saw. His left index finger is attached by only a thin strip of tissue. Classify the wound as a(n): _____.

4. An 11-year-old boy brushed his elbow against a hot clothes iron. He has a burn about 2 inches long by half-inch wide with a blister at one edge of it. Classify the wound as a(n): _____.

5. A two-year-old child fell at daycare and struck the bridge of his nose against the bottom rung of a chair. There is a grape-sized swelling between his eyes. Classify the wound as a(n): _____.

6. An 82-year-old woman fell out of bed, striking her arm on a night table. She has a flap of skin that is pushed back, exposing the tissue beneath. Classify the wound as a(n): _____.

7. A 10-year-old girl was burned when her pajamas caught on fire while she was roasting marshmallows over a campfire. She has an area of charred, leathery-looking skin on the medial aspect of her right forearm. Classify the wound as a(n): _____.

Check Your Recall and Apply Concepts

Select the best possible choice for each of the following questions.

_____ 1. The nerves, blood vessels, and glands of the skin are located primarily in the:
    a. epidermis.
    b. dermis.
    c. subcutaneous layer.
    d. subdermal layer.

_____ 2. A 28-year-old man has a large black-and-blue discoloration on his thigh after being struck with a baseball. The injury is best described as a(n):
    a. abrasion.
    b. hematoma.
    c. contusion.
    d. avulsion

_____ 3. You have responded to a patient who was purposely set on fire as he slept in an alley. The fire has been extinguished. As you approach, you smell an acrid odor, which you associate with burnt hair. The patient is moving his extremities weakly and groaning and has stridorous, wheezing respirations. There is burnt clothing adhering to his wounds, which appear charred. Which one of the following should you do first?
    a. Cool the burns by flushing with copious amounts of cool water.
    b. Open the airway using a head-tilt/chin-lift maneuver.
    c. Start an IV of lactated Ringer's solution and infuse fluids rapidly.
    d. Prepare to administer nitrous oxide for pain.

_____ 4. Your patient is a 30-year-old construction worker whose legs are trapped beneath a massive slab of concrete. He is awake and oriented and complains of surprisingly little pain. He is anxious, but his vital signs are within normal limits, with a heart rate of 88, respirations of 20, and blood pressure of 124/80. His SpO_2 is 99 percent on room air. Which one of the following has the highest priority as the rescue proceeds?

    a. Start an IV of normal saline and begin infusing fluids.

    b. Allow the patient to self-administer nitrous oxide.

    c. Administer 1 mg of IM glucagon.

    d. Give oxygen by nonrebreather mask.

_____ 5. A 26-year-old woman suffered a closed fracture of the tibia and fibula when she was struck by a car as she crossed the street. She is complaining of increasingly severe pain in her leg and tingling sensations. Her leg is swollen and her foot is cool and pale, but she has palpable pedal and posterior tibial pulses. You should suspect:

    a. crush syndrome.   **c.** compartment syndrome.

    b. a severed nerve.   **d.** tetanus.

_____ 6. A 24-year-old male motorcyclist was struck on the right side by a vehicle whose driver did not see him as he merged into the motorcyclist's lane of traffic. The patient's right foot was amputated just above the ankle. The patient is awake and anxious but oriented. He has pale, cool skin but is breathing adequately. He has lost about 500 mL of blood. Your first priority is:

    a. finding the foot and preparing it to be transported with the patient.

    b. applying high-flow oxygen.

    c. starting an IV and infusing 1,500 mL of fluid.

    d. controlling bleeding from the patient's leg.

_____ 7. The care of an open wound to the neck is different from the care of other open wounds in that you must:

    a. avoid direct pressure.

    b. cover the wound with an occlusive dressing.

    c. use a moist, sterile dressing.

    d. apply circumferential direct pressure.

_____ 8. A 16-year-old has a gunshot wound to his right forearm. There is bleeding from what appear to be entrance and exit wounds. Your first attempt to control the bleeding is to:

    a. use a topical hemostatic agent.   **c.** apply direct pressure.

    b. elevate the extremity.   **d.** apply a tourniquet.

_____ 9. Your patient's right hand and arm were burned with steam when he took the radiator cap off of a hot car radiator. He has blistering and redness on his hand and about halfway up his forearm. He is complaining of intense pain. You could use any of the methods below to help relieve pain EXCEPT:

    a. apply an ice pack or chemical cold pack.

    b. apply a dry, sterile dressing.

    c. apply a moist, sterile dressing.

    d. allow the patient to self-administer nitrous oxide.

_____10. You are caring for a patient who was rescued from an apartment fire. He is anxious, but awake and oriented. His skin is flushed, but there are no burns. His heart rate is 92 per minute, respirations are 20 per minute, and blood pressure is 132/90. His SpO$_2$ on room air is 93 percent. As you are asking him questions, he coughs and you see that his sputum contains traces of soot. The patient is at most risk of deterioration over the coming hours to days due to:
   a. carbon monoxide poisoning.
   b. cyanide poisoning.
   c. delayed toxin-induced lung injury.
   d. fluid loss.

Clinical Reasoning

CASE STUDY: A RASH DECISION

Jeff King is celebrating his 21st birthday by taking his new motorcycle for a ride through the mountains. As he descends through a steep incline, he enters a hairpin turn too quickly and loses control of his motorcycle. He skids along with the motorcycle, now on its side, for 20 yards before being separated from it. In the process, his jeans and tee shirt are shredded and he sustains "road rash" along his entire left side, including his arm, shoulder, chest, back, hip, and lower extremity. When you arrive, Jeff is sitting alongside the road in obvious pain. He is oriented to person, place, and time. He tells you it feels like he is on fire and that it hurts to take a deep breath. You can see that the abrasions are accompanied by some areas of avulsed tissue and that there is a large amount of debris, such as pebbles, dirt, and twigs embedded in the injuries.

1. What other injuries should you anticipate based on the mechanism of injury and the patient's presentation?

   _____

   _____

   _____

   _____

2. Once you have identified and managed any threats to life, how can you best manage the patient's abrasions?

   _____

   _____

   _____

   _____

3. What factors should you take into consideration in choosing a transport destination?

_____

_____

_____

_____

_____

Project-Based Learning

Visit the website of the American Burn Association at http://www.ameriburn.org/. Explore the resources to find out where the burn center closest to you is. Review the burn center referral criteria listed on the site. Explore the educational resources to learn more about preventing various types of burns. Select one of the presentations and prepare to deliver it to your study group. Prepare a five-question quiz to give your study group members after the presentation and be ready to discuss the rationales for your answers.

The EMS Professional in Practice

What can you do in your home and in your community to reduce the chances of burn injuries? Make a checklist that you can use to make your home safer. Jot down any additional thoughts in a notebook or journal for discussion in class or in your study group.

Skills Checklist

The following skill checklist covers the major steps of a selected skill from Chapter 35. Review it prior to your laboratory classes. Practice skills only after they have been demonstrated for you in class and only under the supervision of an authorized instructor or clinical preceptor.

Advanced EMT Skill Checklist: *Open Soft-Tissue Injury Management*		
Skill Stimulus: The primary assessment has been completed and an open soft-tissue wound has been identified during the primary or secondary assessment.		
Step	**Performed**	**Not Performed**
Ensure that your personal protective equipment is adequate to the amount of bleeding.		
Use a dressing that is larger than the wound to apply direct pressure to control bleeding.		
If some bleeding continues, place more dressings over the first dressing and continue direct pressure. *Note: If significant bleeding occurs and you cannot control it with direct pressure, use a tourniquet for extremity wounds.*		
Once you have controlled bleeding with direct pressure, check the distal circulation, sensation, and motor function for extremity injuries.		
Secure the dressing in place with tape or a roller bandage.		
Prevent movement of the injured area to reduce bleeding. Immobilize injuries involving the hand with the hand in the position of function by placing a bandage roll in the hand so that the patient's fingers are slightly curved around it.		
Consider slight elevation of injured extremities to reduce pain and swelling.		
Reassess the distal circulation, sensation, and motor function.		
Reassess the patient including checking the bandages for bleeding and checking the distal circulation and motor function.		
Skill Completion: Bleeding is controlled; a dressing covers the wound and is secured in place; the distal neurovascular status has been reassessed.		

36 Musculoskeletal Injuries

Content Area

- Trauma

Advanced EMT Education Standard

- The Advanced EMT applies fundamental knowledge to provide basic and selected advanced emergency care and transportation based on assessment findings for an acutely injured patient.

Summary of Objectives

36.1 Define key terms introduced in this chapter.

Knowing and being able to apply the key terms in each chapter is critical to understanding chapter concepts. Write the list of key terms. Then write the definition of each one in your own words. Check your understanding by confirming the definitions in the textbook glossary. Correct any misunderstandings. Create a study aid by writing each key term on the front of an index card and the definition on the back. Use the cards to quiz yourself or to have someone quiz you. The exercises under Vocabulary and Concept Review below will give you additional practice.

36.2 Describe the structures and functions of the musculoskeletal system, including bones, cartilage, joints, ligaments, skeletal muscle, and tendons.

Bones provide support, shape, protection, and a system of levers to allow movement. Skeletal muscle works with the system of levers comprised of bones to allow movement and provide protection and shape for the body. Tendons connect muscles to bones to allow for movement. Ligaments connect bones to other bones at joints. Cartilage plays a number of roles, including providing nonbony structure to the ears and nose and providing a smooth surface at joints to allow bones to move against each other. Joints are the points at which two or more bones come together. Most joints allow at least some movement, but a few, such as the sutures of the skull, are immovable.

36.3 Give examples of direct, indirect, and twisting forces that can produce musculoskeletal injuries.

Direct forces include severe blows at the site of the fracture, such as might occur in a vehicle collision and gunshot wounds. Indirect forces are transmitted from the point of impact to a distant point in the bone. An example is a fracture of the forearm from falling onto an outstretched hand. Twisting forces cause the bone to rotate around its axis. An example is having a foot planted solidly on the ground and being struck a glancing blow to the upper body, causing rotation that can fracture the femur or tear the ligaments of the knee or ankle.

36.4 Describe each of the following types of injuries: dislocations and subluxations, fractures, sprains, and strains.

Dislocations occur when a bone end is displaced from a joint. A subluxation is a partial dislocation. Fractures are breaks in the continuity of a bone, ranging from cracks, to chips, to clean breaks across a bone, to fragmentation. Sprains are injuries in which ligaments are stretched or torn. Strains are injuries in which muscle fibers are stretched or torn.

36.5 Describe the signs and symptoms associated with injury to the musculoskeletal system.

Signs and symptoms of musculoskeletal injury include pain, swelling, deformity, loss of use, discoloration, crepitus, and exposed bone ends or fragments.

36.6 Explain why fractures of the femur, pelvis, and multiple concomitant long bones are considered critical fractures.

Bones are living tissue that receives blood supply. The large bones of the pelvis and femur and other long bones in the extremities have a rich vascular supply that can be disrupted in a fracture. Such fractures also can damage blood vessels in close proximity to the bone. Bleeding can be severe and is often hidden within the tissues of the pelvis or femur.

36.7 Establish the priority for assessing and treating musculoskeletal injuries with respect to a patient's overall condition.

Musculoskeletal injuries can have a dramatic appearance and be very painful, but most are not life threatening. However, the mechanism of injury that caused the musculoskeletal trauma also may have produced other, potentially life-threatening, injuries. Do not be distracted from the priorities of the airway, breathing, and circulation by the appearance of the injury or the patient's concern over it.

36.8 Describe the rationale for assessing distal circulation, sensation, and motor function before and after splinting a musculoskeletal injury and for frequently reassessing for changes in distal neurovascular function.

Fractures and dislocations can cause damage to adjacent nerves and blood vessels. Splinting can potentially result in movement of bone ends that could result in neurovascular damage. Swelling, especially swelling within a muscle compartment, can impair circulation and nerve function. Early recognition of neurovascular injury is critical to successful treatment. Assessment before and after splinting helps document when a neurovascular injury might have occurred.

36.9 Recognize signs and symptoms of compartment syndrome.

Compartment syndrome is identified by the "5 Ps," although the presence of any one of the signs or symptoms must increase your suspicion of compartment syndrome. The "5 Ps" are: pain (increasing pain out of proportion with the injury), paresthesia (tingling), pallor (paleness), pulselessness (or any signs of decreased perfusion), and paralysis (loss of use).

36.10   Describe the pathophysiology of compartment syndrome.

Compartment syndrome occurs when swelling within the fascia of a skeletal muscle increases the pressure within the compartment. The increased pressure overcomes the pressure within the capillaries, resulting in decreased tissue perfusion. As the pressure increases, pulselessness may occur.

36.11   Consider the need for fluid replacement and pain management in patients with musculoskeletal injuries.

Musculoskeletal injuries can be very painful. Patients whose condition is noncritical with isolated musculoskeletal trauma may be candidates for prehospital analgesia, according to your protocols. Fracture of the femur, pelvis, or multiple long bones can result in hypovolemia, requiring treatment for shock, which includes intravenous fluid infusion.

36.12   Explain the rationale for splinting musculoskeletal injuries.

Splinting reduces motion, which can limit further injury and pain.

36.13   Describe special considerations for splinting pelvic fractures.

Pelvic fracture requires a significant mechanism of injury, so prioritize assessment and management of the airway, breathing, and circulation. Pelvic stabilization may be achieved with a long backboard, pneumatic antishock garment (PASG), or pelvic binder.

36.14   Discuss pitfalls associated with improper splinting.

Improper splinting can lead to excessive motion of the injured part; abnormal positioning, which may result in injury; or compression of blood flow, resulting in ischemia and increased swelling.

36.15   Compare and contrast the characteristics and uses of various types of splints, including formable splints, improvised splints, pressure (air or pneumatic) splints, rigid splints, sling and swathe, long backboard, traction splints, and vacuum splints.

Formable splints can be molded to the shape of the extremity. Improvised splints can be made of suitable materials in the environment when an appropriate commercial splint is not available. Pressure (air or pneumatic) splints are inflatable, and the pressure in them can be adjusted. Suitable for most long-bone fractures, examples of rigid splints include aluminum gutter splints and board splints. Padding is required to fill voids between the extremity and the splint and to prevent tissue pressure from the splint. Sling and swathe are used for upper extremity injuries, including injuries of the shoulder, clavicle, humerus, elbow, forearm, and wrist to suspend the upper extremity and stabilize it against the body. The long backboard is used to splint the spine and in patients in critical condition whose urgency for transport does not allow splinting of individual fractures, it provides a way of minimizing movement of the legs, pelvis, and upper extremities. Traction splints are used for femur fractures and provide counter traction against another point in the extremity. Vacuum splints work by extracting air from the splint so it molds to the contour of the extremity.

36.16   Given a variety of scenarios involving patients with musculoskeletal injuries, manage the injury using general rules of proper splinting.

Refer to the skill checklists at the end of this chapter.

Resource Central

Resource Central offers extra practice and review materials in a variety of media. To access it, follow the directions on the Student Access Card provided with the Student Textbook. If there is no card, go to www.bradybooks.com and follow the Resource Central link to Buy Access.

Vocabulary and Concept Review

Exercise 1

Write the letter of the correct definition in the blank next to the term. (See Resource Central for more vocabulary review.)

1. _____ closed fracture

2. _____ comminuted fracture

3. _____ compartment syndrome

4. _____ dislocation

5. _____ greenstick fracture

6. _____ impacted fracture

7. _____ oblique fracture

8. _____ open fracture

9. _____ spiral fracture

10. _____ sprain

11. _____ strain

12. _____ subluxation

13. _____ transverse fracture

a. Break in a bone that is oriented at a 90-degree angle to its long axis

b. Tearing or stretching of ligaments

c. Fracture accompanied by a break in the skin

d. Fracture in which the skin remains intact

e. Displacement of bone ends from a joint

f. Partial displacement of bone ends from a joint

g. Fracture in which the angle of the break is greater or less than 90 degrees to the long axis of the bone

h. Fracture in which the fracture line "corkscrews" around the bone

i. Stretching or tearing of muscle fibers

j. Fracture that results from compression of the bone along its long axis so that the bone is shortened

k. Partial fracture that occurs in a bone that retains some flexibility, such as in pediatric patients

l. Fracture with multiple fragments

m. Tissue ischemia from swelling within the fascia surrounding a muscle

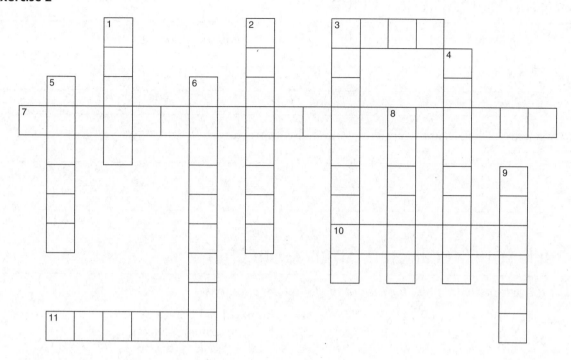

Across

3. Type of bone that includes the femur and humerus.

7. This must be checked before and after splinting musculoskeletal injuries.

10. Connective tissue that secures muscle to bone.

11. This band of material is used along with a sling to secure an injured upper extremity to the body.

Down

1. Type of bone that includes the metacarpals and phalanges.

2. Break in the continuity of a bone.

3. Bands of connectie tissue that provide a connection between bones.

4. Specialized type of splint used for femur fractures.

5. Up to 2000 mL of blood can be lost from a fracture of this ring of bones.

6. Connetive tissue that provides shape to strutures, such as ears and nose, and covers the ends of bones.

8. Device used to immobilize an injured extremity.

9. Membrane that surrounds a skeletal muscle.

Patient Assessment Review

1. What signs and symptoms indicate the possibility of compartment syndrome?

_____

_____

_____

2. What are the signs and symptoms associated with fractures?

_____

_____

_____

Check Your Recall and Apply Concepts

Select the best possible choice for each of the following questions.

_____ 1. Which one of the following is the best example of flat bones?
   a. Tibia, fibula, humerus
   b. Metatarsals, phalanges
   c. Sternum, scapula, ribs
   d. Patella, pisiform

_____ 2. A 19-year-old with a gunshot wound to his left thigh has a femur fracture in which the bone has been splintered into several fragments. This description is most consistent with a(n) _____ fracture.
   a. comminuted
   b. impacted
   c. spiral
   d. oblique

_____ 3. Nine-year-old Matt Delgado fell from a piece of playground equipment and injured his arm. The emergency department physician tells Matt's parents that his radius buckled, but did not break all the way through. This description is most consistent with a(n) _____ fracture.
   a. comminuted
   b. greenstick
   c. spiral
   d. impacted

_____ 4. You are transporting a hiker who fell and fractured his tibia and fibula. It took several hours for a rescue crew to locate the patient and remove him to an area accessible by vehicle. The patient is complaining of severe pain that has increased since the time of injury. When you assess his leg, you find that it is swollen to nearly double the circumference of the uninjured leg. The foot is cool and mottled in color. He has a faint pedal pulse, but has minimal movement and sensation in his foot. He says he has a "pins and needles" sensation in his foot. Which one of the following should you suspect most highly?
   a. Severed artery
   b. Compartment syndrome
   c. Gangrene
   d. Crush syndrome

_____ 5. Your patient is 25 years old and the driver of a vehicle that sustained a lateral impact from an SUV that ran a red light. The driver's side door was pushed into the driver's compartment, compressing the area between the door and the center console to about 15 inches. The patient had to be extricated. She is awake, anxious, and in pain. She is complaining of severe pain in her left hip and thigh. Her skin is pale and she is sweating profusely. Her respirations are 20 per minute and she has a palpable but thready radial pulse of 124 per minute. As soon as the patient is extricated, the first thing you should do is:
   a. perform a rapid trauma examination.
   b. use a pelvic binder to stabilize the pelvis.
   c. place the patient on the stretcher and transport.
   d. start two large-bore IVs of isotonic crystalloid fluid.

_____ 6. Your patient is a 24-year-old woman whose arm was injured when she fell off of a dock and into a boat, landing on her outstretched hand. Her forearm is angulated and the radial pulse is very weak. The patient complains of numbness and tingling in her hand and capillary refill is poor. You have a 45-minute transport time. You should:

    a. splint the arm in the position in which it was found.

    b. allow the patient to support her arm in a position of comfort.

    c. apply a compression bandage to slow bleeding within the arm.

    d. support the arm and gently apply longitudinal traction below the injury site.

_____ 7. You have just applied a traction splint for a fractured femur. The next thing you should do is:

    a. complete the primary assessment.

    b. administer nitrous oxide for pain relief.

    c. check the pedal pulse and neurologic status in the foot.

    d. check the femoral pulse.

_____ 8. A 42-year-old bicyclist who struck a curb and fell off her bike complains of shoulder pain. You see that her clavicle is deformed. The best splint for this injury is a(n):

    a. air splint.   **c.** traction splint.

    b. sling and swathe.   **d.** rigid splint.

_____ 9. A 51-year-old motorcyclist is unresponsive and has several obvious extremity fractures, some of them open. The best way to splint the patient's fractures is to use:

    a. a long backboard.   **c.** a pneumatic antishock garment.

    b. rigid splints.   **d.** formed splints.

_____10. A patient has a fracture at the midshaft humerus. Which one of the following describes the correct immobilization of the injury?

    a. Immobilize so the splint prevents movement at the elbow and shoulder.

    b. Apply a splint that is the same length as the humerus.

    c. Immobilize from the fingers to the shoulder.

    d. Apply a splint that keeps the patient from moving at the shoulder but allows elbow movement.

_____11. A traction splint is used for fractures of the:

    a. tibia.   **c.** femur.

    b. humerus.   **d.** radius and ulna.

_____12. A 32-year-old utility worker fell 20 feet from the elevated basket on the utility truck. He has deformities of the right tibia and right femur. The best way to immobilize the right lower extremity prior to transport is to use a(n):

    a. long backboard.   **c.** vacuum splint.

    b. traction splint.   **d.** formed splint.

Clinical Reasoning

CASE STUDY: THOSE ARE THE BREAKS

Brad Melloy, 30 years old, injured his hand in a fight. The area over his fifth metacarpal on his right hand is swollen, discolored, and painful.

1. What should you do before caring for this injury?

_____

_____

_____

_____

_____

2. How should you splint this injury?

_____

_____

_____

_____

3. How should you check the distal neurovascular status in this injury?

_____

_____

_____

_____

_____

Project-Based Learning

Rotator cuff tears in the shoulder and ligamentous injuries of the knee, such as a torn anterior cruciate ligament, are common. Find out more about those injuries. Draw a diagram of one of the injuries to help you explain it to your study group.

The EMS Professional in Practice

How can you prevent musculoskeletal injuries at work? Jot down your thoughts in a notebook or journal for discussion in class or in your study group.

Skills Checklists

The following skill checklists cover the major steps of selected skills from Chapter 36. Review them prior to your laboratory classes. Practice skills only after they have been demonstrated for you in class and only under the supervision of an authorized instructor or clinical preceptor.

Advanced EMT Skill Checklist: *Long-Bone Splinting*		
Skill Stimulus: The primary assessment has been completed. Secondary assessment reveals signs and symptoms of a long-bone fracture.		
Step	**Performed**	**Not Performed**
Direct manual stabilization of the injured area.		
Check distal neurovascular function.		
Select a splint appropriate to the specific injury and situation.		
Measure the splint. A properly applied splint immobilizes the joint above and below the injury.		
Pad the splint, if necessary.		
Apply the splint, taking care to minimize motion of the injured extremity.		
Secure the splint in place, taking care that it is not applied tightly enough to restrict circulation.		
Reassess distal neurovascular function.		
Elevate the extremity and apply cold packs to reduce swelling.		
Skill Completion: The extremity is immobilized, and the distal neurovascular function has been checked.		

Advanced EMT Skill Checklist: *Splinting an Injured Joint*

Skill Stimulus: The primary assessment has been completed. Secondary assessment reveals signs and symptoms of a joint injury.

Step	Performed	Not Performed
Direct manual stabilization of the injured area.		
Check distal neurovascular function.		
Select a splint appropriate to the specific injury and situation.		
Measure the splint. A properly applied splint immobilizes from the bone below the injury to the bone above it.		
Pad the splint, if necessary.		
Apply the splint, taking care to minimize motion of the injured extremity.		
Secure the splint in place, taking care that it is not applied tightly enough to restrict circulation.		
Reassess distal neurovascular function.		
Elevate the extremity and apply cold packs to reduce swelling.		
Skill Completion: The extremity is immobilized, and the distal neurovascular function has been checked.		

Advanced EMT Skill Checklist: *Applying a Unipolar Traction Splint*		
Skill Stimulus: The primary assessment has been completed. Secondary assessment reveals signs and symptoms of a femur fracture without pelvis or hip injuries or injuries of or distal to the knee.		
Step	**Performed**	**Not Performed**
Direct manual stabilization of the injured area.		
Check distal neurovascular function.		
Select a splint appropriate to the specific injury and situation.		
Place the splint along the medial aspect of the injured leg. Adjust the length so that it extends 4 inches beyond the heel.		
Secure the strap to the thigh.		
Apply the ankle hitch and attach it to the splint.		
Extend the splint to apply traction.		
Secure the splint in place.		
Reassess distal neurovascular function.		
Skill Completion: The extremity is immobilized, and the distal neurovascular function has been checked.		

Advanced EMT Skill Checklist: *Application of a Bipolar Traction Splint*

Skill Stimulus: The primary assessment has been completed. Secondary assessment reveals signs and symptoms of a long-bone fracture.

Step	Performed	Not Performed
Direct manual stabilization of the injured area.		
Check distal neurovascular function.		
Adjust the length of the splint so that it is about 6 inches longer than the uninjured extremity.		
Place the padded ring beneath the leg just inferior to the ischial tuberosity.		
Raise the heel stand of the splint.		
Apply the ischial strap around the proximal thigh at the groin.		
Place the ankle hitch over the patient's foot and attach the ankle hitch to the splint.		
Turn the ratchet mechanism clockwise to pull traction on the leg until the injured leg is approximately equal to the length of the uninjured leg.		
Fasten the support straps.		
Reassess the distal neurovascular function.		
Skill Completion: The extremity is immobilized, and the distal neurovascular function has been checked.		

Chapter 37

Head, Brain, Face, and Neck Trauma

Content Area

• Trauma

Advanced EMT Education Standard

• The Advanced EMT applies fundamental knowledge to provide basic and selected advanced emergency care and transportation based on assessment findings for an acutely injured patient.

Summary of Objectives

37.1 Define key terms introduced in this chapter.

Knowing and being able to apply the key terms in each chapter is critical to understanding chapter concepts. Write the list of key terms. Then write the definition of each one in your own words. Check your understanding by confirming the definitions in the textbook glossary. Correct any misunderstandings. Create a study aid by writing each key term on the front of an index card and the definition on the back. Use the cards to quiz yourself or to have someone quiz you. The exercises under Vocabulary and Concept Review below will give you additional practice.

37.2 Describe the anatomy and function of the eye, facial structures, and structures of the neck.

The face contains specialized sensory structures, including the eyes, nose, and mouth; the face and neck contain the structures of the upper airway. The neck contains several large blood vessels.

37.3 Discuss the relationship between injuries of the scalp, eye, neck, and face and injuries to the spine and brain.

Because the scalp, eye, and face are all part of the head, injuries to these structures can be associated with injuries to the brain. Trauma to the head also can result in excessive forces to the neck, resulting in spine injury.

37.4 Describe the purpose and process of reassessing patients with injuries to the head, face, and neck.

As edema increases, the airway can be obstructed and traumatic brain injuries can become evident as cerebral edema or bleeding within the cranium continues. This means the patient's level of responsiveness, neurologic function, and vital signs can change rapidly and dramatically. Constantly monitor the level of responsiveness and frequently reassess neurologic functions and vital signs.

37.5 Describe the anatomy and physiology of the skull, meninges, meningeal spaces, cerebrospinal fluid, brain, and intracranial blood vessels.

The brain is surrounded by cerebrospinal fluid that cushions and bathes it in a specific chemical environment within the cranial cavity of the skull. The bones of the skull and the membranous layers of the meninges provide additional protection to the brain. From deep to superficial, the layers of the meninges are the pia mater, arachnoid, and dura mater. Blood can accumulate between the layers of the meninges (subdural or subarachnoid bleeding) or above the surface of the dura (epidural bleeding). The blood supply to the brain is provided by the internal carotid arteries (anterior circulation) and vertebral arteries (posterior circulation). The brain itself is the seat of consciousness and controls the sensory, voluntary, and involuntary functions of the body.

37.6 Associate each of the major anatomical portions of the brain with its functions.

The cerebral hemispheres control higher brain functions. Each hemisphere consists of four lobes with complex functions: frontal lobe (conscious thought), parietal lobes (sensory association area), temporal lobes (speech), and occipital lobes (vision). The cerebellum is responsible for motor coordination, and the brainstem controls vital functions.

37.7 Discuss special considerations in the assessment and management of patients with injuries to the head, face, and neck, including airway compromise, profuse bleeding, potential that injuries may be self-inflicted or the result of violence, and patient fears associated with those injuries.

Special considerations for airway compromise include checking for edema, bleeding, loose teeth, and foreign objects. Use manual maneuvers, suction, basic adjuncts, and advanced airways as needed. For profuse bleeding of the face and scalp, which have a rich blood supply and can bleed profusely, use direct pressure to control bleeding. Penetrating injuries to the neck can result in exsanguination or hematoma formation. Cover penetrating injuries to the neck with an occlusive dressing to prevent air from entering the large blood vessels. Because the face and head are often targeted in assaults, including domestic violence, and gunshot wounds to the head may be self-inflicted, consider the potential for self-infliction and violence whenever you see trauma there. Maintain awareness of your own safety and involve law enforcement if needed. Patients may fear disfigurement from facial injuries or loss of vision from eye injuries, so provide reassurance and emotional support.

37.8 Given a variety of scenarios, demonstrate the assessment-based management of patients with injuries to the eye, scalp, face, and neck.

The priorities of care, as always, are scene safety, airway management, ensuring adequate ventilation and oxygenation, and controlling bleeding. If the mechanism of injury is consistent with the potential for spinal-cord injury, use manual restriction of cervical spine motion and consider spinal immobilization.

37.9 **Demonstrate the assessment and management of specific injuries of the eye, scalp, face, and neck, including injury to the orbit, injury to the eyelid, injuries to the globe of the eye, chemical burns to the eye, impaled objects in the eye, extruded eyeball, facial fractures, avulsed tooth, impaled object in the cheek, injury to the nose, injury to the ear, penetrating injury to the neck, and blunt injury to the neck.**

For injury to the orbit, treat associated soft-tissue and globe injuries; cold packs may help reduce swelling. For injury to the eyelid, avoid excessive direct pressure in controlling hemorrhage. Treat injuries to the globe of the eye by covering and bandaging both eyes to prevent movement of the affected eye. Irrigate chemical burns to the eye with water to remove remaining chemicals. Stabilize impaled objects in the eye in place without applying pressure to the eye. Cover the extruded eyeball with a dressing moistened with sterile saline and cover the eye with a cup. Bandage over both eyes to prevent movement.

For facial fractures, assess carefully for airway obstruction, and avoid use of nasopharyngeal airways in midface fractures. For an avulsed tooth, carefully place it in a container of sterile saline for transport.

Remove an impaled object in the cheek if it interferes with the airway. Apply direct pressure to both sides of the injury if removal of the object results in bleeding.

Control epistaxis from injury to the nose by gently pinching the nostrils. To prevent aspiration, elevate the patient's head or allow him to sit up, if there are no contraindications.

For injury to the ear, apply direct pressure to control bleeding, and transport avulsed parts with the patient, if possible.

In penetrating injury to the neck check for subcutaneous air and hematoma formation, control bleeding with direct pressure but do not use a circumferential dressing, and apply an occlusive dressing to prevent air embolism.

In blunt injury to the neck, be alert to the possibility of laryngeal fracture and airway compromise and of hematoma formation, which also can obstruct the airway. Consider requesting ALS or air medical transport if definitive airway management is required.

37.10 **Explain the indications and procedure for removing contact lenses from an injured eye.**

Remove contacts for chemical exposure to the eye. The patient may be able to remove the contacts himself. Otherwise, remove soft contacts by carefully pinching them up and away from the cornea. If hard contact lenses are in the eye, remove them by opening the eyelids wide, exposing the entire contact lens, then gently applying pressure to the eyelids as you close them toward the edges of the lens.

37.11 **Explain the pathophysiology and significance of the following with respect to traumatic brain injury: scalp lacerations and avulsions, open and closed skull fractures, cerebral concussion and diffuse axonal injury, cerebral contusion, coup–contrecoup injury, cerebral and intracranial hematomas, and cerebral hemorrhage.**

- *Scalp lacerations and avulsions:* Suspect underlying brain injury when scalp lacerations and avulsions are present.
- *Open and closed skull fractures:* Both open and closed skull fractures may be associated with varying degrees of underlying traumatic brain injury.
- *Cerebral concussion and diffuse axonal injury:* A concussion occurs without radiologic evidence of injury, yet the function of neurons is temporarily disrupted, often resulting in anterograde amnesia. Diffuse axonal injury is a shearing of the neurons, disrupting their functions.
- *Cerebral contusion:* A bruising of the brain tissue from blunt or penetrating trauma. Associated cerebral edema can increase intracranial pressure.
- *Coup–contrecoup injury:* Traumatic brain injury occurs at the point of impact and opposite the point of impact from a rebound effect due to sudden deceleration.
- *Cerebral and intracranial hematomas:* Both types of bleeding occupy space within the cranium and result in increased intracranial pressure.

37.12 Explain the compensatory mechanisms, and the resulting signs, for increased intracranial pressure.

The cranium is a rigid container of fixed size that cannot accommodate an increase in volume without an increase in the pressure within the container. Swelling and bleeding within the cranium add volume, increasing the pressure within the cranial cavity. As the brain is compressed, neurologic signs can occur. The body attempts to maintain an adequate cerebral perfusion pressure—the difference between mean arterial pressure and intracranial pressure—by increasing the blood pressure, particularly the systolic blood pressure. The heart slows by reflex in response to the hypertension. Signs include altered mental status, unilateral or bilateral fixed and dilated pupils, hypertension, widened pulse pressure, bradycardia, and abnormal response to painful stimuli (posturing).

37.13 Explain the limitations of the compensatory mechanisms for increased intracranial pressure.

Beyond a certain point, an increase in blood pressure cannot exceed intracranial pressure by enough to allow cerebral perfusion. Cerebral hypoxia leads to more cell death and cerebral edema, which increases intracranial pressure even more.

37.14 Describe the pathophysiology and key signs of increased intracranial pressure and brain herniation.

Severely increased intracranial pressure pushes brain tissue along the path of least resistance. Brain tissue may shift from laterally, across the midline, downward, or through the only opening in the skull, the foramen magnum. Signs include unilateral or bilateral fixed dilated pupils, change in the respiratory pattern, and posturing.

37.15 Identify and, where possible, manage factors that can worsen traumatic brain injuries, including: hyperglycemia, hyperthermia, hypoglycemia, hypotension, hypoxia, hypercarbia, and hypocarbia.

For hyperglycemia, check the blood glucose level. For hyperthermia, create conditions that allow for normal body temperature. For hypoglycemia, check the blood glucose level and administer 50 percent dextrose to manage it. For hypotension, administer IV fluids to maintain an adequate mean arterial pressure. For hypoxia, administer oxygen and assist ventilations to maintain an SpO_2 of 95 percent or higher. For hypercarbia, ensure ventilations are adequate to maintain end-tidal CO_2 between 30 and 35 mmHg. For hypocarbia, do not hyperventilate; maintain end-tidal CO_2 between 30 and 35 mmHg.

37.16 Describe the goals of emergency treatment of patients with traumatic brain injuries.

Maintain the patient's airway and assist ventilations to maintain an end-tidal CO_2 between 30 and 35 mmHg and an SpO_2 of 95 percent or greater, administering oxygen as needed. Maintain normal body temperature and blood glucose levels. Control hemorrhage to prevent further loss of oxygen-carrying hemoglobin and administer IV fluids to manage hypotension and maintain an adequate mean arterial pressure. Transport to the closest facility capable of treating the patient's injuries or, if that is not feasible, transport to the closest facility capable of stabilizing the patient for transfer to a trauma center.

37.17 Describe the neurologic assessment of patients with suspected traumatic brain injury.

The Glasgow Coma Scale score is used to assess the severity of traumatic brain injury and predict patient outcomes.

37.18 Discuss the focus of history taking and assessment for patients with injuries to the head.

All aspects of the history of the present illness and SAMPLE history are important in patients with traumatic brain injury.

37.19 Assess and provide emergency treatment of patients with injuries to the head.

Perform a scene size-up, primary assessment, and secondary assessment. Manage the airway, breathing, and circulation; maintain normal end-tidal CO_2 and SpO_2; check the blood glucose level and administer 50 percent dextrose only in cases of hypoglycemia; and maintain the patient's normal body temperature.

37.20 Explain the importance of reassessment of the patient with an injury to the head.

Patients with traumatic brain injury can deteriorate quickly as bleeding or swelling within the cranium continues.

37.21 Document information relevant to the assessment and management of patients with injuries to the head.

Document the mechanism of injury, time the injury occurred, any witnessed loss of consciousness, the patient's initial and subsequent level of responsiveness and neurologic findings, other injuries sustained, baseline and subsequent vital signs and results of monitoring devices, and your treatments.

Resource Central

Resource Central offers extra practice and review materials in a variety of media. To access it, follow the directions on the Student Access Card provided with the Student Textbook. If there is no card, go to www.bradybooks.com and follow the Resource Central link to Buy Access.

Vocabulary and Concept Review

Exercise 1

Write the letter of the correct definition in the blank next to the term. (See Resource Central for more vocabulary review.)

1. _____ basilar skull

   a. Facial fracture that results in a "floating face" due to separation of the facial bones from the cranium

2. _____ brain herniation

   b. Liquid surrounding the brain and spinal cord

3. _____ cerebrospinal fluid

   c. Combination of hypertension, bradycardia, and altered respiratory pattern

4. _____ Cheyne-Stokes respirations

   d. Facial fracture involving the maxillary and nasal bones

5. _____ concussion

   e. Facial fracture involving only the maxilla

6. _____ coup-contrecoup injury

   f. Bones that comprise the floor of the skull

7. _____ Cushing's reflex

   g. Displacement of brain tissue due to increased intracranial pressure

8. _____ Cushing's triad

   h. Bleeding between the innermost and middle layers of the meninges

9. _____ diffuse axonal injury

   i. Nonfocal (widespread) stretching and shearing of neurons in the brain tissue

10. _____ Le Fort I fracture

    j. Collection of blood between the middle and outermost layers of the meninges

11. _____ Le Fort II fracture

    k. Additional brain injury that results from complications of the initial injury and its management

12. _____ Le Fort III fracture

    l. Hypertension that occurs to compensate for increased intracranial pressure, accompanied by reflex bradycardia

13. _____ secondary brain injury

    m. Injury to the brain at two sites—at the point of impact and opposite the point of impact

14. _____ subarachnoid hemorrhage

    n. Temporary dysfunction of the brain due to a blow to the head without radiologic evidence of injury

15. _____ subdural hematoma

    o. Repeated pattern of increasing and decreasing breathing with periods of apnea

Exercise 2

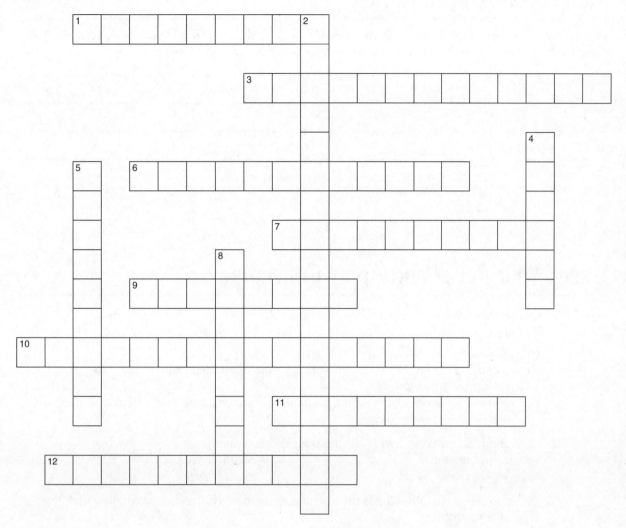

Across

1. Outermost protective membrane surrounding the brain and spinal cord.
3. Hemorrhage within the brain tissue.
6. Hypertension, bradycardia, irregular respirations.
7. Discoloration behind the ears associated with basilar skull fracture.
9. Protective layers surrounding the brain and spinal cord.
10. Collection of blood between the skull and the outermost layer of the meninges.
11. Type of skull fracture in which the bone is pushed inward so that it lies beneath the surface of the skull.
12. increased level of carbon dioxide.

Down

2. Inability to remember events preceding a blow to the head.
4. Clear, outermost surface of the eye.
5. Type of dressing used for open wounds to the neck.
8. Double vision.

Patient Assessment Review

Describe how you recognize increased intracranial pressure. What are the indications that intracranial pressure has increased to the point where brain herniation is imminent?

_____

_____

_____

_____

_____

Check Your Recall and Apply Concepts

Select the best possible choice for each of the following questions.

_____ 1. Your highest priority in the management of patients with facial trauma is:
  a. preventing infection of open wounds.
  b. reassuring the patient by saying it is not possible to determine if the injury is permanently disfiguring.
  c. ensuring an open airway, using manual position, suction, and adjuncts as needed.
  d. providing high-flow oxygen.

_____ 2. The thinnest, weakest portion of the skull is the:
  a. frontal region.   c. occipital area.
  b. basilar skull.   d. parietal region.

_____ 3. Which one of the following is the opening at the base of the skull through which the spinal cord emerges?
  a. Foramen magnum   c. Foramen ovale
  b. Mental foramen   d. Vertebral foramen

_____ 4. The portion of the brain that is just inferior to the cerebrum and plays a role in balance and coordination is the:
  a. temporal lobe.   c. cerebral cortex.
  b. medulla oblongata.   d. cerebellum.

_____ 5. A 19-year-old softball pitcher was struck in the forehead with a softball when a batter hit his pitch. He lost consciousness immediately and fell to the ground. Of the following, you should maintain the highest index of suspicion for associated _____ injury.
  a. abdominal   c. chest
  b. cervical-spine   d. extremity

_____ 6. A 31-year-old woman crashed her vehicle head-on into another vehicle after entering the freeway from an exit ramp and driving in the wrong direction. She was ejected on impact. She has lacerations on her head and extremities and has snoring respirations. When you apply a painful stimulus, she flexes both arms. This response is known as _____ posturing.
  a. pontine   c. decorticate
  b. decerebrate   d. cerebellar

_____ 7. Your patient is a 35-year-old construction worker who fell 15 feet onto concrete, striking his head. He has a laceration on the back of his head and the occipital region of his skull feels soft to palpation. He is unresponsive and has irregular respirations. When you attempt to use a modified jaw-thrust maneuver, you find that his jaws are clenched (trismus) and you are unable to adequately displace the mandible to open his mouth. His pulse is strong at 52 per minute. He has a blood pressure of 172/84 and an SpO_2 of 93 percent on room air. His right pupil is midsized and sluggishly reactive to light; his left pupil is widely dilated and does not respond to light. Which one of the following is the best plan for this patient?
   a. Keep the head and neck in neutral alignment, insert a nasopharyngeal airway, and perform bag-valve-mask ventilations with supplemental oxygen at a rate of 20 to 24 breaths per minute.
   b. Use a head-tilt/chin-lift maneuver, insert a nasopharyngeal airway, and perform bag-valve-mask ventilations with supplemental oxygen at a rate of 16 to 20 breaths per minute.
   c. Use a head-tilt/chin-lift maneuver and perform bag-valve-mask ventilations with supplemental oxygen at a rate of 10 per minute.
   d. Use a triple airway maneuver and perform bag-valve-mask ventilations with supplemental oxygen at a rate of 12 to 15 breaths per minute.

_____ 8. A 21-year-old college student was assaulted as she was walking home from class. The assailant used a knife to cut her throat. She has a laceration across the anterior neck, just below the thyroid cartilage. The laceration is superficial on the left side but deeper, with copious dark red bleeding, on the right side. Bystanders chased the assailant away and one of them immediately applied direct pressure to the wound. The patient is awake and anxious with cool, pale, sweaty skin. Her airway is open and there does not appear to be subcutaneous air in the neck. She is breathing about 24 times per minute and has a radial pulse of 120 per minute. Which one of the following is the next step in the care of this patient?
   a. Apply an occlusive dressing over the neck wound and maintain direct pressure over the deeper end of the laceration to control bleeding.
   b. Apply a pressure dressing to control bleeding from the wound.
   c. Apply an absorbent dressing but do not use pressure to avoid airway and circulatory obstruction.
   d. Maintain direct pressure with your gloved hand, but do not apply a dressing or bandage.

_____ 9. In the management of patients with suspected traumatic brain injury, you should strive to maintain which one of the following physiologic parameters?
   a. Systolic blood pressure of 150 mmHg or higher
   b. Blood glucose level of 50 to 60 mg/dL
   c. SpO_2 of 90 to 95 percent
   d. End-tidal CO_2 of 30 to 35 mmHg

_____ 10. Which one of the following describes the best care of an avulsed tooth?
   a. Wipe off blood and debris with sterile gauze and place the tooth in the pocket between the patient's lower gum and cheek.
   b. If available, place the tooth in a container of whole milk.
   c. Wrap the tooth in sterile gauze moistened with water and place it on ice.
   d. Rinse the tooth with sterile water and place it back in the socket and have the patient bite down lightly to hold it in place.

_____ **11.** A 43-year-old man was grinding a piece of metal but was not wearing protective eyewear. He has a small metal shaving in his left eye. Which one of the following is the best plan for this patient?

   a. Gently flush the eye with sterile saline to attempt to remove the debris, and then bandage both eyes.

   b. Use the corner of a piece of sterile gauze to wipe away the metal shaving, and then bandage both eyes.

   c. Have the patient close his eye, and then apply an eye patch or cup over the eye and bandage it in place.

   d. Have the patient blink rapidly several times to dislodge the shaving, and then apply an eye patch or cup over the eye and bandage it in place.

Clinical Reasoning

CASE STUDY: INJURED MAN IN THE RESERVOIR

You and your partner, Evelyn, are dispatched for an injured person in the water at the reservoir. En route, you learn that bystanders have pulled an unresponsive male from the water. The patient, 28-year-old Artie Blevins, was riding his jet ski at a high rate of speed when he hit the remnants of an old concrete dam. When you arrive, you see frantic bystanders surrounding an unresponsive male whom they have placed on his side. The patient has a large amount of frothy blood coming from his mouth and nose and the bystanders are trying to wipe it away to keep his airway clear. The patient's face is deformed and appears sunken over the midface. You can hear gurgling when the patient breathes.

1. What are the first actions you should take?

_____

_____

_____

_____

_____

2. What injuries do you suspect?

_____

_____

_____

_____

_____

3. How do you anticipate those injuries will affect your care of the patient?

_____

_____

_____

_____

_____

Project-Based Learning

Draw a diagram of the brain, including the right and left hemisphere, the cerebellum, and brainstem. Label each area with the functions it controls. Write what disabilities a person may have with an injury to each area of the brain. Check your answers at the Brain Trauma Foundation website: http://www.braintrauma.org.

The EMS Professional in Practice

What happens to patients with traumatic brain injury in the emergency department and beyond? How does traumatic brain injury affect the lives of those who survive? How can your actions at the scene and en route improve the patient's outcome? Jot down your thoughts in a notebook or journal for discussion in class or in your study group.

Chapter
38 Thoracic Trauma

Content Area

• Trauma

Advanced EMT Education Standard

• The Advanced EMT applies fundamental knowledge to provide basic and selected advanced emergency care and transportation based on assessment findings for an acutely injured patient.

Summary of Objectives

38.1 Define key terms introduced in this chapter.

Knowing and being able to apply the key terms in each chapter is critical to understanding chapter concepts. Write the list of key terms. Then write the definition of each one in your own words. Check your understanding by confirming the definitions in the textbook glossary. Correct any misunderstandings. Create a study aid by writing each key term on the front of an index card and the definition on the back. Use the cards to quiz yourself or to have someone quiz you. The exercises under Vocabulary and Concept Review below will give you additional practice.

38.2 Explain the relationship between an intact thoracic cavity and lungs, and ventilation, oxygenation, and respiration.

A sealed thoracic cavity with contact between the pleural layers is necessary to generate negative pressure when the chest cavity enlarges, allowing inspiration. Inspiration is the active phase of ventilation, the mechanical movement of air in and out of the lungs. Respiration occurs in two phases: external respiration and internal respiration. External respiration is the exchange of oxygen and carbon dioxide between the lungs and blood across the respiratory membrane. Internal respiration is the exchange of oxygen and carbon dioxide at the cellular level.

38.3 Relate mechanism of injury to the potential for specific types of chest trauma.

Determine whether there are penetrating or blunt mechanisms of trauma, keeping in mind the potential for broken ribs, lacerated blood vessels, pneumothorax, hemothorax, traumatic asphyxia, cardiac injuries, and mediastinal injuries.

38.4 Relate assessment findings to suspicion for specific types of chest injuries.

Assessment of the chest includes assessing the level of responsiveness, airway, ventilation, and circulation. Look for indications of respiratory distress, such as use of accessory muscles and cyanosis. The hypoxia that may accompany chest injuries can lead to decreased responsiveness. Use inspection, auscultation, and palpation to detect signs of injury. Look for open and closed injuries, subcutaneous air, paradoxical movement, adequacy and equality of chest expansion; listen for abnormal breathing sounds and the presence and equality of breath sounds bilaterally; and palpate to check for tenderness, crepitus, and chest expansion. Assess the vital signs.

38.5 Explain the pathophysiology and management of the following types of chest injuries: blunt cardiac injury, commotio cordis, flail chest, hemothorax, myocardial contusion, open pneumothorax, penetrating cardiac injury, pericardial tamponade, pulmonary contusion, rib fractures, simple pneumothorax, tension pneumothorax, and traumatic asphyxia.

For all chest injuries, maintain the airway, administer oxygen to maintain an SpO_2 of 95 percent or higher, assist ventilations as needed, administer IV fluids to maintain perfusion but maintain awareness of the risk of pulmonary edema, perform CPR if the patient becomes pulseless, and apply an AED. Immediately cover open wounds to the chest and maintain awareness that the dressing can result in tension pneumothorax if it completely seals the wound and does not allow the escape of air on expiration.

Pathophysiology of specific types of chest injuries is as follows:

- *Blunt cardiac injury:* Blunt force applied to the chest can result in myocardial contusion, commotio cordis, or cardiac rupture. In myocardial contusion, cardiac dysrhythmia, heart failure, and cardiogenic shock can occur.
- *Commotio cordis:* A form of sudden cardiac arrest caused by a blow to the chest during a vulnerable portion of the cardiac cycle. Mortality is high, even with immediate treatment.
- *Flail chest:* Two or more adjacent ribs each fractured in two or more places create a segment of the chest wall that is no longer continuous with the rest of the chest wall. When the chest rises on inspiration, the flail segment collapses. Pain and impaired chest wall motion impair ventilation.
- *Hemothorax:* Laceration of a blood vessel, such as from penetrating trauma or a fractured rib, can cause an accumulation of blood within the thorax. The blood can separate the pleural layers and interfere with ventilation, but the primary problem may be hypovolemia, because each side of the thorax can hold a tremendous amount of blood.
- *Myocardial contusion:* A bruise to the myocardium acts much like a myocardial infarction, impairing the function of the affected portion of the myocardium.
- *Open pneumothorax:* Also called a sucking chest wound; a defect that is two thirds the diameter of the trachea or larger allows atmospheric air to enter through the wound each time negative intrathoracic pressure is generated on inspiration. The amount of air in the thorax can continue to accumulate, worsening ventilatory impairment.
- *Penetrating cardiac injury:* A stab or gunshot wound can result in pericardial tamponade or massive blood loss and decreased cardiac output.
- *Pericardial tamponade:* Accumulation of blood within the relatively inelastic pericardial sac compresses the chambers of the heart and prevents adequate filling, which reduces cardiac output.
- *Pulmonary contusion:* Bruising of the lung tissue can result in a ventilation–perfusion mismatch and hypoxia. The contusion can continue to evolve, causing the patient to deteriorate over time.
- *Rib fractures:* Pain can reduce inspiratory depth, leading to hypoventilation; a fractured rib can lacerate blood vessels or damage lung tissue, leading to hemothorax or pneumothorax.
- *Simple pneumothorax:* Air accumulates within the pleural cavity, causing atelectasis of a portion of the lung.

- *Tension pneumothorax:* A large defect in the lung allows air under pressure to continue to accumulate within the pleural space. Increasing pressure shifts the mediastinal structures, reducing return of blood to the heart. Hypotension occurs, and eventually the opposite lung is compressed, as well.
- *Traumatic asphyxia:* Occurs when sudden compression of the chest causes an abrupt increase in intrathoracic pressure and retrograde blood flow to the upper portion of the body.

Resource Central

Resource Central offers extra practice and review materials in a variety of media. To access it, follow the directions on the Student Access Card provided with the Student Textbook. If there is no card, go to www.bradybooks.com and follow the Resource Central link to Buy Access.

Vocabulary and Concept Review

Exercise 1

Fill in the blank with the most appropriate vocabulary word from the following list.

traumatic asphyxia	Beck's triad
commotio cordis	myocardial contusion
hemoptysis	hemothorax
flail chest	open pneumothorax
paradoxical movement	tracheal deviation

1. The triad of hypotension, jugular vein distention, and muffled heart sounds, indicating pericardial tamponade, is called: _____.

2. Sudden cardiac arrest resulting from a blow to the chest is called: _____.

3. Two or more ribs, each fractured in two or more places, results in a condition known as: _____.

4. The medical term for coughing up blood is: _____.

5. When blood accumulates within the plural space, the condition is called: _____.

6. A bruise to the heart muscle is called a(n): _____.

7. An injury that allows air to enter the pleural cavity from a wound in the chest wall is called a(n): _____.

8. When a section of the chest wall collapses on inspiration instead of rising with the rest of the chest wall, it is known as: _____.

9. Displacement of the windpipe from the midline, which can occur as a sign of tension pneumothorax, is called: _____.

10. Sudden compression of the chest resulting in retrograde blood flow is called: _____.

Exercise 2

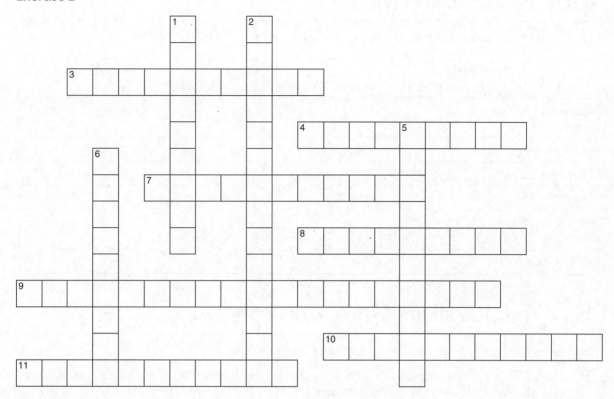

Across

3. Blood in the sputum.
4. Muscle that creates the inferior boundary of the thoracic cavity.
7. Space in the center of the thoracic cavity that holds the heart, great vessels, trachea, and esophagus.
8. Hypotension, JVD, and muffled heart sounds that indicate pericardial teamponade.
9. Accumulation of air under pressure in the the thoracic cavity.
10. Movement in which the flail segment appears to sink as the chest wall expands.
11. Between the ribs.

Down

1. Air trapped beneath the skin is a subcutaneous form of this condition.
2. Smooth membrane layer that adheres to the surface of the lungs.
5. Accumulation of blood in the pleural space.
6. Dressing placed over an open chest wound.

Patient Assessment Review

Fill in the following table to compare and contrast the features of the chest injuries.

	Simple Pneumothorax	Tension Pneumothorax	Open Pneumothorax	Hemothorax
Mechanism of injury				
Breath sounds				
Heart rate				
Blood pressure				
Assessment of the neck				
Level of distress				

Check Your Recall and Apply Concepts

Select the best possible choice for each of the following questions.

_____ 1. A 37-year-old woman has a stab wound to her back between the 11th and 12th ribs on the right side. There is no air movement at the site of injury. The patient is awake and anxious with a chief complaint of difficulty breathing. Her skin is slightly pale, cool, and moist. There is no cyanosis. Her breath sounds seem slightly diminished in the right base as compared to the left. She has a heart rate of 116, respirations of 24 per minute, blood pressure of 122/78, and SpO$_2$ of 95 percent on room air. Which one of the following injuries is most consistent with the mechanism of injury and patient presentation?

    a. Pulmonary contusion   c. Sucking chest wound

    b. Hemothorax   d. Tension pneumothorax

_____ 2. A 22-year-old man has a gunshot wound that appears to have entered the right chest anteriorly at the level of the seventh rib and exited posteriorly on the right side. The entrance wound is about 0.5-inch in diameter and the exit wound about 1 inch in diameter. He responds to painful stimuli. He is pale, cool, and diaphoretic with cyanosis of the lips. Respirations are 30 per minute and shallow, and he has a weak, thready radial pulse of 124 per minute. Which one of the following actions is most appropriate in the care of this patient prior to transport?

    a. Insert an oropharyngeal airway.

    b. Assist ventilations with a bag-valve-mask device.

    c. Apply oxygen by nonrebreather mask.

    d. Start an IV and administer a 2,000-mL fluid bolus.

_____ 3. Your patient, a 50-year-old woman, was the driver of a sedan that was struck in the driver's side door by a pick-up truck. She is responsive to pain and cyanotic with rapid, shallow respirations. She does not have a palpable radial pulse, but her carotid pulse is 130 per minute. While checking the carotid pulse, you notice that her jugular veins are distended. She has a large contusion to the left side of her chest and her breath sounds are absent on the left side. You begin ventilating the patient by bag-valve mask. Which one of the following is most likely to be immediately beneficial in the treatment of this patient?

    a. Request ALS to respond or intercept for needle chest decompression.

    b. Start two large-bore IVs and infuse a 2,000-mL fluid bolus.

    c. Apply CPAP to overcome the pressure within the thorax.

    d. Use a tidal volume of 200 to 300 mL to prevent further accumulation of air in the thoracic cavity.

_____ 4. A 31-year-old male patient was struck several times in the chest with a large wrench during a fight. You suspect he has a pulmonary contusion. Which one of the following should you anticipate as a result of pulmonary contusion?
   a. Tracheal deviation away from the affected side
   b. Hypovolemia
   c. Paradoxical movement of the chest wall
   d. Increasing hypoxia and dyspnea

_____ 5. A 91-year-old woman fell in her living room, striking the left side of her chest on an end table. She is complaining of pain in the left side of her chest at the point of impact and difficulty breathing. She cannot speak more than three to four words without taking a breath. As you inspect and palpate the chest, you notice that a portion of the chest wall on the left side seems to collapse when the rest of the chest expands. The mechanism of injury and findings are most consistent with:
   a. pericardial tamponade.   c. flail chest.
   b. tension pneumothorax.   d. traumatic asphyxia.

_____ 6. A 25-year-old man fell 15 feet from a tree he was trimming, landing on his left side on a log. His brother was going to transport him to the nearest emergency department for treatment of what they assumed to be broken ribs. Within 10 minutes of the fall, the patient began getting short of breath, so his brother called 911. The patient is awake and starting to get nervous about the potential severity of his injury. You find a contusion on the left side of his chest along with some subcutaneous emphysema and crepitus at the site of injury. His breath sounds are diminished on the left side. His heart rate is 92 per minute, respirations are 24 per minute, blood pressure is 112/72, and SpO_2 is 91 percent on room air. Which one of the following is appropriate in your management of the patient?
   a. Apply a circumferential dressing to the chest to splint the injury.
   b. Administer nitrous oxide for pain.
   c. Apply oxygen by nasal cannula.
   d. Apply CPAP.

_____ 7. A 15-year-old boy was kicked in the chest in martial arts class and immediately collapsed. A bystander started CPR. When you arrive, you confirm that the patient is in cardiac arrest. The mechanism and history are most consistent with:
   a. pericardial tamponade.   c. commotio cordis.
   b. flail chest.   d. traumatic asphyxia.

_____ 8. A 29-year-old man has a stab wound to his left anterior chest at the junction of the sternum and fourth rib. He responds to painful stimuli and has pale, cool, diaphoretic skin. He does not have a radial pulse, but his carotid pulse is 134 and weak. As you check the carotid pulse, you notice that he has jugular vein distention. He is breathing 24 times per minute. His breath sounds are clear and equal. The mechanism of injury and presentation are most consistent with:
   a. myocardial contusion.   c. traumatic asphyxia.
   b. pericardial tamponade.   d. tension pneumothorax.

_____ 9. A 37-year-old man was working beneath his car when the jack collapsed and the car fell on his chest, trapping him beneath the car. His son ran to get help and a neighbor used the jack to lift the car off the patient and pulled him from beneath it. When you arrive, you see that the patient's face and tongue are swollen and discolored, and his eyes are bloodshot. He has jugular vein distention, but the trachea is in the midline. Bilateral breath sounds are clear and equal. The mechanism of injury and findings are most consistent with:
   a. commotio cordis.   c. traumatic asphyxia.
   b. pericardial tamponade.   d. tension pneumothorax.

_____ **10.** As you are completing the patient care report on the patient you just delivered to the emergency department, a man supported by two friends walks into the ambulance bay. He is in obvious respiratory distress. He is not wearing a shirt. As the patient stops to lean on your ambulance and catch his breath, you see an open wound with frothy blood on his right side under his arm. Your first action should be to:

  a. go back into the emergency department and get a wheelchair for the patient.

  b. place your gloved hand over the wound.

  c. get your oxygen bag out of the ambulance and apply oxygen by nonrebreather mask.

  d. notify dispatch that you will be out of service longer than anticipated.

Clinical Reasoning

CASE STUDY: THAT COVERS IT

You and your partner, Don, are responding to a city park for an injured person. En route, dispatch notifies you that law enforcement has arrived and found a male patient with a gunshot wound to the chest. When you arrive, you see a male adolescent lying supine on the grass with a police officer applying pressure to a wound on the patient's chest. The patient is awake, agitated, and obviously scared. He is extremely diaphoretic with cool skin. He is breathing 24 times per minute and has a radial pulse of 124. He has a gunshot wound to his left anterolateral chest at the ninth intercostal space.

At your request, the police officer releases pressure so you can inspect the wound. The result is frothy blood that bubbles around the wound with the patient's respirations. You instruct the police officer to cover the wound again and ask your partner to prepare an occlusive dressing.

As you complete your examination, you find that breath sounds are slightly diminished on the left side and there are no other wounds, either anteriorly or posteriorly. The patient's blood pressure is 128/78 and his SpO_2 is 94 percent on room air. You apply oxygen by nonrebreather mask and secure an occlusive dressing over the wound, taping it on three sides.

En route to the trauma center, the patient becomes more short of breath and agitated. His heart rate has increased to 132 per minute and his respirations are 30 per minute, with an SpO_2 of 81 percent despite the nonrebreather mask. You notice distended jugular veins, but the trachea is in the midline.

1. What hypotheses do you have about the cause of the patient's deteriorating condition?

_____

_____

_____

_____

2. Which of your hypotheses do you think is most likely? Why?

_____

_____

_____

_____

_____

3. What is your treatment plan for the patient?

_____

_____

_____

_____

_____

Project-Based Learning

Write five test questions you anticipate your instructor will put on your examination over this chapter. Prepare an answer key. Administer the quiz to a study partner or your study group members, and take the quiz or quizzes they have prepared. By defending your questions and discussing those of your classmates, you will gain a better understanding of chest injuries.

The EMS Professional in Practice

Why is it important that Advanced EMTs be able to differentiate, to a reasonable degree, between different types of chest injuries? Jot down your thoughts in a notebook or journal for discussion in class or in your study group.

39 Abdominal Trauma

Content Area

• Trauma

Advanced EMT Education Standard

• The Advanced EMT applies fundamental knowledge to provide basic and selected advanced emergency care and transportation based on assessment findings for an acutely injured patient.

Summary of Objectives

39.1 Define key terms introduced in this chapter.

Knowing and being able to apply the key terms in each chapter is critical to understanding chapter concepts. Write the list of key terms. Then write the definition of each one in your own words. Check your understanding by confirming the definitions in the textbook glossary. Correct any misunderstandings. Create a study aid by writing each key term on the front of an index card and the definition on the back. Use the cards to quiz yourself or to have someone quiz you. The exercises under Vocabulary and Concept Review below will give you additional practice.

39.2 Describe the gross anatomy of the abdominal cavity and its contents.

The abdominal cavity lies beneath the diaphragm and extends into the pelvis. It is lined by parietal peritoneum, which has folds that cover the organs (visceral peritoneum). The abdomen primarily contains organs of the gastrointestinal tract and accessory organs of digestion. The digestive tract consists of the hollow stomach and small and large intestines. Solid organs include the liver and spleen (part of the hematologic system). The kidneys and major blood vessels (aorta and vena cava) are retroperitoneal.

39.3 Differentiate between the characteristics of solid and hollow organs in the abdomen.

Hollow organs are elastic and have less-dense vasculature than solid organs. When injured, their contents can enter the peritoneal cavity, causing peritonitis. Solid organs are inelastic and highly vascular. Injury often results in massive hemorrhage.

39.4 Give examples of both blunt and penetrating mechanisms of abdominal trauma.

Blunt mechanisms include deceleration injuries, which result from shearing forces, and direct impact to the abdomen. Falls, assaults, and motor vehicle collisions are common causes of blunt abdominal trauma. Penetrating mechanisms include stab wounds, gunshot wounds, and impalements.

39.5 Recognize signs and symptoms associated with injuries to the abdomen.

Bruising, abrasions, punctures, lacerations, and evisceration are indications of abdominal injury; patients may experience abdominal pain or tenderness, along with voluntary or involuntary guarding. True rigidity and distention are indications of massive hemorrhage within the abdominal cavity. Patients with hemorrhage from abdominal injuries may exhibit signs of hypoperfusion.

39.6 Describe the association between abdominal injury and the potential for life-threatening hemorrhage.

The abdomen contains large blood vessels and highly vascular organs. Injury can lead to massive hemorrhage that must be controlled surgically.

39.7 Demonstrate an assessment-based approach to management of the patient with open and closed abdominal injury, including evisceration and impaled objects.

The primary prehospital treatment for patients with abdominal trauma is recognizing the potential for injury and treating for hypoperfusion. Cover eviscerated organs with a sterile, nonadherent dressing soaked in sterile normal saline. Cover the moist dressing with an occlusive material, such as plastic wrap, to help maintain moisture and correct temperature of the exposed organs. Never attempt to replace exposed organs back into the abdominal cavity. Impaled objects are stabilized in place with bulky dressings. If necessary, request resources to shorten objects that are too long to be transported in the ambulance.

39.8 Explain the special considerations for airway management in the care of patients with abdominal injuries.

Patients with abdominal trauma may vomit. Position the patient in anticipation of vomiting and have suction immediately available. A ruptured diaphragm can lead to displacement of the abdominal organs into the thoracic chest cavity, impairing ventilation.

39.9 Explain the process and elements of reassessment of patients with abdominal injuries.

Patients with abdominal trauma can deteriorate due to ongoing bleeding. In addition to other components of reassessment, recheck vital signs, perfusion, and signs of injury to the abdomen (palpation and inspection).

Resource Central

Resource Central offers extra practice and review materials in a variety of media. To access it, follow the directions on the Student Access Card provided with the Student Textbook. If there is no card, go to www.bradybooks.com and follow the Resource Central link to Buy Access.

Vocabulary and Concept Review

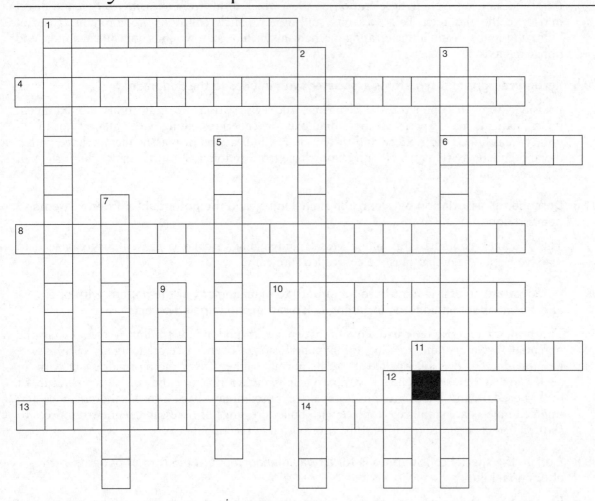

Across

1. Mechanism that creates a blast wave in which a sudden increase in pressure within a hollow organ can cause it to rupture.
4. Smooth membranous lining that covers the abdominal organs.
6. An abdomen that feels stiff, hard, or unyielding is called this.
8. Smooth membranous lining of the abdominal cavity.
10. Pain referred to the left shoulder in splenic injury.
11. An organ that has a cavity or space inside is called this.
13. Upper boundary of the abdominal cavity.
14. An object that penetrates the skin and remains embedded in the abdomen is said to be this.

Down

1. Injury in which abdominal organs protrude through an open wound in the abdominal wall.
2. Ecchymosis of the flanks.
3. Space behind the abdominal cavity that holds organs such as the kidneys.
5. Periumbilical ecchymosis.
7. Quadrant of the abdomen where the liver is located.
9. Large solid organ in the right upper quadrant.
12. Typical skin color in shock.

Patient Assessment Review

Match each assessment finding associated with abdominal trauma with its significance. Write the corresponding letter in the blank. Responses may be used more than once.

> **a.** Normal response to palpation of a painful abdomen
>
> **b.** Muscle spasm associated with peritonitis
>
> **c.** Retroperitoneal bleeding
>
> **d.** Splenic injury

1. _____ Cullen's sign
2. _____ Grey-Turner's sign
3. _____ Kehr's sign
4. _____ voluntary guarding
5. _____ involuntary guarding

Check Your Recall and Apply Concepts

Select the best possible choice for each of the following questions.

_____ 1. The most significant concern following closed injury to a solid abdominal organ is:
   a. peritonitis from organ contents.   **c.** infection.
   b. pain.   **d.** bleeding.

_____ 2. Which one of the following organs is most highly associated with life-threatening hemorrhage when it is injured?
   a. Colon   **c.** Gallbladder
   b. Stomach   **d.** Liver

_____ 3. A 25-year-old man was the driver of a sedan struck in the driver's side door by a vehicle that ran a red light. The patient initially denied injury and refused treatment. As you prepare to leave the scene, a police officer tells you that the patient is complaining of pain in his left shoulder and appears pale and sweaty. Which one of the following injuries is most consistent with the mechanism of injury and patient's presentation?
   a. Dislocation of the left shoulder
   b. Liver laceration
   c. Splenic injury
   d. Pancreatic injury

_____ 4. A 32-year-old woman has a stab wound to her abdomen, just above the umbilicus, from which a loop of bowel is protruding. There has been about 50 mL of blood loss from the wound, but active bleeding has stopped. She is awake and very upset about the incident and the nature of the wound. Her skin is moist but warm with normal color. She is breathing 16 times per minute without difficulty and has a radial pulse of 88 per minute. Her SpO$_2$ is 99 percent on room air. You found no other injuries on your secondary examination. Which one of the following should you do next?
   a. Place an occlusive dressing, such as a piece of plastic wrap, over the wound.
   b. Place a moist, sterile dressing over the wound and cover it with an occlusive dressing.
   c. Start two large-bore IVs.
   d. Administer oxygen by nonrebreather mask.

_____ 5. A 17-year-old boy has a stab wound to the abdomen, about 2 inches inferior to the xiphoid process in the midline of his abdomen. He responds to verbal stimuli and has cool, pale, diaphoretic skin. There is minimal external bleeding and no eviscerated organs. The patient's neck veins are distended, his trachea is in the midline, and his breath sounds are clear and equal bilaterally. The chest expands normally with inspiration. The abdomen is not distended. The patient's respirations are 24 per minute and he has a weak radial pulse of 128 per minute. Of the following injuries, which one is most likely responsible for the patient's presentation?

a. Ruptured diaphragm
b. Pericardial tamponade
c. Lacerated spleen
d. Lacerated aorta

_____ 6. A 20-year-old woman has a small-caliber gunshot wound to her abdomen just below the left costal margin. She responds only to painful stimuli and is pale, cool, and diaphoretic. Her respirations are 24 per minute, and she does not have a palpable radial pulse. Her carotid pulse is weak and thready at about 130 per minute. There is approximately 150 mL of external blood loss. Her neck veins are flat, the trachea is in the midline, and breath sounds are clear and equal bilaterally. Which one of the following is the most likely cause of the patient's presentation?

a. Hemorrhagic shock
b. Pericardial tamponade
c. Tension pneumothorax
d. Ruptured diaphragm

Clinical Reasoning

CASE STUDY: DRIVE-BY SHOOTING

You and your partner are one of four ambulances responding to the scene of a drive-by shooting with multiple patients. When you arrive, the triage officer assigns you to a 13-year-old female patient. She has a large-caliber gunshot wound that appears to have entered from the back on the right side between the 12th rib and the iliac crest and exited just below the umbilicus. She responds to painful stimuli and is pale and diaphoretic with cool skin. Respirations are 28 per minute. There is no palpable radial pulse; the carotid pulse is 134, weak, and thready. There appears to be about 750 mL of external blood loss. A rapid trauma assessment reveals no additional injuries.

1. What are the highest priorities in the management of this patient?

_____

_____

_____

_____

_____

2. What types of injury do you suspect?

_____

_____

_____

_____

_____

3. What complications do you anticipate from the patient's injuries?

_____

_____

_____

_____

_____

Project-Based Learning

Without using a reference, draw the abdominal cavity and the structures within it from memory to help you visualize the location of the organs within the abdomen. Check your work against the artwork in the textbook. If your perceptions of the location of organs was not correct, study the artwork and try the exercise again.

The EMS Professional in Practice

Detecting abnormal abdominal findings takes practice with both normal and abnormal examination findings. During your emergency department clinical rotations, seek patients with abdominal complaints or potential abdominal injury. Have your preceptor guide you through the examination and discuss the results with you. Record your observations in a notebook or journal for discussion in class or in your study group.

40 Spine Injuries

Content Area

• Trauma

Advanced EMT Education Standard

• The Advanced EMT applies fundamental knowledge to provide basic and selected advanced emergency care and transportation based on assessment findings for an acutely injured patient.

Summary of Objectives

40.1 Define key terms introduced in this chapter.

Knowing and being able to apply the key terms in each chapter is critical to understanding chapter concepts. Write the list of key terms. Then write the definition of each one in your own words. Check your understanding by confirming the definitions in the textbook glossary. Correct any misunderstandings. Create a study aid by writing each key term on the front of an index card and the definition on the back. Use the cards to quiz yourself or to have someone quiz you. The exercises under Vocabulary and Concept Review below will give you additional practice.

40.2 Describe the structure and function of the spinal column, spinal cord, and spinal nerves.

The spinal cord is a bundle of nerves that connects the brain and peripheral nervous system. When the spinal cord is damaged, communication between the brain and peripheral nervous system is disrupted. The spinal cord is protected within a bony column comprised of the ringlike vertebrae. Spinal nerve roots enter (afferent nerves) and exit (efferent nerves) the spinal column through openings in the vertebrae called foramina (singular: foramen).

40.3 Use scene size-up, understanding of mechanisms of injury, patient assessment, and patient history to develop an index of suspicion for spine injuries.

Spine injury can occur from direct and indirect trauma, and from penetrating and blunt trauma. Mechanisms that result in bony spine injury, injury to the nerve roots, or spinal cord injury include high-speed motor vehicle collisions, falls from significant heights, direct blows to the spine, axial loading mechanisms (such as football or shallow-water diving injuries), gunshot wounds, and stab wounds. Signs and symptoms include pain anywhere along the spinal column, paresthesia, loss of sensation, motor weakness, and paralysis.

40.4 Describe the incidence of neurologic deficit in patients with injury to the spinal column.

In many cases, there is injury to the vertebrae, ligaments, or intervertebral disks that does not cause neurologic deficit. Such injuries may be stable, meaning they are not prone to disrupting the normal alignment of the spine; or unstable, meaning that injured portions can shift and cause damage to nerves or the spinal cord.

40.5 Explain the threat to ventilation associated with injuries to the spinal cord at the cervical level.

The phrenic nerve, which supplies the motor function of the diaphragm, arises from the levels of C3, C4, and C5. Injuries to the spinal cord above the level of C5 can impair movement of the diaphragm and interfere with ventilation.

40.6 Anticipate the presence of other injuries in patients with mechanisms of injury that can produce spine injury.

Traumatic spine injury is generally associated with significant mechanisms of injury that are likely to produce injuries to other body systems in addition to spine injury. Anticipate problems with the airway and breathing and the potential for significant external and internal hemorrhage from fractures and organ injuries.

40.7 Differentiate between the concepts of spinal column injury and spinal cord injury.

A spinal column injury involves the vertebrae, intervertebral disks, or ligaments of the spine and may or may not involve the spinal cord. A spinal cord injury involves the tissue of the spinal cord itself and is often, but not always, associated with spinal column injury.

40.8 Give examples of forces that would produce each of the following mechanisms of spine injury: compression, distraction, extension, flexion, lateral bending, penetration, and rotation.

- *Compression:* Jumping from a height and landing on the feet, striking the head in a shallow-water diving injury, a hard landing in an airplane.
- *Distraction:* A force that causes the body and head to accelerate at different rates, such as a pedestrian being struck in the torso by a vehicle. This is particularly likely in pediatric patients, who have a relatively large, heavy head. Hanging also can result in distraction injuries.
- *Extension:* Anything that forces the head and neck beyond their normal range of extension, such as striking the forehead against the windshield in a motor vehicle collision, or a rear-end collision without a headrest on the seat.
- *Flexion:* Anything that forces the head and neck beyond their normal range of flexion, such as being struck in the back of the head, or impacting toward the occiput in a shallow-water diving injury.
- *Lateral bending:* A blow to the head from the side or a lateral-impact motor vehicle collision.
- *Penetration:* Gunshot wounds, stab wounds, or impaled objects.
- *Rotation:* Anything that causes the head and neck to exceed their normal limits of rotation, such as a blow to the side of face.

40.9 Describe the concepts of complete and incomplete spinal cord injury.

A complete spinal cord injury affects the transmission of nerve impulses through all of the tracts of the spinal cord. An incomplete injury affects nerve transmission in some tracts, but not others, leaving some functions intact below the point of injury.

40.10 Differentiate between the concepts of spinal shock and neurogenic hypotension.

Spinal shock is a concussive injury to the spinal cord that temporarily disrupts its function. Neurogenic hypotension occurs when nervous control of peripheral vascular diameter is lost due to injury that affects the sympathetic nerves that exit the thoracic level of the spine; usually occurs with high spinal cord injury.

40.11 Recognize signs and symptoms of spinal cord and spinal column injury.

Signs and symptoms include pain, deformity, loss of sensation, loss of movement, paresthesia, and weakness.

40.12 Given a series of scenarios, demonstrate the assessment and management of patients suspected of having an injury to the spine.

Use manual restriction of spinal movement when managing the airway, and provide an adequate airway. A modified jaw-thrust maneuver is preferred, but a head-tilt/chin-lift maneuver is used if a modified jaw-thrust maneuver does not result in an adequate airway. Suction as needed. Ventilations may be impaired, so be prepared to assist breathing with a bag-valve-mask device. Provide oxygen to maintain an SpO_2 of 95 percent or higher. Control external hemorrhage. Lack of sensation below the injury site means that patients are not aware of injuries that would otherwise be painful. Be thorough in your secondary assessment to detect injuries. Use a cervical collar and long backboard to immobilize the spine. Treat other injuries as indicated. Perfusion is not usually inadequate as a result of neurogenic hypotension. Do not assume hypotension is neurogenic, because it may be hypovolemic or obstructive. Treat with IV fluids according to the patient's clinical presentation.

40.13 Describe the importance of padding and filling voids between the patient and spinal immobilization devices.

You must use padding to avoid forcing the spine into an unnatural position and to prevent an increase in tissue pressure over bony areas, which results in pain and possible tissue ischemia that can lead to decubitus ulcers.

40.14 Demonstrate the following skills associated with management of the patient with a suspected spine injury: Inline manual stabilization of the cervical spine to seated and supine patients; modified jaw-thrust maneuver; repositioning the patient; application of a cervical collar; immobilization to a long backboard or other full-body spinal immobilization device; application of a short spinal immobilization device; rapid extrication; spinal immobilization of patients found in seated, standing, supine, and prone positions; managing patients wearing helmets or football equipment; and immobilizing infants and children.

For selected skills, refer to the skill scans in the chapter and the skill checklist at the end of this workbook chapter.

40.15 Describe the purpose and process of reassessing patients with suspected injury to the spine.

You must reassess all patients to detect trends in their conditions. As spinal cord swelling increases, signs and symptoms may appear or worsen, and other injuries can result in the patient's deterioration. Serial neurologic examination is very important to detect any changes in sensory or motor function.

40.16 Discuss current trends and controversies in the assessment and management of patients with suspected spine injuries.

Some EMS services are implementing selective spinal immobilization protocols to reduce indiscriminate use of spinal immobilization. The incidence of spinal cord injury is not as high as often assumed by EMS providers, with the most risk to patients who have significant craniofacial trauma or a GCS of less than 8. Spinal immobilization is not a benign intervention. It can result in pain and tissue damage, especially when the patient is immobilized for prolonged periods.

Resource Central

Resource Central offers extra practice and review materials in a variety of media. To access it, follow the directions on the Student Access Card provided with the Student Textbook. If there is no card, go to www.bradybooks.com and follow the Resource Central link to Buy Access.

Vocabulary and Concept Review

Exercise 1

Fill in the blanks to accurately complete each statement.

1. The spinal tracts that carry nerve impulses from the body to the brain are called:
   _____.

2. The first cervical vertebra is called the: _____ and the second cervical vertebra is called the: _____.

3. An injury that affects one side of the spinal cord but not the other produces signs and symptoms known as: _____ syndrome.

4. The spinal tracts that carry nerve impulses from the brain to the body are called the:
   _____.

5. A mechanism of injury that causes excessive stretching of the spine is called: _____.

6. The low blood pressure associated with high spinal cord injury is known as:
   _____ hypotension.

7. A sign of spine injury in males that is a persistent, abnormal erection of the penis is called: _____.

8. A concussive injury to the spinal cord, resulting in temporary neurologic dysfunction is known as: _____.

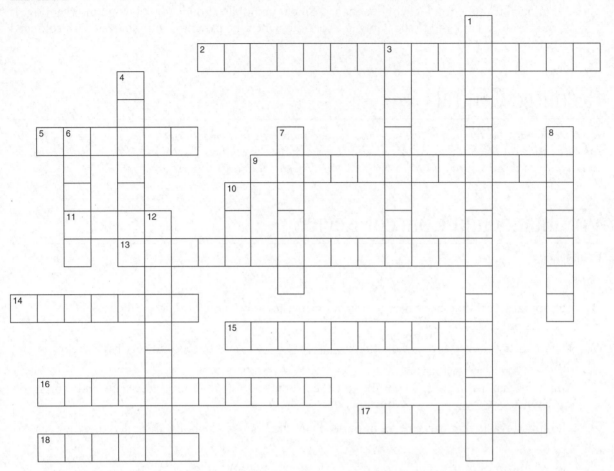

Across

2. Person whose help you should enlist when removing a sports helmet from an injured player.

5. Area of the spine that articulates with the pelvis.

9. Paralysis of the arms and legs.

11. Second cervical vertebra.

13. Rigid device placed around the neck to restrict movement.

14. Bending the neck forward so that the chin is closer to the chest.

15. Paralysis of the lower extremities.

16. Paralysis of the arms and legs.

17. Coordinated maneuver to turn the patient onto his side in order to position a long backboard behind him.

18. Lower-most portion of the spinal column.

Down

1. Procedure used when a patient must quickly be removed from a vehicle but has a possibility of spine injury.

3. Superior-most portion of the spinal column.

4. Nerve that controls movement of the diaphragm.

6. First cervical vertebra.

7. Area of the spine that supports the greatest amount of body weight.

8. Cushioning placed between the patient and the long backboard to fill voids and prevent pressure points.

10. MVCs and other forms of trauma that can damage the spine.

12. Type of injury that occurs from swelling or ischemia after the initial injury to the spine.

Patient Assessment Review

Identify the type of spine injury associated with each of the following assessment descriptions.

1. A 14-year-old man injured in an all-terrain vehicle collision cannot move his lower extremities. From the level of T4 downward, he cannot sense pain or temperature. However, the patient is aware of the position of his legs. _____

2. A 33-year-old man with a stab wound to the back has a loss of movement of the lower extremities on one side, along with a loss of awareness of the position of the extremity on that side. On the opposite side, he has some motor weakness, but cannot sense pain or temperature. _____

3. A 21-year-old woman who was ejected from a motorcycle has extreme weakness in her upper extremities, especially in the hands, with only mild weakness in the lower extremities. She also complains of a burning sensation in her hands. _____

Check Your Recall and Apply Concepts

Exercise 1

Write a "T" next each statement that is true and an "F" next to each statement that is false.

1. _____ Approximately 50 percent of all patients with blunt craniofacial trauma have associated spinal cord injuries.

2. _____ Of the five regions of the spine, the cervical region is the most commonly injured.

3. _____ Ascending spinal tracts carry nerve impulses from the brain to the body.

4. _____ When a patient has a spinal cord injury and has neurologic deficits at the scene, the extent of neurologic damage is immediately apparent.

5. _____ The spinal cord must be completely severed to result in neurologic deficits.

6. _____ Despite hypotension, the skin of a patient with a spinal cord injury may be warm and have normal color, especially below the site of injury.

7. _____ Neurologic hypotension is associated with reflex tachycardia.

8. _____ The recommended procedure is to secure the patient's body to a long backboard first, and then secure the head.

9. _____ The primary indication for the use of a short spinal immobilization device is for rapid extrication.

10. _____ Rapid extrication is used for all trauma patients with suspected spine injury.

Exercise 2

Select the best possible choice for each of the following questions.

_____ 1. A 22-year-old man was snowboarding and fell about 15 feet when he attempted a trick, landing backward on his upper back and then flipping several times. He is awake and scared, complaining that he cannot move or feel anything from his shoulders down. The patient is breathing adequately. He has a radial pulse of 72 per minute. You should suspect an injury at the level of:
   a. C3. c. T8.
   b. C7. d. T12.

_____ 2. A 16-year-old boy jumped from a second-story balcony railing, about 15 feet off the ground, onto asphalt below. He is complaining of pain in both of his lower extremities and in his back at the level of T10. Sensation and movement are present in all extremities. He denies neck pain and all other complaints except leg and back pain. He is alert, but has an odor of alcohol on his breath. The best way to manage this patient is to:
   a. apply full spinal immobilization, including a cervical collar, head immobilization, and a long backboard.
   b. use a cervical collar and short spinal immobilization device.
   c. use a long backboard, securing the torso; but cervical-spine motion restriction is not needed.
   d. use a short spinal immobilization device, but a cervical collar is not needed.

_____ 3. A 35-year-old bicyclist was struck from behind by a car traveling 25 miles per hour and was ejected from her bike. She opens her eyes to verbal stimuli, but does not follow commands to move her extremities and does not respond when you touch her. Her breathing is shallow and rapid with minimal chest movement. Her skin is warm and dry and she has a radial pulse of 80 per minute. Which one of the following is the highest priority in the management of this patient?
   a. Full spinal immobilization
   b. Application of a cervical collar
   c. Ventilation by bag-valve-mask device
   d. Starting two large-bore IVs and administering a 1,500-mL fluid bolus

_____ 4. A 25-year-old football player was tackled during a play, but was unable to get up afterward. He had no movement or sensation from his neck down. You are surprised to learn a month later that he is in rehabilitation and walking with assistance. The patient's initial presentation and outcome are most consistent with:
   a. Brown-Séquard syndrome.   c. anterior cord syndrome.
   b. central cord syndrome.   d. spinal cord concussion.

_____ 5. A 34-year-old woman was the driver of a vehicle that was struck from the rear as she slowed for a stoplight. The difference in speed between her vehicle and the vehicle that struck it was about 20 miles per hour. The patient had a properly adjusted headrest, but is complaining of a stiff neck and pain across her chest from her shoulder harness restraint. She is awake and alert; has no difficulty speaking or breathing; has warm, dry skin; and can move all extremities. The best method of spinal immobilization for this patient is:
   a. rapid extrication.
   b. cervical collar only.
   c. cervical collar, short spinal immobilization device, and long backboard.
   d. cervical collar and carefully moving the patient from the vehicle directly onto a long backboard.

_____ 6. Neurogenic hypotension is a form of _____ shock.
   a. distributive   c. hypovolemic
   b. obstructive   d. cardiogenic

_____ 7. Your patient is a 33-year-old front-seat passenger of a vehicle involved in a frontal collision with a concrete bridge support at a speed of 55 mph. He responds only to painful stimuli; is cyanotic; has rapid, shallow breathing; and has paradoxic motion of the anterior chest wall. The best way to minimize movement of the spine in this patient is:
   a. rapid extrication.
   b. cervical collar only.
   c. cervical collar, short spinal immobilization device, and long backboard.
   d. cervical collar and carefully moving the patient from the vehicle directly onto a long backboard.

Clinical Reasoning

CASE STUDY: INJURED PERSON AT THE FAIRGROUNDS

You are providing special event coverage at the state fair, when you are called for an injured person at the Big Rattler, a popular carnival ride. A 25-year-old man fell 25 feet from the ride as it started down a steep incline. It appears that he struck several support beams on the way down and landed face down on the concrete pad below. He has massive facial trauma with substantial bleeding. He is unresponsive with shallow, rapid, gurgling respirations. He has a radial pulse of 100 per minute. You are not able to establish an adequate airway after suctioning and using a modified jaw-thrust maneuver.

1. What is the risk of spine injury in this patient?

   _____

   _____

   _____

   _____

   _____

2. How should you manage the patient's airway?

   _____

   _____

   _____

   _____

   _____

3. What steps should you take to package this patient for transport?

   _____

   _____

   _____

   _____

   _____

Project-Based Learning

You may already have had the opportunity to be fully immobilized on a long backboard, be rapidly extricated from a vehicle, and be extricated from a vehicle using a short spinal immobilization device. If not, play the role of the patient while classmates perform those procedures. Pay attention to how the procedures affect you. Do you feel anxious at not being able to move? Does the cervical collar feel too tight on your neck or restrict your breathing or ability to open your mouth? What if you had to stay immobilized for 30 or 45 minutes or longer? How will you refine your application of those skills based on your experience as a "patient"? Jot down your observations about your experience and how they affect your thoughts about the skills in your notebook or journal and be prepared to discuss them in your class or study group.

The EMS Professional in Practice

You are working a Sunday shift in the emergency department. A patient on a long backboard is waiting for cervical-spine X-rays. He has been initially evaluated by a surgical resident, who feels the patient probably has a concussion, due to the repetitive questions he is asking, but he is scheduled for a CT scan after his cervical-spine X-ray. In the meantime, he has repeated several times that, "this thing," referring to the cervical collar, "is too tight on my neck." The technician caring for him tells him he needs to leave it alone. As the patient struggles to remove the collar, the technician becomes upset with the patient, and raises his voice, telling him he needs to lie down and be still or he is going to end up being paralyzed. How can you be a patient advocate in this case? Jot down your thoughts in a notebook or journal for discussion in class or in your study group.

Skills Checklists

The following skill checklist covers the major steps of a selected skill from Chapter 40. Review it prior to your laboratory classes. Practice skills only after they have been demonstrated for you in class and only under the supervision of an authorized instructor or clinical preceptor.

Advanced EMT Skill Checklist: Spinal Immobilization: *Long Backboard*		
Skill Stimulus: The primary assessment has been completed with manual cervical-spine motion restriction in place. The patient has indications for spinal immobilization based on the mechanism of injury.		
Step	**Performed**	**Not Performed**
Size and apply a rigid cervical collar.		
Maintaining alignment of the spine, coordinate a log roll on the direction of the EMS provider at the patient's head. Roll the patient slightly past perpendicular to the ground toward the knees of the responders performing the log roll.		
Place the long backboard flat on the ground behind the patient with the foot end of the board at the level of the patient's knees.		
Place a folded blanked along the patient's back and buttocks for padding.		
Coordinate reversing the log roll on the direction of the EMS provider at the patient's head to place the patient supine on the long backboard. Ensure that one EMS provider prevents the board from moving as the patient is rolled into supine position.		
Using longitudinal traction by EMS responders grasping the blanket beneath the patient, pull the patient toward the head of the board and make sure he is centered on the board.		
Apply straps across the body to prevent movement. At a minimum, the straps must secure the patient at the shoulders, hips, and legs. Pad between the body and sides of the board as needed to fill voids and prevent lateral movement.		
Use a head immobilization device or towel rolls and tape to secure the patient's head to the board.		
Skill Completion: The patient is immobilized with the spine in neutral alignment.		

Environmental Emergencies

Content Area

- Trauma

Advanced EMT Education Standard

- The Advanced EMT applies fundamental knowledge to provide basic and selected advanced emergency care and transportation based on assessment findings for an acutely injured patient.

Summary of Objectives

41.1 Define key terms introduced in this chapter.

Knowing and being able to apply the key terms in each chapter is critical to understanding chapter concepts. Write the list of key terms. Then write the definition of each one in your own words. Check your understanding by confirming the definitions in the textbook glossary. Correct any misunderstandings. Create a study aid by writing each key term on the front of an index card and the definition on the back. Use the cards to quiz yourself or to have someone quiz you. The exercises under Vocabulary and Concept Review below will give you additional practice.

41.2 Explain actions you should take to protect your own safety when responding to environmental emergencies.

By their nature, environmental emergencies involve hazards in the environment, necessitating special caution when approaching the patient. Dress for the weather, move the patient and yourself out of an inhospitable environment, and avoid hazards such as water, storms, insects, and animals.

41.3 Describe the scene size-up, primary and secondary assessments, and management of environmental emergencies to include the following: bites and stings by venomous snakes, insects, spiders, and marine animals; deep-water diving injuries; high-altitude sickness; lightning strike; local cold injuries; submersion/drowning; and systemic heat and cold injuries.

- *Bites and stings by venomous snakes, insects, spiders, and marine animals:* Determine if the patient is still at the location where the bite occurred and whether there are still insects or animals in the vicinity. Animal and insect toxins can act locally or systemically, so assess the level of responsiveness, airway, breathing, and circulation. Get a description of the insect or animal involved. Marine animal venom is inactivated by hot water. Snakebites may or may not be envenomated, but constricting bands and ice are contraindicated.
- *Deep-water diving injuries:* There is a high likelihood of impaired airway, breathing, and circulation. Assess them carefully and intervene as needed. Obtain a thorough history of the dive and dives preceding it. Consider transport to a facility with a hyperbaric chamber.
- High-altitude sickness: Altitude sickness can range from mild to severe, with pulmonary or cerebral edema. Manage the airway, breathing, and circulation and move the patient to a lower altitude.
- *Lightning strike:* Multiple patients may be involved, so make sure all patients have been identified. Move to a safe location to treat the patient. Respiratory arrest is the primary cause of cardiac arrest, necessitating attention to the airway and ventilation early in CPR. Multiple injuries are possible, including neurologic, musculoskeletal, and internal organ injuries.
- *Local cold injuries:* Protect yourself from the cold. Assess for hypothermia. Immobilize the affected extremity and anticipate extreme pain as the injury begins to thaw.
- *Submersion/drowning:* Asphyxia is the primary problem, necessitating particular attention to the airway and ventilation during resuscitation. If the incident occurred as a result of a watercraft collision or shallow-water diving, consider spinal immobilization.
- *Systemic heat and cold injuries:* Protect yourself from the environment. Manage the airway and breathing. Cool patients with heat stroke. Patients with heat emergencies require rehydration with isotonic fluids. Prevent further heat loss in patients with cold emergencies and anticipate cardiac dysrhythmia in severe hypothermia.

41.4 Explain the process of thermoregulation, including mechanisms by which the body gains and loses heat.

Thermoregulation is a homeostatic mechanism controlled by the hypothalamus. Under normal circumstances, the heat produced by metabolism is balanced by heat loss to the environment. In some cases, heat loss to the environment can be inadequate or excessive, overcoming the body's mechanisms for preserving or losing heat. Heat is lost from the body by convection, conduction, evaporation, respiration, and radiation.

41.5 Explain the risk factors, pathophysiology, signs, symptoms, assessment, and management of the following: heat cramps, heat exhaustion, heat stroke (classical and exertional), local cold injury, and mild, moderate, and severe hypothermia.

Risk factors for heat- and cold-related emergencies include extreme weather conditions and personal factors, such as age, health status, and medications. Assessment is aimed at obtaining a history of exposure, the presence of risk factors, and identifying signs and symptoms associated with exposure to extreme weather conditions. Management is aimed at ensuring an open airway, adequate breathing, and adequate circulation; preventing further gains or losses in body temperature; and correcting hyperthermia and hypothermia. Localized tissue injury from cold exposure is treated by protecting the extremity from further injury and managing pain.

41.6 Describe the characteristics of common venomous snakes, spiders, insects, and marine animals including the following: brown recluse and black widow spiders, fire ants, freshwater and saltwater marine animals, pit vipers and other venomous snakes, scorpions, and ticks.

- *Brown recluse and black widow spiders:* Brown recluse spiders are brown with a violin-shaped marking on the abdomen. Black widow spiders are shiny black with a red or red-orange hourglass marking on the abdomen.
- *Fire ants:* Small and brownish-orange, fire ants swarm prey aggressively and sting persistently.

- *Freshwater and saltwater marine animals:* Jellyfish are transparent and distinctive-looking saltwater marine animals. Catfish have whiskers (barbels) that give them a characteristic look. They do not have scales and appear smooth. They release stinging proteins from rays on their fins.
- *Pit viper and other venomous snakes:* Pit vipers have hollow fangs, a heat-sensing organ on the head, and elliptical pupils. Coral snakes have alternating bands of red, yellow, and black.
- *Scorpions:* Scorpions have eight legs and a tail that curves upward.
- *Ticks:* Small insects, ticks enlarge as they become engorged with blood.

41.7 Associate bites and stings with the potential for anaphylactic shock.

Hymenoptera, the family to which bees and wasps belong, cause bites and stings most often associated with anaphylaxis.

41.8 Explain the risk factors, pathophysiology, signs, symptoms, assessment, and management of envenomated bites and stings.

Risk factors include being in the environment in which particular venomous animals are found. Various venoms have local or systemic effects. Signs and symptoms include pain and swelling at the site. Systemic effects depend on the type of venom, and may include cardiovascular and neurologic signs and symptoms. Assess and manage the airway, breathing, and circulation. Management depends on whether the effects are local or systemic, and the type of animal that caused the injury.

41.9 Explain the risk factors, pathophysiology, signs, symptoms, assessment, and management of lightning strike injuries.

Lightning strike is usually associated with storms in the area, but may occur some distance from the actual storm. Lightning strike injuries include burns, respiratory arrest, neurologic injuries, and musculoskeletal injuries. In some cases, there are multiple patients. Remove patients from the outdoors as quickly as possible. Manage the airway, breathing, and circulation. Consider the possibility of spine injury. Treat burns.

41.10 Explain the following gas laws as they relate to high altitude and deep-water diving emergencies: Boyle's law, Charles' law, Dalton's law, and Henry's law.

- *Boyle's law:* As the pressure on a given amount of gas decreases, its volume increases. As the pressure increases, the volume decreases. This phenomenon allows gases to accumulate in the blood under pressure. As pressure decreases, the gas must be released through the respiratory system. A sudden decease in pressure results in expansion of gases in the tissues and vascular system.
- *Charles' law:* As the temperature of a given amount of gas increases, so does its volume. As the temperature decreases, so does the volume.
- *Dalton's law:* Also known as the law of partial pressures, Dalton's law is the total pressure of a mixture of a gas is the sum of the partial pressures of each gas in the mixture.
- *Henry's law:* The solubility of a gas in solution is related to the amount of pressure of the gas being exerted in the gas mixture above the solution.

41.11 Explain the risk factors, pathophysiology, signs, symptoms, assessment, and management of high-altitude sickness and dysbarism to include the following: acute mountain sickness, arterial gas embolism, barotrauma, decompression sickness, high-altitude cerebral edema, high-altitude pulmonary edema, and nitrogen narcosis.

- *Acute mountain sickness:* Occurs when a person ascends to an altitude of 6,600 feet too rapidly. Signs and symptoms can be classified as mild or severe, ranging from headache to shortness of breath to altered mental status.

- *Arterial gas embolism:* If ascent occurs too rapidly or if the diver holds his breath during ascent, nitrogen bubbles will form in the arterial bloodstream.
- *Barotrauma:* Occurs when air pressure in the hollow spaces of the body rises too high or drops too low.
- *Decompression sickness:* Occurs as nitrogen gas bubbles are produced and accumulate in the blood and tissues as a result of rapid ascent during a dive.
- *High-altitude cerebral edema:* An increase in intracranial pressure that can occur in conjunction with high-altitude pulmonary edema or acute mountain sickness.
- *High-altitude pulmonary edema:* Noncardiogenic pulmonary edema that occurs at altitudes of 8,200 feet or higher.
- *Nitrogen narcosis:* A state of stupor resulting from nitrogen's effect on cerebral function.

41.12 Explain the risk factors, pathophysiology, signs, symptoms, assessment, and management of submersion incidents/drowning.

Children are at particular risk of drowning, and male adolescents are also at increased risk. Alcohol plays a role in many adolescent and adult drownings. Drowning is a form of asphyxiation that ultimately results in cardiac arrest. Hypothermia can occur, as well. Management is aimed at correcting hypoxia by managing the airway, breathing, and circulation.

41.13 Recognize additional mechanisms of injury and illness that are associated with submersion incidents, such as trauma and hypothermia.

Suspect associated trauma in recreational craft collisions (personal watercraft, boats) and shallow-water diving incidents. Hypothermia can occur quickly in water that is less than 70 degrees Fahrenheit.

41.14 Explain factors that affect the likelihood of survival from submersion incidents.

Factors that affect survival from submersion include the patient's age and health status, the duration of submersion, the type and condition of the water, and the water temperature.

Resource Central

Resource Central offers extra practice and review materials in a variety of media. To access it, follow the directions on the Student Access Card provided with the Student Textbook. If there is no card, go to www.bradybooks.com and follow the Resource Central link to Buy Access.

Vocabulary and Concept Review

Exercise 1

Write the letter of the correct definition in the blank. Notice that there are more definitions than there are terms. (See Resource Central for more vocabulary review.)

1. _____ acute mountain sickness

2. _____ arterial gas embolism

3. _____ Boyle's law

4. _____ Dalton's law

5. _____ evaporation

6. _____ exertional heat stroke

7. _____ heat cramps

8. _____ high-altitude cerebral edema

9. _____ thermolysis

a. Muscle cramping caused by overexertion and dehydration in a hot environment

b. Life-threatening emergency in which core body temperature rises at a rapid rate, prior to the cessation of the sweating mechanism

c. Signs and symptoms due to ascension to an altitude of 6,600 feet or higher at too-rapid a rate

d. Slowed metabolism due to sudden immersion in cold water

e. Loss of heat to the environment

f. Principle that pertains to the relationship of the partial pressures of individual gases in a mixture to the total pressure of a mixture of gases

g. Addresses the inverse relationship between the pressure and volume of a gas

h. Conversion of liquid to a vapor

i. Occlusion of efferent blood vessels by air bubbles

j. Swelling of the brain and increased intracranial pressure due to a sudden increase in elevation

Exercise 2

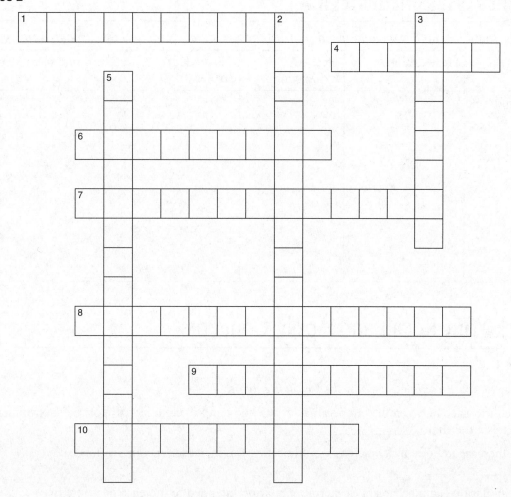

Across

1. This is how heat is lost when you come in contact with a cold object.

4. Law that explains how carbon dioxide is dissolved in a sealed bottle of soda.

6. Heat loss into a still atmosphere.

7. Sickness also called the "bends".

8. Fluid in the lungs from rapid ascension to a high altitude.

9. Severe pain in the ear or sinuses when descending rapidly during a dive are examples of this.

10. Losing heat to air currents moving across the body.

Down

2. Also known as "rapture of the deep."

3. Death due to asphyxia from submersion in a liquid.

5. Mild state of shock that occurs as a result of exposure to a hot environment.

Patient Assessment Review

Fill in the following table to compare and contrast the assessment findings in heat-related emergencies.

	Heat Cramps	Heat Exhaustion	Classic Heat Stroke	Exertional Heat Stroke
Signs and symptoms				

Check Your Recall and Apply Concepts

Exercise 1

Fill in the blank to complete each of the following items.

1. The difference between the temperature of the body and the temperature of the environment creates a thermal _____.

2. An increase in body heat, such as would occur from increased metabolism, is called _____.

3. Vasodilation is a mechanism of thermoregulation intended to increase heat loss by _____.

4. The combination of heat and humidity that makes the temperature feel warmer than it actually is, is called the _____.

5. Five ways in which the body can lose heat are

    _____

    _____

    _____

    _____

6. A term that means body temperature that is above normal is _____.

7. A high school football player who collapses during practice in hot, humid weather and who has hot, wet, flushed skin, altered mental status, and a very high body temperature is most likely suffering from _____.

8. A drop in core body temperature to between 90 and 95 degrees Fahrenheit is classified as _____ hypothermia.

9. In the first stage of hypothermia _____ occurs.

10. When ice crystals form in the tissue cells, the condition is called _____.

11. If delayed transport dictates that you rewarm an extremity with a local cold injury in the prehospital setting, you should use water that is _____ degrees Fahrenheit.

12. When a person asphyxiates as a result of submersion, the condition is known as _____.

13. The general term for injuries resulting from extremes or abrupt changes in atmospheric pressure is _____.

14. The gas law that best explains the formation of nitrogen bubbles in the blood and tissues when a diver rapidly ascends is _____.

15. Altitude-related illnesses can mostly be prevented by allowing for a process of _____.

Exercise 2

Select the best possible choice for each of the following questions.

_____ 1. A 17-year-old girl became ill at track practice. She is complaining of weakness and severe pain in the calf of her right leg. She is alert and oriented. Her skin is warm and moist with good color. Her heart rate is 104 with respirations of 20 and a blood pressure of 108/74. Her SpO_2 is 99 percent with ambient air. Which one of the following would be most beneficial in the treatment of this patient?
   a. Administer oxygen by nasal cannula.
   b. Place cold packs in her axillae and groin.
   c. Allow her to sip a sports drink.
   d. Start an IV of 5 percent dextrose in water.

_____ 2. Your patient is a 21-year-old woman who works at an outdoor car wash. It has been above 90 degrees Fahrenheit for eight consecutive days, with humidity between 80 and 90 percent. She lives in an apartment without air conditioning. When you arrive at her residence, she is lying on the sofa with a wet washcloth on her head. She is complaining of a headache, lightheadedness, near-syncope when she tries to stand up, nausea, and weakness. She is awake but seems lethargic. Her skin is cool, pale, and moist. Her heart rate is 116 and her respiratory rate is 24. Her blood pressure is 96/64. Her SpO_2 is 95 percent on room air. Of the following, which should you do first?
   a. Give oxygen by nonrebreather mask.
   b. Start an IV of lactated Ringer's solution and give a 1,000-mL bolus.
   c. Allow the patient to sip a sports drink.
   d. Place the patient in the back of the ambulance in an air-conditioned environment.

_____ 3. Your patient is a college football player who collapsed at practice in 92-degree-Fahrenheit temperature with high humidity while wearing full protective gear and uniform. Teammates removed the equipment and uniform jersey and have been pouring water over him. He is unresponsive and has hot, wet, flushed skin. Which one of the following should you do first?
   a. Place cold packs in his axillae and groin.
   b. Implement manual spinal motion restriction.
   c. Apply oxygen by nonrebreather mask.
   d. Open the airway with a head-tilt/chin-lift maneuver.

_____ 4. You and your partner have been dispatched just after daybreak for an unresponsive person on a bench in a small park. The temperature is 17 degrees Fahrenheit with a 15 mile per hour wind. It is not known how long the patient has been outside. He is in his 30s and is wearing an unlined jean jacket over a sweater, a stocking cap, jeans, and tennis shoes. The patient has slow, shallow respirations, and his muscles are very rigid. You are barely able to palpate a carotid pulse at a rate of about 36 per minute. You estimate that the patient is in stage _____ hypothermia.
   a. 2
   b. 3
   c. 4
   d. 5

_____ 5. A 15-year-old boy fell through the ice on a pond and was immersed in the water for 10 minutes before his companions were able to pull him out. He is still outside when you arrive. His companions have placed their coats over him and his wet clothing. The patient is shivering uncontrollably, to the point that his is not able to speak clearly. Which one of the following is the highest priority in the management of this patient?
   a. Give warmed IV fluids.
   b. Remove the wet clothing.
   c. Give warmed, humidified oxygen.
   d. Cover him with blankets.

_____ 6. A 16-year-old girl has just returned from an afternoon ice skating outdoors on a frozen pond. She complains that her toes were initially numb, but as she warmed them in front of a heater they began to sting and burn. Her toes are red and warm to the touch and there are no blisters. The patient's presentation is most consistent with:
   a. superficial cold injury.
   b. immersion foot.
   c. deep cold injury.
   d. fourth-degree frostbite.

_____ 7. A recreational diver suddenly ascends from a depth of 50 feet after a bottom time of 15 minutes. He is at greatest risk for:
   a. nitrogen narcosis.
   b. decompression sickness.
   c. ruptured tympanic membranes.
   d. pulmonary edema.

_____ 8. A 42-year-old woman from Florida is visiting her sister in a mountain town at an elevation of 5,900 feet. She complains of weakness, headache, and mild shortness of breath after a short hike. Of the following problems, the one most likely is:
   a. mild acute mountain sickness.
   b. severe acute mountain sickness.
   c. high-altitude pulmonary edema.
   d. high-altitude cerebral edema.

_____ 9. A 23-year-old hiker became ill at an altitude of 8,500 feet. She is very short of breath and has developed a cough. When you perform your assessment, you find that she has crackles (rales) in both lungs, a heart rate of 116, respirations of 28, and an SpO_2 of 88 percent. Of the following, the one most beneficial intervention for this patient is:
   a. consulting with medical direction about giving diuretics.
   b. starting an IV and giving a 500-mL fluid bolus.
   c. administering nitrous oxide.
   d. descending to a lower altitude.

_____ 10. A group of 32 marching band members was injured when lightning struck near the practice field. Most of them have complaints of pain, weakness, numbness, tingling, and dizziness. A few are confused and complaining of dizziness. The most likely mechanism involved is a:
   a. direct lightning strike.
   b. contact strike.
   c. side flash strike.
   d. ground current strike.

Clinical Reasoning

CASE STUDY: BURNING DOWN THE HOUSE

You are part of the rehabilitation sector at fire training exercise in which there is a live burn of an abandoned farmhouse. Despite the relatively mild temperature of 65 degrees Fahrenheit, one of the firefighters seems to be suffering from a heat-related emergency. He is confused, lethargic, and weak. His skin is hot, flushed, and diaphoretic.

1. What heat emergency explains the patient's presentation?

_____

_____

_____

_____

_____

2. What are the initial steps you should take in this patient's management?

_____

_____

_____

_____

_____

3. What complications should you anticipate and be prepared to manage?

_____

_____

_____

_____

_____

Project-Based Learning

Find out what types of venomous animals and insects are in your area. Develop a fact sheet that describes the appearance of each animal or insect, where it is found, how to avoid its bites or stings, signs and symptoms of bites and stings, and what to do if you receive a bite or sting. As a starting place, check the website of your state department of natural resources.

The EMS Professional in Practice

Your EMS service has been dispatched for several submersion incidents at a beach along the river. In one incident, two children and the bystander who tried to save them drowned. What can you do, as a health care provider and community member, to reduce the number of submersion incidents? Jot down your thoughts in a notebook or journal for discussion in class or in your study group.

Multisystem Trauma and Trauma Resuscitation

Content Area

• Trauma

Advanced EMT Education Standard

• The Advanced EMT applies fundamental knowledge to provide basic and selected advanced emergency care and transportation based on assessment findings for an acutely injured patient.

Summary of Objectives

42.1 Define key terms introduced in this chapter.

Knowing and being able to apply the key terms in each chapter is critical to understanding chapter concepts. Write the list of key terms. Then write the definition of each one in your own words. Check your understanding by confirming the definitions in the textbook glossary. Correct any misunderstandings. Create a study aid by writing each key term on the front of an index card and the definition on the back. Use the cards to quiz yourself or to have someone quiz you. The exercises under Vocabulary and Concept Review below will give you additional practice.

42.2 Discuss the increased morbidity and mortality associated with multisystem trauma.

Compromise of more than one system affects the body's ability to compensate for injuries and increases the chances of death substantially.

42.3 Describe the importance of each of the following principles of out-of-hospital multisystem trauma care: ensure safety of rescue personnel and the patient; determine the need for additional resources; understand mechanism of injury; identify and manage life threats; manage the airway while maintaining cervical-spine immobilization; support ventilation and oxygenation; control external hemorrhage and treat for shock; perform a secondary assessment and obtain a medical history; splint musculoskeletal injuries and maintain spinal immobilization; and make transport decisions.

- *Ensure safety of rescue personnel and the patient:* To provide patient care, you must first prevent injury to yourself and your partner, and you must prevent further injury to the patient to provide him with the best chances of recovery.
- *Determine the need for additional resources:* In order for all patients to receive the care they need as quickly as possible, you must recognize what resources you need and request them as soon as possible.
- *Understand mechanism of injury:* Some injuries are not immediately evident by physical examination, but can be anticipated and treated proactively by understanding how various mechanisms of injury affect the body.
- *Identify and manage life threats:* The key to successful resuscitation is immediate recognition and intervention in conditions that affect the airway, breathing, and circulation.
- *Manage the airway while maintaining cervical-spine immobilization:* In cases in which cervical-spine injury is suspected, you must manually stabilize the cervical spine without impairing the ability to maintain a patent airway. In most cases, airway management can be achieved with a modified jaw-thrust maneuver. However, if that maneuver does not allow adequate airflow, you must use a head-tilt/chin-lift maneuver.
- *Support ventilation and oxygenation:* Ventilation and oxygenation can be impaired by airway obstruction, traumatic brain injury, or chest injury. To provide adequate tissue perfusion, you must manage the patient's airway, ventilation, and oxygenation.
- *Control external hemorrhage and treat for shock:* Hemorrhage leads to decreased tissue perfusion. You must control hemorrhage and treat for shock to prevent worsening of perfusion.
- *Perform a secondary assessment and obtain a medical history:* A secondary assessment is required in multisystem trauma patients to find all injuries. The medical history provides information about medications and medical conditions that can affect the patient's ability to compensate and the treatment he needs.
- *Splint musculoskeletal injuries and maintain spinal immobilization:* Splinting decreases pain, bleeding, and additional injury, all of which can worsen the patient's condition. When spinal immobilization is necessary, it is performed to minimize the chances of neurologic injury.
- *Make transport decisions:* Transport decisions are among the most important prehospital patient care decisions for multisystem trauma patients. You must transport the patient without delay to the most appropriate facility for his condition. Depending on the patient's condition, resources available, and other circumstances, this may mean air medical transport, ground ALS transport, transport to the closest facility for stabilization and later transfer, or transport to a trauma center.

Resource Central

Resource Central offers extra practice and review materials in a variety of media. To access it, follow the directions on the Student Access Card provided with the Student Textbook. If there is no card, go to www.bradybooks.com and follow the Resource Central link to Buy Access.

Vocabulary and Concept Review

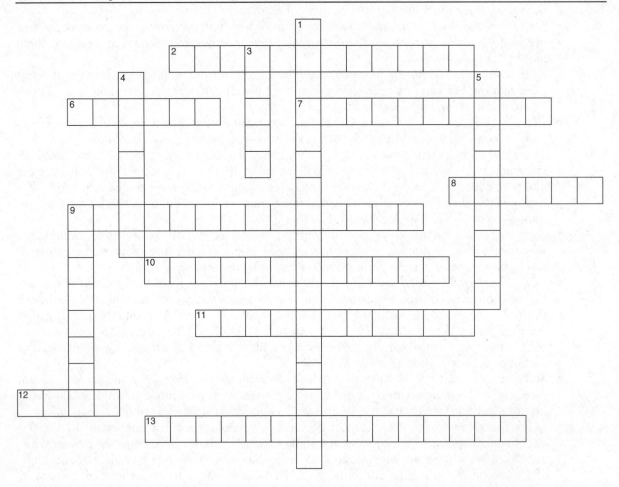

Across

2. Subsequent evaluation of the multisystem trauma patient to detect trends in his condition and the effects of treatment.

6. Management of this is your primary responsibility when caring for a critically injured patient.

7. Bleeding.

8. Your first priority on any emergency scene

9. Method that is effective in controlling most external bleeding.

10. Condition of abnormal blood clotting.

11. Type of trauma that occurs to more than one body structure.

12. Pants-like device sometimes used for patients with pelvic fractures accompanied by shock.

13. Portion of the secondary assessment that is performed in multisystem trauma patients immediately after the primary assessment.

Down

1. Specific traumatic forces applied to the body.

3. State of hypoperfusion

4. Type of assessment in which you identify and treat problems with the airway, breathing, and circulation.

5. Steps taken to prepare a patient for transport, which may include spinal immobilization.

9. Mnemonic for use during rapid trauma assessment.

Patient Assessment Review

Exercise 1

List seven mechanisms of injury that should lead you to suspect multisystem trauma.

_____

_____

_____

_____

_____

_____

_____

Exercise 2

Outline the sequence of patient assessment steps for the multisystem trauma patient.

_____

_____

_____

_____

_____

_____

_____

Check Your Recall and Apply Concepts

Exercise 1

Select the best possible choice for each of the following questions.

_____ 1. When treating a patient with hemorrhagic shock, in addition to managing the airway, breathing, and circulation in the primary assessment, which one of the following interventions is generally recommended for all patients?
   a. PASG
   b. Trendelenburg position
   c. Keeping the patient warm
   d. 3,000-mL to 4,000-mL bolus of isotonic crystalloid IV fluid

_____ 2. You are caring for a patient who was involved in a high-speed motor vehicle collision. You suspect that he has abdominal injuries and a fractured pelvis. He responds to verbal stimuli and has cool, pale, diaphoretic skin. His heart rate is 120 per minute. His respirations are 20 per minute, and he has a blood pressure of 74 by palpation. Which one of the following is the appropriate goal for his systolic blood pressure to guide IV fluid administration?
   a. 80 mmHg   c. 100 mmHg
   b. 90 mmHg   d. 110 mmHg

3. You are considering applying PASG to a patient. Which one of the following conditions should make you decide against applying them?
   a. Evisceration of abdominal organs
   b. Systolic blood pressure below 70 mmHg
   c. Suspected pelvic fracture
   d. Suspected spine injury

4. Your patient was stabbed once in the chest and jumped from a second-story balcony onto a paved surface to escape his attacker. Which one of the following injuries must be specifically managed during the primary assessment?
   a. Open fracture of the distal right tibia
   b. Suspected lumbar spine injury
   c. Suspected fracture of the left forearm
   d. Open wound to the anterior right chest at the fourth intercostal space

Clinical Reasoning

CASE STUDY: HEAD-ON COLLISION

You and your partner have been dispatched for a single-vehicle collision on a rural section of highway. The car left the road, went down an embankment, and rolled over several times. The patient is a 42-year-old man who is unresponsive to verbal and painful stimuli. You suspect head injuries, internal organ injuries, and multiple long bone fractures.

1. What are the priorities of assessment and management for this patient?

   _____
   _____
   _____
   _____

2. What are your goals for managing the airway, breathing, and circulation of this patient?

   _____
   _____
   _____
   _____

3. What factors should you consider in making decisions about when, how, and where to transport the patient?

   _____
   _____
   _____
   _____
   _____

Project-Based Learning

To help familiarize yourself with trends and issues in trauma management and to help you develop skills in critically evaluating research, select three articles on prehospital trauma management that have been published in a peer-reviewed journal within the past three years. Journals to consider are *Prehospital Emergency Care*, *The Journal of Emergency Medicine*, and *The Journal of Trauma*. Share the articles with at least three classmates or members of your study group. Jot down the following questions and your answers in your notebook or journal in preparation for a discussion of the three articles: What was the goal of each study? What were the major findings of each study? Based on the strengths and weaknesses of the study, would you recommend changes in EMS practice based on the outcomes of the study?

The EMS Professional in Practice

There is currently debate in a rural EMS service about whether the best policy is to transport trauma patients directly to a level I trauma center 45 miles away or transport them to a critical access hospital that is within 10 miles of most locations in the county. What issues should be considered in the debate? Jot down your thoughts in a notebook or journal for discussion in class or in your study group.

Chapter 43

Obstetrics and Care of the Newborn

Content Area

- Special Patient Populations

Advanced EMT Education Standard

- Applies a fundamental knowledge of growth, development, and aging and assessment findings to provide basic and selected advanced emergency care and transportation for a patient with special needs.

Summary of Objectives

43.1 Define key terms introduced in this chapter.

Knowing and being able to apply the key terms in each chapter is critical to understanding chapter concepts. Write the list of key terms. Then write the definition of each one in your own words. Check your understanding by confirming the definitions in the textbook glossary. Correct any misunderstandings. Create a study aid by writing each key term on the front of an index card and the definition on the back. Use the cards to quiz yourself or to have someone quiz you. The exercises under Vocabulary and Concept Review below will give you additional practice.

43.2 Describe the anatomy and physiology of the female reproductive system.

The female external genitalia consist of the mons pubis, labia majora, labia minora, and clitoris. The vagina is a hollow tubular passageway that connects the external genitalia with the internal genitalia. The uterus is a small muscular organ lined with endometrium, tissue that thickens each month during the reproductive years in preparation for the possible implantation of a fertilized ovum. The outer portion of each fallopian tube drapes around an ovary, providing a passageway for ova to travel toward the uterus. The ovaries and endometrium undergo cyclical monthly changes under the influence of the endocrine system, called the menstrual cycle.

43.3 Describe the anatomy and physiology of pregnancy, including the following: fertilization of an ovum, gestational age, placenta, umbilical cord, amniotic sac, changes in the reproductive system, changes in the respiratory and cardiovascular systems, changes

in the gastrointestinal and urinary systems, changes in the musculoskeletal system, and normal labor and delivery.

- *Fertilization of an ovum:* An ovum is fertilized by a spermatozoon in the outer third of the fallopian tube during a short window of time near ovulation.
- *Gestational age:* This refers to the duration of pregnancy and is determined from the date of the mother's last menstrual period. Pregnancy normally lasts from 38 to 42 weeks.
- *Placenta:* This is a temporary organ of pregnancy that allows the nutrients and oxygen from the maternal bloodstream to reach the fetal circulation. It also allows fetal wastes to be eliminated through the maternal circulatory system.
- *Umbilical cord:* This contains the umbilical arteries and umbilical vein that allow the maternal and fetal circulation to come into close contact with each other through the placenta.
- *Amniotic sac:* The amniotic sac is part of the fetal membranes and contains the amniotic fluid that surrounds the developing fetus.
- *Changes in the reproductive system:* The corpus luteum persists in the ovary, instead of degenerating, if fertilization occurs and begins secreting hormones to support the pregnancy. Once the fertilized egg is implanted in the uterine lining, it is called an embryo. The uterus expands to accommodate the growing embryo, which is called a fetus after the eighth week of development.
- *Changes in the respiratory and cardiovascular systems:* The maternal blood volume increases substantially and the respiratory rate and depth increase slightly to accommodate the metabolic needs of the developing fetus.
- *Changes in the gastrointestinal and urinary systems:* The activity of the gastrointestinal system slows, and nausea and vomiting are common in early pregnancy. The kidneys must accommodate the increase in metabolic waste created by the fetus. The expanding uterus places pressure on the bladder, resulting in frequent urination, especially in the first and third trimesters.
- *Changes in the musculoskeletal system:* The ligaments soften in response to pregnancy hormones to allow the pelvis to expand. However, the effect on the joints is not selective, making the pregnant woman prone to musculoskeletal injuries.
- *Normal labor and delivery:* True labor is preceded by Braxton-Hicks contractions, which start the process of cervical effacement and dilation. The contractions of true labor are regular and become closer together. Labor progresses through four stages. In the first stage the cervix becomes completely effaced and dilated, in the second stage the fetus is expelled, and in the third stage the placenta is delivered. The fourth stage lasts from expulsion of the placenta to 1 hour after it is expelled. Knowledge of the first three stages is most relevant to prehospital care.

43.4 Elicit a pertinent history from the patient with an obstetric emergency.

A pertinent history includes both a SAMPLE history and an obstetric history, including the date of the last menstrual period, the number of pregnancies, the number of births, history of prenatal care, and any known problems with the current pregnancy.

43.5 Describe the assessment and emergency management of patients with antepartum emergencies, including the following: abruptio placentae, ectopic pregnancy, placenta previa, pre-eclampsia/eclampsia, pregnancy-induced hypertension, ruptured uterus, spontaneous abortion, supine hypotensive syndrome, and trauma in pregnancy.

The management priorities of airway, breathing, and circulation apply to antepartum emergencies in the pregnant patient. Signs of shock can be delayed despite substantial blood loss because of the increase in maternal blood volume. Maintain a lower threshold for treating for shock. In the third trimester, the uterus can compress the vena cava when the patient is supine, so place third-trimester patients on their left sides, rather than supine.

43.6 **Describe the assessment and management of a patient in active labor.**

Determine whether delivery is imminent and whether there is time to transport or if you must prepare for field delivery. Signs and symptoms of imminent delivery include intense, frequent contractions and a sensation of pressure in the pelvis that is sometimes interpreted by the mother as the need to move the bowels. Just prior to delivery, the perineum bulges with contractions and the presenting part of the fetus, usually the head, becomes visible at the vaginal opening, first during contractions and then during and between contractions. The primary responsibilities are to reassure the mother, prevent explosive delivery of the head, clear the infant's airway, clamp and cut the umbilical cord, and dry and warm the infant.

43.7 **Describe the steps of assisting with a prehospital obstetric delivery.**

The steps of assisting with a prehospital delivery include assembling needed equipment and supplies, using Standard Precautions, positioning the mother, controlling delivery of the head, suctioning the mouth and nose of the infant, assisting with delivery of the body, clamping and cutting the umbilical cord, assessing the infant's APGAR score, drying and warming the infant, checking the mother for and managing excessive postpartum hemorrhage, and anticipating delivery of the placenta.

43.8 **Take steps to manage abnormal prehospital obstetric deliveries, including the following: breech and limb presentations, meconium staining, multiple births, preterm labor/ premature rupture of membranes, precipitous delivery, prolapsed umbilical cord, and shoulder dystocia.**

- *Breech and limb presentations:* Breech deliveries can sometimes be accomplished in the prehospital setting, but the head may have difficulty passing beneath the mother's pubic bone, especially in full-term pregnancies. You may need to apply gentle upward traction on the baby's body to assist delivery of the head. If the head does not deliver, you may need to provide an airway for the infant by placing your fingers on either side of his nose and mouth. Limb presentations cannot be managed in the prehospital setting, and the mother must be transported to a hospital with obstetric surgical capabilities.
- *Meconium staining:* Suction the mouth and nose as usual with a bulb syringe. If secretions are copious, additional suctioning with a bulb syringe may be necessary. Consider ALS or air medical transport for infants in respiratory distress.
- *Multiple births:* Multiples are sometimes smaller than in single-fetus pregnancies and may be premature. Warm and dry the infants and be prepared to provide support of the airway, breathing, and circulation.
- *Preterm labor/premature rupture of membranes:* Preterm labor can sometimes be stopped by an infusion of intravenous fluids, but you must check with medical direction and follow your protocols. Consider ALS or air medical transport if a facility with a neonatal intensive care unit is not nearby. If preterm delivery occurs, be prepared to provide treatment for the infant, whose lungs and thermoregulatory mechanisms are not mature.
- *Precipitous delivery:* Be aware of the risk of maternal and fetal injury.
- *Prolapsed umbilical cord:* Place the mother in knee–chest position; administer oxygen; cover the umbilical cord with a moist, sterile dressing; if necessary, keep the presenting part from pressing on the cord; and transport to a facility with obstetric surgery capabilities.
- *Shoulder dystocia:* It may help to have the mother use her hands to pull her knees toward her shoulders with her buttocks at the very edge of the bed and for you to apply pressure just above the pubic bone. If delivery does not occur, transport without delay.

43.9 **Take steps to manage postpartum complications, including the following: postpartum hemorrhage and pulmonary embolism.**

For postpartum hemorrhage, apply direct pressure to external lacerations. Support the body of the uterus with one hand just above the pubic bone and massage the fundus of the uterus through the abdominal wall with the other hand. Allow the infant to nurse. Start an IV and administer fluids for ongoing hemorrhage.

For pulmonary embolism, provide an adequate airway, ventilation, oxygenation, and circulation. Transport without delay.

43.10 Demonstrate the steps of assessing and managing a neonate, including the following: APGAR scoring, assessing breathing and circulation, positioning, preventing heat loss, and suctioning.

In APGAR scoring a value of 0, 1, or 2 is assigned to each of five dimensions represented by the mnemonic APGAR, for a total of up to 10 points. Each dimension is evaluated at 1 minute and 5 minutes after birth.

To assess breathing and circulation you must know that the normal newborn respiratory rate is up to 60 per minute and the newborn should have a strong cry. The normal SpO_2 in a newborn in the first 10 minutes is between 70 and 80 percent.

Position the newborn who is not in distress in his parent's arms. If copious airway secretions continue, temporarily place the newborn on his side with his head just slightly lower than his body may help. If airway management is required, place padding under the infant's shoulders to achieve a neutral position of the head and neck.

To prevent heat loss dry the newborn and wrap him in receiving blankets, making sure to cover the head.

Suction, using a bulb syringe, to clear the infant's mouth and nose.

43.11 Recognize signs that indicate the need for neonatal resuscitation.

The three characteristics of neonates who do not require resuscitation include being full-term gestation, crying or breathing, and having good muscle tone. If any of the characteristics is not present, then one or more of the following steps are taken: dry, warm, and stimulate the newborn; suction the airway; provide oxygen; ventilate; provide chest compressions; and prepare IV or IO access.

43.12 Apply the concepts of the neonatal resuscitation pyramid to the care of neonates in need of resuscitative measures.

In order of relative frequency, the steps needed in neonatal resuscitation are to dry, warm, and stimulate the newborn; suction the airway; provide oxygen; ventilate; provide chest compressions; prepare IV or IO access; and administer medications.

43.13 Effectively communicate to other health care providers a pertinent patient history, assessment findings, and interventions for pregnant patients and neonates.

You must summarize the relevant findings of assessment, including the mother's prenatal history, events surrounding labor and delivery, the 1- and 5-minute APGAR scores, and any resuscitative measures taken.

Resource Central

Resource Central offers extra practice and review materials in a variety of media. To access it, follow the directions on the Student Access Card provided with the Student Textbook. If there is no card, go to www.bradybooks.com and follow the Resource Central link to Buy Access.

Vocabulary and Concept Review

Exercise 1

Write the letter of the correct definition in the blank. (See Resource Central for more vocabulary review.)

1. _____ abortion

2. _____ Braxton-Hicks contractions

3. _____ eclampsia

4. _____ embryo

5. _____ gravida

6. _____ meconium

7. _____ parturition

8. _____ precipitous delivery

9. _____ pre-eclampsia

10. _____ preterm labor

11. _____ spontaneous abortion

12. _____ stillbirth

13. _____ zygote

a. Contents of the first fetal or newborn bowel movement

b. Infant of 20 weeks or less gestation without signs of life

c. A developing human organism from conception to the point of implantation in the uterine lining

d. Hypertensive emergency of pregnancy characterized by the onset of seizures or coma

e. The process of giving birth

f. Pregnancy; the number of pregnancies a woman has had

g. The loss of pregnancy from natural causes prior to 20 weeks gestation

h. Mild, irregular contractions of the uterus noticed during the last trimester of pregnancy

i. Onset of regular contractions prior to 37 weeks gestation

j. Loss of pregnancy from any cause prior to 20 weeks gestation

k. Developing human organism in the first 60 days following conception

l. Birth of a baby within 3 hours of the onset of labor

m. Hypertensive disorder of pregnancy characterized by high blood pressure, edema, protein in the urine, headache, visual disturbances, and hyperactive reflexes

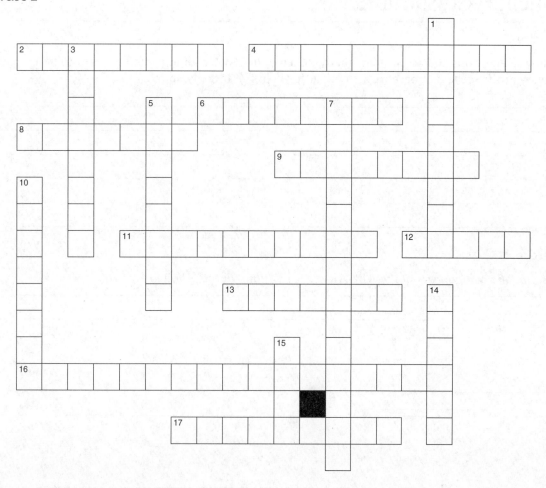

Across

2. Visibility of the presenting part of the fetus at the vaginal opening.

4. Term that describes a woman who has given birth more than once.

6. Condition in which the umbilical cord is the presenting part during labor and delivery.

8. Type of pregnancy in which the embryo is implanted anywhere other than the uterine lining.

9. Temporary organ of pregnancy that allows exchange of oxygen, nutrients, and wastes between the mother and fetus.

11. Point at which the presenting part of the fetus drops into the maternal pelvis.

12. Developing human organism from 60 days gestation to birth.

13. A newborn.

16. Premature separation of the placenta from the uterine wall.

17. Period of time from conception to delivery.

Down

1. Descriptor for a newborn born between 20 and 37 weeks of gestation.

3. A posterior pituitary hormone that causes uterine muscle contraction and stimulates the letdown reflex in lactation.

5. Widening of the diameter of the cervical os in preparation for delivery.

7. Condition in which the placenta partially or completely covers the internal cervical opening.

10. Conditions in which the fetal head delivers but in which the shoulders become wedged behind the public bone.

14. Position in which the baby's buttocks or feet are the presenting part in the birth canal.

15. Term that describes a woman who has given birth to an infant greater than 20 weeks gestation.

Patient Assessment Review

Exercise 1

Write the questions and assessments that will help you in determining whether you should prepare for delivery at the scene or transport the patient for delivery at the hospital.

_____

_____

_____

_____

_____

_____

Exercise 2

Describe the components of the APGAR score by filling in the following chart.

A: _____

0	1	2

P: _____

0	1	2

G: _____

0	1	2

A: _____

0	1	2

R: _____

0	1	2

Check Your Recall and Apply Concepts

Select the best possible choice for each of the following questions.

_____ 1. The correct term for the vaginal opening is:
    a. labia minora.
    b. introitus.
    c. urethral meatus.
    d. cervix.

_____ 2. The lining of the uterus is the:
    a. endometrium.
    b. chorion.
    c. myometrium.
    d. fundus.

_____ 3. Menstrual bleeding marks day _____ of the menstrual cycle.
    a. 1
    b. 14
    c. 21
    d. 28

_____ 4. Which one of the following statements is most accurate regarding the cardiovascular system in pregnancy?
    a. Cardiac output decreases.
    b. Blood pressure normally is 10 to 15 mmHg higher in pregnancy.
    c. The stroke volume increases and the heart rate decreases late in pregnancy.
    d. Signs and symptoms of shock may be delayed until 30 to 35 percent of blood volume is lost.

_____ 5. A patient who is 38 weeks pregnant complains of slight shortness of breath after a 4-hour commercial airline flight to attend a family funeral. You should:
    a. assume that shortness of breath is normal at this stage in pregnancy.
    b. immediately administer high-flow oxygen by nonrebreather mask.
    c. obtain a history and perform a focused secondary assessment.
    d. assume that any increase in respiratory rate is a result of hyperventilation syndrome.

_____ 6. You have just arrived at the home of a 26-year-old woman who is 10 weeks pregnant and suffering from hyperemesis gravidarum. She is otherwise in good health. Her sister states that the patient became pale and sweaty and nearly fainted when she stood up from a lawn chair. The patient is on IV fluids and antiemetics to treat her condition at home. She is lying down but is still slightly pale. She is alert and oriented and complaining of nausea. Which of the following should be highest on your list of hypotheses about the cause of the patient's near-syncopal episode?
    a. Dehydration
    b. Pre-eclampsia
    c. Gestational diabetes
    d. Supine hypotensive syndrome

_____ 7. Stage one of labor is best described by which one of the following statements?
    a. From complete dilation of the cervix to birth of the baby
    b. Irregular, painless contractions that come and go during the last trimester
    c. From delivery of the infant to the delivery of the placenta
    d. The onset of regular contractions to the complete dilation of the cervix

_____ 8. You have responded to a call for a woman in labor. The patient is 37 weeks pregnant and states that this is her fourth child. She says contractions started about 90 minutes ago but she already feels the need to push. Contractions are intense and approximately 2-1/2 minutes apart. As you are getting this information from her, her water breaks. The fluid is clear. Which one of the following should be your greatest concern for complications?
    a. Precipitous delivery
    b. Uterine rupture
    c. Shoulder dystocia
    d. Prematurity of the infant

_____ 9. Which one of the following occurs in fetal circulation?
   a. Blood is shunted from the right ventricle directly to the left ventricle.
   b. The umbilical artery returns blood to the fetal circulation.
   c. Blood is shunted from the pulmonary artery to the aorta.
   d. Blood completely bypasses the fetal kidneys.

_____ 10. Which one of the following is within the range of the normal tidal volume of a newborn?
   a. 10 mL   c. 50 mL
   b. 20 mL   d. 75 mL

_____ 11. A 40-week pregnant patient is complaining about the onset of contractions approximately 2 hours ago. Contractions are regular and are about 8 minutes apart. She is a G2 P1. She denies the sensation of pressure in the pelvic floor. Which one of the following is the best action for the Advanced EMT to take?
   a. Prepare the patient for transport to the hospital of her choice.
   b. Auscultate fetal heart tones.
   c. Inspect the perineum for bulging or crowning.
   d. Prepare for on-scene delivery.

_____ 12. Your patient is 34 weeks pregnant and is complaining of a severe headache and blurred vision. She has edema of the face, hands, and feet. Which of the following signs should you most expect to find?
   a. Bright red, painless vaginal bleeding
   b. Blood pressure that is higher than normal
   c. Irregular pulse
   d. Elevated blood glucose level

_____ 13. A 37-year-old woman, G4, P2, Ab1, is 31 weeks pregnant. She presents with sharp, tearing abdominal pain. She denies vaginal bleeding. Which of the following treatment sequences is in the patient's best interest?
   a. Administer high-flow oxygen by nonrebreather mask, start a saline lock, and transport.
   b. Administer high-flow oxygen by nonrebreather mask, start two large-bore IVs, place the patient supine, and begin transport.
   c. Place the patient in Trendelenburg position, administer oxygen to maintain an SpO_2 of 95 percent or higher, begin transport, and start two large-bore IVs of isotonic crystalloid position.
   d. Place the patient in left lateral recumbent position, administer oxygen to maintain an SpO_2 of 95 percent or higher, begin transport, and start two large-bore IVs of isotonic crystalloid position.

_____ 14. You are assisting with a field delivery and the infant's head has delivered. The umbilical cord is wrapped around the infant's neck, but there is not enough slack in the cord to free it. You should:
   a. instruct the mother not to push and assist her in assuming the knee-chest position. Transport emergently.
   b. immediately clamp the cord in two places and cut it between the clamps.
   c. place your hand over the top of the infant's head to prevent delivery of the body.
   d. instruct the mother to pull her knees toward her chest as far as possible and push.

_____ 15. You have just delivered an infant and have clamped and cut the cord. One minute after birth, he has a pink head and trunk but blue extremities. He cried immediately after birth and is now quietly looking around. His arms and legs are flexed, his heart rate is 152 per minute, and there are no signs of respiratory distress. His respiratory rate is 42 per minute. Which one of the following most accurately represents his APGAR score?
   a. 10   c. 8
   b. 9   d. 7

_____16. Following the delivery of a normal newborn, the mother has approximately 700 mL of bleeding from the vagina. You should immediately:
   a. perform fundal massage.
   b. pack the vagina with sterile gauze.
   c. start two large-bore IVs of isotonic crystalloid and infuse a 1,000-mL bolus.
   d. apply traction to the umbilical cord to deliver the placenta.

_____17. You have arrived at a rural location about 40 minutes from the nearest hospital (a small county hospital) for a woman in labor. She is very upset because one of the baby's feet is protruding from her vagina. You should immediately:
   a. place your hand in the mother's vagina and provide an airway for the baby.
   b. place the mother in knee–chest position and transport by ground.
   c. request air medical transport.
   d. attempt to deliver the second foot.

_____18. In which of the following situations is there a definite need for at least some resuscitative measures?
   a. Baby born at 38 weeks gestation
   b. Baby cries at birth but then stops
   c. Baby is limp and does not have flexion of the extremities
   d. Baby has cyanosis of the hands and feet

_____19. Which one of the following is the most commonly needed resuscitative technique in newborns?
   a. Oxygen
   b. Chest compressions
   c. IV or IO access
   d. Drying, warming, and stimulating the baby

_____20. You should begin chest compressions on a newborn when which of the following occurs?
   a. Central cyanosis
   b. Heart rate below 60 per minute that does not increase with ventilations
   c. Respirations less than 30 per minute
   d. Pulse oximetry less than 90 percent

_____21. A newborn is in respiratory distress. His abdomen is sunken in appearance. Together, those findings are most consistent with:
   a. omphalocele.
   b. choanal atresia.
   c. congenital diaphragmatic hernia.
   d. myelomeningocele.

Clinical Reasoning

CASE STUDY: IT'S A GIRL!

You and your partner have been dispatched for a woman in labor. You arrive just in time to deliver a full-term baby girl.

1. What are the priorities of assessment and management of the newborn?

   _____

   _____

   _____

   _____

   _____

2. What are the priorities of assessment and management of the mother?

   _____

   _____

   _____

   _____

   _____

Project-Based Learning

In anticipation of your labor and delivery clinical rotation, so that you will be better informed and prepared, do some research to find out about some of the things you might encounter. Jot down the answers in your notebook or journal.

1. What are the indications for cesarean section?

2. What can you determine by external fetal monitoring?

3. How do you think the absence of fetal monitoring equipment affects decisions you might make about delivery in the field?

The EMS Professional in Practice

Many EMS providers are nervous about assisting with a newborn delivery. Why do you think that may be the case? What things can you do to decrease any anxiety you may have about the process? Jot down your thoughts in a notebook or journal for discussion in class or in your study group.

44 Pediatric Emergencies

Content Area

• Special Patient Populations

Advanced EMT Education Standard

• Applies a fundamental knowledge of growth, development, and aging and assessment findings to provide basic and selected advanced emergency care and transportation for a patient with special needs.

Summary of Objectives

44.1 Define key terms introduced in this chapter.

Knowing and being able to apply the key terms in each chapter is critical to understanding chapter concepts. Write the list of key terms. Then write the definition of each one in your own words. Check your understanding by confirming the definitions in the textbook glossary. Correct any misunderstandings. Create a study aid by writing each key term on the front of an index card and the definition on the back. Use the cards to quiz yourself or to have someone quiz you. The exercises under Vocabulary and Concept Review below will give you additional practice.

44.2 Discuss the leading reasons that pediatric patients require medical attention.

Acute illnesses, such as infectious diseases, and injury are the most frequent reasons children require medical attention.

44.3 Explain the special considerations in dealing with the caregiver of a sick or injured child.

It is important to both the child and the caregiver to be able to remain together during assessment and management. Consider both the child's needs and the emotional stress of the parents.

44.4 Describe the major anatomic, physiologic, and developmental characteristics of pediatric patients in each of the following age groups: infant, toddler, preschooler, school age, and adolescent.

Infants communicate through crying. Their systems are immature, and organs such as the liver are disproportionately large and less protected than in older children and adults. The head is disproportionally large, the airway is narrow and flexible, and dehydration occurs rapidly.

Toddlers and preschoolers still have relatively large heads for their sizes. They are prone to infectious diseases. Though most diseases are mild in immunized children, bronchiolitis can lead to severe respiratory distress. Airway obstruction is a concern in this age group. Strangers can provoke anxiety in this age group.

School-age children's physical proportions become more adult-like. Approval and acceptance are important. Reasoning skills remain relatively concrete. Children in this age group are beginning to develop an understanding of illness, loss, death, and dying. Modesty and the need for privacy are developing.

Adolescents are physically beginning to be similar to young adults. Immature judgment and the experimentation that emerges during identity development can lead to risky behaviors, including unsafe driving, use of tobacco, alcohol and drugs, and unsafe sexual behavior. Rates of depression and suicide increase in this age group.

44.5 Give examples of modifications of patient assessment and management techniques that increase the likelihood of cooperation by patients in each of the following age groups: infant, toddler, preschooler, school age, and adolescent.

- *Infant*: Allow the parent or caregiver to hold the child while you perform the assessment.
- *Toddler and preschooler*: Allow the child to see and touch the equipment you will be using, if appropriate, or demonstrate what you are going to do on a doll.
- *School age*: Respect modesty and keep the school-age child informed about what you are doing.
- *Adolescent*: Keep in mind the adolescent's possible reluctance to be forthcoming with relevant health information in the presence of family and peers.

44.6 Given a description of vital signs for pediatric patients of various ages, classify the values as normal or abnormal.

In general, the heart and respiratory rates are higher in infancy and gradually decrease toward adult levels in late adolescence. The blood pressure is lower in infancy and gradually increases into adolescence.

44.7 Use the pediatric assessment triangle to determine a pediatric patient's status.

The pediatric assessment triangle uses the patient's general appearance, work of breathing, and circulation to the skin to help you form a general impression of the seriousness of the patient's condition.

44.8 Recognize signs of respiratory distress, respiratory failure, and respiratory arrest in pediatric patients.

Abnormal airway noises, abnormal positioning (such as the tripod position), chest and neck muscle retractions, nasal flaring, abnormal respiratory rate or depth, cyanosis, and altered mental status are signs of respiratory distress and respiratory failure.

44.9 Describe the presentation and assessment-based prehospital management of the following conditions: altered mental status, anaphylaxis, apparent life-threatening emergencies (ALTE), asthma, bronchiolitis, cardiac arrest, complications of cystic fibrosis, congenital heart disease, croup, drowning, epiglottitis, fever, gastrointestinal disorders, meningitis, pneumonia, poisoning, seizures (including status epilepticus), shock, and sudden infant death syndrome (SIDS).

- *Altered mental status:* Use the AEIOU-TIPS mnemonic to search for possible causes. Treat reversible causes such as hypoxia, hypoventilation, hypoglycemia, hypothermia, and hypoperfusion.

- *Anaphylaxis:* Be alert to airway obstruction, bronchospasm, and hypoperfusion and treat with airway management, oxygenation, ventilation, intravenous fluids, and subcutaneous or intramuscular epinephrine.
- *Apparent life-threatening emergencies (ALTE):* Manage the patient's airway and ventilation and provide supplemental oxygen as needed. Be prepared to perform CPR if cardiac arrest occurs.
- *Asthma:* Treat with oxygenation and nebulized bronchodilators (albuterol). Assist ventilations as needed.
- *Bronchiolitis:* Treat wheezing with bronchodilators and administer oxygen as needed. Be prepared for respiratory failure and be ready to assist ventilations. Treat high fever with antipyretics if allowed by protocol and keep the patient dressed lightly.
- *Cardiac arrest:* Consider respiratory causes of cardiac arrest. Perform CPR according to the current American Heart Association Guidelines.
- *Complications of cystic fibrosis:* Respiratory complications are common. Provide oxygen as needed, and consider IV fluids and bronchodilators in consultation with medical direction.
- *Congenital heart disease:* The treatment is aimed at supported oxygenation and perfusion.
- *Croup:* Do not agitate the child with unnecessary assessments and procedures. Albuterol may be of some benefit if approved by medical direction.
- *Drowning:* Manage asphyxia with airway management, ventilation, and oxygenation. Perform CPR and defibrillate as needed. Consider hypothermia.
- *Epiglottitis:* Do not agitate the child with unnecessary assessments and procedures. Anticipate the need for advanced life support.
- *Fever:* Keep the patient dressed lightly, but do not let him become chilled. Administer antipyretics if approved by medical direction.
- *Gastrointestinal disorders:* Assess for dehydration. Start an IV or IO line if the patient is at risk for shock and hypoperfusion.
- *Meningitis:* Treatment is nonspecific and supportive in the prehospital setting. If bacterial meningitis is suspected, wear a mask to prevent exposure to respiratory droplets and follow up to learn if you were exposed to the disease.
- *Pneumonia:* Anticipate hypoxia and support the airway, ventilation, and oxygenation.
- *Poisoning:* Treat supportively to manage the airway, breathing, oxygenation, and circulation. Consult poison control or medical direction and provide the type of poison, amount, route of exposure, and time since exposure.
- *Seizures, including status epilepticus:* Prevent the patient from being injured. Manage the airway, breathing, and circulation. Request advanced life support to manage status epilepticus.
- *Shock:* Maintain the airway, ensure adequate ventilation and oxygenation, start an IV or IO line, and administer fluids according to the type of shock.
- *Sudden infant death syndrome (SIDS):* Perform CPR if indicated; if death is apparent, follow your protocols for contacting law enforcement.

44.10 Demonstrate emergency medical care techniques for pediatric patients including the following: airway management, CPR, fluid resuscitation, management of partial and complete foreign body airway obstruction, medication administration, oxygen administration, and ventilation.

Refer to the skill checklists at the end of this workbook chapter and at the end of Chapter 12 (Medication Administration), Chapter 16 (Airway Management, Ventilation, and Oxygenation), and Chapter 17 (Resuscitation: Managing Shock and Cardiac Arrest).

44.11 Describe special considerations in the scene size-up in suspected SIDS.

Observe the child's environment, location, and position; what clothing he is wearing; objects in the environment; condition of the residence; and others at the scene.

44.12 **Describe special considerations in assisting family members in suspected SIDS.**

Do not treat the parents as if they are at fault in the patient's death. Be careful how you form your questions to avoid implying blame. Do not misinterpret normal signs of death, such as livor mortis or frothy, potentially pink-tinged discharge from the mouth or nose, as signs of abuse. In cases of pediatric resuscitation, allow parents to be in attendance if possible.

44.13 **Describe the importance of the presence of parents during pediatric resuscitation.**

The parents have a strong need to be with their child and to be kept informed about what is happening. In the event that the patient does not survive, the parents are helped to realize that everything that could be done for the child was done.

44.14 **Integrate consideration of a pediatric patient's size and anatomy into the assessment of mechanism of injury.**

The child's proportionally larger and heavier head changes the child's movement in response to impact. The neck is weak for the size of the head, so acceleration of the head away from the body can result in distraction injury of the spine. The abdominal organs are less protected by the ribs and musculature. The bones are more flexible, making fracture less likely despite injury to the organs and tissues surrounding them.

44.15 **Demonstrate removal of a pediatric patient from a child car seat.**

The child is removed using manual restriction of spinal motion. Once a child car seat has been involved in a collision, it is no longer a safe device for transporting the child.

44.16 **Demonstrate proper spinal immobilization of a pediatric patient.**

Use pediatric-size equipment. Pad beneath the shoulders to maintain neutral alignment of the neck and airway.

44.17 **Explain the importance of injury prevention programs to reduce pediatric injuries and deaths.**

Injuries are the leading cause of death in children. The majority of deaths and injuries can be prevented.

44.18 **Recognize indications of child abuse and neglect.**

Among the possible indications are a history of the injury that does not explain the injuries the child has, multiple injuries in various stages of healing, and specific injuries such as "stocking foot" burns, cigarette burns, and injuries that reflect the pattern of a possible weapon such as a handprint or belt buckle impression.

44.19 **Explain special considerations in managing situations in which you suspect child abuse or neglect.**

Do not make accusations, document objectively, and contact law enforcement or make a report according to your protocols.

44.20 **Discuss ways in which you can manage the stress that can be associated with pediatric calls, both during and after the call.**

Being knowledgeable about pediatric emergencies, practicing the application of your skills in lab, and being comfortable with children are all steps in reducing stress prior to pediatric calls. Acknowledge your feelings but temporarily put them aside in order to provide the best care possible to the patient, with the understanding that you will examine the feelings at an appropriate time. Recognize signs of acute stress reaction, cumulative stress, and post-traumatic stress disorder.

Resource Central

Resource Central offers extra practice and review materials in a variety of media. To access it, follow the directions on the Student Access Card provided with the Student Textbook. If there is no card, go to www.bradybooks.com and follow the Resource Central link to Buy Access.

Vocabulary and Concept Review

Exercise 1

Complete each of the following sentences with the correct term. (See Resource Central for more vocabulary review.)

1. An infant's episode that involves some combination of gagging or choking, apnea, change in muscle tone and color change, and which is frightening to the observer is called a(n) _____.

2. A viral illness that results in inflammation and sloughing of the bronchiolar lining and that can lead to respiratory distress in the pediatric population is called _____.

3. _____ is a genetic disease that results in production of thick, viscous mucus and affects the pancreas and lungs.

4. A seizure that occurs in the pediatric population and is caused by a sudden increase in body temperature associated with illness is called a _____ seizure.

5. _____ is an increase in cerebrospinal fluid within the ventricles of the brain due to an imbalance between CSF production and drainage or absorption.

6. The scheme for forming a general impression of the level of distress in a child by evaluating the general appearance, work of breathing, and circulation to the skin is called the _____.

7. Whooping cough is also called _____.

8. One of the primary causes of bronchiolitis is _____

9. The unexpected, unexplained death of an infant younger than 12 months old is classified as _____.

Exercise 2

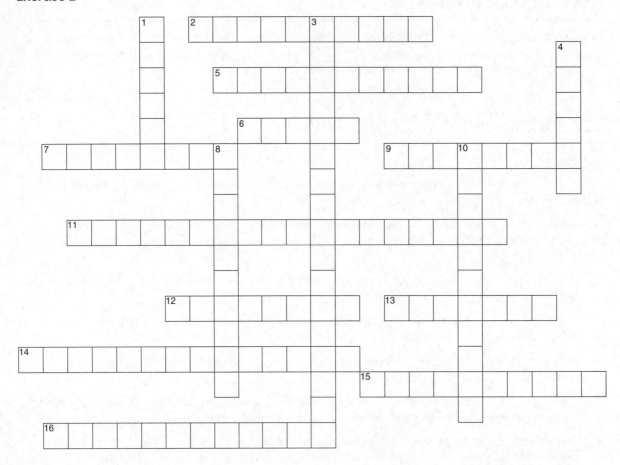

Across

2. Teenager.
5. Pulling in of the tissues above the clavicies and between the ribs; an indication of respiratory distress.
6. Laryngotracheobronchitis.
7. Cause of cardiac arrest and death in drowning.
9. This form of stored energy is limited in the muscles and live of a child, meaning fatigue and deterioration can occur quickly in illness or injury.
11. Condition that should be suspected when the pediatric patient's capillary refill time is greater than 4 seconds.
12. Pulse checked in infants.
13. Child from one to three years old.
14. Cardiac arrest due to a blow to the chest.
15. May be viral or bacterial; inflammation of the lining around the central nervous system structures.
16. Access route for fluid replacement and medication administration in a pediatric patient when an IV cannot be obtained.

Down

1. How oxygen is administered to a child who needs it but does not tolerate a nasal cannula or mask.
3. Severe, prolonged asthma attack that cannot be broken with nebulized beta$_2$ agonists.
4. Child from one month to one year of age.
8. Component of the pediatric assessment triangle determined by the muscle tone, interactiveness, consolability, eye contact, and speech or cry of the patient.
10. Narrowest portion of the infant airway.

Patient Assessment Review

Exercise 1

Write findings in a history and assessment that should make you suspect the pediatric patient is dehydrated.

_____

_____

_____

_____

_____

_____

Exercise 2

Write indications at a scene and in a history and assessment that should make you suspicious of the possibility of child abuse.

_____

_____

_____

_____

_____

_____

Check Your Recall and Apply Concepts

Exercise 1

Select the best possible choice for each of the following questions.

_____ 1. The most common cause of cardiac arrest in pediatric patients is:
a. congenital heart defects.
b. respiratory failure and arrest.
c. traumatic brain injury.
d. febrile seizures.

_____ 2. Which one of the following is an anatomic difference in infants that can affect the ability to compensate, patterns of injury, assessment, or management?
a. The abdominal wall is thin and has less muscle and fat.
b. The ribs are brittle and easily fractured.
c. The airway is short and wide, compared to that of adults.
d. Children have substantial muscle and liver glycogen stores.

_____ 3. A pediatric patient who is challenging of authority, has a sense of invulnerability, and is prone to risky behaviors is most likely to be in the _____ age group.
a. toddler
b. preschooler
c. school-age
d. adolescent

_____ 4. Which one of the following should result in a poor general impression of a pediatric patient when the pediatric assessment triangle is used?
  a. The child maintains eye contact with you.
  b. A lack of nasal flaring with respirations.
  c. The child cries inconsolably.
  d. Flexion of the extremities and ability to hold up the head.

_____ 5. You have arrived on the scene of a reported sick person. You find a school-age child lying in bed. He is unresponsive and does not appear to be breathing normally. Your first action should be to:
  a. look, listen, and feel for breathing.
  b. insert an oral airway and begin ventilations by bag-valve-mask device.
  c. check a carotid pulse.
  d. call for law enforcement.

_____ 6. While assessing a sick infant, you notice that his anterior fontanel is depressed. With which of the following conditions is this finding associated?
  a. Dehydration   c. Meningitis
  b. Traumatic brain injury   d. Hydrocephalus

_____ 7. Which one of the following is an infectious disease that is increasing in incidence among pediatric patients?
  a. Epiglottitis   c. Pertussis
  b. Croup   d. Cystic fibrosis

_____ 8. Which one of the following is the LEAST likely cause of cardiac arrest in an adolescent?
  a. Commotio cordis   c. Left ventricular hypertrophy
  b. Coronary artery disease   d. Cardiac conduction abnormality

_____ 9. The peak incidence of SIDS is in infants aged _____ months.
  a. 8 to 12   c. 5 to 7
  b. 6 to 8   d. 2 to 4

_____ 10. A two-month-old infant turned blue, stopped breathing, became limp, and seemed to be choking, but recovered before you arrived on the scene. This description is most consistent with:
  a. SIDS.   c. status asthmaticus.
  b. foreign body airway obstruction.   d. ALTE.

_____ 11. The triad of sensitivity to light, headache, and stiff neck, particularly when accompanied by fever, are highly suspicious for:
  a. meningitis.   c. hydrocephalus.
  b. febrile seizure.   d. hyperglycemia.

_____ 12. Normal capillary refill time in a pediatric patient is _____ second(s).
  a. more than 4
  b. 2 to 4
  c. less than 2
  d. 1

_____ 13. When shock is suspected in a pediatric patient, you should consider an initial fluid bolus of _____ mL/kg.
  a. 10   c. 50
  b. 20   d. 75

_____ 14. Which one of the following groups has an increased incidence of drowning compared to other pediatric groups?
  a. Toddlers   c. School-age boys
  b. Infants   d. Adolescent girls

_____ 15. A 14-year-old girl was witnessed by her friends to become distressed while swimming and become submerged. As you arrive on the scene, bystanders have recovered the patient and are with her in about 4 feet of water. She is unresponsive and does not appear to be breathing. Which one of the following is the best approach to treatment for this patient?
   a. Immediately remove her from the water, check for a carotid pulse, and if the patient is pulseless, begin chest compressions.
   b. Float a long backboard under the patient while maintaining manual spinal motion restriction, apply a cervical collar, open the airway with a modified jaw-thrust maneuver, and begin ventilations before removing the patient from the water.
   c. Begin rescue breathing in the water, using a modified jaw-thrust maneuver to open the airway, use a long backboard to remove the patient from the water, check for a carotid pulse and, if the patient is pulseless, begin CPR.
   d. Begin chest compressions in the water, and apply an AED as soon as the patient is removed from the water.

Exercise 2

Fill in the following table to show the normal vital signs of pediatric patients in different age groups.

Age Group	Respiratory Rate (per minute)	Heart Rate (per minute)	Systolic Blood Pressure in mmHg	Temperature in °F
Newborn				
Infant				
Toddler				
Preschooler				
School age				
Adolescent				

Clinical Reasoning

CASE STUDY: CHILD WITH DIFFICULTY BREATHING

You and your partner are dispatched at 2330 hours for a 22-month-old female patient with difficulty breathing. When you arrive, the parents are holding the child, who has inspiratory stridor and a cough that sounds like barking. The parents tell you that the child seemed to have a cold when she woke up in the morning. After she had been asleep in bed for about 2-1/2 hours, she woke up with the cough, which seems to be getting worse.

1. What are some illnesses that could explain the child's presentation?

_____

_____

_____

_____

2. Explain what factors would make you lean more toward one hypothesis than another.

_____

_____

_____

_____

_____

3. What treatment should you implement?

_____

_____

_____

_____

_____

Project-Based Learning

During your clinical and field rotations, observe other health care providers' interactions with pediatric patients of different ages. What techniques seem more effective? What techniques seem less effective? Jot down your thoughts in your notebook or journal. Select one of the more effective methods and write a goal for trying it out when the next opportunity arises.

The EMS Professional in Practice

Because EMS providers care for children less often than they care for adult patients, it can be more difficult to remain knowledgeable and proficient about their care. Take an inventory of your knowledge and skills about pediatric patients. Use the results to identify goals for continuing professional development to help you learn more about pediatric patients.

Skills Checklists

The following skill checklists cover the major steps of selected skills from Chapter 44. Review them prior to your laboratory classes. Practice skills only after they have been demonstrated for you in class and only under the supervision of an authorized instructor or clinical preceptor.

Advanced EMT Skill Checklist: *Infant CPR*		
Skill Stimulus: An infant is apparently unresponsive and not breathing or not breathing normally.		
Step	Performed	Not Performed
If you are off duty and alone, perform 2 minutes of CPR before calling 911. If someone else is present, designate a person to call 911 and to retrieve an AED if you are in a facility with a public access defibrillation program.		
Check for a brachial pulse.		
If no pulse is detected within 10 seconds or the pulse is below 60 per minute and the patient has poor perfusion, and an AED is not immediately available, perform 30 chest compressions. Use two fingers over the sternum just below the intermammary line, or encircle the chest with the hands and place your thumbs over the sternum.		
If an AED is immediately available, apply the pads, clear all contact with the patient, and turn on the machine.		
If an AED is not immediately available, open the airway and deliver 2 ventilations. (If you are off duty and do not have the proper equipment, you may perform hands-only CPR.)		
If a defibrillator is not available or following defibrillation, perform CPR with a ratio of chest compressions to ventilations of 30:2 at a compression rate of at least 100 per minute. If two rescuers are present, the ratio is 15:2.		
Keep interruptions in compressions to a minimum.		
Periodically check for return of spontaneous circulation.		
Skill Completion: Patient has return of spontaneous circulation or resuscitative efforts are terminated by physician order.		

Advanced EMT Skill Checklist: *Child CPR*

Skill Stimulus: A child patient is apparently unresponsive and not breathing or not breathing normally.

Step	Performed	Not Performed
If you are off duty and alone, perform 2 minutes of CPR before calling 911. If someone else is present, designate a person to call 911 and to retrieve an AED if you are in a facility with a public access defibrillation program.		
Check for a carotid pulse.		
If no pulse is detected within 10 seconds or the pulse is less than 60 per minute and the patient has poor perfusion, and an AED is not immediately available, perform 30 chest compressions.		
Use one or two hands (depending on the size of the child) over the lower half of the sternum. Depress the chest 2 inches or one third of the anterior–posterior dimension of the chest. Allow complete recoil of the chest between compressions.		
If an AED is immediately available, apply the pads, clear all contact with the patient, and turn on the machine.		
If an AED is not immediately available, open the airway and deliver 2 ventilations. (If you are off duty and do not have the proper equipment, you may perform hands-only CPR.)		
If a defibrillator is not available or following defibrillation, perform CPR with a ratio of chest compressions to ventilations of 30:2 at a compression rate of at least 100 per minute. If two rescuers are performing CPR, the ratio is 15:2.		
Keep interruptions in compressions to a minimum.		
Periodically check for return of spontaneous circulation.		
Skill Completion: Patient has return of spontaneous circulation or resuscitative efforts are terminated by physician order.		

Advanced EMT Skill Checklist: *Relieving Foreign Body Airway Obstruction—Conscious Infant*

Skill Stimulus: A conscious infant patient exhibits signs of complete foreign body airway obstruction, such as sudden inability to speak, cough, or breathe; or severe partial airway obstruction with inadequate breathing.

Step	Performed	Not Performed
Place the patient prone along your forearm so that you are supporting the upper chest with your hand and the patient's legs are straddling your arm. The patient's head should be slightly lower than his body.		
Perform five back blows.		
Sandwich the patient by placing your other arm over his back, supporting the head with your hand and turn him prone while supporting him with the arm placed on his back.		
Perform five chest thrusts.		
Repeat the series of five back blows and five chest thrusts until the obstruction is relieved or the patient becomes unresponsive.		
Skill Completion: Airway obstruction is relieved or the patient becomes unresponsive.		

Advanced EMT Skill Checklist: *Relieving Foreign Body Airway Obstruction—Unresponsive Infant*

Skill Stimulus: An unresponsive infant exhibits signs of complete foreign body airway obstruction, such as apnea and inability to provide artificial ventilation despite manual airway maneuvers; and there is no history that would indicate another cause of obstruction, such as edema from anaphylaxis or airway burns.

Step	Performed	Not Performed
Cradle the infant in a football hold or lay him supine on a firm surface.		
Perform 30 chest thrusts.		
Open the airway in preparation for delivering ventilations and inspect for the presence of the foreign body in the mouth.		
If a foreign body is seen, remove it with a finger sweep.		
Attempt 2 ventilations.		
Continue the cycle of 30 chest compressions to 2 ventilations.		

Skill Completion: The airway obstruction has been relieved as evidenced by the ability to deliver ventilations, or advanced life support personnel are available to use additional measures to establish an airway and ventilation.

Advanced EMT Skill Checklist: *Relieving Complete Foreign Body Airway Obstruction—Conscious Adult or Child*

Skill Stimulus: A conscious adult or child patient exhibits signs of complete foreign body airway obstruction, such as the universal choking sign (grasps the throat with both hands) and sudden inability to speak, cough, or breathe; or severe partial airway obstruction with inadequate breathing.

Step	Performed	Not Performed
Stand behind the patient and reach around him with both arms.		
Place the thumb side of one fist against the patient's abdomen below the diaphragm. Cup your other hand over your fist.		
Deliver a series of firm inward, upward thrusts.		
Continue until the obstruction is relieved or the patient becomes unresponsive.		

Skill Completion: Obstruction is relieved or the patient becomes unresponsive.

Advanced EMT Skill Checklist: *Relieving Foreign Body Airway Obstruction—Unresponsive Adult or Child*

Skill Stimulus: An unresponsive adult or child patient exhibits signs of complete foreign body airway obstruction, such as apnea and inability to provide artificial ventilation despite manual airway maneuvers; and there is no history that would indicate another cause of obstruction, such as edema from anaphylaxis or airway burns.

Step	Performed	Not Performed
Place the patient supine on a firm surface.		
Perform 30 chest compressions.		
Open the airway in preparation for delivering ventilations and inspect for the presence of the foreign body in the mouth.		
If the foreign body is seen, remove it with a finger sweep.		
Attempt to deliver 2 ventilations.		
Continue a cycle of 30 chest compressions to 2 ventilations.		

Skill Completion: The airway obstruction has been relieved as evidenced by the ability to deliver ventilations, or advanced life support personnel are available to use additional measures to establish an airway and ventilation.

Advanced EMT Skill Checklist: *Pediatric Intraosseous Access (EZ IO)*

Skill Stimulus: An IV order is received (standing order or online medical direction); Six Rights of Medication Administration have been confirmed.

Step	Performed	Not Performed
Collect all equipment and supplies needed for the procedure.		
Set up an IV fluid infusion.		
Prefill the extension tubing with saline and leave the syringe attached.		
Locate the insertion site on the anteriomedial tibia, two fingerbreadths below the tibial tuberosity.		
Select the proper needle length for the patient.		
Prepare the site using a povidone-iodine swab.		
Place the needle on the driver.		
Hold the driver at a 90 degree angle to the leg and depress the trigger mechanism to drill the needle into the bone.		
Remove the stylet (guide) from the needle.		
Attach the prefilled extension tubing and flush with saline. Observe for free-flow of fluid and absence of infiltration.		
Attach the IV tubing to the extension tubing and adjust the flow rate.		
Secure the needle and tubing to the leg. Complete and attach the information band.		

Skill Completion: The IO line is patent and secure, the drip is adjusted correctly, and the patient is being monitored.

45

Geriatrics

Content Area

- Special Patient Populations

Advanced EMT Education Standard

- Applies a fundamental knowledge of growth, development, and aging and assessment findings to provide basic and selected advanced emergency care and transportation for a patient with special needs.

Summary of Objectives

45.1 Define key terms introduced in this chapter.

Knowing and being able to apply the key terms in each chapter is critical to understanding chapter concepts. Write the list of key terms. Then write the definition of each one in your own words. Check your understanding by confirming the definitions in the textbook glossary. Correct any misunderstandings. Create a study aid by writing each key term on the front of an index card and the definition on the back. Use the cards to quiz yourself or to have someone quiz you. The exercises under Vocabulary and Concept Review below will give you additional practice.

45.2 Summarize age-related anatomic and physiologic changes for each of the following systems: cardiovascular, endocrine, gastrointestinal, integumentary, musculoskeletal, nervous and sensory, renal, and respiratory.

- *Cardiovascular:* Atherosclerosis develops, changes in cardiac conduction system occur, hypertension occurs, and the risk of stroke, heart attack, dysrhythmia, and heart failure increase. Diminished cardiac output and decreased maximum heart rate occur.
- *Endocrine:* There is decreased homeostatic regulation and decreased glucose regulation and thyroid function.
- *Gastrointestinal:* There is decreased gastrointestinal motility and decreased absorption of nutrients.
- *Integumentary:* Skin thins and becomes more fragile and less pigmented.

- *Musculoskeletal:* Muscle and bone mass decrease, and there is an increased risk of weakness, osteoporosis, and fractures and falls.
- *Nervous and sensory:* Decreases in vision, hearing, taste, smell, and proprioception occur. There is decreased reaction time and slower cognitive processing.
- *Renal:* Glomerular filtration rate decreases and there is decreased efficiency in eliminating drugs and wastes.
- *Respiratory:* Diminished cough and gag reflexes, decreased elasticity of chest wall, decreased ciliary function, and decrease gas exchange occur.

45.3 Relate the anatomic and physiologic changes associated with aging to anticipated differences in complaints and assessment findings for geriatric patients.

Complaints of pain may be more vague, and altered mental status may occur as a sign in illnesses such as pneumonia and myocardial infarction. The patient may attribute pain and decreased function to aging instead of to disease and may not recognize the seriousness of the problem. Patients may not have a fever despite the presence of serious infection.

45.4 Discuss the presentation, assessment, and management of common medical emergencies in the elderly population, including the following: altered mental status; congestive heart failure; COPD; delirium and dementia, including Alzheimer's disease; drug toxicity; environmental emergencies; gastrointestinal problems; HHNC; myocardial infarction; pneumonia; pulmonary embolism; seizures; stroke and TIA; and syncope

In many ways, these illnesses present in the elderly much as they do in younger patients. In some cases, however, complaints may be vague and the history more difficult to determine. Always suspect the potential for serious illness despite vague or multiple complaints, and keep in mind the effects of decreased efficiency of homeostatic mechanisms, such as thermoregulation. Suspect drug toxicity or interactions as an underlying cause of problems such as hypotension and altered mental status. Never assume that altered mental status is "normal" for a patient. In treatment, keep in mind that drugs may not be cleared as quickly by the liver and kidneys and that fluid overload can easily occur.

45.5 Describe the elderly patient's altered response to trauma.

The cardiovascular and respiratory systems are less able to compensate for blood loss, hypoxia, and injury. Typical signs and symptoms of shock, such as cool, diaphoretic skin and tachycardia, may not always be present despite blood loss. Blood clotting mechanisms can be impaired, resulting in more serious hemorrhage.

45.6 Recognize signs and risk factors of elder abuse.

Patient factors include age 80 or older, female, physically or financially dependent on others, immobile, incontinent, dementia, sleep disturbances, and multiple medical problems. Signs and symptoms include a fearful patient, a history that does not match injuries, unexplained injuries, and injuries with a specific pattern, such as bite marks and cigarette burns. Neglect can be indicated by inadequate shelter, food, access to medical care, and hygiene. Abuse also may be of a sexual or financial nature.

45.7 Describe modifications that may be necessary to effectively assess and treat geriatric patients.

You may need to compensate for the patient's difficulty in seeing or hearing, move more slowly, exercise patience, and work with multiple layers of clothing.

Resource Central

Resource Central offers extra practice and review materials in a variety of media. To access it, follow the directions on the Student Access Card provided with the Student Textbook. If there is no card, go to www.bradybooks.com and follow the Resource Central link to Buy Access.

Vocabulary and Concept Review

Exercise 1

Write the term from the vocabulary list next to the statement that best describes it. (See Resource Central for more vocabulary review.)

Alzheimer's disease	confabulation
decubitus ulcer	delirium
incontinence	life span
pathologic fracture	spondylosis

1. An acute state of confusion and agitation due to an underlying medical cause.

   _____

2. Loss of ability to control bowel or bladder function.

   _____

3. Maximum biologically determined amount of time human beings could live under ideal conditions.

   _____

4. A false memory that fills a gap in recall.

   _____

5. A form of arthritis that affects the vertebrae and intervertebral disks, especially in the elderly.

   _____

6. A break that occurs with minimal force in a diseased or weakened bone.

   _____

7. A common form of dementia in which there is a progressive loss of cognitive function.

   _____

8. A pressure sore or bed sore.

   _____

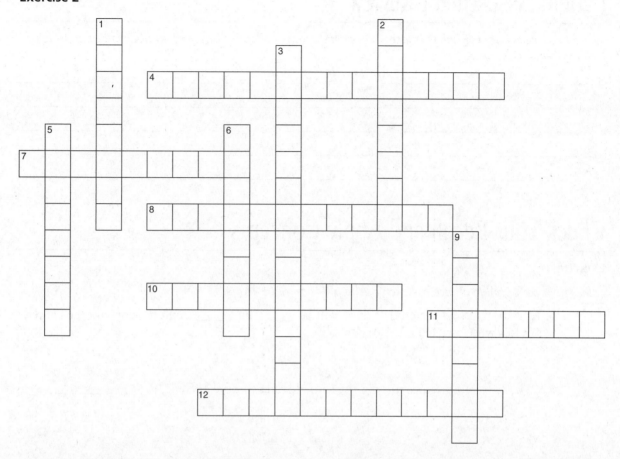

Across

4. Ability to sense the location, orientation, and movement of the body and its parts.

7. Cessation of menstruation.

8. Loss of bone density.

10. Branch of medicine that specializes in treating elderly patients.

11. Person with whom you should first attempt to communicate when responding to a call for an elderly person.

12. Use of multiple medications.

Down

1. Increase in birth rate following World War II.

2. Abnormal curvature of the upper spine.

3. Statistical calculation of the length of time a person can anticipate living based on year of birth and other factors.

5. Program that funds medical care for eligible low-income families and individuals.

6. Progressive, irreversible loss of cognitive function.

9. Clouding of the lens of the eye.

Patient Assessment Review

Write how assessment findings in acute coronary syndrome could differ in an older adult compared to a middle-aged adult.

_____

_____

_____

_____

_____

Check Your Recall and Apply Concepts

Exercise 1

Select the best possible choice for each of the following questions.

_____ 1. By 2015, it is expected that there will be _____ million people in the United States who are aged 65 years and older.
   a. 37
   b. 47
   c. 64
   d. 79

_____ 2. The current life expectancy in the United States, on the average, is _____ years.
   a. 65.4
   b. 77.9
   c. 91
   d. 120

_____ 3. A common age-related change in vision is the loss of ability to see:
   a. distant objects.
   b. in the daylight.
   c. brightly colored objects.
   d. close-up objects.

_____ 4. Which one of the following can make airway management more challenging in the elderly patient?
   a. The airway is short and narrow.
   b. The trachea is flexible and collapses easily.
   c. There is exaggerated curvature of the thoracic spine.
   d. There is increased sensitivity of the gag reflex.

_____ 5. Which one of the following conditions increases the risk of aspiration and foreign body airway obstruction in elderly patients?
   a. Difficulty swallowing
   b. Increased sensitivity of the gag reflex
   c. Hypersensitive cough reflex
   d. Increased salivation

_____ 6. In an elderly patient, a sudden onset of confusion and agitation is generally an indication of:
   a. Alzheimer's disease.
   b. dementia.
   c. delirium.
   d. Wernicke-Korsakoff syndrome.

_____ 7. An elderly patient may be considered oriented to time if he is able to tell you what _____ it is.
   a. hour of the day
   b. day of the week
   c. month
   d. year

_____ 8. Which one of the following conditions should make you maintain a high index of suspicion for acute myocardial infarction in an elderly patient?
   a. Pain in the calf of the leg
   b. High fever
   c. Rhonchi and wheezing in the lungs
   d. Epigastric discomfort described as "indigestion"

_____ 9. A 79-year-old woman presents with a 4-hour history of progressive dyspnea. She is anxious and you can hear crackles (rales) in her lungs without the aid of a stethoscope. She has a cough that is productive of frothy, pink-tinged sputum. Her son tells you that she has been feeling tired for 3 days. Her heart rate is 84 and irregular, respirations are 24 and labored, blood pressure is 182/98, and SpO_2 is 83 percent on room air. Which one of the following interventions would be most beneficial in the prehospital care of this patient?
   a. CPAP
   b. Oxygen by nasal cannula
   c. IV of normal saline at 50 mL/hour
   d. 162 mg of chewable aspirin

_____ 10. A 68-year-old woman presents with a complaint of chest pressure and nausea. She is slightly short of breath and has diaphoretic skin. She states that the pain began while she was getting out of the car from getting groceries about 30 minutes ago and has not stopped since. She is alert with a radial pulse that is regular at a rate of 72 per minute, a respiratory rate of 20, blood pressure of 142/90, and SpO_2 of 96 percent on room air. Which of the following actions should you take first?
   a. Begin immediate transport.
   b. Give 162 mg of chewable aspirin.
   c. Give two 0.4-mg nitroglycerin tablets sublingally.
   d. Start an IV of normal saline at a keep-open rate.

_____ 11. A 70-year-old man in generally good health presents with near syncope and a chief complaint of "burning, tearing pain in his lower back." He is pale, with cool, diaphoretic skin. His radial pulse is weak and thready at 122 per minute, his respirations are 24 per minute, blood pressure is 84 by palpation, and SpO_2 on room air is 93 percent. His lower extremities are cold and mottled. Which one of the following is most consistent with those findings?
   a. Acute myocardial infarction
   b. Septic shock
   c. Aortic dissection
   d. Pulmonary embolism

_____ 12. A disease related to degeneration of dopamine-producing cells in the brain that is more common in patients over the age of 50 and results in postural rigidity, tremors, and loss of facial expression is:
   a. Parkinson's disease.
   b. Alzheimer's disease.
   c. transient ischemic attack (TIA).
   d. Bell's palsy.

_____ 13. A 70-year-old woman with a history of type 2 diabetes presents with a decreased level of responsiveness 2 days after being released from the hospital for surgery on her hip. She responds to painful stimuli and has hot, dry skin with poor turgor. Her breath sounds are clear and equal, and her abdomen is soft. Her heart rate is 116, respirations are 16, blood pressure is 108/76, SpO_2 is 97 percent on room air, and blood glucose level is 810 mg/dL. Which one of the following interventions is most indicated for this patient?
   a. 25 grams 50 percent dextrose, IV
   b. 1 mg glucagon, IM
   c. 15 L/min of oxygen by nonrebreather mask
   d. 1,000 mL of normal saline, IV bolus

_____ 14. An 86-year-old female nursing home resident, with a past history of stroke resulting in paralysis of the left side and speech impairment, presents with a new onset of altered mental status. She opens her eyes to your voice, her skin is mottled and cool, bilateral breath sounds have crackles (rales) bilaterally in the bases, and she has a Foley catheter in place. There is about 450 mL of slightly cloudy, dark urine in the collection bag. Her heart rate is 118, respirations are 20, blood pressure is 72 by palpation, SpO_2 is 88 percent on room air, and blood glucose level is 124 mg/dL. The nursing home staff states the patient is usually alert, although she suffers from mild Alzheimer's disease. The patient has gradually become less responsive over the past 6 hours. The patient has no other significant past medical history. Which one of the following conditions is most consistent with the patient's presentation?

    a. Hyperthermia
                         c. Myxedema coma
    b. Septic shock
                           d. Hyperglycemic nonketotic coma

Exercise 2

Place a "T" next to each statement that is true and an "F" next to each statement that is false. If the statement is false, rewrite it so that it is correct.

1. _____ An irregular pulse is a common finding in elderly patients.

   _____

2. _____ Crackles (rales) heard on auscultation of the lungs can be a normal finding in elderly patients.

   _____

3. _____ Elderly patients should be considered an unreliable source of information.

   _____

4. _____ Pneumonia is rarely a cause of death in the elderly.

   _____

5. _____ Pneumonia can be ruled out in the elderly patient who does not have a fever.

   _____

6. _____ Atrial fibrillation is a risk factor for pulmonary embolism in the elderly.

   _____

7. _____ Hypoglycemia is a common cause of syncope in the elderly.

   _____

8. _____ Vertigo is a sensation of tumbling or spinning, or moving through space even though stationary.

   _____

9. _____ Abdominal pain must be considered a serious complaint in the elderly patient.

   _____

10. _____ Hot tap water can cause severe burns in elderly patients.

   _____

Clinical Reasoning

CASE STUDY: ELDERLY PATIENT WITH DIFFICULTY BREATHING

A 91-year-old man presents with dyspnea and an altered mental status. He lives at home with his wife. He has a history of heart failure, hypertension, vertigo, renal failure, and bowel incontinence and takes several medications. His wife states that he normally is aware of his surroundings and knows what is going on, and though he is weak, uses a walker to get around the house. For the past 12 hours the patient has been lethargic, nauseated, and growing more confused and short of breath. He opens his eyes to your voice but cannot give answers to your questions. He tries to pull away from you when you attempt to check his pulse.

1. What are your initial hypotheses?

   _____

   _____

   _____

   _____

   _____

2. How will you narrow your hypotheses to a shorter list of differential diagnoses?

   _____

   _____

   _____

   _____

   _____

3. What initial treatments should you consider, and why is each one indicated?

   _____

   _____

   _____

   _____

   _____

Project-Based Learning

To help you prepare to care for geriatric patients in your practice as an Advanced EMT, check with your instructor to arrange a clinical rotation in an extended care facility (nursing home) or senior citizen's center. Write a journal entry to describe your experience, listing at least three things that you would not have realized if you had not participated in the clinical rotation.

The EMS Professional in Practice

What if your boss is 70 years old? How would you view him compared to a younger person in the same position? Would you feel he is less competent or more competent than a younger person? Would you be as likely to approach your boss with the same types of issues as you would if he was younger? Jot down your thoughts in a notebook or journal for discussion in class or in your study group.

Chapter 46

Patients with Special Challenges

Content Area

• Special Patient Populations

Advanced EMT Education Standard

• The Advanced EMT applies a fundamental knowledge of growth, development, and aging and assessment findings to provide basic and selected advanced emergency care and transportation for a patient with special needs.

Summary of Objectives

46.1 Define key terms introduced in this chapter.

Knowing and being able to apply the key terms in each chapter is critical to understanding chapter concepts. Write the list of key terms. Then write the definition of each one in your own words. Check your understanding by confirming the definitions in the textbook glossary. Correct any misunderstandings. Create a study aid by writing each key term on the front of an index card and the definition on the back. Use the cards to quiz yourself, or to have someone quiz you. The exercises under Vocabulary and Concept Review below will give you additional practice.

46.2 Explain the importance of understanding the care of patients with special challenges.

Patients with special challenges may experience medical emergencies that are related to their special challenges, requiring you to be familiar with their particular needs.

46.3 Demonstrate empathy and respect when dealing with patients with special challenges.

Treat patients with special challenges and their caregivers with the same empathy and respect as you do all other patients.

46.4 Advocate for the empathetic treatment of patients with a variety of special challenges.

Set a positive example for the empathetic treatment of patients with special challenges and hold your peers to the same level of treatment.

46.5 Give examples of special challenges.

Special challenges include poverty and homelessness, obesity, deafness, blindness, being dependent on a ventilator, and a variety of developmental and physical disabilities.

46.6 Describe the special physiologic, medical, and psychosocial concerns, and accommodations and modifications to patient assessment and management that are required when caring for patients with each of the following types of challenges: abused patients; bariatric patients; brain-injured patients; dialysis patients; homeless/impoverished patients; patients with mental, emotional, or developmental impairments; paralyzed patients; patients with gastrointestinal and genitourinary devices; patients with intraventricular shunts; patients with sensory impairments; technology-dependent patients; and terminally ill patients.

- *Abused patients:* Be aware of indications of possible abuse; do not confront the suspected abuser; make every effort to transport the patient for care; document the scene, the physical examination, and statements of the patient; document who else was present at the scene, their demeanor, and how you reported your suspicions.
- *Bariatric patients:* Pay particular attention to airway and breathing, especially if the patient must be placed in a supine position. Use equipment designed for bariatric patients to prevent injury to yourself and the patient.
- *Brain-injured patients:* These patients may have a variety of disabilities, both cognitive and physical, that affect your assessment and management.
- *Dialysis patients:* Be aware of complications of the dialysis access site and the potential for complications from dialysis, or from missing scheduled dialysis.
- *Homeless/impoverished patients:* These patients' overall health status may be poor, decreasing the ability to compensate for illness and injury.
- *Mental, emotional, or developmental impairments:* Treat the patient with respect and dignity. Interact with the patient first, when possible, rather than the caregivers, to obtain the history. Anticipate a decreased ability to give a specific chief complaint and elaborate on it.
- *Paralyzed patients:* Needs depend on the type of paralysis, whether it involves hemiplegia, paraplegia, or quadriplegia. Needs may range from needing assistance with mobility to needing assistance with ventilation.
- *Patients with gastrointestinal and genitourinary devices:* Use care to avoid dislodging the devices. If the device is malfunctioning or has become dislodged, transport the patient for further care of the device. Keep in mind that the patient and caregiver are very knowledgeable about the device and its management.
- *Patients with intraventricular shunts:* Be alert to the possibility of increased intracranial pressure if the shunt is not functioning properly.
- *Sensory impairments:* Use assisted communication devices or a sign language interpreter for hearing-impaired patients, if available, and make sure he can see your face to assist in understanding what you are saying. Writing messages may help. For vision-impaired patients, tell him what you are going to do before you do it. If a patient has a service animal, allow the service animal to accompany him in the ambulance.
- *Technology-dependent patients:* These patients or their caregivers are often the best source of information about troubleshooting the devices and assisting you in preparing the patient for transport.
- *Terminally ill patients:* Be aware of the five stages of grief and how patients and family members may react in different ways. Respect all legally binding advance directives.

46.7 Describe common types of home medical equipment, including the following: apnea monitors, CPAP and BiPAP, feeding tubes, intraventricular shunts, mechanical ventilators, medical oxygen, ostomy bags, tracheostomy tubes, urinary catheters, and vascular access devices.

- *Apnea monitors:* These are often used in infants at increased risk for ALTE or SIDS.
- *CPAP and BiPAP:* These are used by patients with respiratory illnesses and sleep apnea to provide positive airway pressure.

- *Feeding tubes:* These are used to provide nutrition into the gastrointestinal tract in patients who cannot take food or fluids orally.
- *Intraventricular shunts:* Ventriculostomy shunts are used to drain excess cerebrospinal fluid from the ventricles of the brain.
- *Mechanical ventilators:* These are used in patients with severe disabilities or illnesses that impair breathing.
- *Medical oxygen:* Patients with heart failure or respiratory diseases may use oxygen continuously or as needed at home, and may use portable oxygen concentrators when away from home.
- *Ostomy bags:* These are used to collect contents of the gastrointestinal tract in patients with a temporary or permanent ostomy, or connection of the intestine to the abdominal wall.
- *Tracheostomy tubes:* These are used in patients who are ventilator dependent or who have a high likelihood of needing mechanical ventilation. They provide a passage between the anterior neck and the trachea.
- *Urinary catheters:* These are inserted through the urethra and into the bladder to empty it.
- *Vascular access devices:* These are used for patients who need regular intravenous medications, such as patients who have cancer or other critical illnesses.

46.8 Describe the philosophy of hospice care.

Hospice provides support to the dying patient and his family. Hospice care allows patients to die with dignity, as comfortably as possible, surrounded by loved ones.

Resource Central

Resource Central offers extra practice and review materials in a variety of media. To access it, follow the directions on the Student Access Card provided with the Student Textbook. If there is no card, go to www.bradybooks.com and follow the Resource Central link to Buy Access.

Vocabulary and Concept Review

Exercise 1

Write the letter of the correct definition in the blank next to the term. (See Resource Central for more vocabulary review.)

1. _____ articulation disorder

2. _____ bariatrics

3. _____ BiPAP

4. _____ child abuse

5. _____ domestic abuse

6. _____ language disorder

7. _____ neglect

a. An act or failure to act on the part of a parent or caretaker, which results in harm to a minor

b. Inability to speak clearly

c. Failure of a caregiver to provide proper care to an individual for whom they are responsible

d. Violence used to intimidate a partner to gain power or control

e. Assisted breathing device that provides two levels of pressure: inspiratory positive airway pressure and a lower positive pressure during expiration

f. Inability to understand spoken or written communication

g. Branch of medicine that specializes in the care of obese patients

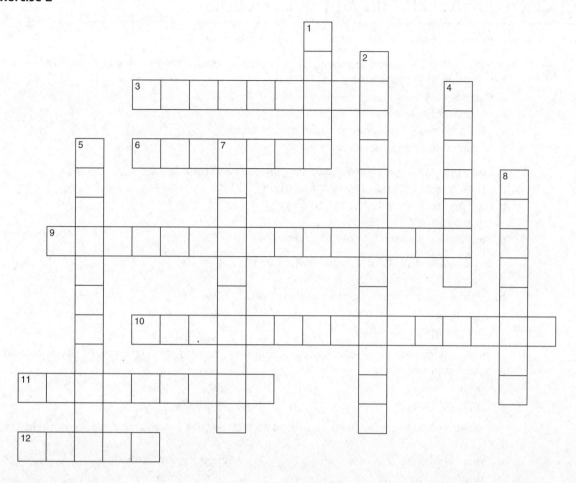

Across

3. Inability to see.
6. Care focused on the needs of terminally ill patients and their families.
9. Surgically placed device that allows some deaf patients to hear.
10. Stuttering speech.
11. Loss of motor ability.
12. Common obstruction to a tracheostomy tube.

Down

1. Significantly overweight.
2. Type of abuse: the willful inflection of mental or emotional anguish through threat, or humiliation through verbal or nonverbal means.
4. Low income resulting in an inability to pay for necessities.
5. Type of tube that is inserted through the nose; it extends through the pharynx and esophagus into the stomach as a route for administering nutrition or medication.
7. Paralysis of the lower extremities.
8. Severe hearing impairment.

Check Your Recall and Apply Concepts

Select the best possible choice for each of the following questions.

_____ 1. Which one of the following techniques is recommended to improve communication with hearing-impaired patients?
   a. Speak very loudly.
   b. Speak very slowly.
   c. Remain where the patient can see your face.
   d. Exaggerate pronunciation of words.

_____ 2. When approaching a vision-impaired patient, you should:
   a. flick a light on and off to get his attention.
   b. snap your fingers to get his attention.
   c. grasp him by the shoulder.
   d. announce yourself as you approach.

_____ 3. A voice production disorder results from:
   a. damage to the vocal cords or larynx.
   b. damage to the speech center in the brain.
   c. deafness.
   d. nerve impulse disorder.

_____ 4. A patient with a cervical-level spinal cord injury, resulting in paralysis of the arms and legs, suffers from:
   a. hemiplegia.   c. paraplegia.
   b. quadriplegia.   d. epiplegia.

_____ 5. All of the following have been identified as factors that increase the risk of homelessness EXCEPT:
   a. mental illness.   c. cigarette smoking.
   b. domestic violence.   d. substance abuse.

_____ 6. Approximately _____ percent of women are victims of domestic violence at least once in their lifetimes.
   a. 15   c. 40
   b. 25   d. 55

_____ 7. Which one of the following child behaviors is a possible indication of child abuse?
   a. Wants his parents to stay with him in the ambulance
   b. Expresses concern that treatment of the injury will hurt
   c. Does not cry when he otherwise would be expected to
   d. Favors one parent over the other when injured

_____ 8. When you suspect that an elderly patient has been abused, which one of the following should be your most immediate priority?
   a. Getting the patient out of the environment
   b. Identifying who committed the abuse
   c. Contacting social services
   d. Identifying all of the risk factors for abuse

_____ 9. The device that is placed in an opening in the neck to provide an airway for mechanical ventilation is called a:
   a. stoma.   c. nasogastric tube.
   b. ventilator circuit.   d. tracheostomy tube.

_____ 10. When a mechanical ventilator gives a high-pressure alarm, you should anticipate any of the following EXCEPT:
   a. an obstruction of the ventilator circuit.
   b. a mucus plug in the airway device.
   c. pulmonary edema.
   d. an air leak in the ventilator circuit.

_____ 11. A J tube is for which one of the following purposes?
   a. Administering nutrition into the small intestine
   b. Draining the bladder of urine
   c. Providing access to the stomach for nutrition and medication administration
   d. Collecting waste from the colon in a pouch outside the body

Clinical Reasoning

CASE STUDY: HOPE FULBRIGHT

Hope Fulbright is a 49-year-old woman who suffered a traumatic brain injury and cervical-spine injury in a motorcycle collision. She is cared for at home, but is dependent on a mechanical ventilator. Her daughter called 911 because the ventilator keeps giving high-pressure alarms. She has suctioned her mother's tracheostomy tube and checked the ventilator circuit for obstructions.

1. What are other possible causes of the high-pressure alarm?

_____

_____

_____

_____

_____

2. What assessments should you perform to detect potential problems?

_____

_____

_____

_____

_____

Project-Based Learning

Ask your instructor to help you arrange a clinical rotation with the respiratory therapy department of a hospital. Write a journal entry to describe your experience, listing at least three things that you would not have realized if you had not participated in the clinical rotation.

The EMS Professional in Practice

Volunteer for an agency that works with the homeless. Jot down your thoughts and feelings about the experience in a notebook or journal for discussion in class or in your study group.

Rescue Operations and Vehicle Extrication

Content Area

• Rescue Operations and Vehicle Extrication

Advanced EMT Education Standard

• The Advanced EMT applies knowledge of operational roles and responsibilities to ensure patient, public, and personnel safety during rescue and vehicle extrication.

Summary of Objectives

47.1 Define key terms introduced in this chapter.

Knowing and being able to apply the key terms in each chapter is critical to understanding chapter concepts. Write the list of key terms. Then write the definition of each one in your own words. Check your understanding by confirming the definitions in the textbook glossary. Correct any misunderstandings. Create a study aid by writing each key term on the front of an index card and the definition on the back. Use the cards to quiz yourself, or to have someone quiz you. The exercises under Vocabulary and Concept Review below will give you additional practice.

47.2 Use scene size-up information to anticipate potential problems in accessing patients.

A good scene size-up of the incident is essential. It will inform the Advanced EMT's decisions related to the type of rescue techniques that are needed for quick and safe access to the patient. A windshield survey plus an on-scene briefing from the rescue unit leader assists in making critical decisions on what personal protective equipment as well as what medical equipment is needed, how the extrication should proceed, and what additional resources are needed to perform a successful rescue with a viable patient.

47.3 Determine what types of resources may be needed in rescue situations.

Perform a thorough scene size-up to determine the need for fire suppression, extrication, law enforcement, animal control, hazardous materials team, utility company, water rescue team, high-angle rescue team, or other specialty resources.

47.4 Explain the integration of medical care and rescue operations through teamwork.

When the patient requires special resources for rescue or extrication, he requires those services as well as medical care. The rescue and medical teams must work together to ensure both goals are accomplished.

47.5 Establish personnel, patient, and public safety as priorities in rescue situations.

Rescue situations can be hazardous to the safety of everyone involved. Do not attempt rescues that you are not trained and equipped to perform, ensure your own safety and that of other personnel before approaching the patient, and take measures to ensure that bystanders are not endangered.

47.6 Recognize equipment used for water, rough terrain, confined space, and vehicle rescue.

A variety of specialized tools are used for rescue situations. You should be familiar with the tools used by the special services that interact with your EMS agency.

47.7 Select appropriate personal protective equipment for use during vehicle extrication.

You must wear a protective helmet, turnout coat, bunker pants, heavy gloves, and boots during extrication.

47.8 Identify the safest, most effective ways of gaining access to patients in given motor vehicle collision scenarios.

Always attempt access through doors first, keeping in mind that they may be locked. It may be necessary to break a window to access the door locks. If the patient cannot be accessed and removed through the doors, consult with the extrication team about the best way to remove the patient from the vehicle, given his condition.

47.9 Protect the patient from further harm during vehicle extrication.

Cover the patient with a protective blanket or tarp during extrication to prevent him from being injured by breaking glass and other debris.

47.10 Explain how to minimize risk of injury from extrication hazards, such as airbags that have not deployed, fuel leaks, traffic, weather, and other hazards.

Ensure that law enforcement has controlled traffic at the scene. Use absorbent material on fluid leaks and disconnect the battery cables to prevent undeployed airbags from deploying. Wear protective equipment to prevent against injury from broken glass and sharp metal.

47.11 Describe the processes used to stabilize a vehicle prior to beginning extrication.

Deflate the tires and use cribbing or chocks to assist in stabilizing the vehicle.

47.12 Discuss the impact on extrication procedures of damage to specific parts of the vehicle.

The amount and type of damage to the doors, roof, and other parts of the vehicle will play a role in how the extrication team decides to approach the extrication procedure.

47.13 Explain specific extrication safety considerations for hybrid vehicles.

You must disable and avoid contact with the high-voltage battery system by turning off the ignition, disconnecting the 12-volt battery, and avoiding contact with the bright orange high-voltage power cables.

47.14 Discuss the uses of particular types of hand and hydraulic extrication tools.

Simple hand tools, such as a spring-loaded window punch, can be used to gain access to vehicles, as well as axes, hammers, pry bars, saws, snipping tools, and mallets. Powerful hydraulic spreaders and lifts, and pneumatic lifting tools may be needed, as well.

Resource Central

Resource Central offers extra practice and review materials in a variety of media. To access it, follow the directions on the Student Access Card provided with the Student Textbook. If there is no card, go to www.bradybooks.com and follow the Resource Central link to Buy Access.

Vocabulary and Concept Review

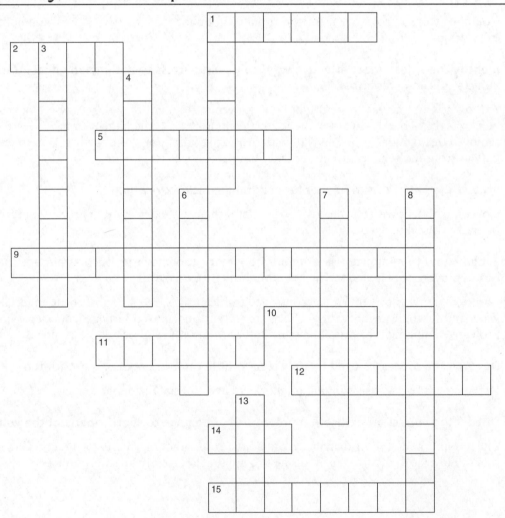

Across

1. Specialized team requested when there is a chemical release.
2. Thin piece of cribbing.
5. Ropes, chains, or webbing used to help stabilize a vehicle.
9. The process of freeing the patient from entrapment.
10. Standards for eyewear that should be met for protection against debris and fluid.
11. First phase of a rescue operation.
12. If not deployed on impact, these vehicle restraint systems must be deactivated before gaining access to the passenger compartment.
14. Should be worn by personnel working on or near water during rescue operations.
15. Prying tool used for auto extrication.

Down

1. Vehicle that uses a combination of fuel and high-voltage electrical energy for power.
3. Jaws of Life is an example of this type of tool.
4. Material used to fill voids between the vehicle and the ground for stabilization.
6. Gloves should be made of this material to protect your hands from jagged metal and broken glass during extrication.
7. Alternative to firefighting turnout coat and pants for use by EMS personnel during extrication.
8. Process of disentangling and removing a patient from a vehicle damaged in a collision.
13. Standards for personal protective equipment that should be met by personnel participating in extrication.

Check Your Recall and Apply Concepts

Exercise 1

Select the best possible choice for each of the following questions.

_____ 1. The vehicle structural support that is between the windshield and the front seat windows of a vehicle is the _____ post.
   a. A
   b. B
   c. C
   d. D

_____ 2. The area of a vehicle from the rear edge of the back door to the rear bumper is the _____ panel.
   a. fender
   b. kick
   c. quarter
   d. rocker

_____ 3. You should wear _____ gloves for protection from glass and metal while assisting with extrication.
   a. latex
   b. leather
   c. cloth
   d. vinyl

_____ 4. After arrival and size-up, the next phase of a rescue operation is:
   a. patient access.
   b. patient packaging.
   c. medical care.
   d. hazard control.

_____ 5. The additional protective equipment needed when entering a hazardous atmosphere is a:
   a. PFD.
   b. SCBA.
   c. Halligan tool.
   d. Porta-power.

Exercise 2

Write a "T" in the space next to each true statement. Write an "F" in the space next to each false statement. If a statement is false, rewrite it to make it correct.

1. _____ Rescuers account for 50 percent of confined space deaths.

   _____

2. _____ A standard hard hat, like those worn in construction work, is recommended for rescuer protection during extrication.

   _____

3. _____ You should remain at least 10 inches away from a nondeployed driver's front airbag when assisting with vehicle extrication.

   _____

4. _____ Rigging is used to fill voids between a vehicle and the ground to stabilize it during extrication.

   _____

5. _____ You should be alert to the possibility of a fuel spill in collisions involving hybrid vehicles.

   _____

6. _____In some cases, the use of hand tools alone is sufficient to gain access to a patient in a damaged vehicle.

   _____

7. _____ Personal protective equipment is not required when only hand tools are used for extrication.

   _____

Clinical Reasoning

CASE STUDY: SWIFT-WATER RESCUE IN THE DESERT

You are watching a 24-hour news channel when the anchor announces live coverage of a person being swept away in an arroyo full of fast-moving water after a sudden, heavy monsoon rain in the desert. The live footage shows a teenaged male, head barely above water, being carried away in the rapidly moving current.

1. What teams and resources are needed for this rescue?

   _____

   _____

   _____

   _____

   _____

2. What is the role of EMS providers in this situation?

_____

_____

_____

_____

_____

3. What factors can affect the outcome of this rescue?

_____

_____

_____

_____

_____

Project-Based Learning

To learn more about various aspects of rescue operations, search for three articles on rescue operations and write an abstract of the main points of the articles. Be prepared to discuss your findings with your study group or in class.

The EMS Professional in Practice

What kind of rescue training would be of benefit to you in your employment? Search out various courses you can take to become more skilled in rescue operations. Jot down your thoughts in a notebook or journal for discussion in class or in your study group.

Content Area

- EMS Operations

Advanced EMT Education Standard

- The Advanced EMT applies knowledge and operational roles and responsibilities to ensure patient, public, and personnel safety.

Summary of Objectives

48.1 Define key terms introduced in this chapter.

Knowing and being able to apply the key terms in each chapter is critical to understanding chapter concepts. Write the list of key terms. Then write the definition of each one in your own words. Check your understanding by confirming the definitions in the textbook glossary. Correct any misunderstandings. Create a study aid by writing each key term on the front of an index card and the definition on the back. Use the cards to quiz yourself, or to have someone quiz you. The exercises under Vocabulary and Concept Review below will give you additional practice.

48.2 Explain the Advanced EMT's role in hazardous materials situations.

An EMS provider's role is to recognize a hazardous materials situation, request appropriate resources to respond, and treat patients after they have been decontaminated by hazardous materials personnel.

48.3 List indications that a hazardous material situation may exist.

Indications include smoke, vapors, fume, particulates or dust, fire, leaking liquids, unusual sounds (hissing, rumbling, tearing metal), an NFPA 704 or DOT placard, unusual odors, and multiple patients.

48.4 Describe the principle dangers and types of damage that can be caused by hazardous materials.

Hazardous materials can cause chemical burns, result in fire, release toxic fumes, explode, and cause toxic effects on the body and environment.

48.5 Given a scenario involving a hazardous materials incident, list specific actions you should take to minimize your chance of exposure to the materials.

Anticipate calls that can involve hazardous materials and approach the scene cautiously. If you identify indications of a hazardous materials incident, retreat to a safe distance and use binoculars to identify any placards that could give additional information. Move upwind and uphill from chemical releases. Use the Emergency Response Guidebook to decide on evacuation distances.

48.6 Explain the U.S. Department of Transportation placard system and the National Fire Protection Association symbols for identifying hazardous materials.

The U.S. Department of Transportation placards recognize nine classes of hazardous materials. Placards are keyed to the Emergency Response Guidebook for recognition of the type of hazard involved. The NFPA system identifies the basic nature of the chemical involved and the level of hazard it poses for fire, health, and explosion.

48.7 Explain the purpose and limitations of shipping papers and material safety data sheets.

Shipping papers and material data safety sheets are often stored or transported in proximity to the hazardous material and may not be accessible.

48.8 Identify resources that can be used in the identification and management of hazardous materials situations.

Recognize placards, use the Emergency Response Guidebook, be aware of material safety data sheets and shipping papers, and contact the hazardous materials team.

48.9 Differentiate among the hazardous materials training levels identified by the Occupational Safety and Health Administration.

In order of increasing levels of complexity, the hazardous materials training levels are First Responder Awareness (no minimum hours), First Responder Operations (8- to 16-hour course), Hazardous Materials Operations (40-hour course), Hazardous Materials Technician (additional training to contain the material), and Hazardous Materials Specialist (additional training in leadership and support of hazardous materials operations).

48.10 Discuss the components of hazardous materials incident management, including the following: preincident planning, considerations in implementing the plan, establishing safety zones, and decontamination.

Effective management of hazardous materials incidents requires planning (identifying risks in the area, training personnel, identifying where hazardous materials response teams should be located, and other factors), assessing specific incidents to determine how to implement the plan, using hazardous materials resources to determine the limits of each safety zone, decontaminating all personnel and patients exposed to the hazardous material, and preventing spread of the hazardous material during decontamination.

48.11 Differentiate between acute and chronic effects of hazardous materials exposure.

Acute effects are the effects that occur within a short period of time, ranging from immediately to hours after contact with the hazardous material. Chronic effects can be effects that linger after an acute exposure, or effects due to lower-level exposure over an extended period of time.

48.12 Describe the integration of patient care with the need for safety and patient decontamination when responding to hazardous materials incidents.

The role of EMS providers is to stay in the cold zone and treat patients who have been decontaminated.

48.13 **Describe special considerations in response to incidents involving radiation exposure and contamination.**

The approach to a patient who has been exposed to radiation is different from the approach to a patient who is contaminated with radiation. An exposure is similar to the patient receiving an X-ray: The radioactive energy enters the body and can cause energy, but the radioactive material itself does not contaminate the patient. Contamination occurs when the patient comes into contact with the actual radioactive material. The patient's injuries and the approach to the contaminated patient depend on the type of radiation involved, the dose, the distance the patient was from the source, and any shielding between the patient and the source.

Resource Central

Resource Central offers extra practice and review materials in a variety of media. To access it, follow the directions on the Student Access Card provided with the Student Textbook. If there is no card, go to www.bradybooks.com and follow the Resource Central link to Buy Access.

Vocabulary and Concept Review

Exercise 1

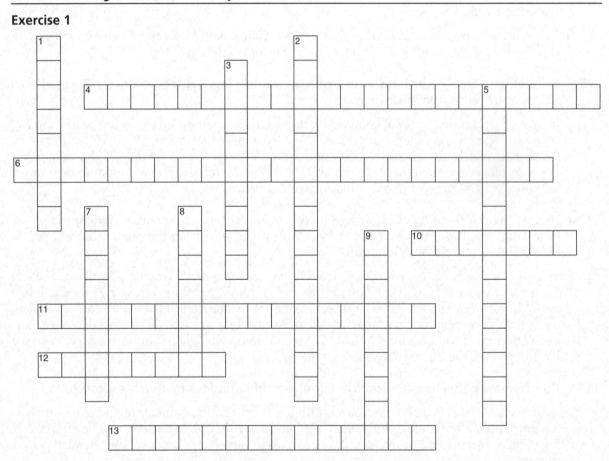

Across

4. Transfer of a hazardous material from contact with an individual or piece of equipment to a person or surface that was not originally affected.

6. Information form created by a chemical manufacturer that describes the physical properties, hazards, and ways of safely handling a hazardous chemical.

10. Diamond-shaped information source on a vehicle or fixed storage facility of hazardous materials.

11. Any substance capable of harming people, property, or the environment.

12. Four digits that identify hazardous substances and products of commercial importance.

13. Documentation containing regulatory information on a particular hazardous material transported by land, sea, or air.

Down

1. Poisonous substance not derived from the metabolism of an organism.

2. Process of reducing or removing hazardous material from someone or something that was exposed to it.

3. Natural process by which energy waves and particles travel through space.

5. Established ingress and egress route for emergency responders on a hazardous materials incident.

7. Area of a hazardous materials incident where triage and treatment take place.

8. Area where a hazardous chemical was released, contaminates the environment, and poses a danger to anyone in that area.

9. Signs and symptoms that occur from exposure to a toxicant.

Check Your Recall and Apply Concepts

Select the best possible choice for each of the following questions.

_____ 1. Using the mnemonic RAIN for actions at the scene of a hazardous material incident, the "R" means you should:
   a. remove the substance.
   b. remove people from the area where the substance is located.
   c. recognize the hazardous material.
   d. respond to the hot zone.

_____ 2. You are approaching the scene of a motor vehicle collision when you notice that one of the vehicles involved is a pick-up truck towing a large cylindrical tank. The tank has jack-knifed and is leaking something from the top hatch. Which one of the following is the best way to identify if the substance poses a hazard?
   a. Ask the pick-up truck driver for the material safety data sheet.
   b. Stop where you are and use binoculars to look for a placard or other identifying information on the tank.
   c. Search the cab of the pick-up truck for the shipping papers.
   d. Try to determine if there is an odor to the substance leaking from the tank.

_____ 3. The red quadrant of an NFPA 704 placard indicates the hazard level related to:
   a. fire.   c. health.
   b. explosion.   d. reactivity.

_____ 4. You approach a storage tank where a person is reported to be injured. You see an NFPA 704 placard in which the blue quadrant has the number 4 and the yellow quadrant has the number 1. The numbers and colors tell you that the substance poses:
   a. extreme fire risk, low health risk.   c. high reactivity risk, low health risk.
   b. high health risk, low fire risk.   d. high health risk, low reactivity risk.

_____ 5. A "W" in the white quadrant of an NFPA placard indicates:
   a. radiation.
   b. the facility is used for chemical storage but is currently empty.
   c. reactivity with water.
   d. a weak chemical.

_____ 6. U.S. Department of Transportation placards are referenced directly to:
   a. the Emergency Response Guidebook.
   b. CHEMTREC.
   c. the National Poison Control Center.
   d. the material safety data sheet.

_____ 7. You have identified a four-digit number from a U.S. DOT placard. When you pick up the appropriate reference book, you should turn to the _____ pages.
   a. white   c. yellow
   b. blue   d. orange

_____ 8. The highest level of OSHA training to deal with hazardous materials incidents is the _____ level.
   a. Awareness   c. Technician
   b. Operations   d. Specialist

_____ 9. Which one of the following is an example of Level D hazardous materials personal protective equipment?
   a. Fully encapsulated suit with SCBA   c. Your regular work uniform
   b. SCBA only   d. A particulate respirator

Clinical Reasoning

CASE STUDY: FIRE AT DAVIS INDUSTRIES

On your way back from an interfacility transfer of a cardiac patient, you and your partner spot a plume of smoke rising from the south end of town, about 2 miles away. You have not heard any radio traffic to indicate the smoke has been reported. Just as you pick up the radio microphone, you see a large fireball rise through the smoke. Your partner says, "You know, that looks like it is coming from Davis Industries. I'm not sure what they do there, but I know the hazmat team gets dispatched whenever there is a fire alarm there."

1. What information should you report to dispatch?

_____

_____

_____

_____

_____

2. What should your next actions be?

_____

_____

_____

_____

Project-Based Learning

Go to the U.S. Environmental Protection Agency (EPA) Web site, http://www.epa.gov/radtown, for an interactive page that helps you identify what types of radiation might be in your community and where they are located. After visiting the site, prepare a list of three to five locations in your community and nearby towns where you would expect to find radiation. Be prepared to compare your list to those of other students in your study group or class to help you identify more possible locations.

The EMS Professional in Practice

What hazardous materials are in your work environment? Look for the material safety data sheets for potentially hazardous materials to learn more about them. Jot down your thoughts in a notebook or journal for discussion in class or in your study group.

Response to Terrorism and Disasters

Content Area

- EMS Operations

Advanced EMT Education Standard

- Knowledge of operational roles and responsibilities to ensure patient, public, and personnel safety.

Summary of Objectives

49.1 Define key terms introduced in this chapter.

Knowing and being able to apply the key terms in each chapter is critical to understanding chapter concepts. Write the list of key terms. Then write the definition of each one in your own words. Check your understanding by confirming the definitions in the textbook glossary. Correct any misunderstandings. Create a study aid by writing each key term on the front of an index card and the definition on the back. Use the cards to quiz yourself, or to have someone quiz you. The exercises under Vocabulary and Concept Review below will give you additional practice.

49.2 Anticipate types of disasters to which you may respond as an Advanced EMT.

You may respond to natural disasters such as earthquakes, tornadoes, floods, and hurricanes; large fires or explosions; and, potentially, acts of terrorism.

49.3 Identify the roles EMS providers play in response to disasters and terrorism incidents.

As always, the primary role of EMS providers is administering emergency care. Because disasters commonly involve multiple casualties, you will most likely be assigned to triage, treatment, or transport of injured patients, working with an incident command system.

49.4 Identify the roles of other types of special teams that may be required in response to disasters and terrorism events.

Specialized search and rescue teams, fire suppression, hazardous materials teams, disaster medical assistance teams (DMAT), and other resources are often involved in disaster response, depending on the exact nature of the disaster.

49.5 Explain considerations in the planning phase of disaster response.

Planning must take into consideration anticipation of specific types of disasters that are possible in a community, as well as resources available and mechanisms for mutual aid.

49.6 Describe the purpose and process of windshield assessment in the response to a disaster.

The windshield assessment is a portion of the scene size-up performed from inside the emergency response vehicle as crews approach the scene to determine what has happened, what is happening, what hazards are present, and what resources are needed.

49.7 Explain the purpose of the National Disaster Medical System.

The National Disaster Medical System is a section of the U.S. Department of Health and Human Services that is responsible for managing the federal medical response to an emergency or disaster. It consists of locally based teams that respond jointly where disaster medical assistance is required.

49.8 Discuss the relationship between multiple casualty incident response and post-traumatic and cumulative stress.

Multiple casualty incidents and disasters often involve disturbing sights, sounds, and smells and witnessing the death and suffering of others on a large scale. Such experiences can lead to post-traumatic stress disorder, or to cumulative stress. Be alert to the signs and symptoms of stress disorders in yourself and others during and after multiple casualty incident and disaster responses.

49.9 Anticipate psychological reactions of disaster survivors.

Disaster survivors may be disoriented and panicked. Anticipate the possibility of behavioral emergencies and the need for psychological support, including activation of disaster mental health services.

49.10 Describe the characteristics of each of the categories of weapons of mass destruction.

Conventional explosives are essentially bombs designed to detonate and create destruction and blast injuries. They may be used as a means of dispersing radiation, shrapnel, or biologic agents. Biologic agents are infectious materials or the toxins they produce and smallpox, anthrax, salmonella, ricin, and many others. Chemical weapons can involve a variety of chemicals, many of them in gas form, such as sarin gas. Chemical weapons include blister agents, cyanide, choking agents, nerve agents, and others. Radiologic agents expose the population to various forms of radiation energy.

49.11 Recognize indications that a response may involve terrorism and weapons of mass destruction.

Explosions, presence of hazardous materials, multiple patients, and patients with similar signs and symptoms are all potential indications of weapons of mass destruction.

49.12 Given a series of scenarios of terrorism involving weapons of mass destruction, anticipate threats to responders, patients, bystanders.

Be alert to secondary attacks on responders, such as secondary explosions or exposures.

49.13 Predict patient injuries associated with various types of disasters and weapons of mass destruction.

Each type of weapon of mass destruction can result in specific sets of signs and symptoms. Anytime multiple patients present with similar signs and symptoms, consider the possibility of a weapon of mass destruction or a multiple casualty incident resulting from accidental exposure to chemicals, radiation, or biological weapons. The nature of a disaster will help you anticipate the types of injuries you may see. A tornado, for example, may involve both blunt and penetrating trauma.

49.14 **Discuss the effects of exposure to various classifications of chemical agents that are likely to be used in a chemical terrorism event.**

Asphyxiants prevent cellular use of oxygen. Choking agents cause respiratory distress, vomiting agents cause coughing and choking, and riot control agents cause irritation of the eyes and mucous membranes.

49.15 **Give examples of biologic agents that are likely to be used in a bioterrorism event.**

Some examples include plague, tularemia, anthrax, smallpox, and hantavirus.

49.16 **Discuss particular concerns with terrorism events involving radiation.**

Radiation incidents can include both exposure, in which tissue injury occurs but in which the patient does not act as a source of radiation to others, or contamination, in which the patient both receives injury and can expose others to radiation. Depending on the dosage, radiation injury can be immediate, or delayed by many hours, days, weeks, or even years.

Resource Central

Resource Central offers extra practice and review materials in a variety of media. To access it, follow the directions on the Student Access Card provided with the Student Textbook. If there is no card, go to www.bradybooks.com and follow the Resource Central link to Buy Access.

Vocabulary and Concept Review

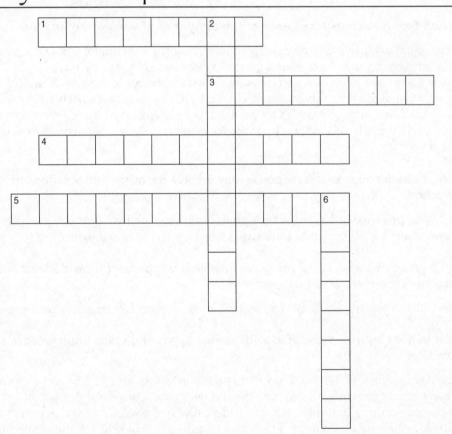

Across

1. Terrorism that involves the intentional, widespread dissemination of anthrax, for example.
3. Terrorism that involves the intentional dispersal of VX or sarin gas, for example.
4. Low-toxicity agent that temporarily incapacitates by irritating the eyes.
5. Type of chemical materials designed to explode or detonate violently.

Down

2. Device used as a weapon that starts a fire.
6. Terrorist who acts by himself and has no long-term affiliation with a group.

Check Your Recall and Apply Concepts

Select the best possible choice for each of the following questions.

_____ 1. A device that is used with the intention of starting a fire is classified as a(n):
  a. dispersal device.
  b. dirty bomb.
  c. conventional explosive.
  d. incendiary device.

_____ 2. Conventional explosives are used primarily to:
  a. detonate violently.
  b. start fires.
  c. disperse radiation.
  d. create smoke.

_____ 3. The most virulent agents of biologic terrorism are classified as category _____ agents.
  a. A
  b. B
  c. C
  d. D

_____ 4. An example of a category A biologic weapon agent is:
  a. psittacosis.
  b. cholera.
  c. plague.
  d. viral encephalitis.

_____ 5. Vessicants are chemicals that act primarily by causing:
  a. cellular asphyxiation.
  b. parasympathetic nervous system stimulation.
  c. blistering and burning of the tissues.
  d. short-term irritation of the eyes.

_____ 6. Which one of the following signs would you most expect in a patient who has been exposed to a nerve agent?
  a. Bradycardia
  b. Dry mucous membranes
  c. Constipation
  d. Blistering of the skin

Clinical Reasoning

CASE STUDY: EF3 IN THE BUSINESS DISTRICT

You and your partner are standing just outside your crew quarters, watching an approaching storm when dispatch broadcasts a tornado warning. Continuing to listen to radio traffic as you move inside your building, you learn within minutes that a tornado is on the ground headed toward an area with several large retail stores and other businesses. Radio traffic picks up with several reports of damage and injuries before the tornado dissipates. You are dispatched to a staging area in the parking lot of a home improvement store.

1. What roles do you expect to play in this situation?

   _____

   _____

   _____

   _____

   _____

2. What types of injuries do you anticipate patients will have?

   _____

   _____

   _____

   _____

3. What dangers should you be alert to?

   _____

   _____

   _____

   _____

4. What other types of problems should you anticipate in accessing, treating, and transporting patients?

   _____

   _____

   _____

   _____

   _____

Project-Based Learning

What is the likelihood of various natural disasters in your community? Use the Internet to search for the history of tornados, hurricanes, floods, and earthquakes in your area. How many people were affected by those events? What kind of damage was done? Jot down notes in your journal or notebook so you can compare your findings to those of your study group or classmates.

The EMS Professional in Practice

What are some of the ways your community would continue to be affected following a natural disaster? What are health, psychosocial, and economic impacts of natural disasters on a community? How will the changes impact your work as an Advanced EMT? Jot down your thoughts in a notebook or journal for discussion in class or in your study group.

WORKBOOK ANSWER KEY

Note: Throughout Answer Key, textbook page references are shown in italic.

Chapter 1: Introduction to Advanced Emergency Medical Technician Practice

VOCABULARY AND CONCEPT REVIEW KEY

1. m   *p. 4*
2. a   *p. 3*
3. g   *p. 4*
4. i   *p. 8*
5. c   *p. 4*
6. f   *p. 8*
7. d   *p. 3*
8. k   *p. 3*
9. b   *p. 8*
10. e   *p. 8*

CHECK YOUR RECALL KEY

1. c   *p. 3*
2. c   *p. 7*
3. b   *p. 10*
4. a   *p. 11*
5. b   *p. 12*

CLINICAL REASONING CASE STUDY: HEALTH CAREERS DAY AT WASHINGTON MIDDLE SCHOOL

1. Students should learn what EMS is, how it fits with the health care system, public safety, and public health; the levels of EMS providers, including the training involved and scopes of practice; and the roles, responsibilities, and professional characteristics of EMS providers.
2. Explain the role of EMRs in arriving quickly and providing basic care measures at the scene, the role of EMTs in transporting patients and providing basic care that can be provided with the equipment typically provided on an ambulance, the role of Advanced EMTs in providing basic and limited advanced assessments and interventions, and the role of paramedics in providing complex assessments and interventions.
3. The National Registry of EMTs website (http://www.nremt.org) and the website of your state EMS office are good resources to give lay public information about EMS.

Chapter 2: Emergency Medical Services, Health Care, and Public Health Systems

VOCABULARY AND CONCEPT REVIEW KEY

1. certificate,   *p. 23*
2. on-line,   *p. 26*
3. continuous quality improvement (CQI),   *p. 26*
4. National EMS Information System (NEMSIS),   *p. 26*
5. critical access hospital,   *p. 26*
6. enhanced 911,   *p. 25*
7. license,   *p. 22*
8. public safety answering point,   *p. 25*
9. third,   *p. 23*
10. reciprocity,   *p. 25*

CHECK YOUR RECALL AND APPLY CONCEPTS KEY

EXERCISE 1

p. 18

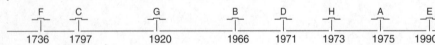

F	C	G	B	D	H	A	E
1736	1797	1920	1966	1971	1973	1975	1990

EXERCISE 2

1. g   *p. 21*
2. e   *p. 21*
3. c   *p. 21*
4. h   *p. 21*
5. f   *p. 21*
6. a   *p. 21*
7. d   *p. 21*
8. b   *p. 21*

CLINICAL REASONING CASE STUDY: TRAINING NIGHT AT MOUNT PLEASANT EMS

1. As a health care professional, competence and patient safety are ethical obligations. Refresher education is important in maintaining current skills and knowledge to ensure patient safety. Continuing education is necessary to increase awareness of changes in knowledge and practice to help ensure the best patient care possible, based on research.
2. Information to plan refresher and continuing education should be based on CQI and emerging research, as well as state and national blueprints for mandatory educational content.
3. In addition to scheduled face-to-face classes, you can obtain refresher and continuing education through journal articles (usually with associated quizzes), professional conferences, and opportunities for computer software-based and web-based education, including websites and podcasts.

Chapter 3: Workforce Wellness and Personal Safety

VOCABULARY AND CONCEPT REVIEW KEY

EXERCISE 1

1. c   p. 51
2. k   p. 45
3. i   p. 50
4. g   p. 43
5. d   p. 39
6. m   p. 45
7. a   p. 36
8. e   p. 37
9. b   p. 36
10. l   p. 46
11. f   p. 51
12. j   p. 50
13. h   p. 35

EXERCISE 2

Across

6. Physical and psychological exhaustion from over-exposure to stress. [BURNOUT]   *p. 38*

7. Released from the anterior pituitary and acts on the adrenal glands. [ACTH]   *p. 36*

10. Using good posture and proper lifting techniques to prevent injury. [BODYMECHANICS]   *p. 41*

11. A biological substance that can cause harm or disease. [BIOHAZARD]   *p. 49*

13. Disease that can be transmitted directly or indirectly from one person to another. [COMMUNICABLEILLNESS]   *p. 43*

Down

1. Hormone responsible for the fight or flight response. [EPINEPHRINE]   *p. 36*

2. Type of infection acquired in a health care setting. [NOSOCOMIAL]   *p. 46*

3. Contact between non-intact skin and potentially infectious body fluids of another person. [EXPOSURE]   *p. 50*

4. Physiologic equilibrium. [HOMEOSTASIS]   *p. 37*

5. Disease-causing microorganism. [PATHOGEN]   *p. 43*

8. Occurs immediately in response to a stressor and may last up to four weeks. [ACUTESTRESS]   *p. 37*

9. Type of exercise that increases heart rate to between 74% and 88% of its maximum. [VIGOROUS]   *p. 54*

12. A state of complete wellness and not just the absence of disease. [HEALTH]   *p. 33*

CHECK YOUR RECALL AND APPLY CONCEPTS KEY

1. d	*p. 36*	**6.** c	*p. 43*	**11.** a	*p. 0*
2. c	*p. 36*	**7.** c	*p. 43*	**12.** d	*p. 44*
3. a	*p. 38*	**8.** b	*p. 33*	**13.** d	*p. 41*
4. b	*p. 40*	**9.** a	*p. 35*	**14.** a	*p. 44*
5. c	*p. 45*	**10.** d	*p. 54*	**15.** a	*p. 49*

CLINICAL REASONING CASE STUDY: EMPLOYEE WELLNESS AT CITY AMBULANCE

Possible answers:

1. Regular health screenings, such as weight, body mass index, blood pressure, blood glucose, and cholesterol levels. Increased body weight, body mass index, blood pressure, and cholesterol and diabetes are all risk factors for serious health problems, such as cardiovascular disease.

2. Psychological services. Stress can have negative impact on performance in the short term and long term and can have negative effects on health.

3. Buying equipment to furnish an exercise room. Regular exercise improves weight, strength, and endurance and reduces stress.

4. Referrals for personal health counseling for weight loss, smoking cessation, and other health issues. Improving health behaviors reduces risks for a number of illnesses such as cancer, cardiovascular disease, and diabetes.

Chapter 4: Ethical and Medical/Legal Considerations in Advanced EMT Practice

VOCABULARY AND CONCEPT REVIEW KEY

EXERCISE 1

1. e	*p. 66*	**5.** i	*p. 70*	**9.** f	*p. 70*
2. d	*p. 62*	**6.** b	*p. 70*	**10.** c	*p. 70*
3. a	*p. 69*	**7.** h	*p. 70*		
4. j	*p. 63*	**8.** g	*p. 69*		

EXERCISE 2

1. assault,	*p. 66*	**7.** EMTALA,	*p. 61*
2. ethics,	*p. 60*	**8.** nonfeasance,	*p. 69*
3. tort law,	*p. 61*	**9.** malfeasance,	*p. 69*
4. livor mortis,	*p. 69*	**10.** plaintiff,	*p. 69*
5. misfeasance,	*p. 69*		
6. Good Samaritan aws,	*p. 72*		

EXERCISE 3

1. (Across) SLANDER
2. (Down) DEFAMATION
3. (Across) DEFENDANT
4. (Across) ETHICS
5. (Down) CERTIFICATION
6. (Across) COMPETENT / CAPACITY
7. (Down) ASSAULT
8. (Down) BATTERY
9. (Down) REGISTRATION
10. (Across) RES IPSA LOQUITUR
11. (Across) LIABLE
12. (Across) DUTY TO ACT
13. (Across) ABANDONMENT

1. Defamation by spoken word. [SLANDER] *p. 70*
3. Person against whom a claim of legal wrongdoing is made. [DEFENDANT] *p. 61*
4. Principles of proper professional conduct. [ETHICS] *p. 60*
6. Has the capacity to make decisions. [COMPETENT] *p. 62*
10. Being self-evident. [RESIPSALOQUITUR] *p. 69*
11. Being legally responsible. [LIABLE] *p. 70*
12. Obligation to provide services. [DUTYTOACT] *p. 69*
13. Ending patient care without appropriate transfer to a qualified health care provider when the patient is still need of care. [ABANDONMENT] *p. 66*

2. Harming the reputation of another person by giving malicious false information. [DEFAMATION] *p. 70*
5. Recognition of accomplishment that can be provided by any party of agency. [CERTIFICATION] *p. 62*
7. An act that places a patient in fear of harm. [ASSAULT] *p. 66*
8. Physical contact without consent of reasonable expectation of physical contact. [BATTERY] *p. 66*
9. Having your name listed in a database. [REGISTERED] *p. 62*

CHECK YOUR RECALL AND APPLY CONCEPTS KEY

EXERCISE 1

1. Disturb as little as possible. Follow the same path out of the crime scene as you took into it and have all providers take the same path. Use the minimum number of providers needed to care for the patient. Avoid cutting through holes in clothing. If the patient is dead, do not enter the crime scene. If you must remove anything from the scene, notify law enforcement. Document your observations and actions. *p. 72*
2. That you had (a) a duty to act, (b) breached that duty, (c) damages occurred, (d) your actions or omissions caused the harm. *p. 69*
3. (a) animal bites, (b) child abuse, (c) elder abuse, (d) gunshot and knife wounds, (e) communicable diseases *p. 73*
4. (a) if a patient consents to the release of information, (b) for billing purposes, (c) to other health care providers who need to have the information to care for the patient, (d) under court order, (e) information may be released to the patient *p. 71*

EXERCISE 2

1. d	*p. 60*	5. b	*p. 61*	9. a	*p. 66*
2. d	*p. 60*	6. c	*p. 62*	10. b	*p. 66*
3. b	*p. 70*	7. b	*p. 63*	11. a	*p. 67*
4. a	*p. 61*	8. d	*p. 63*	12. b	*p. 70*

CLINICAL REASONING CASE STUDY: MR. STRUMPH'S DENIAL

1. Determine the patient's level of responsiveness and obtain a more detailed assessment of his mental status. Speak to the patient's wife to determine if the patient's mental status seems impaired in any way. Check for the possibility that the patient is under the influence of drugs or alcohol. Ask questions of the patient to see if he understands the seriousness of his condition and the possible consequences of refusing care.
2. Make sure the patient understands the seriousness of his situation and the possible consequences of refusing treatment and transport. Find out if there is a particular reason the patient is reluctant to be transported and try to address it to the best of your ability. Involve family members at the scene and contact on-line medical direction for assistance. Document all conversation between you and the patient to record your attempts to get the patient to consent. Follow your protocols for refusal of treatment, and complete any checklists and forms required. Have the patient sign the form and, if possible, get a witness to the refusal. Inform the patient that he or his wife can call again at any time if he changes his mind.
3. It is always possible to be sued for negligence, but in this case you have a good defense against the claim, as long as you made every reasonable effort to convince the patient to be treated, to make sure he understood his condition and the possible consequences of refusing care; and followed all policies and procedures, not just to the letter, but in spirit as well. You had a duty to act, and you upheld that duty. You acted in accordance with the reasonable person standard. Harm did occur to the patient, but it would be difficult to establish a causal link.

Chapter 5: Ambulance Operations and Responding to EMS Calls

VOCABULARY AND CONCEPT REVIEW KEY

EXERCISE 1

1. c	*p. 95*	6. j	*p. 87*	11. o	*p. 81*
2. h	*p. 96*	7. g	*p. 96*	12. k	*p. 100*
3. f	*p. 83*	8. e	*p. 83*	13. m	*p. 81*
4. a	*p. 99*	9. d	*p. 83*	14. n	*p. 86*
5. b	*p. 95*	10. i	*p. 83*	15. l	*p. 85*

Crossword grid (answers):

Across: 1 TRIAGEDESK, 4 BARIATRIC, 7 AIRPLANE, 8 STAROFLIFE, 11 MECHANISMOFINJURY, 13 PACKAGING, 16 DEFENSIVE, 17 SPOTTER

Down: 2 EXTRICATION, 3 LATERALRECUMBENT, 5 CHIEFCOMPLAINT, 6 HELICOPTER, 9 SUPINE, 10 EMERGENCY, 12 FOWLERS, 14 ACUTE, 15 SIZEUP

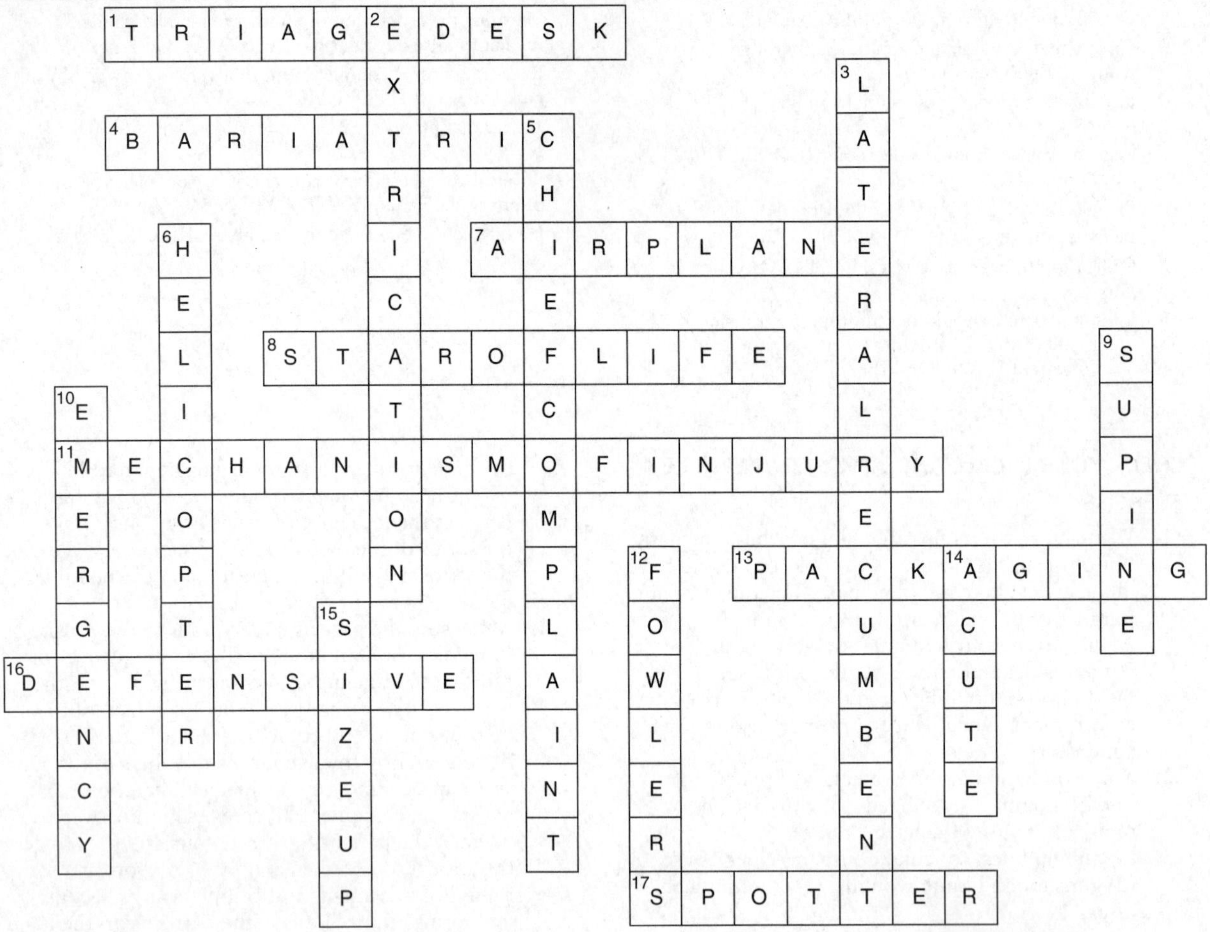

Across

1. Point in the emergency department where arriving patients are usually first evaluated and assigned a priority for care. [TRIAGEDESK] *p. 80*

4. Medical issues related to obesity. [BARIATRIC] *p. 99*

7. Fixed-wing aircraft. [AIRPLANE] *p. 102*

8. Figure with the Rod of Asciepius at the center that is used to represent emergency medical services. [STAROFLIFE] *p. 84*

11. Means by which energy is transmitted to the body, producing the potential for trauma. [MECHANISMOFINJURY] *p. 94*

13. Process of preparing a patient for transport. [PACKAGING] *p. 80*

16. Type of driving that improves safety by anticipating adverse conditions and actions of other drivers. [DEFENSIVE] *p. 85*

17. Person who provides instructions and guidance to assist another individual and avoid obstacles while moving a patient or driving a vehicle. [SPOTTER] *p. 87*

Down

2. Process of removing a patient from entrapment, such as from a damaged vehicle. [EXTRICATION] *p. 102*

3. Position in which the patient is lying on his side. [LATERALRECUMBENT] *p. 96*

5. Reason a patient states he is requesting medical help. [CHIEFCOMPLAINT] *p. 95*

6. Rotor-wing aircraft. [HELICOPTER] *p. 102*

9. Lying on one's back. [SUPINE] *p. 96*

10. Type of move used when a patient is in immediate jeopardy. [EMERGENCY] *p. 95*

12. Position in which a patient is sitting straight up. [FOWLERS] *p. 95*

14. Having a sudden onset. [ACUTE] *p. 81*

15. What is done at the scence to look for potential hazards and determine the nature of the incident. [SIZEUP] *p. 93*

CHECK YOUR RECALL AND APPLY CONCEPTS KEY

1. c *p. 97–99*
2. a *p. 97–99*
3. d *p. 97–99*
4. b *p. 97–99*
5. c *p. 97–99*

ANSWERS TO CLINICAL REASONING
CASE STUDY: DISPATCH FOR AN INJURED PATIENT ON A HIKING TRAIL

1. Terrain limits the type of device that is safe for the patient, and the patient has an isolated knee injury; therefore, a long backboard is not warranted. A stair chair or wheeled stretcher would be difficult to maneuver on anything but a solid, relatively smooth surface. A basket stretcher is an excellent choice.

2. The direct ground lift is the safest way to lift this patient. The extremity lift would be painful considering her injured knee.

3. This patient is stable and does not warrant emergency transport or air medical transport. A slow and smooth transport would be the least painful for the patient.

Chapter 6: Communication and Teamwork

VOCABULARY AND CONCEPT REVIEW KEY

EXERCISE 1

1. d *p. 113*
2. f *p. 122*
3. a *p. 121*
4. i *p. 122*
5. k *p. 112*
6. j *p. 122*
7. m *p. 112*
8. n *p. 113*
9. g *p. 121*
10. b *p. 125*
11. o *p. 112*
12. l *p. 121*
13. c *p. 125*
14. h *p. 122*
15. e *p. 112*

EXERCISE 2

5. Record of an event. [DOCUMENTATION] *p. 123*
9. Ability to exchange information between different communication systems. [INTEROPERABILITY] *p. 114*
11. Disruption in the transmissions of a message. [INTERFERENCE] *p. 113*
14. Type of radio mounted in a vehicle. [MOBILE] *p. 115*
15. "You said you had some health problems a few months ago. Tell me more about what happened." [FACILITATION] *p. 122*
17. Type of listening in which you listen beyond the speaker's words for the meaning's behind them. [ACTIVE] *p. 113*
19. Medium through which a message can be sent. [CHANNEL] *p. 113*
20. Type of question that influences the patient's answer. [LEADING] *p. 121*

1. Seeking feedback to make sure you understand what the patient tells you. [CLARIFICATION] *p. 122*
2. Pointing out inconsistencies in the information a patient gives you.[CONFRONTATION] *p. 122*
3. "The patient complains of nausea but denies vomiting. [PERTINENTNEGATIVE] *p. 125*
4. Believability. [CREDIBILITY] *p. 112*
6. Communication through facial expressions for example. [NONVERBAL] *p. 112*
7. Unit of power used to measure the strength of a radio transmitter.[WATT] *p. 116*
8. High-power two-way radio in a fixed location. [BASESTATION] *p. 114*
10. Echoing the patient's words back to him. [REFLECTION] *p. 122*
12. Possible answers to this type of question are predetermined. [CLOSEDENDED] *p. 121*
13. Understanding the situation of another person. [EMPATHY] *p. 112*
16. Message about a message. [FEEDBACK] *p. 112*
18. Person who initiates a message. [SENDER] *p. 112*

CHECK YOUR RECALL AND APPLY CONCEPTS KEY

EXERCISE 1

1. b   *p. 120*
2. d   *p. 125*
3. b   *p. 118*
4. c   *p. 121*
5. d   *p. 117*
6. c   *p. 121*
7. a   *p. 126*
8. b   *p. 118*

EXERCISE 2

1. Any four of the following: Sit next to the patient in the ambulance, not behind him where he cannot see you; do not interrupt the patient while he is answering your questions; do not be distracted by other people or activities; repeat back what the patient has told you; ask questions relative to what he has told you; look at the patient when he is speaking.
2. Summarize the information given in your radio report; add any relevant information; advise receiving staff of any additional treatment given; relate changes in the patient's condition.

CLINICAL REASONING CASE STUDY: A WELL-MEANING MOM

1. Say something like: "I know you have information for me, but I need to hear the answers to these questions from her."
2. You need to tactfully separate the teenager from her mother, so you might try sending the mother to collect her physician information or medications.
3. To gain her trust, you need to be able to interview her without family members present. Teenagers are often embarrassed about their bodies and are reluctant to discuss health issues.

Chapter 7: Medical Terminology

VOCABULARY AND CONCEPT REVIEW KEY

EXERCISE 1

1. d   *p. 139*
2. c   *p. 139*
3. g   *p. 135*
4. a   *p. 135*
5. f   *p. 135*
6. e   *p. 135*
7. b   *p. 135*

EXERCISE 2

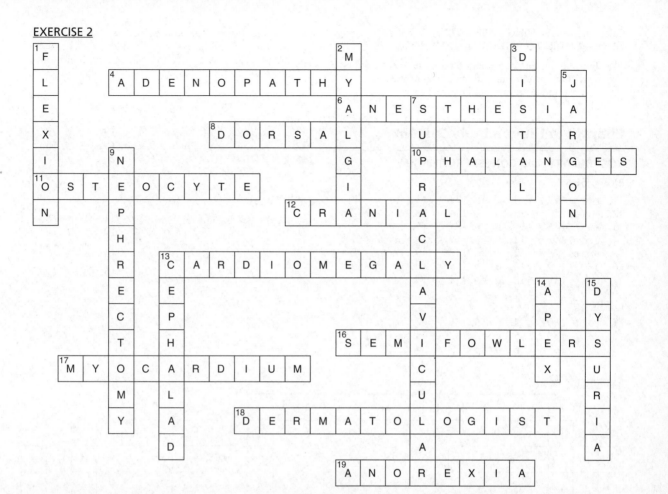

Across

4. Disease process of a gland. [ADENOPATHY] *p. 144*
6. Lack of sensation. [ANESTHESIA] *p. 144*
8. Pertaining to the back of the body or body structure. [DORSAL] *p. 141*
10. Finger bones. [PHALANGES] *p. 139*
11. Bone cell. [OSTEOCYTE] *p. 138*
12. Term that refers to the body cavity that houses the brain. [CRANIAL] *p. 142*
13. Enlargement of the heart. [CARDIOMEGALY] *p. 136*
16. Position in which the patient is partially sitting up. [SEMIFOWLERS] *p. 136*
17. Heart muscle. [MYOCARDIUM] *p. 136*
18. Physician who specializes in treatment of skin disorders. [DERMATOLOGIST] *p. 136*
19. Loss of appetite. [ANOREXIA] *p. 144*

Down

1. Action of bending a joint. [FLEXION] *p. 141*
2. Muscle pain. [MYALGIA] *p. 138*
3. Location of the fingers with reference to the wrist. [DISTAL] *p. 141*
5. Acronyms and idiomatic expressions that are not understood outside a particular group. [JARGON] *p. 139*
7. Above the clavicle. [SUPRACLAVICULAR] *p. 137*
9. Surgical removal of a kidney. [NEPHRECTOMY] *p. 138*
13. Toward the head. [CEPHALAD] *p. 141*
14. The tip of a structure. [APEX] *p. 141*
15. Difficult or painful urination. [DYSURIA] *p. 137*

CHECK YOUR RECALL AND APPLY CONCEPTS KEY

EXERCISE 1

1. suffix, *p. 135*
2. prefix, *p. 135*
3. the study of, *p. 136*
4. root word, *p. 136*
5. combining vowel, *p. 135*
6. root word, *p. 135*
7. prefix, *p. 136*
8. suffix, *p. 138*
9. suffix, *p. 138*
10. root word, *p. 135*

EXERCISE 2

1. dyspnea, *p. 144*
2. WNL, *p. 148*
3. sub, *p. 137*
4. without change, *p. 147, 148*
5. keep the vein open, *p. 148*
6. coronary artery bypass graft, *p. 145*
7. apnea, *p. 144*
8. pupils equal and reactive to light, *p. 147*
9. as needed (PRN), *p. 147*
10. rule out acute myocardial infarction, *pp. 148, 145*

CLINICAL REASONING CASE STUDY: PATIENT TRANSPORTED TO REHABILITATION HOSPITAL

1. This patient has been diagnosed with an enlarged heart but has chronic inflammation of the heart valves and tissue surrounding the heart.

2. He was probably given the antiemetic to prevent motion sickness on his trip. Traveling backward in an ambulance is difficult for patients with motion sickness.

Chapter 8: Human Body Systems

VOCABULARY AND CONCEPT REVIEW KEY

EXERCISE 1

1. f *p. 158*	8. r *p. 174*	15. t *p. 157*
2. l *p. 157*	9. q *p. 154*	16. d *p. 157*
3. k *p. 158*	10. b *p. 185*	17. o *p. 158*
4. g *p. 157*	11. i *p. 185*	18. m *p. 155*
5. p *p. 174*	12. s *p. 157*	19. e *p. 158*
6. a *p. 159*	13. c *p. 156*	20. j *p. 160*
7. h *p. 159*	14. n *p. 155*	

EXERCISE 2

1. i *p. 180*	4. n *p. 175*	7. o *p. 173*
2. s *p. 180*	5. t *p. 167*	8. m *p. 172*
3. c *p. 167*	6. d *p. 177*	9. e *p. 162*

(continued, right column)

10. j *p. 162*	14. g *p. 174*	18. r *p. 176*
11. f *p. 155*	15. p *p. 174*	19. q *p. 166*
12. l *p. 167*	16. a *p. 173*	20. b *p. 173*
13. k *p. 174*	17. h *p. 176*	

EXERCISE 3

1. g *p. 166*	6. j *p. 201*	11. i *p. 185*
2. f *p. 153*	7. c *p. 176*	12. d *p. 191*
3. n *p. 185*	8. m *p. 185*	13. a *p. 155*
4. e *p. 188*	9. b *p. 202*	14. k *p. 191*
5. l *p. 155*	10. o *p. 178*	15. h *p. 199*

EXERCISE 4

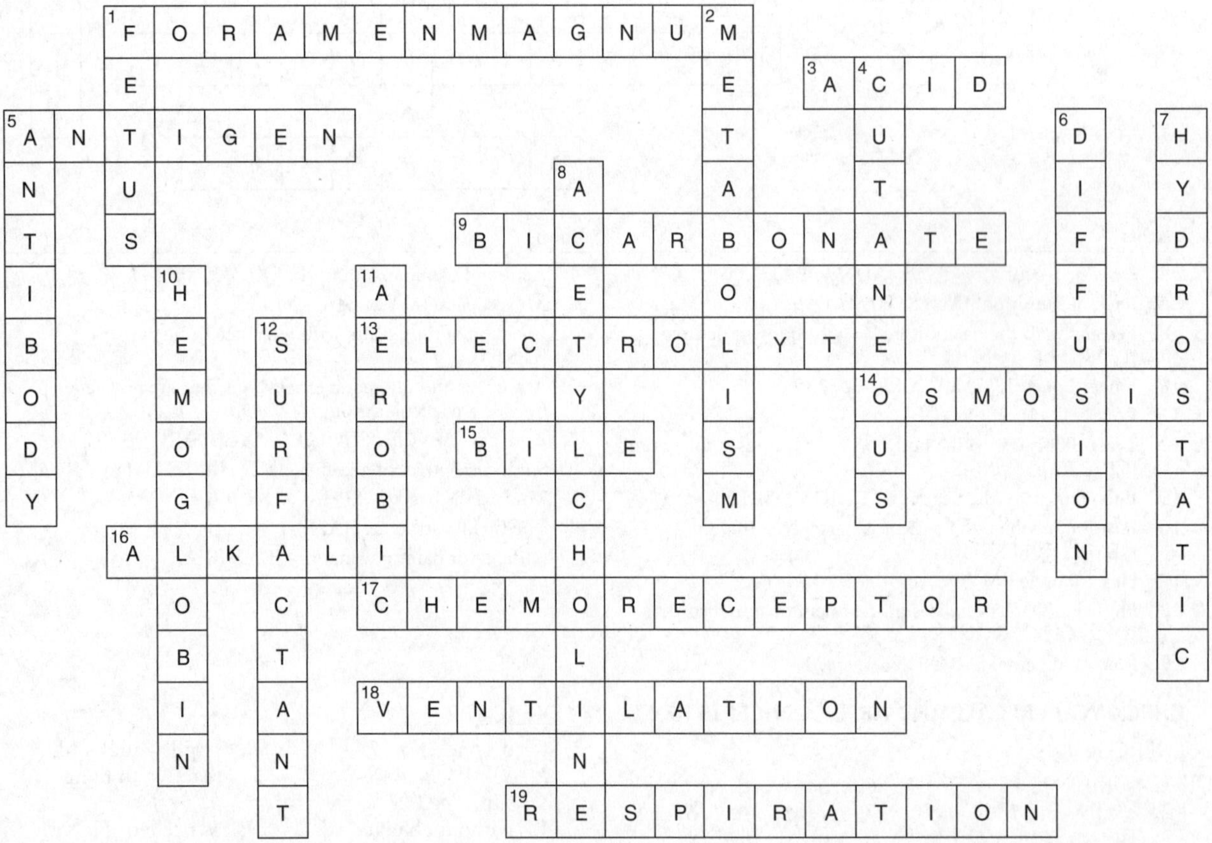

Crossword answer key:

Across:
1. FORAMEN MAGNUM
3. ACID
5. ANTIGEN
9. BICARBONATE
13. ELECTROLYTE
14. OSMOSIS
15. BILE
16. ALKALI
17. CHEMORECEPTOR
18. VENTILATION
19. RESPIRATION

Down (selected):
2. METABOLISM
4. CUTANEOUS
5. ANTIBODY
6. DIFFUSION
7. HYDROSTATIC
10. HEMOGLOBIN
12. SURFACTANT

Across	Down
1. Large opening at the base of the skull. [FORAMENMAGNUM] *p. 167*	1. Human organism from the eighth week of gestation to birth. [FETUS] *p. 206*
3. Substance that gives up hydrogen ions in a solution. [ACID] *p. 158*	2. Sum of all chemical and physical changes in the body. [METABOLISM] *p. 157*
5. Any substance recognized by the body as foreign. [ANTIGEN] *p. 180*	4. Pertaining to the skin. [CUTANEOUS] *p. 172*
9. Increased amount in the blood indicates alkalosis. [BICARBONATE] *p. 174*	5. Substance synthesized by immune system that recognizes a foreign material and initiates a specific immune response against it. [ANTIBODY] *p. 180*
13. Substances that dissosiates into ions when placed in a solution. [ELECTROLYTE] *p. 154*	6. Movement of solutes from an area of higher concentration to an area of lower concenteation. [DIFFUSION] *p. 174*
14. Movement of water across a semipermeable membrane to achieve equilibration of solute concentration. [OSMOSIS] *p. 155*	7. Type of pressure exerted by water. [HYDROSTATIC] *p. 155*
15. Bitter fluid that breaks down fats in the digestive tract. [BILE] *p. 203*	8. Preganglionic sympathetic nervous system neurotransmitter. [ACETYLCHOLINE] *p. 193*
16. Substance that accepts hydrogen ions in a solution. [ALKALI] *p. 158*	10. Iron-containing protein molecule that carries oxygen within red blood cells. [HEMOGLOBIN] *p. 174*
17. Sensory cells that respond to chemical changes in the body. [CHEMORECEPTOR] *p. 177*	11. Phase of metabolism that occurs when oxygen is present at the cellular level. [AEROBIC] *p. 157*
18. Movement of air in and out of the lungs. [VENTILATION] *p. 173*	12. Substance that acts to prevent collapse of the alveoli. [SURFACTANT] *p. 176*
19. Exchange of oxygen and carbon dioxide between the body and the environment. [RESPIRATION] *p. 173*	

CHECK YOUR RECALL AND APPLY CONCEPTS KEY

EXERCISE 1

1. c *p. 156*   5. a *p. 158*   9. b *p. 180*
2. c *p. 157*   6. d *p. 171*   10. a *p. 183*
3. b *p. 157*   7. d *p. 157*
4. a *p. 157*   8. a *p. 156*

EXERCISE 2

A. 1. chromatin, *p. 160*
2. nucleolus, *p. 160*
3. nuclear envelope, *p. 160*
4. centriole, *p. 160*
5. free ribosomes, *p. 160*
6. cytoplasm, *p. 160*
7. lysosome, *p. 160*
8. rough endoplasmic reticulum, *p. 160*
9. nucleus, *p. 160*
10. mitochondrion, *p. 160*
11. smooth endoplasmic reticulum, *p. 160*
12. nuclear pore, *p. 160*
13. ribosome, *p. 160*
14. cell membrane, *p. 160*
15. cell coat, *p. 160*
16. Golgi body, *p. 160*

B. 1. coronal or frontal plane, *p. 163*
2. transverse or horizontal plane, *p. 163*
3. midsagittal plane, *p. 163*

C. 1. skull, *p. 169*
2. cervical spine, *p. 169*
3. manubrium, *p. 169*
4. sternum, *p. 169*
5. xiphoid process, *p. 169*
6. thoracic spine, *p. 169*
7. costal cartilage, *p. 169*
8. lumbar spine, *p. 169*
9. iliac crest, *p. 169*
10. pelvis, *p. 169*
11. femoral head, *p. 169*

12. acetabulum, *p. 169*
13. pubis, *p. 169*
14. ischium, *p. 169*
15. clavicle, *p. 169*
16. scapula, *p. 169*
17. ribs, *p. 169*
18. humerus, *p. 169*
19. elbow, *p. 169*
20. ulna, *p. 169*
21. radius, *p. 169*
22. femur, *p. 169*
23. patella, *p. 169*
24. tibia, *p. 169*
25. fibula, *p. 169*
26. tarsals, *p. 169*
27. metatarsals, *p. 169*
28. phalanges, *p. 169*

D. 1. frontal bone
2. sphenoid bone
3. nasal bone
4. lacrimal bone
5. ethmoid bone
6. maxillary bone
7. zygomatic bone
8. parietal bone
9. temporal bone
10. occipital bone
11. external auditory canal
12. mastoid bone
13. styloid process
14. zygomatic process
15. temporal process
16. mandible

E. 1. superior vena cava, *p. 183*
2. aorta, *p. 183*
3. pulmonary trunk, *p. 183*
4. right atrium, *p. 183*
5. pulmonary valve, *p. 183*

6. tricuspid valve, *p. 183*
7. right ventricle, *p. 183*
8. inferior vena cava, *p. 183*
9. left atrium, *p. 183*
10. aortic valve, *p. 183*
11. mitral valve, *p. 183*
12. left ventricle, *p. 183*
13. endocardium, *p. 183*
14. myocardium, *p. 183*
15. epicardium, *p. 183*

F. 1. rectum, *p. 206*
2. prostate gland, *p. 206*
3. bulbourethral gland, *p. 206*
4. urinary bladder, *p. 206*
5. seminal vesicle, *p. 206*
6. symphysis pubis, *p. 206*
7. vas deferens, *p. 206*
8. urethra, *p. 206*
9. epididymus, *p. 206*
10. glans penis, *p. 206*
11. testis, *p. 206*

G. 1. cervix, *p. 207*
2. vagina, *p. 207*
3. fallopian tube, *p. 207*
4. ovary, *p. 207*

Chapter 9: Life Span Development and Cultural Considerations

VOCABULARY AND CONCEPT REVIEW KEY
EXERCISE 1

1. fontanel, *p. 218*
2. preschooler, *p. 216*
3. school-age child, *p. 216*
4. life span, *p. 216*

5. rectouterine pouch, *p. 207*
6. uterus, *p. 207*
7. urinary bladder, *p. 207*
8. urethra, *p. 207*
9. clitoris, *p. 207*
10. labia minora, *p. 207*
11. vaginal orifice, *p. 207*

CLINICAL REASONING CASE STUDY: DROWNING AT MOSQUITO LAKE

1. Drowning is a form of asphyxia, which prevents ventilation. Without ventilation, respiration cannot occur. The cells can engage in anaerobic metabolism for a short time, but at the cost of decreased energy production and accumulation of cellular wastes. Without knowing what led to the drowning, you must also suspect other underlying problems, such as trauma or medical problems (hypoglycemia or seizures, for example).
2. In the absence of oxygen, there is decreased energy production and accumulation of lactic acid. Without adequate energy and in the presence of acidosis the cellular sodium/potassium fails. Excess sodium in the cell promotes water entry into the cell and cellular lysis.

5. hospice, *p. 226*
6. adolescent, *p. 216*
7. grief, *p. 226*
8. life expectancy, *p. 216*
9. toddler, *p. 216*
10. bereavement, *p. 226*
11. palliative care, *p. 229*
12. proprioception, *p. 223*
13. mourning, *p. 226*
14. infant, *p. 216*

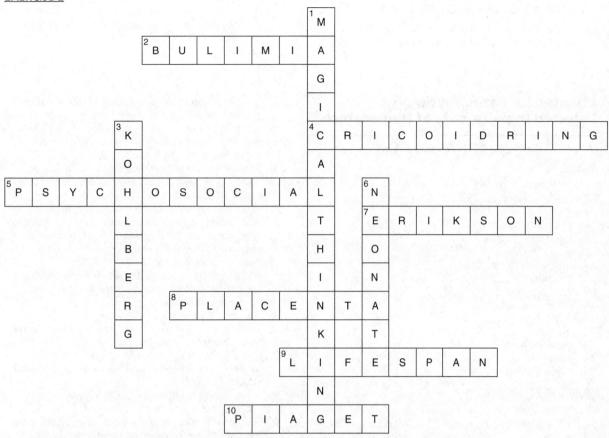

Across

2. Eating disorder characterized by binging and purging. [BULIMIA] *p. 222*

4. Narrowest part of the infant airway. [CRICOIDRING] *p. 219*

5. Type of development based on psychological maturation through interactions in a social context. [PSYCHOSOCIAL] *p. 214*

7. His eight-stage theory of development is based on the resolution of conflicts at various stages of life from birth through old age. [ERIKSON] *p. 214*

8. It allows maternal antibodies to be passed to a fetus before birth. [PLACENTA] *p. 220*

9. About 120 years for human beings. [LIFESPAN] *p. 216*

10. His theory of development explains how people develop cognitively up to adulthood. [PIAGET] *p. 214*

Down

1. Toddlers use this to explain things they cannot yet understand. [MAGICALTHINKING] *p. 221*

3. His theory of development explains the moral reasoning behind actions. [KOHLBERG] *p. 215*

6. Individual from birth to one month of age. [NEONATE] *p. 215*

CHECK YOUR RECALL AND APPLY CONCEPTS KEY

EXERCISE 1

1.	T	*p. 223*	9. F	*p. 218*
2.	F	*p. 214*	10. F	*p. 219*
3.	F	*pp. 214, 215*	11. T	*p. 220*
4.	T	*p. 216*	12. F	*p. 224*
5.	F	*p. 216*	13. T	*p. 225*
6.	T	*p. 216*	14. T	*p. 226*
7.	T	*p. 216*	15. F	*p. 229*
8.	F	*p. 218*		

EXERCISE 2

1. adolescent, *pp. 221, 222*
2. school-age child, *p. 221*
3. older adult, *pp. 223, 224*
4. middle-age adult, *p. 222*
5. young adult, *p. 222*
6. toddler, *pp. 220, 221*
7. infant, *pp. 216–220*
8. preschooler, *pp. 220, 221*
9. young adult, *p. 222*
10. adolescent *pp. 221, 222*

1. Pain perception decreases with age and even serious injury and illness may not produce the expected degree of pain.

Chapter 10: Pathophysiology: Selected Impairments of Homeostasis

VOCABULARY AND CONCEPT REVIEW KEY

EXERCISE 1

1. atelectasis, *p. 243*
2. defibrillation, *p. 245*
3. pathology, *p. 234*
4. pyruvate, *p. 238*
5. hypoxia, *p. 234*
6. sign, *p. 234*
7. anaphylaxis, *p. 234*
8. symptom, *p. 234*
9. cardiomyopathy, *p. 251*
10. shock, *p. 235*
11. ischemia, *p. 237*
12. apoptosis, *p. 239*
13. pneumothorax, *p. 243*
14. hyperpyrexia, *p. 258*
15. asphyxiation *p. 245*

EXERCISE 2

1. f	*p. 251*	6. j	*p. 234*	11. k	*p. 250*
2. i	*p. 250*	7. m	*p. 234*	12. g	*p. 245*
3. h	*p. 258*	8. a	*p. 244*	13. l	*p. 245*
4. n	*p. 245*	9. o	*p. 244*	14. b	*p. 245*
5. c	*p. 250*	10. d	*p. 227*	15. e	*p. 250*

EXERCISE 3

1. It is the portion of the airway in which gases are present but there is no mechanism for exchange of gases with the blood. *p. 239*

2. Teens can have a sense of invulnerability. This, along with immature judgment and the experimentation that emerges during identity development, can lead to risky behaviors, including unsafe driving.

2. It is the preliminary determination of the patient's problem based on the patient's history, signs, and symptoms and the application of the EMS provider's knowledge and process of clinical reasoning to the problem. *p. 234*

3. It is a state of inadequate cellular perfusion in which the body can no longer maintain perfusion to the vital organs. *p. 250*

4. It is a state of inadequate cellular perfusion in which the body can make adjustments to maintain perfusion to the vital organs, but at the cost of decreased circulation and oxygenation of the peripheral tissues. *p. 250*

5. It is a hyperglycemic diabetic emergency in which the patient suffers from dehydration, acidosis, and electrolyte imbalance. *p. 246*

6. It is a state of shock in which, even with proper resuscitation, the patient ultimately cannot survive the amount of tissue damage done. *p. 249*

7. It is the chemical formed from pyruvate in anaerobic metabolism, and the cause of acidosis in shock. *p. 238*

8. It is a decreased blood pH and decrease in bicarbonate. *p. 238*

9. It is the obstruction of the pulmonary circulation by a blood clot or other material, resulting in ventilation of a nonperfused area of the lung and decreased oxygenation. *p. 244*

10. It is a condition in which either pulmonary circulation or alveolar ventilation is impaired. *p. 243*

EXERCISE 4

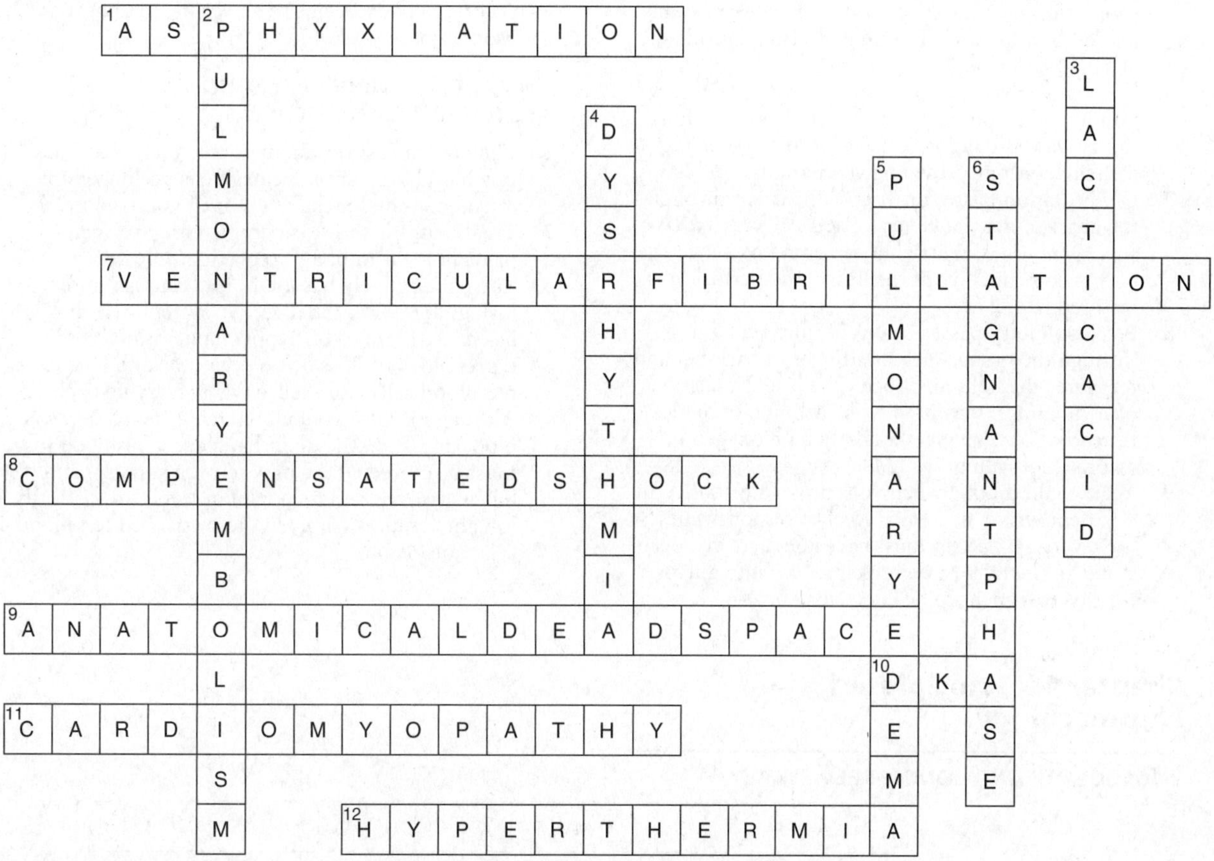

Crossword grid answers:

Across:
- 1. ASPHYXIATION
- 7. VENTRICULARFIBRILLATION
- 8. COMPENSATEDSHOCK
- 9. ANATOMICALDEADSPACE
- 11. CARDIOMYOPATHY
- 12. HYPERTHERMIA
- 10. DKA

Down words shown in grid: PULMONOEDEMA, DYSRHYTHMIA, LACTICACID, PULMONARYEMBOLISM, STAGNATPHASE, VARY, COMB..., etc.

Across

1. Suffocation. [ASPHYXIATION]   *p. 245*

7. Lethal cardiac dysrhythmia in which there is chaotic, ineffective electrical activity. [VENTRICULARFIBRILLATION]   *p. 245*

8. Perfusion is inadequate but the blood pressure is normal. [COMPENSATEDSHOCK]   *p. 250*

9. Portion of the airway where air is present but gas exchange cannot occur. [ANATOMICALDEADSPACE]   *p. 239*

5. State of hyperglycemia, dehydration, and acidosis in a patient with diabetes.[DKA]   *p. 246*

6. Type of enlargement of the heart that results in inadequate heart function.[CARDIOMYOPATHY]   *p. 251*

7. High body temperature due to exposure to a hot environment.[HYPERTHERMIA]   *p. 258*

Down

2. Blood clot that obstructions circulation through the lungs. [PULMONARYEMBOLISM]   *p. 244*

3. Byproduct of anaerobic metabolism.[LACTICACID]   *p. 238*

4. Abnormal heartbeat.[DYSRHYTHMIA]   *p. 251*

5. Increase in interstitial fluid in the lungs that interferes with gas exchange.[PULMONARYEDMA]   *p. 234*

6. Stage of shock in which both the precapillary and postcapillary sphincters are closed.[STAGNATPHASE]   *p. 250*

CHECK YOUR RECALL AND APPLY CONCEPTS KEY

1. The increased amount of insulin quickly facilitates the entry of the available glucose into cells. Without an additional source of glucose from the digestive tract, the blood glucose level quickly falls.   *p. 235*

2. Carbon monoxide binds to hemoglobin, preventing oxygen from binding to it. Oxygen is not delivered to the cellular level, impairing cellular metabolism and the patient becomes hypoxic.   *p. 235*

3. Without enough glucose circulating in the blood, the cells are unable to create enough energy to power the body.   *p. 235*

4. A ruptured bleb, or weakened area of lung tissue, causes a spontaneous pneumothorax in which air enters the pleural cavity and travels upward, beginning collapse of the lung from the top.   *p. 242*

5. Fluid that collects between the alveoli and capillaries, preventing normal exchange of oxygen and carbon dioxide. The fluid also may invade the alveolar sacs. *p. 243*

6. Supportive measures for patients with respiratory failure and respiratory arrest include maintaining the airway, providing supplemental oxygen, and assisting with or providing ventilations. *p. 243*

7. Defibrillation passes an electrical current through the heart to disrupt chaotic electrical activity. If successful, the sinoatrial node again takes over the pacemaker function of the heart, and perfusion is restored. *p. 245*

8. Pulse oximetry passes beams of infrared light through the tissue (such as a finger or earlobe) and measures the light absorbed. The bright red color of hemoglobin saturated with carbon monoxide instead of oxygen gives a falsely high oxygen saturation reading. *p. 244*

9. You would do this when you cannot start an IV in a patient with a decreased level of responsiveness; however, the patient must have adequate glycogen stores in the liver to be broken down into glucose for this treatment to be effective. *p. 246*

10. When the core temperature drops below a certain point, the body begins to shiver increase heat production. *p. 258*

CLINICAL REASONING CASE STUDY: CALL TO PHYSICIAN'S OFFICE

1. The patient is suffering hypovolemic shock. The low blood pressure indicates he is no longer able to compensate for the amount of volume lost.

2. Treatment for shock is administering oxygen, providing warmth, and replacing fluids.

3. The patient likely has a GI bleed and is rapidly losing blood into the digestive system, which has caused him to be hypovolemic. Blood loss represents both loss of fluid volume and loss of red blood cells and their oxygen-carrying capacity. Although fluids may help increase the patient's blood pressure, the underlying cause of blood loss must be corrected (he may require surgery) and if his hematocrit and hemoglobin levels are critically low, he requires whole blood or packed red blood cell transfusion.

Chapter 11: Principles of Pharmacology

VOCABULARY AND CONCEPT REVIEW KEY

Across:
2. PARASYMPATHOLYTIC
6. INOTROPY
9. IDIOSYNCRATIC
13. IATROGENIC
15. CONTRAINDICATION
17. TOLERANCE
19. ABSORPTION
20. AGONIST
21. DROMOTROPY

Down:
1. FIBRINOLYTIC
3. THERAPEUTIC
4. HYPERSENSITIZATION
5. ANTITUSSIVE
7. POTENTIATION
8. DIURESIS
11. OTC
12. CHOLINERGIC
14. INDICATION
16. AFFINITIES
18. NASODYNAMIC

Across

2. Opposes the effects of acetylcholine. [PARASYMPATHOLYTIC] *p. 272*

6. Property that affects the strength of cardiac contraction. [INOTROPY] *p. 274*

9. Drug reaction that is unique to a given individual. [IDIOSYNCRATIC] *p. 278*

11. Acetaminophen is an example. [OTC] *p. 267*

13. Adverse reaction caused by medical treatment. [IATROGENIC] *p. 280*

15. A reason a drug must not be given. [CONTRAINDICATION] *p. 267*

17. The need for a larger dose of a drug to get the same effect as before. [TOLERANCE] *p. 280*

19. How a drug moves from the site of administration to the circulation. [ABSORPTION] *p. 270*

20. Drug that stimulates a specific action in the body. [AGONIST] *p. 272*

21. Property that affects the speed of cardiac conduction. [DROMOTROPY] *p. 274*

Down

1. Drug that acts to break down a blood clot. [FIBRINOLYTIC] *p. 274*

3. Causes harm to a fetus. [TERATOGENIC] *p. 269*

4. Results in an allergic reaction. [HYPERSENSITIVITY] *p. 280*

5. Drug that prevents blood from clotting. [ANTICOAGULANT] *p. 274*

7. Enhances the effect of another drug. [POTENTIATES] *p. 280*

8. Drug that increases urination. [DIURETIC] *p. 274*

12. Increases the function of the parasympathetic nervous system. [CHOLINERGIC] *p. 272*

14. A reason a drug is given. [INDICATION] *p. 267*

16. Degree of attraction between a drug and receptor. [AFFINITY] *p. 278*

18. Ibuprofen is an example. [NSAID] *p. 272*

CHECK YOUR RECALL AND APPLY CONCEPTS KEY

1.	b	*p. 270*	**5.**	c	*p. 271*	**9.**	a	*p. 278*
2.	c	*p. 267*	**6.**	d	*p. 273*	**10.**	d	*p. 272*
3.	a	*p. 267*	**7.**	b	*p. 274*	**11.**	c	*p. 280*
4.	d	*p. 270*	**8.**	c	*p. 275*	**12.**	c	*p. 278*

CLINICAL REASONING CASE STUDY: MRS. MILLER'S MEDICATION

1. You can explain to Mrs. Miller that the mechanism of action is the way that the drug works to have its effect in the body.

2. You can tell Mrs. Miller that an idiosyncratic reaction means an unexpected, unique reaction that is not anticipated. In an idiosyncratic reaction, a person has signs and symptoms other than the known side effect of the drug.

3. Mrs. Miller should understand that alcohol can increase or enhance the effects of the drug and that it may not be safe to consume alcohol while she is taking the drug.

4. Mrs. Miller can benefit from reliable sources of drug information intended for patients. For example, WebMD (http://www.webmd.com/drugs/) has information intended for consumers. Also let Mrs. Miller know that she should call or visit her pharmacy or call her physician's office if she has questions about her medications.

VOCABULARY AND CONCEPT REVIEW KEY

Across

1. Pertaining to the gastrointestinal tract. [ENTERNAL] *p. 286*
9. Substance that causes fever. [PYROGEN] *p. 313*
11. IV tubing that provides 1 mL per 60 gtts. [MICRODRIP] *p. 293*
12. Metric base unit for volume. [LITER] *p. 290*
15. Inserting a needle into a vein. [VENIPUNCTURE] *p. 309*
16. Gaseous analgesic. [NITROUSOXIDE] *p. 298*
17. Administration of medication by an intravenous drip. [INFUSION] *p. 287*
18. Diameter of a needle. [GAUGE] *p. 300*
19. Metric base unit for volume. [KILO] *p. 290*
20. Without infection. [ASEPTIC] *p. 296*
21. Muscle in which volumes of medication exceeding 2 mL can be injected. [GLUTEUS] *p. 288*
22. The type of container in which used sharps are properly disposed of. [BIOHAZARD] *p. 297*

Down

2. Refers to the front of the arm. [ANTECUBITAL] *p. 309*
3. Point at which two branches merge into a single vein. [BIFURCATION] *p. 310*
4. Drug that regulates the heartbeat. [ANTIDYSRHYTHMIC] *p. 286*
5. Escape of interavenous fluid into the surrounding tissue. [INFILTRATION] *p. 310*
6. Can be used in place of alcohol to prepare the skin for an IV. [POVIDONEIODINE] *p. 296*
7. One of the Six Rights of Medication Administration. [DOCUMENTATION] *p. 285*
8. Medication routes that go through the skin. [PERCUTANEOUS] *p. 286*
9. Inflammation of a vein. [PHLEBITIS] *p. 313*
10. Denominator in the standard drip rate calculation formula. [TIME] *p. 293*
13. Device that converts liquid medication to a fine mist. [NEBULIZER] *p. 298*
14. Medication route in which medicine is placed beneath the tongue. [SUBLINGUAL] *p. 287*
19. Metric prefix meaning one thousand. [KILO] *p. 291*

CHECK YOUR RECALL AND APPLY CONCEPTS KEY

1.	c	*p. 285*	5.	c	*p. 297*	9.	b	*p. 291*
2.	d	*p. 289*	6.	b	*p. 291*	10.	b	*p. 292*
3.	a	*p. 288*	7.	c	*p. 291*	11.	d	*p. 292*
4.	c	*p. 290*	8.	c	*p. 291*	12.	d	*p. 292*

CLINICAL REASONING CASE STUDY: NIGHT SHIFT IN THE PRESBYTERIAN HOSPITAL EMERGENCY DEPARTMENT

1. There are several possible complications of IV therapy. It will be helpful if you find out from the patient's nurse what prompted the call for your help. The problem could be that the constricting band was left in place after the IV was started, a clamp on the tubing could be closed, the tubing could be bent or pinched, or the patient's arm could be placed in position that is obstructing flow. The tip of the catheter may be against a valve in the vein, the catheter may be obstructed by a blood clot, the IV could be infiltrated, or the IV bag may not be high enough above the level of the patient's heart. Other problems, such as infection or pyrogenic reaction, are possible, but they would cause other signs and symptoms and would not be as likely to be reported as a problem with the way the IV is working.

2. Start by checking for simple problems that are easily corrected without having to discontinue the IV and start another one. Check above the site to see if the constricting band was left in place, check all of the clamps on the tubing, and examine the length of the tubing for problems. Check the height of the IV bag. Examine the IV site. If it is cool, firm, and swollen, suspect infiltration. If it is warm, red, and tender or painful, suspect infection. If the patient has systemic signs and symptoms, such as fever, chills, and back pain, he may be having a pyrogenic reaction.

3. If you suspect infiltration, infection, or pyrogenic reaction, discontinue the IV. Report the problem to the provider in charge of the patient's care. If troubleshooting the IV does not reveal a correctable problem, you should discontinue it and start an IV at another site.

4. When starting any IV, be sure you understand the reason the IV is needed. If the patient needs large volumes of fluid, a 16- or 14-gauge IV catheter is appropriate. Patients who will receive blood or blood products need at least an 18-gauge IV. If large volumes of medications or thick, viscous medications like dextrose solutions will be given, give an 18-gauge or larger catheter. For routine fluid administration or medications, an 18- or 20-gauge catheter is appropriate. Patients with small or fragile veins and pediatric patients may require a smaller catheter, such as a 22 gauge. The selection of tubing (or a saline lock) depends on the rate at which fluids will be administered. In the hospital setting, patients receiving medicine by IV infusion generally have an IV pump, for which special IV tubing is supplied. If a pump is not available and the patient will be receiving medication, use 60-gtt/mL tubing.

Chapter 13: Medications

VOCABULARY AND CONCEPT REVIEW KEY

Across

4. Solution with an osmolarity that is higher than that of plasma. [HYPERTONIC] *p. 322*

7. Substance that imitates the effects of epinephrine and norepinephrine in the body. [SYMPATHOMIMETIC] *p. 325*

9. Indication for 1:1000 epinephrine. [ANAPHYLAXIS] *p. 325*

12. Condition in which lactated Ringer's solution is contraindicated. [CRUSHSYNDROME] *p. 322*

16. It is indicated to reverse respiratory depression from narcotic overdose. [NALOXONE] *p. 326*

17. Aspirin is given to prevent aggregation of these. [PLATELETS] *p. 324*

19. Beta₂ selective bronchodilator administered by nebulizer or metered-dose inhaler. [ALBUTEROL] *p. 324*

20. Reason why a medication would be given for treatment. [INDICATION] *p. 322*

Down

1. This is given in a concentration of 50 percent to treat hypoglycemia in adults. [DEXTROSE] *p. 325*

2. Solution that contains small particles, such as electrolytes or dextrose. [CRYSTALLOID] *p. 322*

3. Acetyl salicylic acid. [ASPIRIN] *p. 324*

5. Solution that contains large protein molecules. [COLLOID] *p. 322*

6. 0.9% sodium chloride solution. [NORMALSALINE] *p. 322*

8. Therapeutic effect of nitroglycerin. [VASODILATION] *p. 327*

10. You must complete a thorough one of these before giving any drug. [ASSESSMENT] *p. 322*

11. Medication that provides pain relief. [ANALGESIC] *pp. 324, 327, 328*

13. NSAID that is used as an antipyretic in adults and children. [IBUPROFEN] *p. 328*

14. What can happen when too much IV fluid is given. [OVERLOAD] *p. 322*

15. Solution with an osmolarity that is in the same range as that of plasma. [ISOTONIC] *p. 322*

16. IV rate of 30 mL/hour. [TKO] *Chapter 7*

CHECK YOUR RECALL AND APPLY CONCEPTS KEY

EXERCISE 1

1. activated charcoal, *p. 328*
2. albuterol, *p. 324*
3. aspirin, *p. 324*
4. 50 percent dextrose, *p. 325*
5. epinephrine 1:1,000, *p. 325*

6. glucagon, *p. 326*
7. lactated Ringer's solution, *p. 323*
8. naloxone, *p. 326*
9. nitroglycerin, *p. 327*
10. nitrous oxide, *p. 327*
11. normal saline, *p. 323*

EXERCISE 2

1. a   *p. 323*
2. a   *p. 323*
3. b   *p. 323*
4. c   *p. 324*
5. c   *p. 324*
6. d   *p. 324*
7. a   *p. 324*
8. c   *p. 327*
9. a   *p. 325*
10. c   *p. 325*
11. d   *p. 325*
12. a   *p. 326*
13. a   *p. 326*
14. d   *p. 327*
15. b   *p. 327*

CLINICAL REASONING CASE STUDY: MEDICATION MYSTERY

1. You can carry a small print medication reference in your pocket, or download a medication resource onto your smart phone so that the information is readily at hand when you need it. Some of the electronic references (such as *Medscape* and *epocrates*) are free or have free trial versions. The advantage of an electronic resource is that it usually can be easily updated at little or no cost.

2. Doxazosin (Cardura) is an alpha blocker prescribed for the treatment of benign prostatic hypertrophy (BPH) in men and for the treatment of hypertension. (Remember: Alpha sympathetic stimulation causes vasoconstriction; blocking alpha effects decreases vasoconstriction and lowers the blood pressure.) Finasteride (Proscar) is another medication for BPH with a different mechanism of action. Flecainide (Tambocor) is an antidysrhythmic that is used to treat atrial fibrillation. Simvastatin (Zocor) is used to lower blood cholesterol levels, and azithromycin (Zithromax) is an antibiotic. Zithromax is used for several types of infections, including pneumonia and bronchitis, as well as some skin and throat infections.

3. You should suspect that the alpha blocker can lead to orthostatic hypotension by decreasing vasoconstriction, which could explain weakness and near syncope. However, the patient also seems to have a history of cardiac dysrhythmia, which also could explain his symptoms. The patient also appears to have a history of high cholesterol, which is a risk factor for cardiovascular disease. Sepsis also is a possibility, particularly if the antibiotic has been ineffective in treating the source of the patient's infection.

Chapter 14: General Approach to Patient Assessment and Clinical Reasoning

VOCABULARY AND CONCEPT REVIEW KEY

1.	c	p. 333	11.	f	p. 338
2.	g	p. 341	12.	s	p. 339
3.	k	p. 341	13.	i	p. 338
4.	a	p. 333	14.	o	p. 333
5.	n	p. 339	15.	e	p. 334
6.	d	pp. 341,342	16.	p	p. 341
7.	j	p. 333	17.	m	p. 334
8.	q	p. 341	18.	r	p. 334
9.	b	p. 337	19.	h	p. 334
10.	l	p. 333			

CHECK YOUR RECALL AND APPLY CONCEPTS

1.	a	p. 334	5.	c	p. 334
2.	c	p. 337	6.	d	p. 343
3.	d	p. 339	7.	a	pp. 337,342
4.	c	p. 340			

CLINICAL REASONING CASE STUDY: BREAKFAST AT GARCIA'S DINER

1. Even though you were not dispatched to the scene, you must approach it like you would any other scene. Look for potential hazards. Because you are in the kitchen, there may be a threat of being burned, sharp objects, or a slippery floor. Like any other scene, bystanders can pose a hazard, too. See if you can obtain additional information about the nature of the problem from someone who witnessed what happened. Determine if you need additional resources and request them. You have obtained the information that helps you form a general impression: The patient has an airway obstruction and inadequate breathing.

2. You can see that the patient is responsive, though he cannot speak. He has an airway obstruction, and cyanosis and lack of air movement tell you he has inadequate or absent breathing. From those findings, you can determine that he is a critical patient.

3. You must correct the problems with the patient's airway and breathing before moving on to the secondary assessment. However, once you have cleared the airway and the patient is breathing adequately, you must not neglect to perform a secondary assessment.

Chapter 15: Scene Size-Up and Primary Assessment

VOCABULARY AND CONCEPT REVIEW KEY

EXERCISE 1

1.	d	p. 360	6.	o	p. 359	11.	l	p. 359
2.	i	p. 360	7.	e	p. 354	12.	k	p. 359
3.	f	p. 359	8.	m	p. 361	13.	g	p. 359
4.	a	p. 350	9.	h	p. 350	14.	b	p. 360
5.	n	p. 354	10.	c	p. 359	15.	j	p. 359

EXERCISE 2

Across

3. Manual device used to deliver positive pressure ventilations. [BAGVALVEMASK] *p. 359*

6. Refers to the higher mental abilities, such as reasoning and problem-solving. [COGNITIVE] *p. 356*

7. Device that analyzes the cardiac rhythm in unresponsive, pulseless patients and delivers an electrical shock, if indicated. [AED] *p. 358*

8. Paleness of the skin. [PALLOR] *p. 361*

9. A patient should be situated like this if he is breathing spontaneously but is at risk for aspirating secretions in the airway. [RECOVERYPOSITION] *p. 359*

11. Patient's level of responsiveness and level of cognitive function. [MENTALSTATUS] *p. 356*

Down

1. Type of simple airway adjunct inserted through the nares and into the throat to provide a channel for air movement through the upper airway. [NASOPHARYNGEAL] *p. 358*

2. Yellowish discoloration of the skin, often due to liver disease. [JAUNDICE] *p. 354*

4. Muscles in the neck and abdomen that are not used in normal breathing, but are used to assist breathing in respiratory distress. [ACCESSORY] *p. 359*

5. Wide band placed circumferentially around an extremity to compress the blood vessels and control severe hemorrhage. [TOURNIQUET] *p. 361*

10. Scale used to assess the level of responsiveness.[GCS] *p. 355*

CHECK YOUR RECALL AND APPLY CONCEPTS KEY

1. b	*p. 350*	**6.** c	*p. 361*	**11.** b	*p. 358*
2. a	*p. 350*	**7.** d	*p. 353*	**12.** c	*p. 355*
3. c	*p. 351*	**8.** a	*p. 350*	**13.** b	*p. 356*
4. b	*p. 353*	**9.** b	*p. 350*	**14.** c	*p. 357*
5. a	*p. 360*	**10.** d	*p. 357*		

CLINICAL REASONING CASE STUDY: THE EVENING NEWS

1. As you approach the patient, look for information that helps you with a general impression. Look at the patient's position, apparent level of responsiveness, skin color, indications of injuries or obvious signs of illness (such as vomiting or loss of bladder control), and indications of breathing. Listen for abnormal breathing sounds. The patient's apparent decreased responsiveness, pale skin color, and difficulty breathing should result in a poor general impression.

2. As the team leader, ensure your team takes the actions you want them to. For example, "McKenzie, check his level of responsiveness. Kent, check his pulse for me."

3. The first question to ask is, "What happened?"

4. The primary assessment reveals problems with the patient's level of responsiveness, breathing, and perfusion. Even though the patient's airway is open, the decreased level of responsiveness means that the patient is at risk of airway obstruction. The information tells you that the patient is a high priority for transport, but that you must first ensure a patent airway.

5. Use a head-tilt/chin-lift maneuver and if tolerated, a nasopharyngeal airway. If the patient is able tolerate it, his breathing should be assisted with a bag-valve-mask device and supplemental oxygen. Otherwise, use a nonrebreather mask to administer oxygen and keep monitoring the

respiratory status. There is no obvious bleeding and the patient has a pulse, but there are signs of poor perfusion. As you are completing the tasks

of the primary assessment, ensure that one of your team members is retrieving the stretcher in preparation for transport.

Chapter 16: Airway Management, Ventilation, and Oxygenation

VOCABULARY AND CONCEPT REVIEW KEY

EXERCISE 1

1. laryngospasm, *p. 375*
2. hypoxia, *p. 383*
3. peak expiratory flow rate (PEFR), *p. 389*
4. pulmonary edema, *p. 377*

5. tracheostomy, *p. 393*
6. Yankauer, *p. 393*
7. bronchospasm, *p. 379*
8. capnometry, capnography, *p. 388*
9. French (Fr.), *p. 394*
10. hypercapnia, hypocapnia, *p. 388*
11. continuous positive airway pressure (CPAP), *p. 401*
12. pulse oximetry, *p. 386*
13. spirometry, *p. 389*
14. ventilation, *p. 372*

EXERCISE 2

Across

3. Artificial ventilation by forcing air into the airway. [POSITIVEPRESSURE] *p. 391*
5. Airway adjunct inserted into the mouth to prevent the tongue from occluding the airway. [OROPHARYNGEAL] *p. 376*
8. Measurement and graphic representation over time of the level of carbon dioxide in an exhaled air sample. [CAPNOGRAPHY] *p. 388*
9. Device that delivers a constant level of air pressure to the airway through a mask sealed tightly on the face. Hint: Abbreviation. [CPAP] *p. 401*
11. Narrowing of a bronchiole passageway. [BRONCHOCONSTRICTION] *p. 379*
13. Decreased level of carbon dioxide in the blood. [HYPOCAPNEA] *p. 388*
14. Volume of air that actually reaches the alveoli each minute. [ALVEOLARVENTILATION] *p. 377*

Down

1. Units of measure for the diameter of suction catheters. [FRENCH] *p. 394*
2. Airway adjunct inserted through the nose to prevent the tongue from occluding the airway. [NASOPHARYNGEAL] *p. 376*
4. Movement of air into and out of the lungs. [VENTILATION] *p. 372*
6. Increased level of carbon dioxide in the blood. [HYPERCAPNEA] *p. 388*
7. Measurement of the level of carbon dioxide in an exhaled air sample. [CAPNOMETRY] *p. 388*
10. Measurement of various lung volumes and flow rates. [SPIROMETRY] *p. 389*
12. Decreased level of oxygen at the cellular level. [HYPOXIA] *p. 383*

PATIENT ASSESSMENT REVIEW KEY

Scenario 1: Confirm the patient's mental status (confusion may indicate hypoxia, for example), carefully look and listen for signs of respiratory distress that may not be obvious at first glance, such as increased respiratory rate or effort, difficulty speaking, peripheral cyanosis (such as cyanosis of the nail beds), or wheezing that may be apparent as you get closer to the patient. Apply oxygen if signs of respiratory distress become evident.

Scenario 2: Confirm the mental status, identify the degree of distress by looking at the patient's position, assessing ability to speak, looking at the respiratory rate and effort, looking for cyanosis, and listening for abnormal sounds. Apply oxygen and, if ventilations are inadequate, assist ventilations with a bag-valve-mask device or, if indicated, CPAP.

Scenario 3: Confirm level of responsiveness. Look, listen, and feel for air movement to assess whether or not the airway is patent. If there are signs of airway obstruction, such as snoring or decreased or absent air movement, use manual maneuvers to open the airway (head-tilt/chin-lift or modified jaw-thrust maneuver). If necessary, insert an oropharyngeal airway (if the patient does not have a gag reflex) or nasopharyngeal airway to keep the airway open. Assess the rate and depth of ventilation. If ventilation is adequate, apply oxygen by nonrebreather mask. If ventilation is inadequate or absent, assist with or provide ventilations with a bag-valve-mask device. If partial airway obstruction is present, do not intervene to relieve the obstruction. If complete airway obstruction is present, use abdominal thrusts (responsive patient) or chest compressions (unresponsive patient) to relieve the obstruction.

Scenario 4: Confirm level of responsiveness. Look, listen, and feel for air movement to assess whether the airway is patent. If there are signs of airway obstruction, such as snoring or decreased or absent air movement, use manual maneuvers to open the airway (head-tilt/chin-lift or modified jaw-thrust maneuver). If necessary, insert an oropharyngeal airway (if the patient does not have a gag reflex) or nasopharyngeal airway to keep the airway open. Assess the rate and depth of ventilation. If ventilation is adequate, apply oxygen by nonrebreather mask. If ventilation is inadequate or absent, assist with or provide ventilations with a bag-valve-mask device. If partial airway obstruction is present, do not intervene to relieve the obstruction. If complete airway obstruction is present, use abdominal thrusts (responsive patient) or chest compressions (unresponsive patient) to relieve the obstruction.

Scenario 5: Check the carotid pulse. If no pulse is detected in 10 seconds, begin chest compressions. After 30 compressions, open the airway and deliver 2 ventilations and continue the cycle of 30 compressions to 2 ventilations while preparing an AED. If the patient has a pulse, open the airway using a manual maneuver and, if necessary, a basic airway adjunct. If the patient is not breathing after the airway has been opened, or if breathing is inadequate, assist with or provide ventilations by bag-valve-mask device with supplemental oxygen.

CHECK YOUR RECALL AND APPLY CONCEPTS KEY

1.	b	*p. 383*	10.	b	*p. 380*	19.	a	*p. 399*
2.	c	*p. 372*	11.	c	*p. 380*	20.	c	*p. 399*
3.	a	*p. 375*	12.	b	*p. 404*	21.	c	*p. 401*
4.	c	*p. 373*	13.	d	*p. 392*	22.	b	*p. 406*
5.	b	*p. 377*	14.	d	*p. 392*	23.	a	*p. 406*
6.	d	*p. 385*	15.	c	*p. 393*	24.	c	*p. 407*
7.	a	*p. 380*	16.	c	*p. 394*	25.	a	*p. 411*
8.	c	*p. 392*	17.	b	*p. 394*			
9.	a	*p. 380*	18.	b	*p. 397*			

CLINICAL REASONING CASE STUDY: AN INTERFACILITY TRANSFER

1. Mr. Thompson is in respiratory failure. Despite his increased respiratory rate and effort, he is unable to maintain an adequate SpO_2. His hypoxia is further evidenced by his altered mental status and inability to speak more than one to two words at a time. Mr. Thompson is a critical patient and is likely unstable.

2. Respiratory failure can quickly progress to respiratory arrest. Given the two-day history of increasing shortness of breath and the fact that he has not received treatment, Mr. Thompson could very well deteriorate into respiratory arrest and cardiac arrest in the 75 minutes it will take to transport him.

3. Advanced EMTs have the tools and training to treat respiratory failure and arrest in the short term, in patients presenting in the prehospital setting. However, those abilities do not represent definitive treatment of the patient in respiratory failure or respiratory arrest. The patient's treatment needs to be based on additional information and feedback about interventions that are not available in the prehospital setting, such as blood gas analysis. CPAP, judicious use of IV fluids, and a sympathetic beta$_2$ agonist may improve Mr. Thompson's condition, but he also may continue to deteriorate despite treatment because the underlying cause of his problem cannot be treated in the prehospital setting.

4. This situation presents a dilemma. Mr. Thompson has not received simple treatment that could improve his condition enough to determine if he is stable enough for ground transport to a different facility. Transporting a patient who has not been stabilized can place you in legal jeopardy. However, if the physician does not provide appropriate care, the patient will certainly deteriorate, even if he is not transported. A place to start would be to speak with the physician directly and ask if he has any orders to be carried out during transport. If the hospital is not your medical direction hospital, contact your medical director for guidance. You also must notify your supervisor of the situation. As with all dilemmas, there is not an easy answer. You must collect as much relevant information as quickly as you can and determine what is in the patient's best interests.

Chapter 17: Resuscitation: Managing Shock and Cardiac Arrest

VOCABULARY AND CONCEPT REVIEW KEY

EXERCISE 1

1. c   *p. 423*
2. e   *p. 426*
3. f   *p. 436*
4. d   *p. 423*
5. g   *p. 435*
6. b   *p. 435*
7. a   *p. 433*
8. i   *p. 417*
9. j   *p. 435*
10. h   *p. 447*

EXERCISE 2

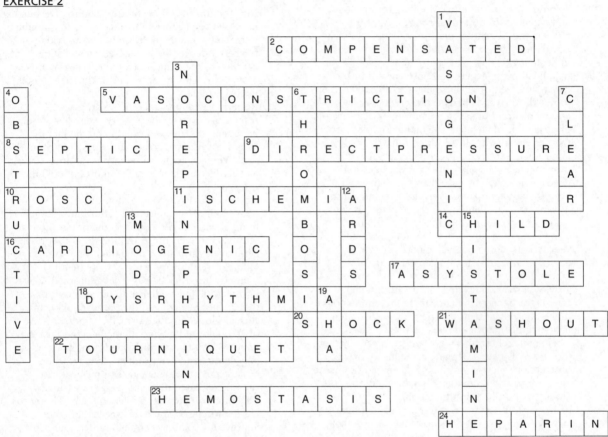

Across	Down

Across

2. A stage of shock that may be difficult to detect because the blood pressure is normal. [COMPENSATED] *pp. 419, 422*

5. First step in the response to laceration of a blood vessel. [VASOCONSTRICTION] *p. 428*

8. Type of shock that occurs from overwhelming infection. [SEPTIC] *p. 424*

9. Method that is effective in controlling most external bleeding. [DIRECTPRESSURE] *p. 428*

10. Abbreviation that means the pulse has come back in a patient who was in cardiac arrest. [ROSC] *p. 443*

11. State of decreased or absent blood flow to tissues. [ISCHEMIA] *p. 423*

14. For CPR purposes, a patient between one and eight years old. [CHILD] *p. 437*

16. Type of shock that occurs when the heart fails. [CARDIOGENIC] *p. 420*

17. Absence of electrical activity in the heart. [ASYSTOLE] *p. 435*

18. Abnormal heart beat. [DYSRHYTHMIA] *p. 435*

20. State in which perfusion is inadequate to meet the demands of cellular metabolism. [SHOCK] *p. 418*

21. Phase of shock in which micro-emboli are released from the capillary beds. [WASHOUT] *p. 419*

22. Device for stopping severe, uncontrollable bleeding in an extremity.[TOURNIQUET] *p. 431*

23. Process of stopping bleeding. [HEMOSTASIS] *p. 428*

24. Injectable anticoagulant that can result in excessive bleeding. [HEPARIN] *p. 430*

Down

1. Way to describe the mechanism behind distributive shock. [VASOGENIC] *p. 418*

3. An adrenal medullary hormone. [NOREPINEPHRINE] *p. 418*

4. Tension pneumothorax is a cause of this kind of shock. [OBSTRUCTIVE] *p. 420*

6. One of the "Five Ts" that can be an underlying cause of cardiac arrest. [THROMBOSIS] *p. 447*

7. What you must instruct all personnel to do before delivering a defibrillation shock to a patient. [CLEAR] *p. 443*

12. Abbreviation for a condition of noncardiogenic pulmonary edema. [ARDS] *p. 423*

13. Abbreviation for a complication of shock in which several body systems are damaged and fail. [MODS] *p. 423*

15. Primary cheminal mediator of anaphylactic reactions that causes vasodilation. [HISTAMINE] *p. 424*

19. Abbreviation for the organization that establishes national guidelines for CPR and emergency cardiac care. [AHA] *p. 432*

CHECK YOUR RECALL AND APPLY CONCEPTS KEY

1.	a	*p. 418*	6.	c	*p. 435*	11.	c	*p. 436*
2.	c	*p. 419*	7.	d	*p. 439*	12.	a	*p. 442*
3.	c	*p. 431*	8.	a	*p. 420*	13.	b	*p. 437*
4.	a	*p. 433*	9.	c	*p. 420*			
5.	b	*p. 433*	10.	d	*p. 420*			

CLINICAL REASONING CASE STUDY: TROUBLE IN THE MEADOW

1. The worst-case scenario is that the patient is in anaphylactic shock from bee sting allergy. The remote distance and long response and transport times make it critical that the patient has an epinephrine auto-injector to treat his condition while awaiting help. If anaphylaxis is severe, the patient could suffer airway obstruction, respiratory failure, or cardiovascular collapse prior to your arrival.

2. Mr. Shaffer's signs and symptoms are due to the release of histamine and other substances in reaction to mast cell degranulation that occurs when there is an antibody–antigen (in this case, a protein in wasp venom) interaction. Histamine causes vasodilation and smooth-muscle constriction in the respiratory and gastrointestinal tracts. The pale, cool, sweaty skin is due to poor perfusion and activation of the sympathetic nervous system. His rapid heart rate is a compensatory mechanism that, unfortunately, is not working. The itchy throat is an indication of upper airway swelling, and wheezing indicates bronchiolar constriction. With continued swelling, airway obstruction and respiratory failure will lead to hypoxia. Without treatment to cause vasoconstriction and replace fluids lost from the vascular space, poor perfusion will lead to cellular dysfunction and death and the patient may die.

3. Although the patient is wheezing and complains of an itchy throat, he is speaking and, therefore, has an airway and is able to breathe. The cause of difficulty breathing is constriction of the bronchioles, which must be reversed. The best way to improve the patient's circulatory status is to combat vasodilation and hypovolemia. Giving intramuscular epinephrine will cause vasoconstriction, which will limit upper airway swelling, relax bronchiolar smooth muscle to improve airflow in the lungs, and constrict the peripheral vasculature to raise the blood pressure and improve perfusion. The patient should immediately receive 0.3 to 0.5 mg of 1:1,000 epinephrine, IM. Apply oxygen if the SpO_2 is below 95 percent. Start an IV of isotonic crystalloid and infuse at a rate that replaces the vascular volume. If wheezing continues, an inhaled sympathetic beta$_2$ agonist, such as albuterol, may be indicated. The half-life of epinephrine is short, and repeated doses may be needed because of the prolonged transport time.

Chapter 18: Vital Signs and Monitoring Devices

VOCABULARY AND CONCEPT REVIEW KEY

EXERCISE 1

1. capillary refill time, *p. 454*
2. fever, *p. 465*
3. vital signs, *p. 454*
4. systolic blood pressure, *p. 458*
5. anisocoria, *p. 468*
6. hyperthermia, *p. 465*
7. hyperpyrexia, *p. 465*
8. hypoglycemia, *p. 470*
9. sphygmomanometer, *p. 454*
10. turgor, *p. 466*

11. antecubital fossa, *p. 455*
12. auscultate, *p. 460*
13. capnometry, *p. 469*
14. cyanosis, *p. 463*
15. palpate, *p. 454*
16. pulse oximetry, *p. 454*
17. pulsus paradoxus, *p. 459*
18. tympanic, *p. 465*
19. icterus, *p. 466*
20. Cushing reflex, *p. 457*
21. electrocardiogram, *p. 471*
22. hypertension, *p. 457*
23. pulse pressure, *p. 458*
24. crackles (rales), *p. 464*
25. tachycardia, *p. 456*

EXERCISE 2

Across	Down

Across

3. Yellow discoloration of the skin resulting from liver disease. [JAUNDICE] *p. 466*

7. Listening to sounds inside the body, usually wih the aid of a stethoscope. [AUSCULTATE] *p. 460*

9. An abnormality in the electrical activity of the heart in which it departs from the rules that define normal sinus rhythm. [CARDIACDYSRHYTHMIA] *p. 471*

12. Blood glucose level that is lower than normal. [HYPOGLYCEMIA] *p. 470*

14. Yellow discoloration of the sclera of the eye resulting from liver disease. [ICTERUS] *p. 466*

15. Bluish or purplish discoloration of the skin and tissues when there is an increased amount of desaturated hemoglobin in the blood. [CYANOSIS] *p. 463*

16. 16. The amount of CO_2 in exhaled air at the end of expiration. [ENDTIDAL] *p. 470*

Down

1. A higher-than-normal blood glucose level. [HYPERGLYCEMIA] *p. 471*

2. Measurement of CO_2 in expired air. [CAPNOMETRY] *p. 469*

4. Coarse, rumbling sounds heard on auscultation, indicating the presence of secretions in the bronchi. [RHONCHI] *p. 464*

5. High blood pressure. [HYPERTENSION] *p. 457*

6. A slower than normal heart rate, which is a heart rate less than 60 per minute in adults. [BRADYCARDIA] *p. 456*

8. A condition in which the pupils are unequal. [ANISOCORIA] *p. 468*

10. Fine crackling, popping sounds ausculated on inspiration, indicating fluid at the level of the terminal bronchioles and alveoli. [RALES] *p. 464*

11. 11. High-pitched whistling sounds that can be heard on exhalation when the bronchioles are constricted. [WHEEZES] *p. 464*

13. A physical examination in which the examiner uses his hands to feel for signs of illness or injury, or to obtain the pulse. [PALPATE] *p. 454*

CHECK YOUR RECALL AND APPLY CONCEPTS KEY

1. c *p. 463*	9. a *p. 460*	17. d *p. 454*
2. d *p. 454*	10. c *p. 465*	18. a *p. 457*
3. c *p. 454*	11. b *p. 466*	19. b *p. 457*
4. d *p. 454*	12. d *p. 469*	20. b *p. 462*
5. a *p. 457*	13. c *p. 470*	21. a *p. 455*
6. c *p. 457*	14. c *p. 454*	22. a *p. 464*
7. c *p. 459*	15. b *p. 454*	23. d *p. 465*
8. d *p. 458*	16. a *p. 455*	

CLINICAL REASONING CASE STUDY: A TOUCH OF LIGHTHEADEDNESS

1. The history of vomiting and diarrhea, especially with an episode of near syncope (near fainting) should lead you to think that Mrs. Hebert has lost a considerable amount of fluid. You should anticipate an increased heart rate and, possibly, a decreased blood pressure. If the cause of vomiting and diarrhea is infectious, you also might find an elevated body temperature. The respiratory rate might or might not be affected. If there is a change in respirations, they most likely would be slightly increased.

2. Orthostatic vital signs are assessed when it is unclear whether or not the patient might have decreased fluid volume. In this case, Mrs. Hebert nearly lost consciousness when she stood up, indicating that she has lost enough fluid that she cannot compensate when she changes positions. It is not safe to have her stand for minutes to assess orthostatic vital signs.

3. It is not known whether or not the patient has a history of diabetes, but the near syncopal episode and history of vomiting and diarrhea should prompt you to obtain a blood glucose level. Pulse oximetry will be useful in this patient and, if allowed in your scope of practice, you should consider cardiac monitoring.

VOCABULARY AND CONCEPT REVIEW KEY

EXERCISE 1

1. f   *p. 491*
2. b   *p. 494*
3. i   *p. 481*
4. e   *p. 491*
5. h   *p. 500*
6. c   *p. 486*
7. l   *p. 501*
8. j   *p. 487*
9. a   *p. 501*
10. g   *p. 487*
11. d   *p. 491*
12. k   *p. 486*

EXERCISE 2

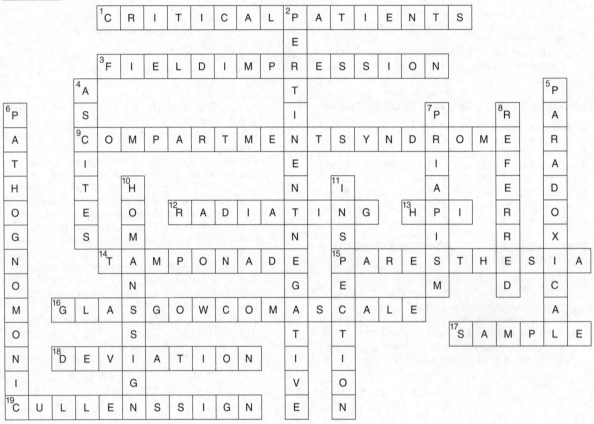

1. They are reassessed every 5 minutes. [CRITICALPATIENTS] *p. 483*

2. When a patient with an injury to his head says he did not lose consciousness, you document that information as a(n)_____. [PERTINENTNEGATIVE] *p. 486*

3. Understanding of the patient's immediate problems, used to make patient care decisions. [FIELDIMPRESSION] *p. 481*

4. A collection of fluid in the abdominal cavity. [ASCITES] *p. 504*

9. What you should suspect in an extremity that has the five Ps: pain, paralysis, pallor, paresthesia, and pulselessness. [COMPARTMENTSYNDROME] *p. 502*

5. Type of movement in which the chest wall moves in the opposite direction than expected. [PARADOXICAL] *p. 500*

12. Type of pain that arises in one location and travels to another, secondary, location. [RADIATING] *p. 487*

6. A sign that is so characteristic of a certain disorder that it is considered diagnostic. [PATHOGNOMONIC] *p. 491*

13. An elaboration of the events surrounding the patient's current problem. [HPI] *p. 487*

7. Involuntary penile erection that can indicate spinal cord injury. [PRIAPISM] *p. 501*

14. A heart condition that should be suspected when the jugular veins are distended. [TAMPONADE] *p. 495*

8. Type of pain that arises somewhere other than the location of the underlying problem. [REFERRED] *p. 487*

15. Tingling sensation. [PARESTHESIA] *p. 501*

16. Assessment tool that assigns a numerical score to the patient's level of responsiveness. [GLASGOWCOMASCALE] *p. 503*

10. Pain in the calf with dorsiflexion of the foot; an indication of deep vein thrombosis. [HOMANSSIGN] *p. 502*

17. Mnemonic used as a checklist to ensure you have obtained a thorough medical history. [SAMPLE] *p. 486*

11. Visualizing the body or a part of it to look for signs of illness or injury. [INSPECTION] *p. 491*

18. What can happen to the trachea when there is a tension pneumothorax. [DEVIATION] *p. 495*

19. Periumbilical ecchymosis. [CULLENSSIGN] *p. 500*

CHECK YOUR RECALL AND APPLY CONCEPTS KEY

1. b	*p. 481*	7. b	*p. 487*	13. b	*p. 492*
2. c	*p. 484*	8. d	*p. 481*	14. a	*p. 485*
3. d	*p. 482*	9. b	*p. 491*	15. c	*p. 487*
4. a	*p. 484*	10. a	*p. 491*	16. c	*p. 492*
5. c	*p. 486*	11. a	*p. 495*	17. d	*p. 493*
6. a	*p. 486*	12. d	*p. 501*	18. c	*p. 495*

CLINICAL REASONING CASE STUDY: 49-YEAR-OLD MAN WITH CHEST PAIN

1. Because Mr. Knight is sitting up and speaking, he does not have an immediate problem with his level of responsiveness, airway, breathing, or circulation. However, you must consider and further investigate any complaint of chest pain potentially serious. In this case, it is prudent to classify the patient's condition as potentially critical and expect to transport without undue delay, keeping a careful watch for changes in the patient's condition.

2. You must efficiently gather more information about the patient's chief complaint and obtain a relevant history, vital signs, and focused examination to direct your treatment. Ideally, you have enough resources to simultaneously prepare the patient for transport and initiate needed interventions. Be prepared to revise priorities based on the results of assessment and reassessment.

EXERCISE 1

Across

1. Inflammation of the voice box, resulting in hoarseness or loss of voice. [LARYNGITIS] *p. 527*
8. Collapsed alveoli. [ATELECTASIS] *p. 523*
10. Lung collapse with progressive accumulation of air under pressure in the thoracic cavity. [TENSIONPNEUMOTHORAX] *p. 526*
14. Sore throat. [PHARYNGITIS] *p. 527*
16. Impairment of either ventilation or circulation to the lung, resulting in hypoxia. [VQMISMATCH] *p. 523*
18. Its chronic form results from smoking and causes increased mucus production. [BRONCHITIS] *p. 519*
19. Type of chest pain that is often sharp in nature and worsened by inspiration. [PLEURITIC] *p. 523*
20. Collapse of the lung in the absence of trauma. [SPONTANEOUSPNEUMOTHORAX] *p. 525*

Down

2. Severe, prolonged bronchospasm that cannot be broken with repeated doses of beta$_2$ agonsists. [STATUSASTHMATICUS] *p. 522*
3. A cold is one type. [URI] *p. 527*
4. Genetic disease in which mucus is thick and sticky, which can affect the lungs and gastrointestinal tract. [CYSTICFIBROSIS] *p. 530*
5. Coughing up blood. [HEMOPTYSIS] *p. 523*
6. Condition in which minute volume of respiration exceeds metabolic needs. [HVS] *p. 526*
7. Condition that encompasses three types of long-standing lung disease that results in poor ventilation and gas exchange. [COPD] *p. 515*
9. Laryngotracheobronchitis. [CROUP] *p. 527*
11. Tingling sensation. [PARESTHESIA] *p. 526*
12. Expectoration. [COUGHING] *p. 521*
13. Severe lung and organ failure, often fatal, resulting from contact with infected excrement of deer mice. [HPS] *p. 527*
15. Progressive lung disease characterized by loss of elasticity of the airways and destruction of alveoli. [EMPHYSEMA]
17. Noncardiogenic pulmonary edema from lung injury. [ARDS] *p. 524*

EXERCISE 2

1. internal respiration, *p. 510*
2. external respiration, *p. 510*
3. aerobic metabolism, *p. 512*
4. lactic acid, *p. 512*
5. sympathetic beta$_2$, *p. 512*
6. carbon dioxide, *p. 510*
7. Hering–Breuer reflex, *p. 513*
8. dyspnea, *p. 514*
9. apnea, *p. 514*
10. smoking, *p. 519*
11. exacerbation, *p. 519*
12. pulmonary embolism, *p. 523*
13. carpopedal spasm *p. 526*

PATIENT ASSESSMENT REVIEW

Problem	Common Features
Pneumonia, *p. 527*	Fever, productive cough, can occur at any age. Likely to hear rhonchi in affected areas. Commonly affects a single lobe of one lung. Patient may show signs of dehydration and have a history of recent URI or bronchitis.
Cardiogenic pulmonary edema, *p. 528*	History of heart failure, heart attack, or high blood pressure. Medications may include diuretics. Onset is usually sudden and may begin while the patient is supine (often occurs at night). There may be crackles (rales) in both lungs, starting at the bases, but throughout the lungs in severe cases. There may be frothy, pink sputum in severe cases. There also may be signs of right heart failure (lower extremity edema).
Asthma, *p. 521*	Wheezing, usually expiratory, is a prominent feature. There is usually a history of asthma. Patient usually has medications to treat asthma (including inhalers). There may be a history of a trigger (pollen, exercise, or other factors). Can affect patients of all ages.
Emphysema/chronic bronchitis exacerbation, *p. 521*	Occurs in people of middle age and older. The patient usually gives a history of COPD and has medications (including nebulizers and inhalers) to treat COPD. May be on oxygen. Often a history of several hours or days of progressing dyspnea. Lung sounds may include wheezing and rhonchi scattered throughout the lung fields.
Pulmonary embolism, *p. 523*	Sudden onset of dyspnea with breath sounds that are initially clear and equal. Can occur in young, middle-age, and elderly patients. Risk factors include immobilization (including casts or splints on extremities), prolonged air travel, recent major surgery, deep vein thrombosis (DVT), hormonal birth control, and cancer. The patient also may have sharp chest pain.
Simple pneumothorax, *p. 525*	Occurs suddenly, often in patients with a history of lung disease, but can also affect young, tall, thin males. There may be a history of onset of dyspnea during exertion (such as lifting). There may be sharp chest pain or painless onset of shortness of breath. Shortness of breath may progress as the accumulation of air increases. Breath sounds will be absent in the affected area of a lung, but sounds transmitted from other lung areas can be heard, making this hard to determine.
Tension pneumothorax, *p. 526*	The onset and risk factors are similar to that of simple pneumothorax, but dyspnea continues to increase and signs of obstructive shock (hypotension, jugular venous distention [JVD]) and tachycardia (pale, cool skin) occur.

CHECK YOUR RECALL AND APPLY CONCEPTS KEY

1. c *p. 512*
2. b *p. 512*
3. a *p. 512*
4. a *p. 517*
5. b *p. 519*
6. a *p. 512*
7. d *p. 521*
9. b *p. 525*
8. c *p. 517*
10. b *pp. 525, 526*
11. d *p. 517*
12. b *p. 527*

CLINICAL REASONING CASE STUDY: DIFFICULTY BREATHING AT A NURSING HOME

1. Mr. Maloney is at risk for several respiratory problems. Because he resides in a nursing home and has reduced mobility, he is at risk for pneumonia. He also has indications of heart failure. His immobility also puts him at risk for pulmonary embolism. If the irregular heartbeat is chronic, that also could increase his risk of pulmonary embolism.

2. You should obtain a complete history, using SAMPLE and OPQRST. The medical record at the nursing home will help, but Mr. Maloney's dementia and acutely increased confusion may limit information about his current symptoms. Your goal for a patient with possible multiple problems is not necessarily to select one problem over another, but to make sure you do not miss any potential problems.

3. It may not be possible to select a field impression of pneumonia versus pulmonary edema in this patient, and he likely has some degree of both problems. Treating the dehydration of pneumonia could exacerbate the heart failure, while treating pulmonary edema could complicate pneumonia. The highest priority is to increase the patient's SpO$_2$, which you should attempt to do by switching him to a nonrebreather mask with 12 to 15 L/min of oxygen. You should obtain IV access but avoid aggressive fluid administration. The patient may or may not respond to bronchodilators, but you should check with medical direction about a possible albuterol treatment. The patient's diagnosis and treatment will be complicated. You should transport without undue delays so he can receive the appropriate workup and treatment.

Chapter 21: Cardiovascular Disorders

VOCABULARY AND CONCEPT REVIEW KEY

EXERCISE 1

1. b p. 555
2. i p. 547
3. f p. 558
4. l p. 554
5. d p. 542
6. a p. 557
7. k p. 539
8. g p. 551
9. c p. 542
10. j p. 539
11. h p. 540
12. e p. 546

EXERCISE 2

(Crossword grid — answers shown below)

1 ATHEROSCLEROSIS 3 SYNCOPE
5 ARTERIOLES 7 PRELOAD
11 ATRIUM
12 ANGINALEQUIVALENT 13 CPAP
15 FIBRILLATION
16 PALPITATIONS
18 PLASMA
19 BICUSPID
20 NITROGLYCERIN
21 DISSECTION

Down: 2 EJECTIONFRACTION, 4 NORMALSINUS, 6 INFARCTION, 8 PLATELETS, 9 SINOATRIALNODE, 10 CARDIACOUTPUT, 14 PERICARDIUM, 17 ASPIRIN

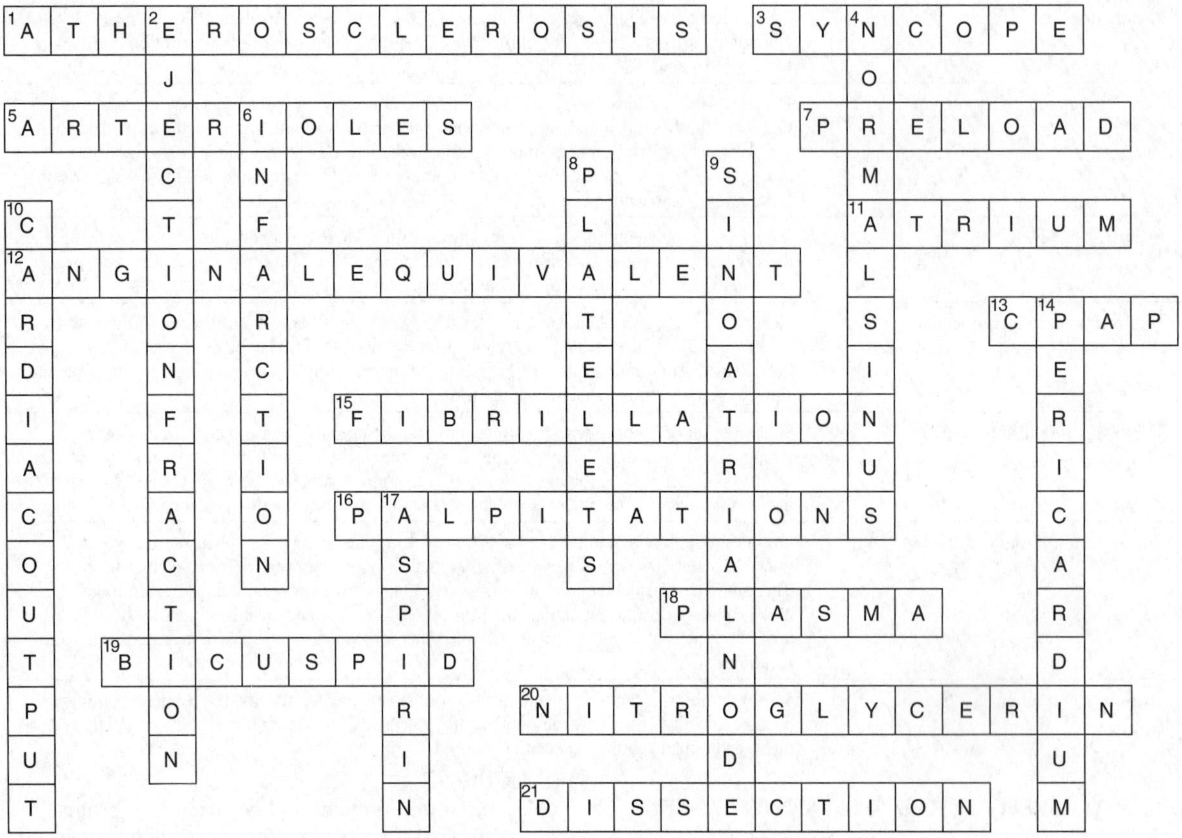

Across

1. Unhealthy condition of the arteries in which plaque narrows the lumen of the vessel. [ATHEROSCLEROSIS] *p. 546*

3. Fainting, sometimes because of dysrhythmia. [SYNCOPE] *p. 546*

5. Smallest of the arteries. [ARTERIOLES] *p. 538*

7. End-diastolic volume. [PRELOAD] *p. 539*

11. One of the two upper chambers of the heart. [ATRIUM] *p. 535*

12. Sign or symptom, other than chest pain, that represents myocardial ischemia. [ANGINALEQUIVALENT] *p. 548*

13. Treatment that produces PEEP to improve ventilation and oxygenation in pulmonary edema. [CPAP] *p. 557*

15. Lethal ventricular dysrhythmia. [FIBRILLATION] *p. 553*

16. Subjective sensation of the heart beating in the chest. [PALPITATIONS] *p. 542*

18. Fluid transport medium for blood cells. [PLASMA] *p. 538*

19. Heart valve that is also called the mitral valve. [BICUSPID] *p. 536*

20. Medication given in suspected ACS to relax vascular smooth muscle. [NITROGLYCERIN] *p. 546*

21. Condition in which blood separates the layers of the aorta. [DISSECTION] *p. 558*

Down

2. Stroke volume expressed as a portion of the end-diastolic volume. [EJECTIONFRACTION] *p. 539*

4. Rhythm seen on the ECG when the heart is healthy and has a properly functioning electrical system. [NORMALSINUS] *p. 543*

6. Tissue death due to ischemia. [INFARCTION] *p. 537*

8. When activated, they clump together at the site of injury in a blood vessel. [PLATELETS] *p. 539*

9. Heart's primary pacemaker. [SINOATRIALNODE] *p. 539*

10. Stroke volume times heart rate. [CARDIACOUTPUT] *p. 540*

14. Tough, fibrous sac that surrounds the heart. [PERICARDIUM] *p. 535*

17. Medication given in suspected ACS to reduce platelet aggregation. [ASPIRIN] *p. 546*

PATIENT ASSESSMENT REVIEW KEY

EXERCISE 1

1. You may find cardiac medications, the patient may be holding his hand over his chest to indicate chest pain, or the patient may be in cardiac arrest.
2. Look for all of the signs of potential danger that you would on any call to a residence, such as indications of violence, objects that could pose a trip or fall hazard, and traffic.
3. Do not assume that the caller's report of a possible heart attack is accurate. Hypoxia can sometimes result in combative or violent behavior.

EXERCISE 2

1. A chief complaint of chest pain or discomfort, dyspnea, or anginal equivalents (arm, shoulder, back, epigastric, or jaw pain; generalized weakness) could all indicate acute coronary syndrome. As with all patients, you must confirm the level of responsiveness and assess the airway, breathing, and circulation.
2. Dyspnea, especially with crackles (rales) in the lungs or frothy sputum, could be an indication of heart failure with pulmonary edema. A patient who is pale, cool, and diaphoretic or who has an altered mental status may be hypoxic (such as from pulmonary edema) or have hypoperfusion, which could be caused by cardiogenic shock or

EXERCISE 3

1. You must explore the chief complaint using the OPQRST mnemonic. Check for complaints and history that are consistent with the risk factors and pathophysiology of cardiac disease. Use the SAMPLE mnemonic to ensure you collect a thorough history. The patient's past medical history and medications can be helpful in your clinical reasoning process, but lack of a prior history of cardiovascular disease does not rule out the possibility of a current cardiac problem. If your clinical reasoning process is leading toward ACS, check in particular if the patient is allergic to aspirin and whether there are any contraindications to administering nitroglycerin. Do not get tunnel vision because the call was dispatched as a "possible heart attack." You must consider other causes of chest pain and dyspnea, as well. Also ask questions that help you differentiate between cardiac and noncardiac causes of those complaints to help you refine your hypotheses.
2. Vital signs provide an overall assessment of the patient's perfusion status. Signs of poor perfusion may be due to cardiogenic shock or hypovolemia associated with aortic aneurysm or dissection. Other indications of a cardiac problem include bradycardia, tachycardia, and an irregular pulse. Hypertension often accompanies left-sided heart failure with pulmonary edema.
3. Pulse oximetry is an important measure of oxygenation and, if permitted in your scope of practice, cardiac monitoring provides information

EXERCISE 4

Reassess patients whose status is critical every 5 minutes and reassess patients whose status is noncritical every 15 minutes. Include

4. You may be able to control some hazards, such as agitated family members, with professional communication techniques.
5. If the patient is combative, you may need additional resources, such as law enforcement, to assist you at the scene.
6. An overall poor impression, such as pallor or cyanosis, and apparent altered mental status all indicate a critical patient.

an aortic aneurysm or dissection. Tachycardia, bradycardia, or an irregular pulse also may be present in cardiac emergencies.
3. You must clear and open the airway if it is not patent. If ventilations are inadequate, you must assist them. If there is significant external bleeding, you must control it.
4. Severe abdominal or back pain may indicate aortic aneurysm or dissection.
5. The transport priority is initially high for any patient with altered mental status or problems with airway, breathing, or circulation. However, you must take immediate action to correct problems with the airway, breathing, oxygenation, and circulation.

about the electrical activity of the heart. If the patient is diabetic or has an altered mental status, obtain the blood glucose level.
4. You should perform a focused physical examination based on the chief complaint and history. Auscultate the breath sounds and check for pedal edema. If the patient complains of abdominal pain or other symptoms consistent with an aortic aneurysm or dissection, gently palpate the abdomen. In suspected aortic aneurysm or dissection, check the pulses in all extremities and compare them. If hypertensive encephalopathy is suspected, perform a neurological examination.
5. Signs and symptoms that increase the suspicion of ACS include chest pain or discomfort; arm, shoulder, back, neck, or jaw discomfort; cool, clammy skin; pale or ashen appearance; diaphoresis; nausea, vomiting, lightheadedness, or weakness; and anxiety or a sense of impending doom.
6. Signs and symptoms consistent with left-sided heart failure include severe dyspnea; a cough that might produce pink, frothy sputum; pale, cool, diaphoretic skin; cyanosis; crackles (rales) in the breath sounds; agitation; or decreased level of responsiveness. The patient may have a history of heart failure with a history of orthopnea and paroxysmal nocturnal dyspnea. Medications can include angiotensin-converting enzyme inhibitors, diuretics, and beta blockers. The patient may have a history of atrial fibrillation. The patient may have pedal edema and ascites.

reassessment of the mental status, airway, breathing, circulation, complaints, and vital signs. If nitroglycerin is given for chest pain, reassess the patient's pain level.

CHECK YOUR RECALL AND APPLY CONCEPTS KEY

EXERCISE 1

1.	d	*p. 536*	5.	c	*p. 543*	9.	a	*p. 557*
2.	q	*p. 538*	6.	c	*p. 547*	10.	c	*p. 557*
3.	b	*p. 539*	7.	d	*p. 551*	11.	b	*p. 561*
4.	b	*p. 540*	8.	b	*p. 551*	12.	d	*p. 561*

EXERCISE 2

1. True *p. 535*
2. True *p. 536*
3. False. Average cardiac output in an adult is 5.25 L/min. *p. 539*
4. True *p. 546*
5. False. Most protocols require that a patient's systolic blood pressure is 90 mmHg or higher to administer nitroglycerin. *p. 551*

CLINICAL REASONING CASE STUDY: 80-YEAR-OLD MAN WITH DIFFICULTY BREATHING

1. A history of sudden nocturnal dyspnea and the presence of crackles (rales) that do not go away with a few deep breaths, along with the patient's age, suggest left-sided heart failure with pulmonary edema. The pedal edema suggests that the patient may have pre-existing right-sided heart failure.
2. Mr. Phillips has taken an important step in his own treatment by sitting up. Gravity will allow excess fluids to pool in the extremities. He requires oxygen to maintain an SpO$_2$ of at least 95 percent. Because he is in mild distress, you might accomplish this with a nasal cannula, which the patient would better tolerate. However, you must continue to monitor his SpO$_2$ and be prepared to use a nonrebreather mask if his

6. False. Because rest, oxygen, and nitroglycerin cannot relieve the obstruction of a coronary artery, they do not relieve chest pain from ACS. *p. 547*
7. False. The most common initial rhythms in cardiac arrest are the lethal ventricular dysrhythmias: ventricular fibrillation and ventricular tachycardia. *p. 553*
8. False. Cor pulmonale is right-sided heart failure associated with lung disease. *p. 555*
9. False. The patient with left-sided heart failure cannot handle the addition of fluid to the cardiovascular system, and IV fluids are not indicated in their management. *p. 556*
10. False. Aortic dissection is a separation of the aortic layers by blood, and aortic aneurysm is a ballooning out of a weakened area of aorta. *p. 560*

SpO$_2$ does not increase to 95 percent or higher. Currently, his level of distress does not warrant use of CPAP or assisted ventilation, but that could change, making frequent reassessment of respiratory status critical. You can consider IV access, but the patient should not receive IV fluids because his perfusion is adequate and he already has pulmonary edema. Because of the mild level of distress, additional orders from medical direction are not likely, but you will call ahead to notify the hospital that you are transporting a patient with a chief complaint of dyspnea.

3. A differential diagnosis to keep in mind is pneumonia. Although there are no indications of fever, the elderly can have severe pneumonia without having a fever. Being in a nursing home is a risk factor for pneumonia.

Chapter 22: Neurologic Disorders

VOCABULARY AND CONCEPT REVIEW KEY

1. Condition in which there are recurrent seizures. [EPILEPSY] *p. 579*

5. Subjective sensation of spinning or moving while stationary; dizziness. [VERTIGO] *p. 584*

6. Period of altered mental status following a seizure. [POSTICTAL] *p. 580*

7. Abbreviation of transient ischemic attack. [TIA] *p. 577*

9. Lack of blood flow to an area of tissue, such as in the brain. [ISCHEMIA] *p. 575*

10. Abnormal sensation that precedes some seizures and migraine headaches. [AURA] *p. 580*

11. Point where two nerve cells communicate with each other. [SYNAPSE] *p. 568*

12. Abbreviation of arteriovenous malformatin. [AVM] *p. 576*

13. Motor activity produced by a generalized seizure. [TONICCLONIC] *p. 579*

14. Signs reflective of inflammation of the meninges. [MENINGISMUS] *p. 582*

1. Mass, which may be a blood clot or other matter, that moves through the bloodstream and may cause an obstruction. [EMBOLUS] *pp. 575, 576*

2. Hypersensitivity of the eyes to light. [PHOTOPHOBIA] *p. 582*

3. Almost fainting. [NEARSYNCOPE] *p. 575*

4. Loss of coordinaion, often presenting as difficulty walking. [ATAXIA] *p. 586*

7. Blood clot that causes obstruction of a blood vessel at the site where it forms. [THROMBUS] *pp. 575, 576*

8. Consider a low level of this important cellular nutrient as a cause of altered mental status. [GLUCOSE] *pp. 572, 575, 576*

PATIENT ASSESSMENT REVIEW KEY

Sign of Stroke	Patient Activity *p. 573*	Interpretation *p. 573*
Facial droop	Have the patient look up at you, smile, and show his or her teeth.	Normal: Symmetry to both sides. Abnormal: One side of the face droops or does not move symmetrically.
Arm drift	Have the patient lift arms up and hold them out with eyes closed for 10 seconds.	Normal: Symmetrical movement in both arms. Abnormal: One arm drifts down or asymmetrical movement of the arms.
Abnormal speech	Have the patient say, "You can't teach an old dog new tricks."	Normal: The correct words are used and no slurring of words is noted. Abnormal: The words are slurred, the wrong words are used, or the patient is aphasic.
Kothari, R. U., Pancioli, A., Liu, T., & Broderick, J. (1999). Cincinnati Prehospital Stroke Scale: Reproducibility and validity. *Annals of Emergency Medicine*, 33, 373–378.		

CHECK YOUR RECALL AND APPLY CONCEPTS KEY

1. c   *p. 575*   3. a   *p. 581*   5. a   *p. 582*
2. b   *p. 579*   4. d   *p. 585*

CLINICAL REASONING CASE STUDY: A SHAKING FEELING

1. Airway. It is the first step in the primary assessment of all patients and it is of paramount importance in the neurologic conditions due to their inability to maintain a gag reflex.

2. Blood glucose. Seizures can be caused by hypoglycemia and, in that case, can be easily rectified.

3. After a seizure, patients enter a postictal state, which is characterized by an unresponsive state.

Chapter 23: Endocrine Disorders

VOCABULARY AND CONCEPT REVIEW KEY

EXERCISE 1

1. h   *p. 605*   10. o   *p. 604*   19. l   *p. 605*
2. k   *p. 605*   11. d   *p. 604*   20. e   *p. 605*
3. b   *p. 598*   12. z   *p. 600*   21. g   *p. 600*
4. r   *p. 605*   13. v   *p. 603*   22. q   *p. 603*
5. w   *p. 598*   14. n   *p. 600*   23. x   *p. 604*
6. i   *p. 600*   15. y   *p. 604*   24. u   *p. 593*
7. a   *p. 593*   16. c   *p. 593*   25. f   *p. 598*
8. s   *p. 594*   17. m   *p. 600*   26. p   *p. 598*
9. j   *p. 594*   18. t   *p. 601*

The completed crossword contains the following answers:

Across: 4. POLYPHAGIA, 7. HORMONE, 8. DEXTROSE, 11. ENDOCRINE, 13. PANCREAS, 14. PITUITARY

Down: 1. DIURESIS, 2. ISLETS, 3. ADRENAL, 5. POSTERIOR, 6. POLYDIPSIA, 9. RECEPTOR, 10. NEGATIVE, 12. ALPHA

Across

4. Excessive hunger. [POLYPHAGIA] *p. 601*
7. Chemical messenger of the endocrine system. [HORMONE] *p. 591*
8. A 50% solution of this is administered intravenously to unresponsive hypoglycemic patients. [DEXTROSE] *p. 598*
11. System of ductless glands. [ENDOCRINE] *p. 592*
13. Secretes insulin, glucagon, and somatostatin. [PANCREAS] *p. 593*
14. Two-part endocrine gland that communicates with the hypothalamus. [PITUITARY] *p. 593*

Down

1. Effect on the kidneys when the blood glucose level is extremely high. [DIURESIS] *p. 601*
2. Clumps of endocrine tissue in the pancreas. [ISLETS] *p. 595*
3. Glands that secrete epinephrine and norepinephrine. [ADRENAL] *p. 605*
5. This part of the pituitary gland releases antidiuretic hormone and oxytocin. [POSTERIOR] *p. 593*
6. Excessive thirst. [POLYDIPSIA] *p. 601*
9. Site on a cell that is selective for a specific hormone. [RECEPTOR] *p. 592*
10. This type of feedback mechanism works like a thermostat. [NEGATIVE] *p. 593*
12. Pancreas cells that secrete glucagon. [ALPHA] *p. 595*

PATIENT ASSESSMENT REVIEW KEY

SCENE SIZE-UP

1. Look for all of the signs of potential danger that you would on any call to a residence, such as indications of violence, objects that could pose a trip or fall hazard, or traffic. Do not assume that the caller's report of a patient with diabetes is accurate. Altered mental status and behavioral changes can be due to many causews, including drug overdose and behavioral emergencies.
2. Medical emergencies can pose several scene hazards. A number of medical emergencies can cause violent behavior; there may be agitated bystanders or items that can cause you to trip or fall.
3. If the patient has diabetes, hypoglycemia can sometimes result in combative or violent behavior.
4. Therapeutic communication can be helpful in dealing with bystanders, but it is difficult to reason with a patient whose brain is not functioning as it should because of inadequate glucose. If the patient is violent, make sure you allow yourself a means of escape.
5. If the patient is combative, you may need additional resources, such as law enforcement, to assist you at the scene.
6. An overall poor impression, such as pallor or cyanosis, apparent altered mental status, obvious blood loss, or critical mechanism of injury all indicate a critical patient.

PRIMARY ASSESSMENT

7. As with all patients, you must confirm the level of responsiveness and assess the airway, breathing, and circulation.

8. Deep, rapid ventilations or an odor of ketones on the breath could indicate diabetic ketoacidosis. Unresponsiveness or altered mental status are also indications of possible hypoglycemia or hyperglycemia.

9. You must clear and open the airway if it is not patent. If ventilations are inadequate, you must assist them. If there is significant external bleeding, you must control it.

10. If history and signs point to a high probability of hypoglycemia, correcting hypoglycemia can quickly improve the patient's status.

11. The transport priority is initially high for any patient with altered mental status or problems with airway, breathing, or circulation.

SECONDARY ASSESSMENT

12. If it is confirmed that the patient has a history of diabetes, ask how the patient treats his disease (insulin or oral medications), if medications have been taken as directed, when they were taken, when the patient last ate, when the patient was last seen well, whether illness occurred suddenly or gradually, what signs and symptoms have been noted (specifically, excessive thirst, urination, or hunger), and whether there have been recent illnesses or injuries. Ask other basic questions such as the presence of allergies, any other medications the patient takes, and any other medical problems the patient might have.

13. Vital signs give a general indication of the patient's status and, in particular, may give information about dehydration (tachycardia, hypotension), and acidosis (Kussmaul's respirations).

CHECK YOUR RECALL AND APPLY CONCEPTS KEY

EXERCISE 1

1. F	p. 593	6. F	p. 595	11. T	p. 594
2. T	p. 592	7. T	p. 593	12. F	p. 596
3. T	p. 593	8. T	p. 593	13. T	p. 599
4. F	p. 602	9. T	p. 593	14. F	p. 598
5. F	p. 600	10. F	p. 594	15. F	p. 602

EXERCISE 2

Presentation	Hypoglycemia	Hyperglycemia
Acetone breath		✓
High insulin level		✓
Thirst		✓
Seizure	✓	
Dehydration		✓
Acute onset	✓	
Dry, warm skin		✓
Bizarre behavior	✓	
Diaphoretic skin	✓	

14. Blood glucose determination is mandatory in all patients with altered mental status and can quickly give information about a possible hypoglycemic or hyperglycemic emergency. Pulse oximetry is also useful in all critical patients.

15. Physical examination is particularly important if you cannot determine the nature of the problem by history, vital signs, and blood glucose determination. It may reveal another cause of the patient's signs and symptoms. If the patient became agitated and combative during a hypoglycemic episode, you must assess him for possible injuries.

16. Hyperglycemia is consistent with findings of gradual onset; excessive urination and thirst; warm, dry skin; signs of dehydration; tachycardia; hypotension; increased respirations; and a blood glucose level above 140 mg/dL.

17. Hypoglycemia is consistent with findings of sudden onset, taking insulin or antihyperglycemic medications; inadequate or delayed food intake after insulin or other diabetic medications; pale, cool, moist skin; altered mental status; and a BGL less than 60 mg/dL.

REASSESSMENT

18. Reassess patients whose status is critical every 5 minutes and reassess patients whose status is noncritical every 15 minutes. Include reassessment of the mental status, airway, breathing, circulation, complaints, and vital signs. If you administer glucose, dextrose, or glucagon, reassess the blood glucose level.

CLINICAL REASONING CASE STUDY: PATIENTS WITH DIABETES KEY

1. This patient likely took her insulin but failed to eat, causing hypoglycemia.

2. While she is breathing slowly with snoring respirations, you should not place a supraglottic airway. After you administer D50, she should wake up fairly rapidly and having a tube in her throat could cause a problem.

3. Because she is breathing slowing with snoring respirations, you could place an NPA and use a bag-valve mask to ventilate her.

Chapter 24: Abdominal Pain and Gastrointestinal Disorders

VOCABULARY AND CONCEPT REVIEW KEY

1. k	*p. 614*	9. h	*p. 618*	17. b	*p. 614*
2. r	*p. 612*	10. x	*p. 614*	18. l	*p. 615*
3. i	*p. 614*	11. s	*p. 614*	19. f	*p. 612*
4. v	*p. 612*	12. c	*p. 614*	20. n	*p. 619*
5. a	*p. 614*	13. j	*p. 619*	21. w	*p. 612*
6. d	*p. 614*	14. p	*p. 621*	22. q	*p. 614*
7. t	*p. 614*	15. u	*p. 614*	23. e	*p. 618*
8. o	*p. 618*	16. g	*p. 619*	24. m	*p. 621*

PATIENT ASSESSMENT REVIEW KEY

Abdominal Region	Organs, *p. 613*	Sources of Referred Pain, *p. 613*
Right upper quadrant	Liver, gallbladder	Pneumonia or pleuritis (right pleural cavity)
Epigastric region	Stomach, pancreas	AMI, appendicitis
Left upper quadrant	Spleen, part of pancreas	Pneumonia or pleuritis (left pleural cavity)
Umbilical and hypogastric	Small intestine, large intestine, aorta, urinary bladder, in females: uterus	Bowel obstruction, appendicitis
Right lower quadrant	Appendix, ascending colon, in females: right ovary and fallopian tube	
Left lower quadrant	Descending colon (diverticula usually are located in the descending colon)	

CHECK YOUR RECALL AND APPLY CONCEPTS KEY

EXERCISE 1

1. c	*p. 611*	4. a	*p. 613*
2. c	*p. 609*	5. b	*p. 623*
3. b	*p. 613*		

EXERCISE 2

1. epigastric, *p. 613*
2. hepatitis, *p. 614*
3. bilirubin, *p. 613*
4. pneumonia, *p. 613*
5. abdominal aortic aneurysm, *p. 616*

6. retroperitoneal, *p. 609*
7. ileostomy, *p. 614*
8. gastrointestinal, *p. 614*
9. hollow, *p. 616*
10. visceral, *p. 616*

CLINICAL REASONING CASE STUDY: FAST FOOD FIASCO

1. Cholecystitis (gallstones)
2. Have you had your gallbladder removed and has this ever happened before?
3. IV, possible pain medication, transport in position of comfort

Chapter 25: Renal, Genitourinary, and Gynecologic Disorders

VOCABULARY AND CONCEPT REVIEW KEY

EXERCISE 1

1. m	*p. 636*	8. k	*p. 639*	15. t	*p. 643*
2. a	*p. 641*	9. b	*p. 635*	16. q	*p. 639*
3. g	*p. 638*	10. e	*p. 644*	17. r	*p. 636*
4. i	*p. 634*	11. p	*p. 634*	18. j	*p. 638*
5. c	*p. 645*	12. o	*p. 634*	19. l	*p. 638*
6. f	*p. 647*	13. n	*p. 643*	20. h	*p. 643*
7. d	*p. 645*	14. t	*p. 639*		

EXERCISE 2

1. intrinsic renal failure, *p. 636*
2. Fournier's gangrene, *p. 643*
3. systemic lupus erythematosus, *p. 637*
4. prerenal renal failure, *p. 637*
5. hemolytic uremic syndrome, *p. 638*
6. parity, *p. 645*
7. renal calculus, *p. 641*
8. postrenal renal failure, *p. 637*
9. renal colic, *p. 641*
10. gravidity, *p. 645*
11. nocturia, *p. 637*
12. phimosis, *p. 643*
13. nephritis, *p. 635*

The crossword grid contains the following completed answers:

Across
- 2. ANEMIA
- 4. NEPHRON
- 7. NEPHROLOGIST
- 8. ECTOPI (C)
- 12. LUPUS
- 13. CHLAMYDIA
- 14. SEPSIS

Down
- 1. SICKLECELLDISEASE
- 3. UROLOGIST
- 5. ENDOMETRIUM
- 6. PERINEUM
- 9. CORTEX
- 10. FLANK
- 11. THRILL

Grid letters as shown:

- 1 (down) S
- 2 ACROSS: A N E M I A
- 3 (down) U
- 4 ACROSS: N E P H R O N
- Column under 1: C K L E C
- 5 (down) E N D O M E T R I U M
- 6 (down) P E R I N E U M
- 7 ACROSS: N E P H R O L O G I S T
- 8 ACROSS: E C T O P I
- 10 (down) F
- 11 (down) T H R I L L
- 12 ACROSS: L U P U S
- Column under 10: F L A N K
- 13 ACROSS: C H L A M Y D I A
- 14 ACROSS: S E P S I S

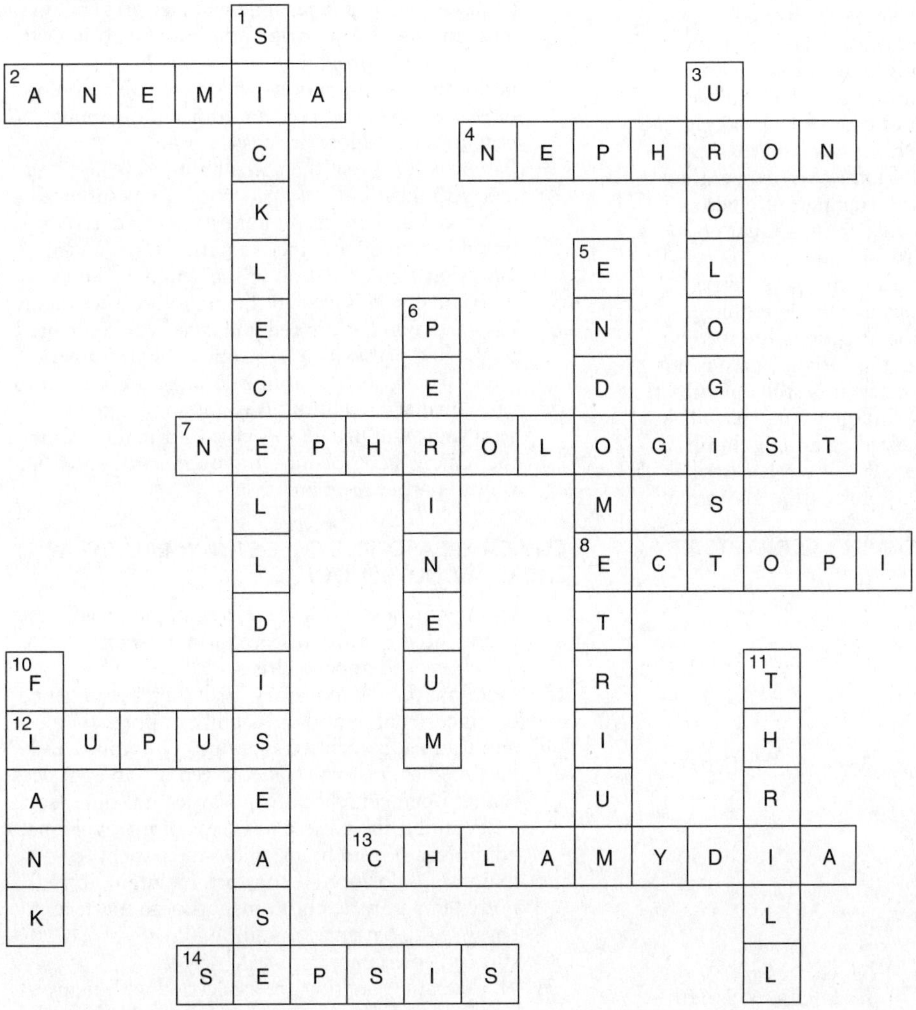

Across

2. Complication of renal failure due to decreased erythropoietin production [ANEMIA] p. 634

4. Microscopic unit of the kidney that produces urine [NEPHRON] p. 630

7. Physician who specializes in treating kidney diseases. [NEPHROLOGIST] p. 630

8. Type of pregnancy that is implanted outside of the uterine cavity. [ECTOPIC] p. 645

12. Autoimmune disease that can affect the kidneys. [LUPUS] p. 637

13. Cause of pelvic inflammatory disease. [CHLAMYDIA] pp. 645, 646

14. Life-threatening complication of an untreated urinary tract infection. [SEPSIS] p. 634

Down

1. Most common non-traumatic cause of priapism. [SICKLECELLDISEASE] p. 633

3. Physician who specializes in treating problems of the male genitalia. [UROLOGIST] p. 630

5. Tissue that is shed during menstruation. [ENDOMETRIUM] p. 632

6. Area of skin between the genitals and anus. [PERINEUM] p. 632

9. Outer layer of the kidney. [CORTEX] p. 630

10. Where the pain associated with a kidney stone is often experienced. [FLANK] p. 634

11. What you will feel if you lightly palpate a properly functioning shunt graft in a hemodialysis patient. [THRILL] p. 639

PATIENT ASSESSMENT REVIEW KEY

1. Patient #1: (a) Ask if the patient has had similar episodes and if so, what caused them. Ask the patient and dialysis center staff if there were any concerns or complications during dialysis. Ask the patient what medications he is taking. (b) Check the patient's heart rate and rhythm and blood pressure. Check the skin temperature (and, if possible, check the temperature with a thermometer). (c) Knowing about similar episodes may help find an underlying cause. Syncope and lightheadedness are side effects of several medications. Vital signs will help determine if hypovolemia or infection are possibilities.

2. Patient #2: (a) Although the patient's pain is not typical of ectopic pregnancy, it is still a possibility. Ask about the patient's last menstrual period. Ask about unusual vaginal bleeding and discharge. (b) Palpate the abdomen. Perform a heel strike test. Take vital signs. (c) Information about the patient's menstrual history and any usual bleeding or discharge help determine whether pregnancy is a possibility. A heel strike test and palpation of the abdomen will provide information about possible peritoneal inflammation. The heart rate and blood pressure provide important information about potential blood loss or sepsis.

3. Patient #3: (a) Ask the patient about his medications. Find out if the patient has suffered any trauma. Also keep phimosis in mind as a possibility in uncircumcised patients. (b) Take vital signs. Examination of the genitalia is not warranted in this case in the prehospital setting. (c) A medication list can tell you if he is being treated for benign prostatic hypertrophy (BPH). Other medications, such as antihistamines, are known to cause urinary retention. It is not anticipated that vital signs will provide specific information about the patient's complaint, but you must be sure there is not another problem.

CHECK YOUR RECALL AND APPLY CONCEPTS KEY

EXERCISE 1

1. kidneys, *p. 630*
2. twelfth, *p. 630*
3. nephron, *p. 630*
4. 30 to 40, *p. 630*
5. bladder, *p. 630*
6. vas deferens, *p. 632*
7. parasympathetic, *p. 632*
8. endometrium, *p. 632*
9. fundus, cervix, *p. 632*
10. sepsis, *p. 634*

EXERCISE 3

1. T *p. 635*
2. T *p. 635*
3. F *p. 635*
4. F *p. 641*
5. T *p. 641*
6. F *p. 641*
7. T *p. 642*
8. T *pp. 639, 640*
9. T *p. 636*
10. F *p. 636*

CLINICAL REASONING CASE STUDY: CALL TO A LOCAL MIDDLE SCHOOL

1. Dysmenorrhea, mittleschmerz, ectopic pregnancy, pelvic inflammatory disease, urinary tract infection, and appendicitis are all possibilities.

2. Obtain a thorough history, including the patient's last menstrual period, possibility of pregnancy, any trauma, associated signs and symptoms, and past medical history. Give oxygen for an SpO_2 less than 95 percent, check orthostatic vital signs, start an IV and if the patient has signs of hypovolemia, administer a fluid bolus, allow the patient to maintain a position of comfort, maintain normal body temperature, and transport without delay, because the patient's condition may involve a surgical emergency.

3. Nausea and vomiting are associated with many conditions. Unfortunately, they do not help in this case in narrowing the differential diagnoses.

Chapter 26: Hematologic Disorders

VOCABULARY AND CONCEPT REVIEW KEY

EXERCISE 1

1. e *p. 652*
2. c *p. 652*
3. h *p. 654*
4. j *p. 657*
5. a *p. 652*
6. k *p. 654*
7. g *p. 657*
8. d *p. 652*
9. l *p. 657*
10. i *p. 659*
11. b *p. 657*
12. f *p. 657*

EXERCISE 2

Across

2. Percentage of blood by volume that is composed of formed elements. [HEMATOCRIT] *p. 653*

5. Disease in which hemoglobin takes on an abnormal shape in low-oxygen conditions. [SICKLECELL] *p. 659*

7. Microhemorrhages. [PETECHIAE] *p. 657*

8. Source of histamine and heparin. [MASTCELL] *p. 653*

9. Nutrient that is important in blood clotting. [VITAMINK] *p. 654*

10. Bone marrow cancer in which large numbers of abnormal white blood cells are produced. [LEUKEMIA] *p. 659*

Down

1. Type of fracture that occurs due to a disease process that weakens the bone. [PATHOLOGICAL] *p. 659*

3. Lacks a nucleus when mature; contains hemoglobin. [REDBLOODCELL] *p. 652*

4. Blotchy, hemorrhagic rash. [PURPURA] *p. 657*

6. Liquid part of blood. [PLASMA] *p. 652*

PATIENT ASSESSMENT REVIEW KEY

EXERCISE 1

The signs and symptoms that you should look for include: pain in any areas affected by vaso-occlusive crisis, abdominal pain, signs and symptoms of stroke, renal failure, blindness, and abdominal pain (left upper quadrant with spleen involvement; right upper quadrant with gallstones/cholecystitis, fever).

EXERCISE 2

You should look for signs and symptoms of a transfusion reaction including flushing, pain at the infusion site, chest pain, back or flank pain, restlessness, anxiety, nausea, fever, chills, and renal failure (decreased urine output, back/flank pain).

CHECK YOUR RECALL AND APPLY CONCEPTS KEY

EXERCISE 1

1. deep vein thrombosis (DVT), *p. 660*
2. disseminated intravascular coagulation, *p. 661*
3. multiple myeloma, *p. 659*
4. polycythemia, *p. 658*
5. AB positive, *p. 655*
6. Rh immune globulin (Rhogam), *p. 656*
7. analgesics, *p. 655*
8. sickle cell crisis, *p. 659*
9. pale, tachycardic (fast), *p. 658*
10. pernicious, *p. 658*
11. lymphoma, *p. 659*

EXERCISE 2

1. Aplastic anemia, iron deficiency anemia, pernicious anemia
2. The abnormal shape of sickle cells makes it difficult for them to move through capillaries. The tissues supplied by the obstructed capillaries become ischemic, resulting in pain and microinfarction of tissues.
3. Their cells can regain normal shape when re-oxygenated, but the changes in shape of the cell damage it, decreasing its life span.
4. Acute lymphoblastic leukemia, acute myelogenous leukemia, chronic lymphocytic leukemia, chronic myelogenous leukemia
5. Bruising, gastrointestinal bleeding, hemorrhagic stroke, epistaxis

CLINICAL REASONING CASE STUDY: AIR TRAVEL

1. Shortness of breath can have several different causes. Consider heart failure and acute coronary syndrome (ACS), as well as chronic pulmonary diseases, such as asthma and COPD; infections, such as pneumonia; anemia; and pulmonary embolism. The absence of a prior history of heart and lung problems, as well as her clear breath sounds, makes asthma, COPD, heart failure, and pneumonia unlikely. The onset of distress was acute, also making those problems unlikely. The patient has three significant risk factors for pulmonary embolism: an immobilized lower extremity from a recent injury, her age, and air travel. The decreased SpO_2 is suspicious for pulmonary embolism. However, always consider ACS in a patient of this age who complains of sudden shortness of breath.

2. The source of a possible pulmonary embolism in this patient is most likely the immobilized extremity. Warmth, redness, pain, tenderness, and a positive Homan's signs would all point to pulmonary embolism. Chest pain might or might not be present in both ACS and pulmonary embolism. When chest pain is present in pulmonary embolism, it is usually sharp in nature, rather than the dull pain or pressure sensation often associated with ACS. The heart rate, respiratory rate, and blood pressure might or might not be affected in both ACS and pulmonary embolism. The vital signs are important in determining the patient's overall condition, but it will not necessarily help you distinguish between the two problems.

3. Administer oxygen to treat the patient's mild hypoxia, but be prepared to intervene to assist ventilations if respiratory failure develops. Both pulmonary embolism and ACS are critical events that make IV access important. If the patient has chest pain and no signs of DVT, medical direction may recommend treating the patient for ACS with nitroglycerin and aspirin. Allow the patient to maintain a position of comfort, unless it is otherwise indicated by her condition. Transport without delay and reassess the patient frequently.

Chapter 27: Immunologic Disorders

VOCABULARY AND CONCEPT REVIEW KEY

<u>EXERCISE 1</u>

1. b *p. 668*   4. f *p. 665*   7. c *p. 667*
2. e *p. 665*   5. d *p. 665*
3. a *p. 669*   6. g *p. 671*

<u>EXERCISE 2</u>

The crossword solution grid:

Across:
1. LYMPHOCYTES
6. IMMUNOGLOBULINE
8. EPINEPHRINE
9. VASODILATION
10. MASTCELL
11. ALBUTEROL
12. ANAPHYLAXIS

Down:
2. COLLAGENVASCULAR
3. HIVES
4. IMMUNITY
5. ANGIOEDEMA
6. INFLAMMATION
7. AUTOINJECTOR

Across

1. White blood cells that carry out the immune response.
   [LYMPHOCYTES] *p. 665*
6. Antibody that plays a role in allergic reactions.
   [IMMUNOGLOBULINE] *p. 665*
8. Drug that is indicated in the treatment of anaphylactic shock. [EPINEPHRINE] *p. 665*
9. Cause of hypotension in anaphylaxis.
   [VASODILATION] *p. 668*
10. Basophil that has migrated into the tissues.
    [MASTCELL] *p. 668*
11. Suitable medication for a patient with an allergic reaction who is wheezing but who does not have severe respiratory distress or hypotension.
    [ALBUTEROL] *p. 670*
12. Life-threatening allergic reaction.
    [ANAPHYLAXIS] *p. 665*

Down

2. Systemic lupus erythematosus and rheumatoid arthritis are in this classification of autoimmune diseases.
   [COLLAGENVASCULAR] *p. 671*
3. Common name for urticaria. [HIVES] *p. 667*
4. Ability for the body to defend itself against specific antigens.
   [IMMUNITY] *p. 665*
5. Response to certain medications that can present as anaphylaxis. [ANGIOEDEMA] *p. 669*
6. Nonspecific response to tissue injuries and antigens.
   [INFLAMMATION] *p. 665*
7. Check to see if a patient with a history of anaphylaxis carries one of these. [AUTOINJECTOR] *p. 669*

	Mild Allergic Reaction, *p. 669*	Anaphylaxis, *p. 669*
Onset	Usually slower and more gradual than anaphylaxis	Usually rapid, often within 30 to 60 seconds of exposure, but up to 1 hour
Skin	Itching, hives	Itching and hives, may be widespread; diaphoresis; may be flushed; cyanosis with severe respiratory involvement
Angioedema	Mild	May be severe enough to cause airway obstruction; stridor indicates significant partial airway obstruction
Mental status	Normal, may be anxious	Anxiety, confusion, decreased responsiveness
Lungs	May have mild or scattered wheezing	May have significant wheezing in all lung fields
Vital signs	Normal	Hypotension, tachycardia, weak peripheral pulses, tachypnea, respiratory distress
Gastrointestinal system	Nausea, increased peristalsis	Nausea, vomiting, diarrhea

CHECK YOUR RECALL AND APPLY CONCEPTS KEY

EXERCISE 1

1. phagocytosis, *p. 665*
2. immunity, *p. 665*
3. lymphocytes, *p. 665*
4. antigen, *p. 665*
5. antibodies, *p. 665*
6. immunoglobulin E (IgE), *p. 665*
7. 30 to 60 seconds, *p. 665*
8. epinephrine, *p. 670*
9. 10 to 20 minutes, *p. 668*
10. hypersensitivity, *p. 668*

EXERCISE 2

1. Any four, including: tachycardia, tremors, chest pain, headache, nausea and vomiting, anxiousness, dizziness, *p. 668*
2. Any four, including: hypotension, edema, respiratory distress, wheezing, uticaria, stridor, acute onset, diarrhea, *p. 669*
3. Any four, including: injection, absorption, inhalation, and ingestion, *p. 668*
4. Any four, including: rheumatoid arthritis, psoriasis, systemic lupus erythematosus, Grave's disease, Crohn's disease, multiple sclerosis, *p. 671*
5. Any four, including: peanuts, shellfish, eggs, milk, fruits, sesame seeds, chocolate, *p. 668*

CLINICAL REASONING CASE STUDY: DISPATCH FOR RESPIRATORY DISTRESS

1. Stridor indicates obstruction, likely due to swelling, of the upper airway. Wheezing indicates narrowing of the bronchioles. With no history of asthma or COPD, those two possibilities are unlikely. The combination of wheezing and stridor, particularly with a sudden onset, are more likely due to an acute infection, inhalation of an irritant, or an allergic reaction. An acute infection leading to both wheezing and stridor in a patient of her age is unlikely. Inhalation of an irritant and allergic reaction should be high on your list of possible hypotheses, and you must explore both possibilities.

2. Your initial pass at a SAMPLE history should focus on things that help you immediately determine the nature of the problem. Find out about symptoms that would help you narrow your hypotheses, such as presence of a fever or other indications of infection, such as a productive cough; whether the patient has any known allergies to food, medication, or other substances; whether she has serious medical problems; what medications she takes (which could give a clue to an allergic reaction or underlying medical problem); what she last had to eat or drink (which could help determine if allergic reaction is a possibility); and what she was doing prior to the onset of signs and symptoms (which could help determine if there was exposure to a respiratory irritant or allergen). Is she taking any new medications? Explore the OPQRST of the chief complaint. The history of taking an antibiotic is suspicious for anaphylaxis, and there are no factors that increase your suspicion of asthma, infection, or toxic exposure. Your suspicion should be increased by the presence of urticaria and the patient's vital signs. Although a food allergy is possible, it has been a few hours since the patient ingested food, making food allergy unlikely, given the severity of the patient's signs and symptoms.

3. You have begun oxygen administration, which is important, but it will not correct the underlying problem. The airway is your first priority. If the airway obstruction worsens, it will be difficult to ventilate the patient, even with basic or advanced airway devices. In fact, continued airway swelling may make it impossible to place an airway device. The only way to reverse her airway obstruction will be with epinephrine, and you must administer it without delay. You will administer 0.3 to 0.5 mg of 1:1,000 epinephrine, IM. You also should obtain IV access. The patient's blood pressure is difficult to interpret on its own (because the patient's normal blood pressure is unknown), but accompanied by the increased heart rate and other indications of anaphylaxis, you must have IV access to allow for fluid administration if hypotension persists after administration of epinephrine. If wheezing persists after epinephrine administration, you may consider albuterol based on medical direction approval. If allowed in your scope of practice, medical direction also might order diphenhydramine. This patient requires transport without delay, and you should consider calling for paramedic backup in case the patient needs to be intubated or needs a surgical airway.

Chapter 28: Infectious Illnesses

VOCABULARY AND CONCEPT REVIEW KEY

EXERCISE 1

1. i   *p. 677*
2. e   *p. 676*
3. b   *p. 677*
4. k   *p. 681*
5. h   *p. 677*

6. m   *p. 677*
7. a   *p. 679*
8. f   *p. 677*
9. n   *p. 677*
10. l   *p. 676*

11. c   *p. 687*
12. o   *p. 676*
13. g   *p. 676*
14. j   *p. 676*
15. d   *p. 677*

EXERCISE 2

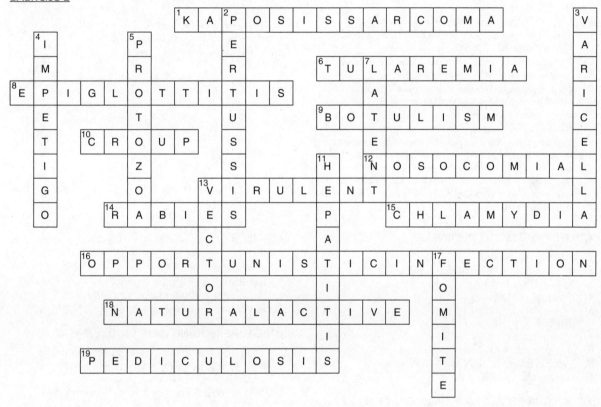

Across

1. Unusual cancer that is seen in immunocompromised patients, such as those with HIV/AIDS. [KAPOSISSARCOMA] *p. 680*

6. Rare in humans, this disease is highly infectious and carries high morbidity, making it a possible weapon of bioterrorism. [TULAREMIA] *p. 684*

8. Relatively rare infection, reduced due to widespread HiB vaccine, that can cause upper airway obstruction. [EPIGLOTTITIS] *p. 683*

9. Usually thought of as a form of food poisoning, it also can cause skin infection, particularly in IV drug abusers. [BOTULISM] *p. 685*

10. Laryngotracheobronchitis. [CROUP] *p. 683*

12. Type of infection acquired in the health care system. [NOSOCOMIAL] *p. 687*

13. Pathogens that are very strong and able to overcome body defenses. [VIRULENT] *p. 676*

14. Viral infection, transmitted from animals to humans, that causes hypersalivation and fear of water. [RABIES] *p. 684*

15. Very common sexually transmitted infection. [CHLAMYDIA] *p. 677*

16. Infection that occurs only under conditions of immune compromise or because antibiotics have altered normal flora. [OPPORTUNISTICINFECTION] *p. 676*

18. Type of immunity that occurs as a result of having an infectious illness. [NATURALACTIVE] *p. 676*

19. Infestation with lice. [PEDICULOSIS] *p. 686*

Down

2. Whooping cough. [PERTUSSIS] *p. 682*

3. Virus that can manifest as chickenpox or shingles. [VARICELLA] *p. 683*

4. Oozing, streptococcal infection of the skin that is more common in children than in adults. [IMPETIGO] *p. 686*

5. Single-celled animals capable of producing disease. [PROTOZOA] *p. 677*

7. Period when disease is present but not causing signs and symptoms. [LATENT] *p. 677*

11. There are at least six different types of this viral illness, some of which are bloodborne and some that spread through the fecal–oral route. [HEPATITIS] *p. 680*

13. Flea that carries the bubonic plague from rodents to humans is one of these. [VECTOR] *p. 684*

17. An unsterilized surgical instrument is an example of one. [FOMITE] *p. 676*

PATIENT ASSESSMENT REVIEW KEY

1. meningitis, *p. 684*
2. tuberculosis or HIV/AIDS, *p. 681*
3. HIV/AIDS, *p. 680*
4. hepatitis, *p. 680*
5. tuberculosis, *p. 681*
6. pertussis, *p. 682*
7. croup, *p. 683*
8. shingles, *p. 683*
9. Lyme disease, *p. 684*
10. ringworm, *p. 686*

CHECK YOUR RECALL AND APPLY CONCEPTS KEY

EXERCISE 1

1. airborne, *p. 681*
2. bloodborne, *p. 680*
3. airborne, *p. 681*
4. food/water borne, *p. 680*
5. sexually transmitted, *p. 685*
6. vectorborne, *p. 677*
7. food/waterborne, *p. 677*
8. direct, *p. 686*
9. airborne, *p. 682*
10. airborne, *p. 682*
11. airborne, *p. 682*
12. vectorborne, *p. 684*
13. direct, *p. 684*
14. vectorborne, *p. 684*
15. food/waterborne, *p. 685*

EXERCISE 2

1. Rabies, *p. 684*
2. antiemetic, *p. 685*
3. Botulism, *p. 685*
4. botulinum and tularemia, *pp. 684, 685*
5. Impetigo, *p. 686*

CLINICAL REASONING CASE STUDY: MRSA

1. The patient in that room is in isolation due to MRSA. It also means that you will need to take additional Standard Precautions.

2. You need to know in what body system the MRSA is located. If it is located in the respiratory tract, you need to take respiratory precautions, which would include an N-95 respirator. If it bloodborne, you need to take the same precautions that you take for any bloodborne pathogen. Some MRSA is located on the skin, usually in a wound. This would not require respiratory precautions, but would require gloves and a gown because it is spread by direct contact.

3. Absolutely, always take your cue from the staff if you have a question about what precautions to take. If she has a gown on, there is a reason for it. Ask the staff specifically about the source of the MRSA and the required Standard Precautions to take. Be sure to properly dispose of or sterilize any materials or equipment used on a patient with MRSA.

Chapter 29: Nontraumatic Musculoskeletal and Soft-Tissue Disorders

VOCABULARY AND CONCEPT REVIEW KEY

EXERCISE 1

1.	i	p. 695	7.	f	p. 695	13.	c	p. 697
2.	e	p. 697	8.	o	p. 696	14.	j	p. 698
3.	l	p. 695	9.	a	p. 698	15.	d	p. 698
4.	n	p. 695	10.	m	p. 694	16.	g	p. 699
5.	p	p. 695	11.	h	p. 695			
6.	b	p. 695	12.	k	p. 696			

EXERCISE 2

Across

1. Most superficial layer of the skin. [EPIDERMIS] *p. 693*
8. Breakdown of muscle tissue with release of muscle cell contents. [RHABDOMYOLYSIS] *p. 698*
9. It is evidenced by tea- or cola-colored urine. [MYOGLOBINEMA] *p. 699*
10. Pigment in the skin. [MELANIN] *p. 693*

Down

2. Syndrome in which 10 percent or less of total body surface area is affected by epidermal detachment. [STEVENSJOHNSON] *p. 696*
3. Decubitis ulcer. [BEDSORE] *p. 695*
4. Fluid-filled cushion that protects the soft tissues from ligaments and tendons. [BURSA] *p. 694*
5. Decrease in bone mass. [OSTEOPENIA] *p. 697*
6. Lateral curvature of the spine. [SCOLIOSIS] *p. 699*
7. Muscle compartment. [FASCIA] *p. 695*

CHECK YOUR RECALL AND APPLY CONCEPTS KEY

1.	T	p. 698	5.	F	p. 695	9.	T	p. 698
2.	F	p. 693	6.	T	p. 696	10.	F	p. 699
3.	T	p. 693	7.	T	p. 697	11.	T	p. 699
4.	F	p. 695	8.	F	p. 698	12.	F	p. 693

1. Take care to make her as comfortable as possible. You need to examine her deformities and plan for appropriate padding to ensure her comfort.
2. You could call ahead to the hospital and explain the physical limitations of your patient so they can prepare to clear her cervical spine as soon as possible.
3. Because her pain is in her neck and upper back, you could consider using a KED or short spine board and allow her to remain in a seated position for transport. However, you should clear this through medical direction first.

Chapter 30: Disorders of the Eye, Ear, Nose, Throat, and Oral Cavity

VOCABULARY AND CONCEPT REVIEW KEY

EXERCISE 1

1. f   *p. 708*   5. h   *p. 709*   9. j   *p. 705*
2. k   *p. 708*   6. a   *p. 705*   10. i   *p. 709*
3. g   *p. 708*   7. c   *p. 709*   11. b   *p. 709*
4. d   *p. 708*   8. e   *p. 705*

EXERCISE 2

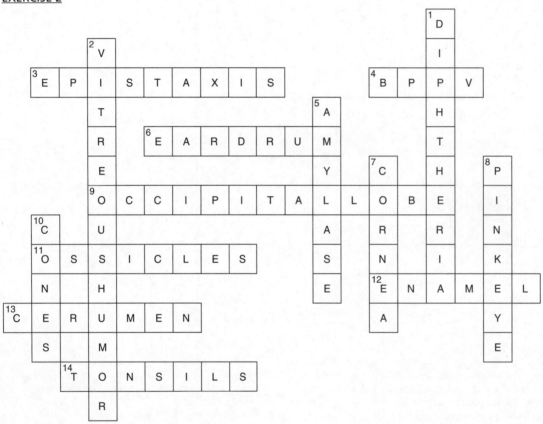

Across

3. Nosebleed. [EPISTAXIS]   *p. 710*
4. Condition in which dizziness results from head movements. [BPPV]   *p. 709*
6. Common name for the tympanic membrane. [EARDRUM]   *p. 705*
9. Location of the visual cortex. [OCCIPITALLOBE]   *p. 704*
11. Tiny bones of the middle ear. [OSSICLES]   *p. 705*
12. Hard, outer layer of a tooth. [ENAMEL]   *p. 706*
13. Ear wax. [CERUMEN]   *p. 709*
14. Clumps of lymphatic tissue in the pharynx. [TONSILS]   *p. 707*

Down

1. Bacterial infection that can cause a pseudomembrane in the respiratory tract. [DIPHTHERIA]   *p. 711*
2. Semisolid gel in the posterior chamber of the eye. [VITREOUSHUMOR]   *p. 704*
5. Enzyme in saliva that breaks down complex carbohydrates. [AMYLASE]   *p. 706*
7. Clear outer layer of the eye that receives oxygen from tears. [CORNEA]   *p. 704*
8. Common name for conjunctivitis. [PINKEYE]   *p. 708*
10. Color-sensitive pigmented cells in the retina. [CONES]   *p. 705*

PATIENT ASSESSMENT REVIEW KEY

1. Glaucoma
2. Stroke, retinal artery occlusion, detached retina, atypical migraine
3. Foreign body in the ear, otitis externa, otitis media
4. Pharyngitis, tonsillitis, peritonsillar abscess, epiglottitis, Ludwig's angina

CHECK YOUR RECALL AND APPLY CONCEPTS KEY

1. a *p. 708*   3. b *p. 706*   5. d *p. 709*
2. c *p. 705*   4. c *p. 708*   6. a *p. 710*

CLINICAL REASONING CASE STUDY: DENTON BLACKSTONE

1. The complaint and presentation are very concerning for orbital cellulitis, but you should consider periorbital cellulitis, as well. Of the two, orbital cellulitis is potentially more serious.
2. Obtain a SAMPLE history and explore the OPQRST of chief complaint, tailoring your questions to the patient's age and getting information from the parents. Obtain vital signs and check for signs of fever and dehydration.
3. Denton does not require specific prehospital treatment, but needs to be transported without delay to the emergency department for evaluation and treatment.

Chapter 31: Mental Illness and Behavioral Emergencies

VOCABULARY AND CONCEPT REVIEW KEY

EXERCISE 1

1. b *p. 718*   6. h *p. 721*   11. q *p. 718*
2. n *p. 719*   7. k *p. 719*   12. l *p. 718*
3. g *p. 716*   8. j *p. 721*   13. p *p. 718*
4. i *p. 716*   9. o *p. 720*   14. a *p. 719*
5. c *p. 720*   10. e *p. 722*   15. d *p. 720*

EXERCISE 2

3. This syndrome in self-harm or producing false signs and symptoms is motivated by the desire to assume the sick role; there is no external gain. [MUNCHAUSEN] *p. 720*

5. Disorder involving impulsive stealing. [KLEPTOMANIA] *p. 720*

6. Mental state in which reality is distorted. [PSYCHOTIC] *p. 721*

8. American Psychological Association guide to identifying mental illnesses. [DSM] *p. 721*

9. Syndrome that occurs due to withdrawal from alcohol in a person who is physically dependent. [DELIRIUMTREMENS] *p. 722*

10. Problem characterized by maladaptive ways of perceiving, thinking, and relating to others. [PERSONALITYDISORDER] *p. 721*

11. Eating disorder characterized by dietary restrictions and severely limited food intake. [ANOREXIA] *p. 720*

1. Psychotic disorder with disordered thinking, often with delusions, hallucinations, and flat affect. [SCHIZOPHRENIC] *p. 721*

2. Alcoholic syndrome that affects the brain, first reversibly, then irreversibly. [WERNICKEKORSAKOFF] *p. 722*

4. An intermediate breakdown product of alcohol. [ACETALDEHYDE] *p. 722*

7. Mood disorder characterized by loss of interest in things, disordered sleep, and feelings of worthlessness or guilt. [DEPRESSION] *p. 720*

8. Patients with this disorder are preoccupied with a physical defect not apparent to others. [DYSMORPHIC] *p. 720*

PATIENT ASSESSMENT REVIEW KEY

1. Yelling, crying, pacing, violent behavior, disordered environment, bizarre dress or appearance, unusual mannerisms

2. Decreased level of responsiveness, airway obstruction, or decreased respirations could indicate an overdose or poisoning. Tachypnea or tachycardia could indicate a panic attack. Obvious bleeding could be due to self-harm.

3. Injuries (old or new) that may be self-inflicted, flat affect, excessive talkativeness, grandiose ideas, disorganized thoughts, abnormal vital signs (could indicate overdose or substance abuse)

4. Changes in mental status or vital signs that could indicate deterioration, perhaps due to an undetected physical problem or overdose that the patient did not disclose

CHECK YOUR RECALL AND APPLY CONCEPTS KEY

EXERCISE 1

1. F *p. 716*   3. T *p. 717*   5. F *p. 721*
2. F *p. 720*   4. T *p. 718*

EXERCISE 2

1. c *p. 719*   3. c *p. 720*   5. b *p. 721*
2. a *p. 720*   4. d *p. 720*   6. a *p. 721*

CLINICAL REASONING CASE STUDY: MANDY PARKER

1. Treat the patient with respect and empathy, but do not go along with her delusions. Be clear that you are there to help. Avoid pulling the sister aside for a private conversation, because the patient may view this as suspicious behavior. Although the patient has not threatened violence, her behavior could change and you must be alert to that possibility.

2. Ensure an open airway and adequate breathing and circulation. Assess the patient's mental status. Inquire about any complaints and perform a focused physical examination as dictated by the patient's complaints. Obtain a complete set of baseline vital signs. Reassess the patient en route to the hospital.

3. Be prepared to spend time to gain the patient's trust and cooperation. If possible, transport to a hospital with a psychiatric emergency department or inpatient psychiatric care.

Chapter 32: Toxicologic Emergencies

VOCABULARY AND CONCEPT REVIEW KEY

EXERCISE 1

1. myoclonus, *p. 744*
2. toxin, *p. 728*
3. toxidrome, *p. 728*
4. Nystagmus, *p. 737*
5. scombroid fish poisoning, *p. 738*
6. ataxic, *p. 737*
7. confabulation, *p. 737*
8. cardiac glycosides, *p. 733*
9. half-life, *p. 735*

The completed crossword puzzle:

3 Across (with 1 Down, 2 Down, 4 Down): POISONCONTROLCENTER

1 Down: JIMSONWEED

2 Down: ORGANOPHOSPHATE

4 Down: CYANIDE

5 Down: SYRUPOFIPECAC

6 Down: NALOXONE

7 Across: BENZODIAZEPINE / **7 Down:** BLACKWIDOW

8 Down: ISOPROPANOL

9 Across: SSRI

10 Down: CAUSTICS

11 Down: COCAINE

12 Across: ACETAMINOPHEN

13 Down: INHALATION

14 Down: METHANOL

15 Across: PITVIPER

16 Across: CIGUATERA

17 Across: AMANITA

18 Across: ACTIVATEDCHARCOAL

19 Across: CARBONMONOXIDE

Across

3. One of more than 60 specialized organizations staffed by toxicology experts 24 hours a day, 7 days a week. [POISONCONTROLCENTER] *p. 728*

7. Class of drugs used to reduce anxiety; diazepam is an example. [BENZODIAZEPINE] *p. 743*

9. Common class of antidepressants that includes citalopram and sertraline. [SSRI] *p. 744*

12. Over-the-counter analgesic that causes hepatotoxicity in relatively small doses. [ACETAMINOPHEN] *p. 742*

15. Classification to which most poisonous snakes belong. [PITVIPER] *p. 741*

16. Toxin that accumulates in older fish in some species as a result of them ingesting organisms called dinoflagellates.[CIGUATERA] *p. 738*

17. Most poisonous mushrooms are from this class. [AMANITA] *p. 739*

18. Used in some cases of poisoning by ingestion to adsorb toxins to prevent them from being absorbed into the body.[ACTIVATEDCHARCOAL] *p. 732*

19. Odorless gas produced by incomplete combustion that has a higher affinity for hemoglobin than oxygen does. [CARBONMONOXIDE] *p. 733*

Down

1. Plant that can result in anticholinergic signs and symptoms when smoked or ingested as a tea for the purposes of intoxication. [JIMSONWEED] *p. 738*

2. Atropine and pralidoxime are antidotes to this kind of poisoning. [ORGANOPHOSPHATE] *p. 732*

4. Toxin found in many forms, including a gas emitted from burning synthetic household items, and acts as a cellular asphyxiant. [CYANIDE] *p. 735*

5. Medication no longer recommended to induce vomiting in the treatment of poisoning by ingestion, but can still be obtained in small quantities over the counter.[SYRUPOFIPECAC] *p. 732*

6. Used to reverse respiratory depression associated with narcotic overdose. [NALOXONE] *p. 732*

7. Shiny, black spider whose venom is a potent neurotoxin. [BLACKWIDOW] *p. 740*

8. Toxic alcohol found in mouthwash and other readily available products that sometimes is used as an ethanol substitute. [ISOPROPANOL] *p. 737*

10. Strong acids and alkalis are in this category of toxins. [CAUSTICS] *p. 735*

11. White powder derived from leaves of the coca plant. [COCAINE] *p. 745*

13. Route of poison exposure in which toxins enter the body through the respiratory system. [INHALATION] *p. 728*

14. Toxic alcohol that is used to manufacture methamphetamine and causes severe metabolic acidosis and blindness when ingested. [METHANOL] *p. 737*

	Cholinergic, *p. 729*	Anticholinergic, *p. 729*	Narcotic, *p. 729*	Sympathomimetic, *p. 729*
Nervous system	Constricted pupils, blurred vision	Dilated pupils, blurred vision, delirium, ataxia, seizures, hyperthermia	Decreased responsiveness, respiratory depression; some substances, such as heroin, cause pinpoint pupils	Euphoria, agitation, seizures
Respiratory system	Bronchoconstriction, increased bronchial secretions		Respiratory depression	
Cardiovascular system	Tachycardia or bradycardia		Bradycardia, hypotension	Hypertension, chest pain, cardiac dysrhythmias, stroke
Musculoskeletal system	Muscle twitches			
Gastrointestinal system	Salivation, gastric distress, emesis, diarrhea	Decreased gastrointestinal activity, dry mouth		
Skin	Sweating	Dry, flushed, hot		

CHECK YOUR RECALL AND APPLY CONCEPTS KEY

EXERCISE 1

1. Ingestion, *p. 728*
2. Cholinergic, *p. 729*
3. Constricted pupils, blurred vision, bronchoconstriction, increased bronchial secretions, salivation, lacrimation, increased urination, vomiting, gastrointestinal distress, diarrhea, muscle twiticing, sweating; increased or decreased heart rate. *p. 729*
4. Muscle spasm, rigidity, or tremor; oculogyric crisis; torticollis; neuroleptic malignant syndrome (hyperthermia), *p. 729*
5. Pulse oximetry measures the saturation of hemoglobin, but does not differentiate whether hemoglobin is saturated with oxygen, or with carbon monoxide, which has a higher affinity than oxygen for hemoglobin. *p. 735*
6. Residential fires, *p. 735*
7. Gasoline, butane, kerosene, lamp oils, mineral oil, toluene, laundry stain removers, spray lubricants (such as WD-40) glues, paints, and aerosol propellants, *p. 736*
8. Pesticides, *p. 736*
9. Neurologic, cardiovascular, and gastrointestinal complications; cirrhosis; increased risk of some cancers; testicular atrophy; pancreatitis; decreased blood clotting, *p. 737*
10. Flushing of the upper half of the body, severe headache, nausea, vomiting, diarrhea, abdominal cramps, palpitations, hives, dizziness, dry mouth, angioedema, bronchospasm, *p. 738*

EXERCISE 2

1.	d	*p. 728*	9.	a	*p. 735*	17. d	*p. 741*
2.	c	*p. 728*	10.	d	*p. 735*	18. b	*p. 742*
3.	b	*p. 728*	11.	b	*p. 736*	19. a	*p. 742*
4.	a	*p. 731*	12.	c	*p. 736*	20. c	*p. 743*
5.	d	*p. 732*	13.	a	*p. 736*	21. d	*p. 744*
6.	c	*p. 733*	14.	c	*p. 737*	22. c	*p. 745*
7.	a	*p. 733*	15.	b	*p. 740*	23. a	*p. 746*
8.	d	*p. 735*	16.	a	*p. 740*		

CLINICAL REASONING CASE STUDY: MAN DOWN AT THE BUS STOP

1. Although the patient seems to have a history of drug abuse, do not assume that the current problem is a drug overdose. Perform a rapid physical examination and when time permits, a thorough head-to-toe examination. Note any unusual odors, such as alcohol or ketones, that can provide clues to the problem. Obtain baseline vital signs and as much history as is available. Determine the blood glucose level. Frequent reassessment is essential for this patient.
2. Knowledge of the history of the present illness and information about the past medical history are important. Bystanders may be able to give a history of the present illness.
3. Maintain the patient's airway, using basic adjuncts as needed. Administer oxygen if indicated by pulse oximetry. Start an IV. If the patient is hypoglycemic, give 50 percent dextrose. Consider giving naloxone because of the patient's decreased ability to maintain his airway and strong indications of narcotic use. Take measures to maintain normal body temperature. Treat any other conditions or injuries that you find during the secondary assessment and transport the patient.

Chapter 33: Trauma Systems and Incident Command

VOCABULARY AND CONCEPT REVIEW KEY

EXERCISE 1

1. primary triage, *p. 759*
2. incident command system (ICS), *p. 757*
3. triage, *p. 756*

EXERCISE 2

4. multiple-casualty incident, *p. 756*
5. national incident command system (NIMS), *p. 756*
6. safety officer, *p. 758*
7. secondary triage, *p. 759*
8. singular command, *p. 758*
9. logistics section, *p. 758*
10. information officer, *p. 758*

Across

4. Incident command section that analyzes data to improve future responses. [PLANNING] *p. 757*
6. Modified triage approach used for pediatric patients. [JUMPSTART] *p. 762*
9. Person who coordinates activities of the incident command system with outside agencies. [LIAISONOFFICER] *p. 758*
10. Strategy for injury prevention that focuses on legislation. [ENFORCEMENT] *p. 754*

Down

1. Opportunity to practice the implementation of the response to multiple-casualty incidents and use of the incident command system. [DISASTERDRILL] *p. 757*
2. Organizational structure used to ensure coordination and effective communication among all agencies responding to a disaster. [NIMS] *p. 756*
3. Patient priority denoted by a red triage tag. [IMMEDIATE]
5. Triage tag color assigned to the walking wounded. [GREEN] *p. 760*
7. Quick sorting process to establish patient priorities for treatment and transport. [TRIAGE] *p. 756*
8. Event in which the number of patients exceeds the available resources. [MCI] *p. 756*

PATIENT ASSESSMENT REVIEW KEY

1. Red
2. Red
3. Yellow
4. Black
5. Green

CHECK YOUR RECALL AND APPLY CONCEPTS KEY

1. b *p. 754*   3. b *p. 755*   5. a *p. 759*
2. a *p. 754*   4. c *p. 756*   6. d *p. 758*

1. The incident commander is on the scene with visual information about the best way to approach. Over-riding the decision can result in an inability for transporting vehicles to leave the scene and can cause confusion.

2. You will most likely be part of the operations section, initially assigned to triage.

3. You will follow a standard triage scheme used by your service, which is likely to be or be similar to the START and JumpSTART triage methods to classify patients according to the urgency for treatment and transport.

Chapter 34: Mechanisms of Injury, Trauma Assessment, and Trauma Triage Criteria

VOCABULARY AND CONCEPT REVIEW KEY

EXERCISE 1

1. e   p. 782
2. c   p. 776
3. b   p. 767
4. a   p. 768
5. d   p. 768
6. i   p. 771
7. f   p. 769
8. g   p. 779
9. j   p. 779
10. h   p. 779

EXERCISE 2

Completed crossword — solution:

Across:
- 3. GLASGOW
- 9. PRIMARY BLAST INJURY
- 10. ROAD RASH
- 11. VELOCITY

Down:
- 1. LATERAL IMPACT
- 2. BLUNT
- 4. DISTRIBUTION
- 5. KINETIC
- 6. REAR IMPACT
- 7. PENETRATING
- 8. TRAUMA

Across	Down

Across

3. Coma scale used to assign a score from 3 to 15 to the patient's neurologic status.[GLASGOW] *p. 781*

9. Ruptured ear drums from an explosion is an example of this. [PRIMARYBLASTINJURY] *p. 779*

10. Severe abrasions obtained in a motorcycle collision caused by friction of the body against the pavement. [ROADRASH] *p. 778*

11. Factor in kinetic energy commonly represented by the speed of the object. [VELOCITY] *p. 769*

Down

1. Sometimes called a T-bone collision.[LATERALIMPACT] *p. 775*

2. Result of being struck by a baseball bat, for example. [BLUNTTRAUMA] *p. 769*

4. Assessment term that refers to neurologic deficit, including decreased level of responsiveness.[DISABILITY] *p. 781*

5. Type of energy possessed by an object in motion.[KINETIC] *p. 767*

6. Collision in which a vehicle is struck from behind. [REARIMPACT] *p. 775*

7. Trauma resulting from being impaled by a screwdriver, for example. [PENETRATING] *p. 769*

8. Injury produced by external forces applied to the body. [TRAUMA] *p. 767*

PATIENT ASSESSMENT REVIEW KEY

EXERCISE 1, *P. 787*

1. No
2. No
3. Yes
4. Yes

EXERCISE 2, *P. 782*

1. E-4, V-5, M-6 (15)
2. E-4, V-4, M-6 (14)
3. E-1, V-1, M-2 (4)
4. E-3, V-3, M-5 (11)

CHECK YOUR RECALL AND APPLY CONCEPTS KEY

1. d *p. 768*
2. b *p. 769*
3. d *p. 769*
4. a *p. 770*
5. b *p. 774*
6. a *p. 780*
7. d *p. 782*

CLINICAL REASONING CASE STUDY: LUCA HANEY

1. The law of inertia applies in that Luca was continuing to move in one direction at a given speed until another force was applied, changing the direction and velocity of his movement. He continued to move in that direction until he struck the ground. The law of conservation of energy applies in that the energy of the SUV was not destroyed on impact, but it changed form from kinetic energy to sound and tissue deformity. The total amount of energy applied to Luca's body depends on the mass of the SUV and its speed, with the speed of the SUV being the more significant of the two factors. The force applied to Luca's body also depends on the rate at which it first accelerated in a different direction upon being struck and then decelerated upon striking the ground.

2. The speed and mass of the SUV and the relative lack of protection of Luca's body should lead you to suspect severe, multisystem injuries. Even though his helmet provides some protection against direct impact, the brain is subject to acceleration and deceleration forces, which can produce shearing injuries to the inelastic brain tissue. Energy from the initial impact with the SUV and the secondary impact with the ground most likely has produced severe blunt force injuries to the tissues (including the bones, because open fractures were immediately obvious). The organs and their attachments have also been subject to significant acceleration and deceleration forces.

3. Do not let the obvious, severe injuries distract you from your priorities. Ensure that the scene is safe before rushing to the patient's side. The forces applied could have resulted in cervical-spine injury, so use manual inline stabilization of the head and neck to restrict spinal motion. If Luca does not appear to be breathing, check the pulse. If the pulse is absent, whether you begin CPR depends on your protocols for resuscitation of blunt trauma victims. Open the airway using a modified jaw-thrust maneuver. If that is not effective, use a head-tilt/chin-lift maneuver to ensure the patient has an open airway. Use suction if necessary. Assess Luca's breathing and assist ventilations if necessary. Note the pulse rate and quality and control bleeding.

Chapter 35: Soft-Tissue Injuries and Burns

VOCABULARY AND CONCEPT REVIEW KEY

EXERCISE 1

1. hemostatic agent, *p. 801*
2. epistaxis, *p. 802*
3. hematoma, *p. 796*
4. abrasion, *p. 797*
5. crush injury, *p. 796*
6. dressing, *p. 802*
7. impaled object, *p. 798*
8. scald, *p. 805*
9. traumatic rhabdomyolysis, *p. 796*
10. avulsion, *p. 797*
11. zone of stasis, *p. 804*
12. rule of nines, *p. 807*

EXERCISE 2

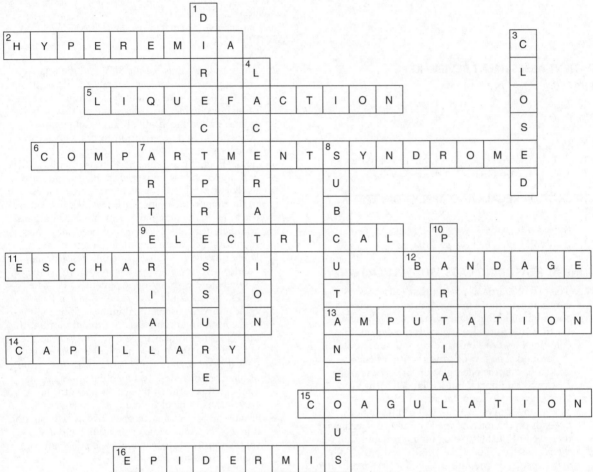

Across	Down

Across

2. Outermost zone of a burn in which there is increased blood flow. [HYPEREMIA] *p. 804*

5. Type of necrosis that occurs when tissues are exposed to a strong alkali substance. [LIQUEFACTION] *p. 812*

6. Increased pressure within the fascia due to swelling, which interferes with perfusion. [COMPARTMENTSYNDROME] *p. 796*

9. Type of burn injury that occurs from lightning strike or contact with high-voltage power lines. [ELECTRICAL] *p. 805*

11. Thick, inelastic tissue resulting from full-thickness burns. [ESCHAR] *p. 805*

12. Material that is applied to secure a dressing in place. [BANDAGE] *p. 803*

13. Condition in which a body part is severed from the body. [AMPUTATION] *p. 797*

14. Source of slow, steady oozing bleeding, usually minor in nature. [CAPILLARY] *p. 800*

15. Type of tissue necrosis produced by exposure to strong acids. [COAGULATION] *p. 812*

16. Outermost layer of the skin. [EPIDERMIS] *p. 794*

Down

1. Compressing the tissues as a method of controlling bleeding. [DIRECTPRESSURE] *p. 801*

3. Contusions and hematomas are examples of this type of soft-tissue injury. [CLOSED] *p. 795*

4. Cut or tear in the skin. [LACERATION] *p. 799*

7. Source of bright red bleeding under pressure. [ARTERIAL] *p. 801*

8. Deepest layer of the skin, in which adipose tissue predominates. [SUBCUTANEOUS] *p. 794*

10. Sometimes called a second-degree burn, this thickness of burn presents with blisters, redness, and pain. [PARTIAL] *p. 806*

PATIENT ASSESSMENT REVIEW KEY

1. abrasion, *p. 797*
2. laceration, *p. 799*
3. partial amputation, *p. 797*
4. partial-thickness burn, *p. 806*
5. hematoma, *p. 796*
6. avulsion, *p. 797*
7. full-thickness burn, *p. 807*

CHECK YOUR RECALL AND APPLY CONCEPTS KEY

1.	b	*p. 794*	5.	c	*p. 796*	9.	a	*p. 810*
2.	c	*p. 795*	6.	d	*p. 801*	10.	c	*p. 810*
3.	b	*p. 795*	7.	b	*p. 799*			
4.	a	*p. 796*	8.	c	*p. 801*			

CLINICAL REASONING CASE STUDY: A RASH DECISION

1. The patient's impact on his left side and complaint of pain with inspiration should make you suspect rib fractures with the potential for underlying organ injury, plus extremity fractures and other musculoskeletal injuries. You must perform a detailed head-to-toe examination on this patient because the pain of the abrasions could distract him from other injuries.

2. Treat extensive abrasions such as those sustained by the patient like burns because much of the skin is damaged, just as it would be in extensive burns. These wounds make the patient prone to impaired thermoregulation, fluid loss, and infection. Irrigate away gross debris and cover the patient with a sterile burn sheet. If the patient's condition allows, treat for pain. Establish IV access and infuse fluids in consultation with medical direction.

3. A burn center is the best destination for this patient. Depending on your distance from a burn center and your protocols, you may transport the patient directly to a burn center, request air medical transportation, or transport to another facility for initial stabilization prior to transfer to burn center.

Chapter 36: Musculoskeletal Injuries

VOCABULARY AND CONCEPT REVIEW KEY

EXERCISE 1

1. d	p. 828	6. j	p. 828	11. i	p. 835
2. l	p. 828	7. g	p. 828	12. f	p. 832
3. m	p. 829	8. c	p. 828	13. a	p. 828
4. e	p. 832	9. h	p. 828		
5. k	p. 828	10. b	p. 832		

EXERCISE 2

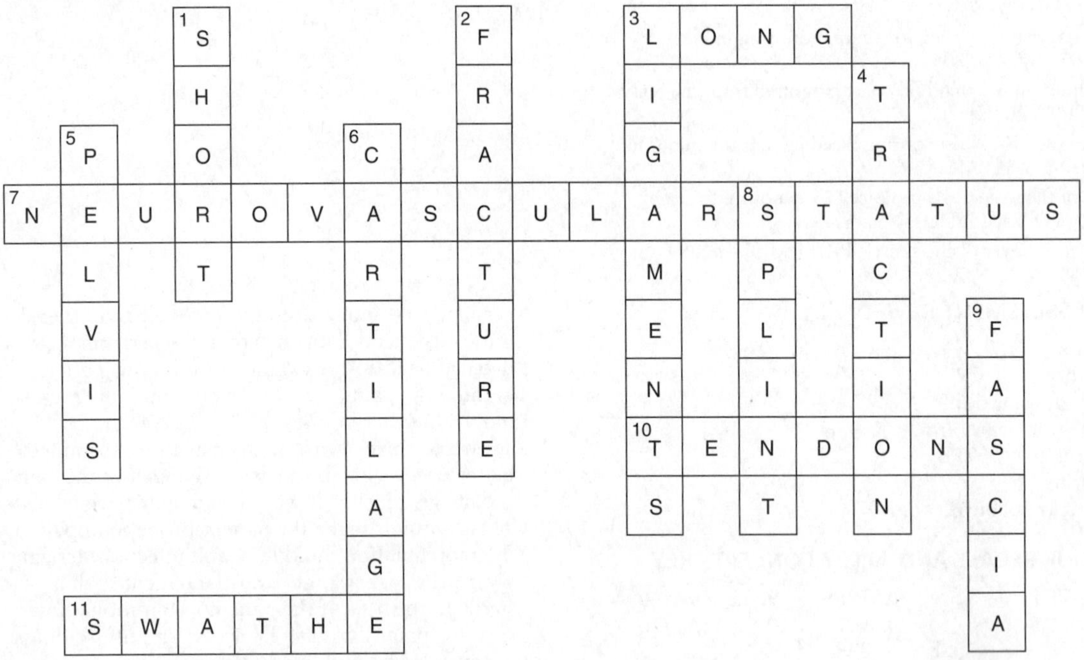

The crossword puzzle answers:

1 (down): S H O R T

2 (down): F R A C T U R E

3 (across): L O N G

3 (down): L I G A M E N T S

4 (down): T R A C T I O N

5 (down): P E L V I S

6 (down): C A R T I L A G E

7 (across): N E U R O V A S C U L A R S T A T U S

8 (down): S P L I C T N N C ... (SPLINT)

9 (down): F A S C I A

10 (across): T E N D O N S

11 (across): S W A T H E

Across

3. Type of bone that includes the femur and humerus. [LONG] *p. 819*
7. This must be checked before and after splinting musculoskeletal injuries. [NEUROVASCULARSTATUS] *p. 822*
10. Connective tissue that secures muscle to bone. [TENDONS] *p. 819*
11. This band of material is used along with a sling to secure an injured upper extremity to the body. [SWATHE] *p. 824*

Down

1. Type of bone that includes the metacarpals and phalanges. [SHORT] *p. 819*
2. Break in the continuity of a bone. [FRACTURE] *p. 827*
3. Bands of connective tissue that provide a connection between bones. [LIGAMENTS] *p. 819*
4. Specialized type of splint used for femur fractures. [TRACTION] *p. 827*
5. Up to 2000 mL of blood can be lost from a fracture of this ring of bones. [PELVIS] *p. 831*
6. Connective tissue that provides shape to strutures, such as ears and nose, and covers the ends of bones. [CARTILAGE] *p. 819*
8. Device used to immobilize an injured extremity. [SPLINT] *p. 823*
9. Membrane that surrounds a skeletal muscle. [FASCIA] *p. 829*

PATIENT ASSESSMENT REVIEW KEY

1. pain, paresthesia, pallor, pulseless, paralysis, *p. 829*
2. Signs and symptoms include pain, deformity, swelling, crepitus, loss of use, and discoloration. *p. 822*

CHECK YOUR RECALL AND APPLY CONCEPTS KEY

1. c	p. 819	5. a	p. 822	9. a	p. 824
2. a	p. 828	6. d	p. 830	10. a	p. 831
3. b	p. 828	7. c	p. 827	11. c	p. 827
4. b	p. 829	8. b	p. 824	12. a	p. 824

CLINICAL REASONING CASE STUDY: THOSE ARE THE BREAKS

1. You must complete a primary and secondary assessment to check for any other injuries sustained in the fight. The format of the secondary assessment (focused or head to toe) depends on whether the patient has other complaints or obvious injuries, information about the nature of the fight, and the patient's mental status.

2. You must splint the hand in the position of function, as if the patient is holding a baseball. Use a roll of gauze in the palm of the patient's hand to achieve this position. Immobilize the fingers and the wrist.

3. Check for sensation in the patient's fingers, especially the fifth digit, and check capillary refill.

Chapter 37: Head, Brain, Face, and Neck Trauma

VOCABULARY AND CONCEPT REVIEW KEY

EXERCISE 1

1. f	p. 841	6. m	p. 848	11. d	p. 850
2. g	p. 846	7. l	p. 846	12. a	p. 850
3. b	p. 842	8. c	p. 846	13. k	p. 846
4. o	p. 848	9. i	p. 848	14. h	p. 848
5. n	p. 847	10. e	p. 850	15. j	p. 848

EXERCISE 2

Crossword answers:

Across:
1. DURA MATER
3. INTRACEREBRAL
6. CUSHING TRIAD
7. BATTLE SIGN
9. MENINGES
10. EPIDURAL HEMATOMA
11. DEPRESSED
12. HYPERCAPNIA

Down:
2. RETROGRADE
4. CORNEA
5. OCCLUSIVE
8. DIPLOPIA

1. Outermost protective membrane surrounding the brain and spinal cord. [DURAMATER] *p. 842*

3. Hemorrhage within the brain tissue. [INTRACEREBRAL] *p. 848*

6. Hypertension, bradycardia, irregular respirations. [CUSHINGTRIAD] *p. 846*

7. Discoloration behind the ears associated with basilar skull fracture. [BATTLESIGN] *p. 845*

9. Protective layers surrounding the brain and spinal cord. [MENINGES] *p. 842*

10. Collection of blood between the skull and the outermost layer of the meninges. [EPIDURALHEMATOMA] *p. 848*

11. Type of skull fracture in which the bone is pushed inward so that it lies beneath the surface of the skull. [DEPRESSED] *p. 845*

12. Increased level of carbon dioxide. [HYPERCAPNIA] *p. 846*

2. Inability to remember events preceding a blow to the head. [RETROGRADEAMNESIA] *p. 847*

4. Clear, outermost surface of the eye. [CORNEA] *p. 842*

5. Type of dressing used for open wounds to the neck. [OCCLUSIVE] *p. 853*

8. Double vision. [DIPLOPIA] *p. 850*

PATIENT ASSESSMENT REVIEW KEY

A history consistent with traumatic brain injury, headache, altered mental status, vomiting, hypertension, and bradycardia can indicate increased intracranial pressure. Suspect herniation with trismus, abnormal breathing patterns, posturing, and unilateral or bilateral dilated, unresponsive pupils.

CHECK YOUR RECALL AND APPLY CONCEPTS KEY

1. c *p. 844*   5. b *p. 844*   9. d *p. 847*
2. b *p. 841*   6. c *p. 846*   10. b *p. 852*
3. a *p. 841*   7. b *p. 844*   11. a *p. 851*
4. d *p. 842*   8. a *p. 853*

CLINICAL REASONING CASE STUDY: INJURED MAN IN THE RESERVOIR

1. The patient's airway is the highest priority. Initially leave the patient on his side and begin suctioning to clear the airway. Once the airway is clear, the best option may be an advanced airway, which will reduce the chances that the patient will aspirate blood. Consider the possibility of cervical-spine injury and restrict motion of the head and neck. Once an airway is established, assess the respiratory status and be prepared to assist ventilations, using supplemental oxygen to maintain an SpO_2 of 95 percent or above. If the source of bleeding is accessible, control it with direct pressure, being careful not to apply too much pressure over unstable bones or depressed fractures. Perform a rapid trauma examination to check for additional life-threatening injuries.

2. The patient may have a Le Fort fracture, among other facial and skull fractures, and may have cervical-spine injuries. Traumatic brain injury is highly likely. Ejection from the jet ski may have resulted in pelvic or femur fractures as the lower body struck the handlebars. Chest and abdominal injuries are possible, as well.

3. The patient is at high risk for airway compromise, hypoxia, and shock. Hypoxia from airway or breathing compromise will lead to secondary brain injury, as will hypoperfusion from shock. Management goals are to maintain adequate oxygenation, normal carbon dioxide levels, and adequate cerebral perfusion.

Chapter 38: Thoracic Trauma

VOCABULARY AND CONCEPT REVIEW KEY

EXERCISE 1

1. Beck's triad, *p. 869*
2. commotio cordis, *p. 867*
3. flail chest, *p. 863*
4. hemoptysis, *p. 860*
5. hemothorax, *p. 865*
6. myocardial contusion, *p. 867*
7. open pneumothorax, *p. 862*
8. paradoxical movement, *p. 863*
9. tracheal deviation, *p. 865*
10. traumatic asphyxia, *p. 866*

EXERCISE 2

Across

3. Blood in the sputum. [HEMOPTYSIS] *p. 860*
4. Muscle that creates the inferior boundary of the thoracic cavity. [DIAPHRAGM] *p. 858*
7. Space in the center of the thoracic cavity that holds the heart, great vessels, trachea, and esophagus. [MEDIASTINUM] *p. 858*
8. Hypotension, JVD, and muffled heart sounds that indicate pericardial teamponade. [BECKTRIAD] *p. 868*
9. Accumulation of air under pressure in the thoracic cavity. [TENSIONPNEUMOTHORAX] *p. 865*
10. Movement in which the flail segment appears to sink as the chest wall expands. [PARADOXICAL] *p. 863*
11. Between the ribs. [INTERCOSTAL] *p. 858*

Down

1. Air trapped beneath the skin is a subcutaneous form of this condition. [EMPHYSEMA] *p. 865*
2. Smooth membrane layer that adheres to the surface of the lungs. [VISCERALPLEURA] *p. 858*
5. Accumulation of blood in the pleural space. [HEMOTHORAX] *p. 865*
6. Dressing placed over an open chest wound. [OCCLUSIVE] *p. 862*

	Simple Pneumothorax, *p. 864*	Tension Pneumothorax, *p. 865*	Open Pneumothorax, *p. 862*	Hemothorax, *p. 865*
Mechanism of Injury	Blunt trauma (rib fracture) or penetrating trauma	Blunt trauma (sudden chest compression against a closed glottis, rib fracture); may occur with penetrating trauma	Penetrating trauma	Blunt or penetrating trauma
Breath Sounds	Diminished on affected side, but decrease may be difficult to detect due to transmitted breath sounds from unaffected portions of the lung	Diminished first on affected side, but transmitted breath sounds may be present; decreased on opposite side as condition progresses	Air movement may be heard at the site of an open chest wound; diminished breath sounds on affected side, but transmitted breath sounds may be heard	Decreased on affected side, depending on degree of atelectasis, but a significant degree of blood loss is required to diminish breath sounds substantially
Heart Rate	May be increased if degree of pneumothorax is significant, resulting in hypoxia	Tachycardia as a compensatory mechanism as cardiac output decreases	May be increased if hypoxia is significant	Tachycardia may occur as a compensatory mechanism for hypovolemia
Blood Pressure	Usually unaffected	Hypotension	Usually unaffected unless accompanied by tension pneumothorax	Hypotension
Assessment of the Neck	Generally no abnormal findings	Jugular vein distension; tracheal deviation away from the affected side as a late sign	Generally no abnormal findings	Flat jugular veins
Level of Distress	Mild to severe, depending on degree of atelectasis	Severe with continuing deterioration	Mild to severe, depending on degree of atelectasis	Mild to severe, depending on amount of blood loss

CHECK YOUR RECALL AND APPLY CONCEPTS KEY

1. b   *p. 865*
2. b   *p. 859*
3. a   *p. 865*
4. d   *p. 864*
5. c   *p. 863*
6. c   *p. 859*
7. c   *p. 867*
8. b   *p. 860*
9. c   *p. 866*
10. b   *p. 862*

CLINICAL REASONING CASE STUDY: THAT COVERS IT

1. Possible causes of the patient's deterioration include hypovolemia, hemothorax, tension pneumothorax, and pericardial tamponade.
2. The existence of an open pneumothorax that was sealed with an occlusive dressing, along with sudden deterioration that includes decreasing SpO$_2$ and jugular venous distention, makes tension pneumothorax a likely cause, but you cannot rule out other problems.
3. Lift the occlusive dressing, which may have become sealed to the wound by blood. As air continues to leak from the injured lung, it may not be able to escape if the occlusive dressing is not open on one side. Air movement out of the wound and improvement in the patient's condition upon lifting the dressing increase the suspicion of tension pneumothorax. Replace the occlusive dressing after exhalation.

Chapter 39: Abdominal Trauma

VOCABULARY AND CONCEPT REVIEW KEY

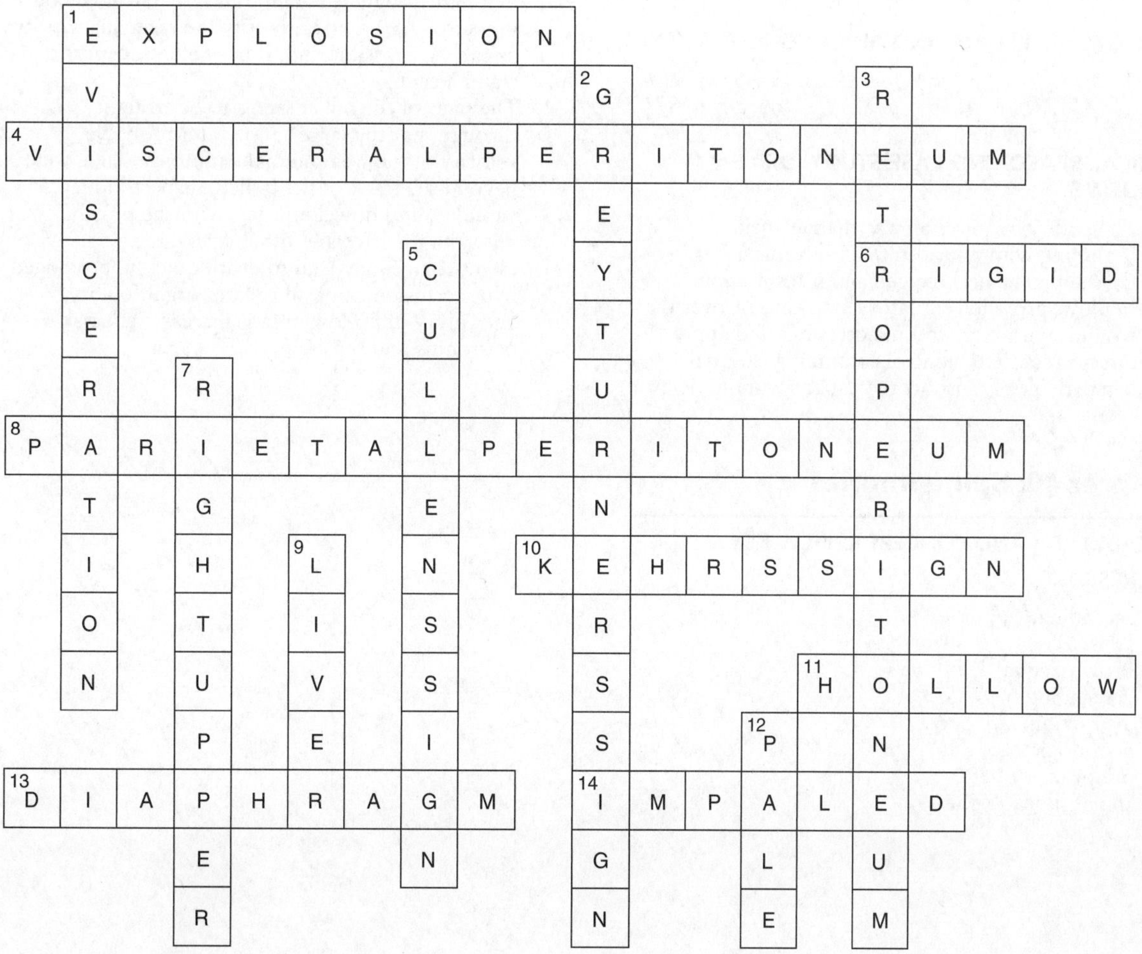

The crossword puzzle grid contains the following answers:

Across

1. **EXPLOSION** — Mechanism that creates a blast wave in which a sudden increase in pressure within a hollow organ can cause it to rupture. *p. 879*
4. **VISCERALPERITONEUM** — Smooth membranous lining that covers the abdominal organs. *p. 872*
6. **RIGID** — An abdomen that feels stiff, hard, or unyielding is called this. *p. 875*
8. **PARIETALPERITONEUM** — Smooth membranous lining of the abdominal cavity. *p. 873*
10. **KEHRSSIGN** — Pain referred to the left shoulder in splenic injury. *p. 875*
11. **HOLLOW** — An organ that has a cavity or space inside is called this. *p. 873*
13. **DIAPHRAGM** — Upper boundary of the abdominal cavity. *p. 872*
14. **IMPALED** — An object that penetrates the skin and remains embedded in the abdomen is said to be this. *p. 877*

Down

1. **EVISCERATION** — Injury in which abdominal organs protrude through an open wound in the abdominal wall. *p. 877*
2. **GREYTURNERSSIGN** — Ecchymosis of the flanks. *p. 875*
3. **RETROPERITONEUM** — Space behind the abdominal cavity that holds organs such as the kidneys. *p. 873*
5. **CULLENSSIGN** — Periumbilical ecchymosis. *p. 875*
7. **RIGHTUPPER** — Quadrant of the abdomen where the liver is located. *p. 873*
9. **LIVER** — Large solid organ in the right upper quadrant. *p. 873*
12. **PALE** — Typical skin color in shock. *p. 875*

PATIENT ASSESSMENT REVIEW KEY

1. c *p. 875*   3. d *p. 875*   5. b *p. 875*
2. c *p. 875*   4. a *p. 875*

CHECK YOUR RECALL AND APPLY CONCEPTS KEY

1. d *p. 873*   3. c *p. 873*   5. b *p. 876*
2. d *p. 873*   4. b *p. 877*   6. a *p. 875*

CLINICAL REASONING CASE STUDY: DRIVE-BY SHOOTING

1. The patient requires airway management, beginning with a head-tilt/chin-lift maneuver. Give supplemental oxygen and if respirations are shallow, provide ventilatory assistance. Cover the wounds with large trauma dressings and apply direct pressure to control continuing external hemorrhage. Transport the patient without delay. Keep her warm and start two large-bore IVs. Administer fluids according to your protocol. A common goal for prehospital fluid resuscitation in a patient with these injuries is a systolic blood pressure of 80 mmHg. Notify the receiving facility as early as possible and, if possible, transport to a trauma center.
2. The path of the bullet seems to be straight through, but the large caliber and probable velocity of the weapon make injury possible well beyond the track of the bullet. Suspect kidney, vascular, and bowel injuries, with the possibility of injury to the liver and other structures.
3. Hemorrhage may lead to death quickly, prolonged hypoperfusion can lead to later organ failure, and injury of hollow organs increases the risk of peritonitis and sepsis.

Chapter 40: Spine Injuries

VOCABULARY AND CONCEPT REVIEW KEY

EXERCISE 1

1. ascending, *p. 885*
2. atlas, axis, *p. 884*
3. Brown-Séquard, *p. 888*
4. descending, *p. 885*
5. distraction, *p. 886*
6. neurologic, *p. 886*
7. priapism, *p. 890*
8. spinal shock, *p. 888*

Across

2. Person whose help you should enlist when removing a sports helmet from an injured player. [ATHLETICTRAINER] *p. 903*

5. Area of the spine that articulates with the pelvis. [SACRAL] *p. 884*

9. Paralysis of the arms and legs. [QUADRIPLEGIA]

11. Second cervical vertebra. [AXIS] *p. 884*

13. Rigid device placed around the neck to restrict movement. [CERVICALCOLLAR] *p. 892*

14. Bending the neck forward so that the chin is closer to the chest. [FLEXION] *p. 887*

15. Paralysis of the lower extremities. [PARAPLEGIA]

16. Paralysis of the arms and legs. [TETRAPLEGIA]

17. Coordinated maneuver to turn the patient onto his side in order to position a long backboard behind him. [LOGROLL] *p. 897*

18. Lower-most portion of the spinal column. [COCCYX] *p. 884*

Down

1. Procedure used when a patient must quickly be removed from a vehicle but has a possibility of spine injury. [RAPIDEXTRICATION] *p. 901*

3. Superior-most portion of the spinal column. [CERVICAL] *p. 883*

4. Nerve that controls movement of the diaphragm. [PHRENIC] *p. 885*

6. First cervical vertebra. [ATLAS] *p. 884*

7. Area of the spine that supports the greatest amount of body weight. [LUMBAR] *p. 884*

8. Cushioning placed between the patient and the long backboard to fill voids and prevent pressure points. [PADDING] *p. 896*

10. MVCs and other forms of trauma that can damage the spine. [MOI] *p. 886*

12. Type of injury that occurs from swelling or ischemia after the initial injury to the spine. [SECONDARY] *p. 886*

PATIENT ASSESSMENT REVIEW KEY

1. Anterior cord syndrome, *p. 888*
2. Brown-Séquard syndrome, *p. 888*
3. Central cord syndrome, *p. 888*

CHECK YOUR RECALL AND APPLY CONCEPTS KEY

EXERCISE 1

1.	F *p. 883*	5.	F *p. 886*	9.	F *p. 898*
2.	T *p. 883*	6.	T *p. 889*	10.	F *p. 901*
3.	F *p. 885*	7.	F *p. 888*		
4.	F *p. 886*	8.	T *p. 896*		

1. b	p. 886	4. d	p. 886	6. a	p. 888
2. a	p. 889	5. c	p. 892	7. a	p. 901
3. c	p. 889				

CLINICAL REASONING CASE STUDY: INJURED PERSON AT THE FAIRGROUNDS

1. Studies indicate that between 3.7 and 7.8 percent of patients with craniofacial trauma and a GCS less than 8 have a cervical-spine injury, but only a subset of those patients have spinal cord injury. It is not possible to know in the prehospital setting which patients with those injuries have spinal column and spinal cord injuries, so avoid unnecessary movement.

2. If a modified jaw-thrust maneuver has been not been effective, a head-tilt/chin-lift maneuver can be used, but the patient's unresponsiveness and bleeding from facial trauma mean that you must insert an advanced airway at the appropriate time.

3. The patient requires initial cervical-spine motion restriction followed by application of a cervical collar and complete immobilization to a long backboard.

Chapter 41: Environmental Emergencies

VOCABULARY AND CONCEPT REVIEW KEY

EXERCISE 1

1. c	p. 922	4. f	p. 920	7. a	p. 912
2. i	p. 921	5. h	p. 909	8. j	p. 923
3. g	p. 919	6. b	p. 913	9. e	p. 909

EXERCISE 2

```
1                          2                    3
C O N D U C T I O N       N                    D
                          I        4
                          T        H E N R Y S
             5            R                    O
             H            R                    W
             E        6                        N
             R A D I A T I O N                 I
             T            G                    N
          7                                    G
             D E C O M P R E S S I O N
             X            N
             H            N
             A            A
          8
             P U L M O N A R Y E D E M A
             S            C
             T        9
             I            B A R O T R A U M A
          10             S
             C O N V E C T I O N
             N            S
```

1. This is how heat is lost when you come in contact with a cold object. [CONDUCTION] *p. 909*
4. Law that explains how carbon dioxide is dissolved in a sealed bottle of soda. [HENRYS] *p. 920*
6. Heat loss into a still atmosphere. [RADIATION] *p. 909*
7. Sickness also called the bends. [DECOMPRESSION] *p. 921*
8. Fluid in the lungs from rapid ascension to a high altitude. [PULMONARYEDEMA] *p. 922*
9. Severe pain in the ear or sinuses when descending rapidly during a dive are examples of this. [BAROTRAUMA] *p. 920*
10. Losing heat to air currents moving across the body. [CONVECTION] *p. 909*

2. Also known as "rapture of the deep." [NITROGENNARCOSIS] *p. 922*
3. Death due to asphyxia from submersion in a liquid. [DROWNING] *p. 917*
5. Mild state of shock that occurs as a result of exposure to a hot environment. [HEATEXHAUSTION] *p. 913*

PATIENT ASSESSMENT REVIEW KEY

	Heat Cramps	Heat Exhaustion	Classic Heat Stroke	Exertional Heat Stroke
Signs and symptoms	Cramps in large muscle groups Weakness Dizziness	Possible increase in body temperature Pale, cool, skin Weakness Headache Dizziness	Flushed, hot skin Elevated body temperature Altered mental status Cessation of sweating Possible seizures	Flushed, hot, wet skin Elevated body temperature Altered mental status Possible seizures

CHECK YOUR RECALL AND APPLY CONCEPTS KEY

EXERCISE 1

1. gradient, *p. 909*
2. thermogenesis, *p. 909*
3. radiation, *p. 909*
4. heat index, *p. 910*
5. conduction, convection, radiation, evaporation, respiration, *p. 909*
6. hyperthermia, *p. 912*
7. exertional heat stroke, *p. 913*
8. mild, *p. 915*
9. shivering, *p. 915*
10. frostbite, *p. 916*
11. 100 to 104, *p. 917*
12. drowning, *p. 917*
13. dysbarism, *p. 919*
14. Henry's, *p. 919*
15. acclimatization, *p. 922*

EXERCISE 2

1. c	*p. 913*	5. b	*p. 915*	9. d	*p. 922*
2. d	*p. 913*	6. a	*p. 916*	10. d	*p. 923*
3. d	*p. 913*	7. b	*p. 921*		
4. c	*p. 915*	8. a	*p. 922*		

CLINICAL REASONING CASE STUDY: BURNING DOWN THE HOUSE

1. The combination of altered mental status, increased body temperature, and a history of exertion in an extremely hot environment are consistent with exertional heat stroke. Heat emergencies tend to be progressive. If the patient's signs and symptoms had not been recognized when they were, it is likely that he would have become unresponsive.
2. The primary concerns are ensuring an open airway and adequate ventilation. Cool the patient by removing heavy clothing, removing him from the hot environment, and using an active cooling method, such as placing a wet sheet over him and fanning him or placing cold packs in the groin and axillae. Replace lost fluid volume intravenously.
3. Anticipate seizures, and consider requesting advanced life support. Watch for shivering, which indicates you are cooling the patient too quickly. Shivering generates heat and will increase the body temperature, worsening the patient's condition.

Chapter 42: Multisystem Trauma and Trauma Resuscitation

VOCABULARY AND CONCEPT REVIEW KEY

<u>EXERCISE 1</u>

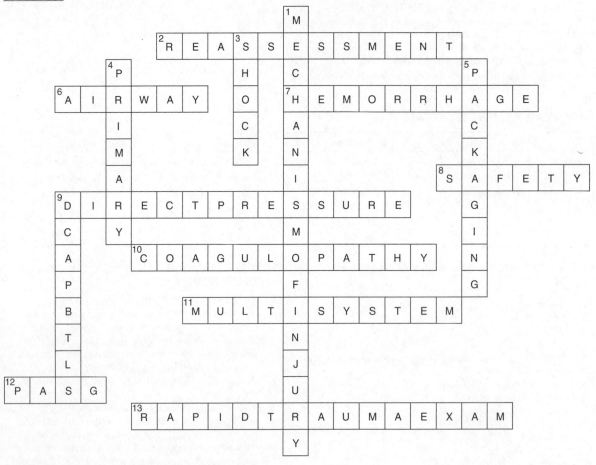

Across

2. Subsequent evaluation of the multisystem trauma patient to detect trends in his condition and the effects of treatment. [REASSESSMENT] *p. 930*

6. Management of this is your primary responsibility when caring for a critically injured patient. [AIRWAY] *p. 929*

7. Bleeding. [HEMORRHAGE]

8. Your first priority on any emergency scene. [SAFETY] *p. 928*

9. Method that is effective in controlling most external bleeding. [DIRECTPRESSURE] *p. 929*

10. Condition of abnormal blood clotting. [COAGULOPATHY] *p. 933*

11. Type of trauma that occurs to more than one body structure. [MULTISYSTEM] *p. 927*

12. Pants-like device sometimes used for patients with pelvic fractures accompanied by shock. [PASG] *p. 932*

13. Portion of the secondary assessment that is performed in multisystem trauma patients immediately after the primary assessment. [RAPIDTRAUMAEXAM] *p. 930*

Down

1. Specific traumatic forces applied to the body. [MECHANISMOFINJURY]

3. State of hypoperfusion. [SHOCK]

4. Type of assessment in which you identify and treat problems with the airway, breathing, and circulation. [PRIMARY] *p. 929*

5. Steps taken to prepare a patient for transport, which may include spinal immobilization. [PACKAGING] *p. 930*

9. Mnemonic for use during rapid trauma assessment. [DCAPBTLS]

PATIENT ASSESSMENT REVIEW KEY

EXERCISE 1

Ejection from a vehicle, pedestrian struck by a vehicle, fall from significant height (greater than 10 feet for an adult), motorcycle and rider separation in a motor vehicle collision (MVC), high-speed MVC (greater than 40 mph), explosion, multiple penetrating injuries, *p. 928*

EXERCISE 2

Scene size-up, primary assessment, rapid trauma examination, vital signs, head-to-toe examination, history, reassessment, *p. 928*

CHECK YOUR RECALL AND APPLY CONCEPTS KEY

1. c *p. 929*
2. b *p. 932*
3. a *p. 932*
4. d *p. 929*

CLINICAL REASONING CASE STUDY: HEAD-ON COLLISION

1. The general priorities are to ensure scene safety and determine if additional resources are needed and if there are additional patients. Cervical-spine injury is possible with this mechanism of injury, so open the airway with a modified jaw-thrust maneuver while manually restricting the motion of the cervical spine. However, if for some reason a modified jaw-thrust maneuver does not allow adequate airflow, use a head-tilt/chin-lift maneuver and plan for insertion of an advanced airway device at the appropriate point in treatment. If breathing is not adequate, assist ventilations with a bag-valve-mask device. With or without adequate ventilations, use supplemental oxygen to maintain an SpO_2 of 95 percent or higher. Control external bleeding. Anticipate shock and the need to improve perfusion.

2. The patient must have a patent airway. An advanced airway device such as a supraglottic airway or Combitube is a good option, especially if transport is prolonged. Ventilate the patient at a rate of 10 to 12 per minute unless there are signs of impending herniation, in which case you should consider a short period of slight hyperventilation. Maintain an SpO_2 of 95 percent or higher and try to achieve a systolic blood pressure of 90 mmHg. If the patient has suspected traumatic brain injury, consider a systolic blood pressure of 100 mmHg. However, you must consider the possibility of internal hemorrhage and the effects of increased systolic blood pressure.

3. Factors affecting transport decisions include the patient's condition, available resources, and the distance to various levels of care.

Chapter 43: Obstetrics and Care of the Newborn

VOCABULARY AND CONCEPT REVIEW KEY

<u>EXERCISE 1</u>

1. j	*p. 951*	6. a	*p. 954*	11. g	*p. 950*
2. h	*p. 945*	7. e	*p. 946*	12. b	*p. 951*
3. d	*p. 952*	8. m	*p. 962*	13. c	*p. 942*
4. k	*p. 941*	9. l	*p. 952*		
5. f	*p. 950*	10. i	*p. 946*		

<u>EXERCISE 2</u>

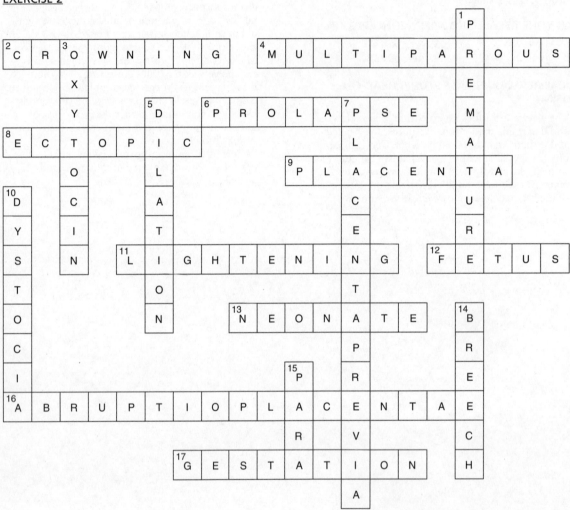

Across	Down
2. Visibility of the presenting part of the fetus at the vaginal opening. [CROWNING] *p. 946*	1. Descriptor for a newborn born between 20 and 37 weeks of gestation. [PREMATURE] *p. 966*
4. Term that describes a woman who has given birth more than once. [MULTIPAROUS] *p. 946*	3. A posterior pituitary hormone that causes uterine muscle contraction and stimulates the letdown reflex in lactation. [OXYTOCIN] *p. 945*
6. Condition in which the umbilical cord is the presenting part during labor and delivery. [PROLAPSE] *p. 960*	5. Widening of the diameter of the cervical os in preparation for delivery. [DILATION] *p. 945*
8. Type of pregnancy in which the embryo is implanted anywhere other than the uterine lining. [ECTOPIC] *p. 951*	7. Condition in which the placenta partially or completely covers the internal cervical opening. [PLACENTAPREVIA] *p. 953*
9. Temporary organ of pregnancy that allows exchange of oxygen, nutrients, and wastes between the mother and fetus. [PLACENTA] *p. 943*	10. Conditions in which the fetal head delivers but in which the shoulders become wedged behind the public bone. [DYSTOCIA] *p. 960*
11. Point at which the presenting part of the fetus drops into the maternal pelvis. [LIGHTENING] *p. 954*	14. Position in which the baby's buttocks or feet are the presenting part in the birth canal. [BREECH] *p. 959*
12. Developing human organism from 60 days gestation to birth. [FETUS] *p. 943*	15. Term that describes a woman who has given birth to an infant greater than 20 weeks gestation. [PARA] *p. 950*
13. A newborn. [NEONATE] *p. 940*	
16. Premature separation of the placenta from the uterine wall. [ABRUPTIOPLACENTAE] *p. 953*	
17. Period of time from conception to delivery. [GESTATION] *p. 943*	

PATIENT ASSESSMENT REVIEW

EXERCISE 1

Indications that the mother is in the second stage of labor, particularly with multiparous women. If contractions are frequent and intense, determine if the mother feels an urge to push and check for crowning. The mother feels an urge to bear down or push, or feels pressure similar to that felt when needing to have a bowel movement. If the mother complains of those symptoms, check for crowning. Perineal bulging or crowning are indications of imminent delivery.

EXERCISE 2

A – Appearance		
0	1	2
Cyanotic head, body, and extremities	Head and body pink, extremities cyanotic	Completely pink
P – Pulse		
0	1	2
Absent	Less than 100	Over 100
G – Grimace		
0	1	2
No reaction to stimuli	Grimaces in response to stimuli	Cries
A – Activity		
0	1	2
Limp	Some flexion of extremities	Active movement
R – Respirations		
0	1	2
Absent	Weak or irregular	Strong cry

1. b	*p. 940*	8. a	*p. 962*	15. b	*p. 963*
2. a	*p. 940*	9. c	*p. 946*	16. a	*p. 958*
3. a	*p. 940*	10. b	*p. 948*	17. c	*p. 959*
4. d	*p. 944*	11. a	*p. 955*	18. c	*p. 962*
5. c	*p. 948*	12. b	*p. 952*	19. d	*p. 962*
6. a	*p. 944*	13. d	*p. 953*	20. b	*p. 965*
7. d	*p. 945*	14. b	*p. 956*	21. c	*p. 967*

CLINICAL REASONING CASE STUDY: IT'S A GIRL

1. You will need to suction the newborn's mouth and nose, clamp and cut the umbilical cord, dry her, and wrap her in a receiving blanket. You will perform APGAR scores at 1 minute and 5 minutes after complete delivery.

2. You will get a complete history from the mother, assess her vital signs, watch for signs of excessive postpartum bleeding, and anticipate delivery of the placenta, although you do not need to wait for delivery of the placenta to transport.

Chapter 44: Pediatric Emergencies

VOCABULARY AND CONCEPT REVIEW KEY

EXERCISE 1

1. apparent life-threatening event, *p. 985*
2. bronchiolitis, *p. 975*
3. cystic fibrosis, *p. 984*
4. febrile, *p. 986*
5. Hydrocephalus, *p. 986*
6. pediatric assessment triangle, *p. 976*
7. pertussis, *p. 983*
8. respiratory syncytial virus, *p. 983*
9. sudden infant death syndrome, *p. 976*

EXERCISE 2

Across	**Down**

Across

2. Teenager. [ADOLESCENT] *p. 975*

5. Pulling in of the tissues above the clavicles and between the ribs; an indication of respiratory distress. [RETRACTIONS] *p. 976*

6. Laryngotracheobronchitis. [CROUP] *p. 983*

7. Cause of cardiac arrest and death in drowning. [ASPHYXIA] *p. 991*

9. This form of stored energy is limited in the muscles and live of a child, meaning fatigue and deterioration can occur quickly in illness or injury. [GLYCOGEN] *p. 981*

11. Condition that should be suspected when the pediatric patient's capillary refill time is greater than 4 seconds. [DECOMPENSATEDSHOCK] *p. 990*

12. Pulse checked in infants. [BRACHIAL] *p. 977*

13. Child from one to three years old. [TODDLER] *p. 975*

14. Cardiac arrest due to a blow to the chest. [COMMOTIOCORDIS] *p. 984*

15. May be viral or bacterial; inflammation of the lining around the central nervous system structures. [MENINGITIS] *p. 985*

16. Access route for fluid replacement and medication administration in a pediatric patient when an IV cannot be obtained. [INTRAOSSEOUS] *p. 982*

Down

1. How oxygen is administered to a child who needs it but does not tolerate a nasal cannula or mask. [BLOWBY] *p. 978*

3. Severe, prolonged asthma attack that cannot be broken with nebulized beta$_2$ agonists. [STATUSASTHMATICUS] *p. 982*

4. Child from one month to one year of age. [INFANT] *p. 973*

8. Component of the pediatric assessment triangle determined by the muscle tone, interactiveness, consolability, eye contact, and speech or cry of the patient. [APPEARANCE] *p. 976*

10. Narrowest portion of the infant airway. [CRICOIDRING] *p. 974*

PATIENT ASSESSMENT REVIEW KEY

EXERCISE 1

Decreased oral intake, vomiting, diarrhea, poor skin turgor (tenting), no or few wet diapers or infrequent urination, no tears when crying, sunken-appearing eyes, dry mucous membranes, sunken anterior fontanel, lethargy, tachycardia, tachypnea, or pale, cool, skin, *p. 987*

CHECK YOUR RECALL AND APPLY CONCEPTS KEY

EXERCISE 1

1.	b	*p. 977*	**6.**	a	*p. 981*	**11.**	a	*p. 985*
2.	a	*p. 973*	**7.**	c	*p. 983*	**12.**	c	*p. 990*
3.	d	*p. 975*	**8.**	b	*p. 984*	**13.**	b	*p. 990*
4.	c	*p. 976*	**9.**	d	*p. 985*	**14.**	a	*p. 991*
5.	c	*p. 977*	**10.**	d	*p. 985*	**15.**	a	*p. 991*

EXERCISE 2

History that is inconsistent with injuries; lack of interest in surroundings; unusual patterns of bruising; injuries that would be unusual in a child, or that have an unusual pattern or location; significant bruising or cuts, burns, welts; bruising to the torso, thighs, or buttocks; injuries with the pattern of an object or handprint; multiple injuries in various stages of healing, *p. 991*

EXERCISE 2, *P. 980*

Age Group	Respiratory Rate (per minute)	Heart Rate (per minute)	Systolic Blood Pressure in mmHg	Temperature in °F
Newborn	30–60	100–180	70–90	98–100
Infant	25–40	100–160	70–90	98–100
Toddler	24–30	80–130	72–100	98.6–99.6
Preschooler	22–34	80–120	78–104	98.6–99.6
School age	18–30	70–110	80–115	98.6
Adolescent	12–20	60–105	88–120	98.6

CLINICAL REASONING CASE STUDY: CHILD WITH DIFFICULTY BREATHING

1. Croup and epiglottitis are consistent with inspiratory stridor. Bronchiolitis is another possibility.

2. If the child has had all recommended vaccinations, epiglottitis and pertussis are unlikely. Bronchiolitis and croup are not prevented by vaccines and both are common in this age group. Auscultation of the breath sounds will most likely reveal wheezes and crackles (rales) in bronchiolitis, whereas croup would not produce those sounds.

3. Avoid unnecessary procedures that might agitate the child and make her condition worse. If the SpO$_2$ is less than 95 percent administer oxygen by the blow-by method. Humidified oxygen is preferred. Check with medical direction about administering a nebulized beta$_2$ agonist.

Chapter 45: Geriatrics

VOCABULARY AND CONCEPT REVIEW KEY

EXERCISE 1

1. delirium, *p. 1008*
2. incontinence, *p. 1009*
3. life span, *p. 998*
4. confabulation, *p. 1004*
5. spondylosis, *p. 1010*
6. pathologic fracture, *p. 1009*
7. Alzheimer's disease, *p. 1008*
8. decubitus ulcer, *p. 999*

EXERCISE 2

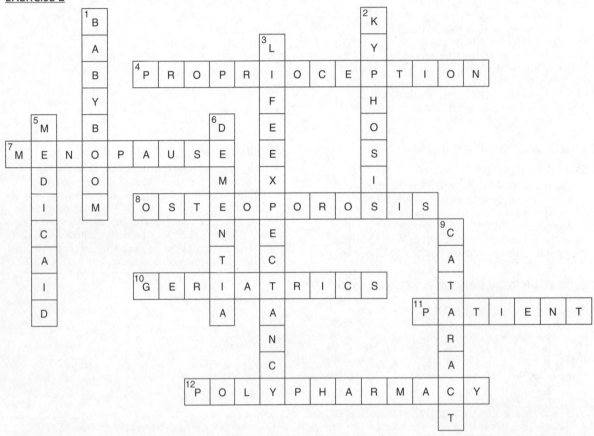

Across

4. Ability to sense the location, orientation, and movement of the body and its parts. [PROPRIOCEPTION] *p. 1001*
7. Cessation of menstruation. [MENOPAUSE] *p. 998*
8. Loss of bone density. [OSTEOPOROSIS]
10. Branch of medicine that specializes in treating elderly patients. [GERIATRICS] *p. 998*
11. Person with whom you should first attempt to communicate when responding to a call for an elderly person. [PATIENT] *p. 1002*
12. Use of multiple medications. [POLYPHARMACY] *p. 1004*

Down

1. Increase in birth rate following World War II. [BABYBOOMJ *p. 998*
2. Abnormal curvature of the upper spine. [KYPHOSIS] *p. 1002*
3. Statistical calculation of the length of time a person can anticipate living based on year of birth and other factors. [LIFEEXPECTANCY] *p. 998*
5. Program that funds medical care for eligible low income families and individuals. [MEDICAID] *p. 1001*
6. Progressive, irreversible loss of cognitive function. [DEMENTIA] *p. 1001*
9. Clouding of the lens of the eye. [CATARACT] *p. 1005*

PATIENT ASSESSMENT REVIEW KEY

Instead of chest pain, the patient may present with generalized weakness, shortness of breath, a general complaint of not feeling well, dizziness, or altered mental status.

CHECK YOUR RECALL AND APPLY CONCEPTS KEY

EXERCISE 1

1. b   *p. 998*
2. b   *p. 998*
3. d   *p. 998*
4. c   *p. 1002*
5. a   *p. 1001*
6. c   *p. 1008*
7. d   *p. 1004*
8. d   *p. 1008*
9. a   *p. 1007*
10. b   *p. 1008*
11. c   *p. 1008*
12. a   *p. 1008*
13. d   *p. 1009*
14. b   *p. 1009*

CLINICAL REASONING CASE STUDY: ELDERLY PATIENT WITH DIFFICULTY BREATHING

1. Initial hypotheses include causes of hypoxia and poor brain perfusion. The combination of dyspnea and altered mental status is suspicious for heart failure and pneumonia. You should consider other possibilities, such as medication interactions, stroke, sepsis, and progression of renal failure with fluid and electrolyte imbalance, as well.
2. The patient's breath sounds and vital signs will be especially helpful in trying to narrow potential causes of the problem. The medications, any history of trauma, and recent changes in the patient's condition will also be helpful. Because

EXERCISE 2

1. T,   *p. 1003*
2. T,   *p. 1006*
3. F, Many elderly patients can give a good history.   *p. 1002*
4. F, Pneumonia is a common cause of death in the elderly.   *p. 1007*
5. F, The elderly may be very ill with infectious diseases, including pneumonia, without having a fever.   *p. 1007*
6. T,   *p. 1007*
7. F, Hypoglycemia can cause altered mental status, but is unlikely to resolve spontaneously as syncope does. You must strongly consider cardiovascular causes in elderly patients with syncope and near syncope.   *p. 1008*
8. T,   *p. 1008*
9. T,   *p. 1009*
10. T,   *p. 1011*

the patient is confused, a thorough head-to-toe assessment can give additional information, such as the presence of decubitus ulcers, signs of trauma, edema, abdominal masses, and other signs.

3. Because the patient is dyspneic, consider administering oxygen based on the patient's SpO_2. Obtain IV access, using the patient's lung sounds and hydration status as guides to the amount of fluid (if any) that is needed. Position the patient for comfort and airway management, protect him from injury, and transport. If additional information indicates a specific underlying cause, you can consider additional treatment.

Chapter 46: Patients with Special Challenges

VOCABULARY AND CONCEPT REVIEW KEY

EXERCISE 1

1. b   *p. 1018*
2. g   *p. 1019*
3. e   *p. 1024*
4. a   *p. 1021*
5. d   *p. 1021*
6. f   *p. 1018*
7. c   *p. 1021*

Across

3. Inability to see. [BLINDNESS] *p. 1017*
6. Care focused on the needs of terminally ill patients and their families. [HOSPICE] *p. 1029*
9. Surgically placed device that allows some deaf patients to hear. [COCHLEARIMPLANT] *p. 1017*
10. Stuttering speech. [FLUENCYDISORDER] *p. 1018*
11. Loss of motor ability. [PARALYSIS] *p. 1019*
12. Common obstruction to a tracheostomy tube. [MUCUS] *p. 1024*

Down

1. Significantly overweight. [OBESE] *p. 1019*
2. Type of abuse: the willful inflection of mental or emotional anguish through threat, or humiliation through verbal or nonverbal means. [PSYCHOLOGICAL] *p. 1021*
4. Low income resulting in an inability to pay for necessities. [POVERTY] *p. 1020*
5. Type of tube that is inserted through the nose; it extends through the pharynx and esophagus into the stomach as a route for administering nutrition or medication. [NASOGASTRIC] *p. 1027*
7. Paralysis of the lower extremities. [PARAPLEGIA] *p. 1019*
8. Severe hearing impairment. [DEAFNESS] *p. 1017*

CHECK YOUR RECALL AND APPLY CONCEPTS KEY

1.	c	*p. 1017*	7.	c	*p. 1022*
2.	d	*p. 1017*	8.	a	*p. 1022*
3.	a	*p. 1018*	9.	d	*p. 1024*
4.	b	*p. 1019*	10.	d	*p. 1025*
5.	c	*p. 1019*	11.	a	*p. 1027*
6.	b	*p. 1021*			

CLINICAL REASONING CASE STUDY: HOPE FULBRIGHT

1. In addition to a mucus plug in the tracheostomy tube and an obstruction of the ventilator circuit, possible causes include pneumothorax, pulmonary edema, bronchospasm, the patient coughing during the inspiratory phase of the ventilator, pneumonia, ventilator settings (tidal volume is too high, expiratory phase is too short), and atelectasis.
2. Assess the patient's SpO_2 and breath sounds, check for fever, and obtain vital signs.

VOCABULARY AND CONCEPT REVIEW KEY

```
                              1
                              H  A  Z  M  A  T
2     3                       Y
S     H     I     M           B
      Y           4           R
      D           C
      R     5     R  I  G  G  I  N  G
      A           B           D
      U           B     6     L      7           8
      L           I     E     J           E
9
D  I  S  E  N  T  A  N  G  L  E  M  E  N  T
      C           G     T     P           R
                        H     10          I
                              A  N  S  I
           11                             C
           S  I  Z  E  U  P        U
                              R     12
                                    A  I  R  B  A  G  S
                        13                T           T
                        N                             I
                   14                                 O
                   P  F  D
                        P
                   15
                   H  A  L  L  I  G  A  N
```

Across

1. Specialized team requested when there is a chemical release. [HAZMAT] *p. 1035*
2. Thin piece of cribbing. [SHIM] *p. 1040*
5. Ropes, chains, or webbing used to help stabilize a vehicle. [RIGGING] *p. 1040*
9. The process of freeing the patient from entrapment. [DISENTANGLEMENT] *p. 1035*
10. Standards for eyewear that should be met for protection against debris and fluid. [ANSI] *p. 1034*
11. First phase of a rescue operation. [SIZEUP] *p. 1035*
12. If not deployed on impact, these vehicle restraint systems must be deactivated before gaining access to the passenger compartment. [AIRBAGS] *p. 1039*
14. Should be worn by personnel working on or near water during rescue operations. [PFD] *p. 1034*
15. Prying tool used for auto extrication. [HALLIGAN] *p. 1041*

Down

1. Vehicle that uses a combination of fuel and high-voltage electrical energy for power. [HYBRID] *p. 1040*
3. Jaws of Life is an example of this type of tool. [HYDRAULIC] *p. 1042*
4. Material used to fill voids between the vehicle and the ground for stabilization. [CRIBBING] *p. 1040*
6. Gloves should be made of this material to protect your hands from jagged metal and broken glass during extrication. [LEATHER] *p. 1034*
7. Alternative to firefighting turnout coat and pants for use by EMS personnel during extrication. [JUMPSUIT] *p. 1034*
8. Process of disentangling and removing a patient from a vehicle damaged in a collision. [EXTRICATION] *p. 1033*
13. Standards for personal protective equipment that should be met by personnel participating in extrication. [NFPA] *p. 1034*

CHECK YOUR RECALL AND APPLY CONCEPTS KEY

EXERCISE 1

1. a *p. 1037*
2. c *p. 1037*
3. b *p. 1034*
4. d *p. 1035*
5. b *p. 1037*

EXERCISE 2

1. T *p. 1037*
2. F, A compact structural firefighting helmet with a four-point suspension system should be used for rescuer protection during extrication. *p. 1033*
3. T *p. 1039*
4. F, Rigging uses ropes or chains to stabilize the vehicle. Cribbing is placed between the vehicle and the ground. *p. 1040*
5. T *p. 1040*
6. T *p. 1041*
7. F, Personal protective equipment is needed any time you must extricate a patient from a vehicle to protect you from injury by sharp metal or broken glass. *p. 1041*

CLINICAL REASONING CASE STUDY: SWIFT-WATER RESCUE IN THE DESERT

1. This rescue requires, at minimum, a swift-water rescue team and EMS.
2. EMS providers must anticipate the types of injuries the patient may have. He may be hypothermic, he may become submerged before he can be rescued and suffer asphyxia, he may become pinned by or struck by debris in the water, there may be drugs or alcohol involved in the situation that led the patient to be in the arroyo during rainfall, or the patient may have jumped from a bridge. Once the patient is rescued, EMS personnel must obtain a thorough history and perform a thorough assessment.
3. Many factors can impact the outcome of the rescue operation, including how long it takes the swift-water rescue team to respond and prepare, how fast the current is carrying the patient, the patient's injuries, the safety equipment, and precautions taken by rescue personnel.

Chapter 48: Hazardous Materials

VOCABULARY AND CONCEPT REVIEW KEY

Crossword answers:

4. SECONDARY CONTAMINATION
6. MATERIAL SAFETY DATA SHEET
10. PLACARD
11. HAZARDOUS MATERIAL
12. UN NUMBER
13. SHIPPING PAPERS

Down answers include: TOXIC, DECONTAMINATION, RADIATION, CARCINOGEN, ACCESS CORRIDOR, COLD ZONE, HOT ZONE, IONIZATION, TOXIN, TOXRODROM, HOTZONE

Across	Down

Across

4. Transfer of a hazardous material from contact with an individual or piece of equipment to a person or surface that was not originally affected. [SECONDARYCONTAMINATION] *p. 1054*

6. Information form created by a chemical manufacturer that describes the physical properties, hazards, and ways of safely handling a hazardous chemical. [MATERIALSAFETYDATASHEET] *p. 1050*

10. Diamond-shaped information source on a vehicle or fixed storage facility of hazardous materials. [PLACARD] *p. 1048*

11. Any substance capable of harming people, property, or the environment. [HAZARDOUSMATERIAL] *p. 1046*

12. Four digits that identify hazardous substances and products of commerical importance. [UNNUMBER] *p. 1049*

13. Documentation containing regulatory information on a particular hazardous material transported by land, sea, or air. [SHIPPINGPAPERS] *p. 1050*

Down

1. Poisonous substance not derived from the metabolism of an organism. [TOXICANT] *p. 1055*

2. Process of reducing or removing hazardous material from someone or something that was exposed to it. [DECONTAMINATION] *p. 1055*

3. Natural process by which energy waves and particles travel through space. [RADIATION] *p. 1056*

5. Established ingress and egress route for emergency responders on a hazardous materials incident. [ACCESSCORRIDOR] *p. 1053*

7. Area of a hazardous materials incident where triage and treatment take place. [COLDZONE] *p. 1052*

8. Area where a hazardous chemical was released, contaminates the environment, and poses a danger to anyone in that area. [HOTZONE] *p. 1053*

9. Signs and symptoms that occur from exposure to a toxicant. [TOXIDROME]

CHECK YOUR RECALL AND APPLY CONCEPTS KEY

1. c   *p. 1047*
2. b   *p. 1048*
3. a   *p. 1048*
4. d   *p. 1048*
5. c   *p. 1048*
6. a   *p. 1052*
7. c   *p. 1050*
8. d   *p. 1054*
9. d   *p. 1054*

CLINICAL REASONING CASE STUDY: FIRE AT DAVIS INDUSTRIES

1. Right now, you do not have specific information about the source of the fire, but you should report what you saw and that you believe it to be in the area of Davis Industries, but make it clear that you are a couple of miles away and cannot confirm the source of the fire.

2. You will likely be needed in the area, but you have not been dispatched yet. Stay upwind of the smoke and be prepared to respond to a staging area designated by incident command.

Chapter 49: Response to Terrorism and Disasters

VOCABULARY AND CONCEPT REVIEW KEY

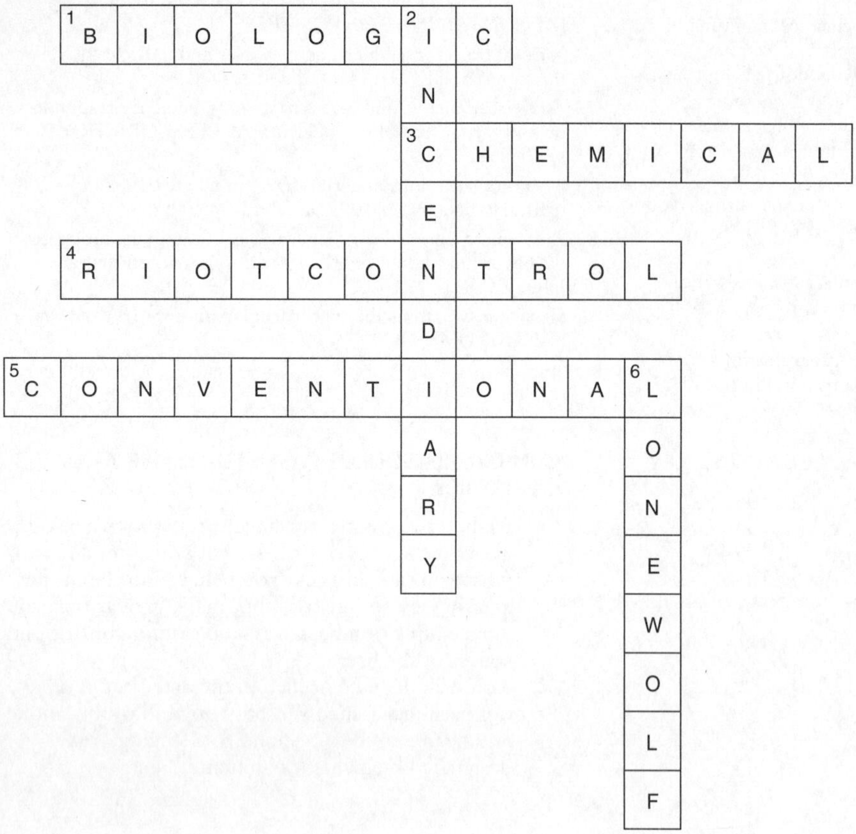

Across

1. Terrorism that involves the intentional, widespred dissemination of anthrax, for example. [BIOLOGIC] *p. 1064*
3. Terrorism that involves the intentional dispersal of VX or sarin gas, for example. [CHEMICAL] *p. 1064*
4. Low-toxicity agent that temporarily incapacitates by irritating the eyes. [RIOTCONTROL] *p. 1064*
5. Type of chemical materials designed to explode or detonate violently. [CONVENTIONAL] *p. 1063*

Down

2. Device used as a weapon that starts a fire. [INCENDIARY] *p. 1063*
6. Terrorist who acts by himself and has no long-term affiliation with a group. [LONEWOLF] *p. 1063*

CHECK YOUR RECALL AND APPLY CONCEPTS KEY

1. d *p. 1063*
2. a *p. 1063*
3. a *p. 1064*
4. c *p. 1064*
5. c *p. 1065*
6. a *p. 1065*

CLINICAL REASONING CASE STUDY: EF3 IN THE BUSINESS DISTRICT

1. You should be prepared to triage, treat, and transport patients.

2. Patients may have lacerations from flying debris and may have severe blunt trauma from debris, building collapse, or being propelled into objects by the tornado.

3. Tornadoes can result in downed electrical lines, hazards from debris and unstable buildings, and natural gas leaks. Anticipate behavioral emergencies and remember that the storm that spawned the tornado can cause additional winds, tornadoes, lightning, heavy rain, and hail.

4. You may have trouble reaching patients or transporting them due to blocked roads, the number of patients may exceed the treatment resources available, and the closest hospitals may also have been damaged or be having power outages.